Handbook of Forensic Anthropology and Archaeology

WORLD ARCHAEOLOGICAL CONGRESS
RESEARCH HANDBOOKS IN ARCHAEOLOGY

Sponsored by the World Archaeological Congress

Series Editors:
George Nicholas (*Simon Fraser University*)
Julie Hollowell (*Indiana University*)

The World Archaeological Congress's (WAC) *Research Handbooks
in Archaeology* series provides comprehensive coverage of
a range of areas of contemporary interest to archaeologists. Research
handbooks synthesize and benchmark an area of inquiry by providing
state-of-the-art summary articles on the key theories, methods, and practical
issues in the field. Guided by a vision of an ethically embedded, multivocal,
global archaeology, the edited volumes in this series—organized and written
by scholars of high standing worldwide—provide clear, in-depth information on
specific archaeological themes for advanced students, scholars, and professionals
in archaeology and related disciplines. *All royalties on these volumes go
to the World Archaeological Congress.*

Bruno David and Julian Thomas (eds.), *Handbook of Landscape Archaeology*

Soren Blau and Douglas Ubelaker (eds.), *Handbook of Forensic Anthropology
and Archaeology*

Jane Lydon and Uzma Rizvi (eds.), *Handbook of Postcolonialism and
Archaeology*

Handbook of Forensic

Anthropology and Archaeology

Soren Blau and Douglas H. Ubelaker

Editors

Left Coast Press inc.

Walnut Creek, California

LEFT COAST PRESS, INC.
1630 North Main Street, #400
Walnut Creek, California 94596
http://www.LCoastPress.com

Left Coast Press is committed to preserving ancient forests and natural resources. We elected to print this title on 30% post consumer recycled paper, processed chlorine free. As a result, for this printing, we have saved:

10 Trees (40' tall and 6-8" diameter)
3,788 Gallons of Wastewater
7 million BTU's of Total Energy
486 Pounds of Solid Waste
913 Pounds of Greenhouse Gases

Left Coast Press made this paper choice because our printer, Thomson-Shore, Inc., is a member of Green Press Initiative, a nonprofit program dedicated to supporting authors, publishers, and suppliers in their efforts to reduce their use of fiber obtained from endangered forests.

For more information, visit www.greenpressinitiative.org

Environmental impact estimates were made using the Environmental Defense Paper Calculator. For more information visit: www.papercalculator.org

Copyright © 2009 by Left Coast Press, Inc.

ISBN 978-1-59874-074-5 hardcover

Library of Congress Cataloging-in-Publication Data

Handbook of forensic anthropology and archaeology / Soren Blau and Douglas H. Ubelaker, editors.
p. cm.—(World Archaeological Congress research handbooks in archaeology)
Includes bibliographical references and index.
ISBN 978-1-59874-074-5 (hardcover : alk. paper)
1. Forensic anthropology—Handbooks, manuals, etc. 2. Forensic anthropology—Case studies. I. Blau, Soren. II. Ubelaker, Douglas H.
GN69.8.H34 2008
614'.17—dc22
2008032123

Printed in the United States of America

The paper used in this publication meets the minimum requirements of American National Standard for Information Sciences—Permanence of Paper for Printed Library Materials, ANSI/NISO Z39.48—1992.

09 10 11   5 4 3 2 1

CONTENTS

Part Three. Forensic Anthropology

Part Four. The Crime and Disaster Scene: Case Studies in
Forensic Archaeology and Anthropology

FIGURES

TABLES

SERIES EDITORS' FOREWORD

Julie Hollowell and George Nicholas

We are pleased to introduce the *Handbook of Forensic Anthropology and Archaeology*, a volume that reflects the origins, methodological breadth, and increasing global reach of the multidisciplinary field of forensic studies in archaeology and anthropology. Over the past decades, this specialized field of research and practice, whose practitioners make significant contributions in medico-legal contexts and often work in extraordinary and challenging social circumstances, has established itself as a vital, extremely valued, and relevant discipline with high standards for practice and training.

There is often an immediacy in forensic studies that distinguishes it from other aspects of archaeology and anthropology. The identification of accident victims for bereaved relatives, the resolution of historical mysteries and missing persons cases, and the persecution of war criminals all fall within its scope.

This volume documents the state of the discipline today, pointing the way toward future developments in method and technology and identifying new challenges faced by practitioners in different world regions and frames of practice. Increasingly, forensic archaeologists and anthropologists are looking beyond internal standards and practices to the broader social implications of their work, making the legal and ethical issues that surround forensics science in practice a topic ripe for further study. Indeed, the discipline seems poised to become more reflexive and critical while at the same time evolving rigorous and innovative techniques to restore identity, dignity, and—all too often—justice to the dead and their descendants. Forensic research not only captures the public's attention and imagination but also has the potential to serve as a powerful tool for social justice and reconciliation (Colwell-Chanthaphonh 2007). We hope that this book sparks many conversations about the past, present, and future of forensic studies and leads to additional insights for us all.

Finally, we take this opportunity to thank members of our editorial board who shared the task of reviewing the volume at several stages: Wendy Ashmore, Jane Buikstra, Ian Lilley, Rasmi Shoocongdej, and Patty Jo Watson. Thanks also to Amy Mundorf and Marina Elliot, who each supplied a thorough initial review, and to Mitch Allen and Jennifer Collier of Left Coast Press for their steady stream of advice and encouragement. We were very pleased to once again work with Stacey C. Sawyer, who has an uncanny and unwavering ability to whip everything into shape. Our deepest appreciation and gratitude go to Soren Blau and Douglas Ubelaker, volume editors, for their persistence and good nature in the face of the many challenges of seeing a major undertaking such as this through to the end. Their work in making this volume a reality marks an historical moment when forensic anthropology and archaeology have attained new levels of public and scholarly recognition.

All royalties generated by sales of books in this series go directly to the World Archaeological Congress. Since its inception, WAC has nurtured the growth of archaeological communities and discussions and has supported participation in meetings in cases where economic and political conditions make this hard to sustain. One way WAC accomplishes this is through the donation of royalties from WAC-related publications. In addition, Left Coast Press donates 50 copies of each volume produced in the Research Handbook Series to WAC's Global Libraries Project, for distribution to libraries around the world.

Acknowledgments

Soren Blau and Douglas Ubelaker would like to thank the series editors, Julie Hollowell and George Nicholas, for their patience and support in the process of seeing this volume through to publication. We would also like to thank Stacey C. Sawyer for her timeless energy devoted to copy editing and project management and Sage Publications, India, for their excellent attention to composition. We acknowledge the time provided by Caroline Rosenberg (Victorian Institute of Forensic Medicine) to improving the resolution of many of the images. Thanks to Tim Denham for endless useful advice. We are extremely grateful to Robin Blau for drawing the symbol used on the chapter title pages; this drawing was based on the 1974 photograph by Charles Wilp and Joseph Beuys of a drawing in sand entitled *Skeleton*, now in the Museum of Contemporary Art in Sydney, Australia. Soren Blau would also like to sincerely thank the Victorian Institute of Forensic Medicine for providing an environment of support and vision for casework, research, and publication.

USE OF IMAGES OF HUMAN REMAINS

This volume presented us, as series editors, with a particular challenge in regard to the use of illustrations that included human remains. We fully understand that a volume on forensics would normally contain numerous images of human remains of a wide variety, and it could be argued that, given the subject of the book, such images are integral for teaching and learning purposes. Nevertheless, for a series sponsored by the World Archaeological Congress (WAC), we believed it was important to make every effort to comply with the Tamaki Makau-rau Accord on the Display of Human Remains and Sacred Objects (WAC 2006), as well as other codes and accords promulgated by WAC. The Tamaki Makau-rau Accord, developed in New Zealand in 2005 and adopted in Osaka in 2006, states that those wishing to publish or otherwise display human remains or images of human remains should first seek permission from affiliated descendants or descendant communities.

Knowing that this was likely quite different from the protocols used in forensic contexts, we brought this issue to the attention of the volume editors. They responded positively and without hesitation to our request that each author whose chapter included images of human comply—or at least attempt to comply—with the Accord and be able to affirm that appropriate permissions sought or received for use of any illustrations containing photographs of human remains. Images in this volume that fall under the Accord range from photographs of a single human bone to several portraying victims of mass genocide to photomicroscopic images of human bone tissue.

In the process, we learned that those working in the field of forensic anthropology have a very well-defined and distinctive interpretation of ethics regarding the use of images portraying human remains. The main criterion is that permission for any use or display is absolutely required whenever the image portrayed is that of an *identifiable* person—which makes good sense, given the major role that identity and personhood play in the discipline. To our initial chagrin, the editors and authors interpreted the Tamaki Makau-rau Accord in this light, and thus it was their understanding that they had indeed complied. Here is a brief statement from volume editor Soren Blau, sent to us after we inquired further about how the Accord had been interpreted:

Access to and use of images of deceased individuals is an important part of the professional forensic anthropologist's casework and/or research. It is understood as part of the forensic anthropologist's professional ethical code of practice that when depicting aspects of the case, the deceased individual must be de-identified (i.e., there is nothing that can identify the person).

Consequently, in all cases in this volume where human remains (whether complete or partial, macroscopic or histology section) are depicted to illustrate a point there are no identifying features on the image. All research based on deceased individuals (whether identified or not), including the use of images, has research ethical approval.

After careful consideration, we decided that the best approach would be to share openly and transparently the approaches that were taken, describing the request for compliance and the interpretation of the Accord by those working in a forensic context. We have also made an effort to advise readers of images that may contain sensitive material. In light of this, all photographs of human remains are identified by an asterisk in the list of figures immediately following the Contents.

This volume has certainly provided an interesting case of practical applications of the Accord and some of the complexities that arise in the process. More than anything else, we have found that approaching authors with the need to comply with the Tamaki Makau-rau Accord has created opportunities for us all to learn from and become sensitive to other ways of thinking when it comes to images of human and ancestral remains. We hope that the experiences here will encourage reflection on these issues and the implications they may have for others, whether in a forensic context or elsewhere.

References

Colwell-Chanthaphonh, C. 2007. *History, Justice, and Reconciliation*, in *Archaeology as a Tool of Civic Engagement*, B. J. Little and P. A. Shackel, pp. 23–46. Lanham, MD: AltaMira Press.

World Archaeological Congress (WAC). 2006. Tamaki Makau-rau Accord on the Display of Human Remains and Sacred Objects, www.worldarchaeologicalcongress.org/site/about_ethi.php

1

FORENSIC ANTHROPOLOGY AND ARCHAEOLOGY: INTRODUCTION TO A BROADER VIEW

Soren Blau and Douglas H. Ubelaker

Over the last ten years interest in the disciplines of forensic anthropology and archaeology has exploded. Despite this increased interest, confusion still exists about what exactly it is that forensic anthropologists do. This problem is exemplified by comments such as "I thought anthropologists studied ants" (comment from Australian Transport and Safety Board inspector, crash site, Victoria, Australia, 2005) and "What the bl***y h*ll do we want an anthropologist for? There are no tribes still to be found in Glasgow!" (Black 2006a). Whether the fascination in forensic anthropology is a result of media hype surrounding anything "forensic" (e.g., Black 2000: 491) or a genuine desire to contribute to forensic investigations, students must have an accurate understanding of the role that forensic anthropologists and forensic archaeologists play in investigations and a solid foundation in both the practical and ethical components of the disciplines.

Forensic anthropology has been diversely defined by practitioners across the world:

- "that branch of physical anthropology, which, for forensic purposes, deals with the identification of more-or-less skeletonised remains known to be, or suspected of being, human" (Stewart 1979: ix);

- "a multidisciplinary field combining physical anthropology, archaeology and other fields of anthropology with the forensic sciences, including forensic dentistry, pathology and criminalistics" (İşcan 1981: 10);

- "a subdiscipline of physical anthropology that applies the techniques of osteology and biomechanics to medicolegal problems" (Reichs 1998a: 13);

- "the identification of the human, or indeed the remains of the human, for medico-legal purposes" (Black 2006b);

- "the application of knowledge and techniques of physical anthropology to problems of medicolegal significance" (Ubelaker 2006: 4);

- "the application of physical anthropology to the forensic context" (Cattaneo 2007: 185).

These definitions range from the broad to the specific and reflect the complexity of the discipline and the somewhat fluid nature of the applications of forensic anthropology (Cattaneo 2007). Although all definitions acknowledge the importance of the legal aspects of the work, practitioners have moved from examinations of "more or less skeletonised" remains (Stewart 1979: ix) to those that involve the living person (Black 2006b). The wide-ranging applications of forensic anthropology are reflected in the contributions to this volume.

Forensic archaeology is defined as the application of archaeological principles and techniques within a medico-legal and/or humanitarian context involving buried evidence. In North America, archaeology has typically fallen under the general umbrella of "anthropology." In Britain, and now increasingly in the United States, there is a push to distinguish archaeology and anthropology as separate disciplines. The distinct yet heavily connected contributions made by the two disciplines to forensic investigations are well illustrated in this volume.

Since the increasing formalisation of forensic anthropology there have been various examining the history of its development (e.g., İşcan 1988, 1999, 2000, 2001; Rodriguez 1994; Snow 1982; Ubelaker 2000, 2004, 2006), textbooks, and a wealth of peer-reviewed journal articles (too numerous to list) demonstrating and critiquing technical methodologies, particularly as related to refining and developing population specific techniques (e.g., Cox and Mays 2000; Hunter, Roberts, and Martin 1996; Krogman and İşcan 1986; Reichs 1998b; Schmitt, Cunha, and Pinheiro 2006; Stewart 1979), and papers detailing case studies (e.g., Fairgrieve 1999; Komar 2003; Rathbun and Buikstra 1984; Steadman 2003). Typically, volumes have dealt separately with forensic anthropology and forensic archaeology at the regional level (e.g., Cox and Mays 2000 for Britain; Steadman 2003 for the United States). The aim of this book is to provide the reader with a comprehensive work that includes a compilation of histories of the discipline from several different (although unfortunately not totally representative) parts of the world, technical aspects of analyses, and examples of current practice (case studies) in one volume.

To demonstrate the scope of the disciplines, this volume draws together contributions from a diverse range of highly experienced forensic anthropology and forensic archaeology practitioners. Authors were invited to contribute a chapter for their subject area expertise and to provide an international perspective throughout the volume.[1] The contributors present descriptive and critical evaluations of standard techniques in addition to discussing new and innovative methodologies.

Organisation of the Volume

The book is divided into five sections that cover the depth and breadth of forensic anthropology and archaeology. Part I, History of the Disciplines, provides overviews of the development and current state of forensic anthropology from different regional perspectives including European (British—Margaret Cox; Italian—Cristina Cattaneo; French—Eric Baccino, and Spanish—José Prieto); North and South American (Douglas Ubelaker, Mark Skinner and Kristina Bowie, and Luis Fondebrider); Australian (Denise Donlon); and Indonesian (Etty Indriati). These contributions include historical perspectives detailing the contributions made by early practitioners, discussions about the development of education and training, as well as presentations of case studies illustrating some of the strengths and weaknesses in approaches to casework and research in different regions. Part I illustrates the different ways in which the discipline has developed reflecting diverse social and political contexts.

The ability of the forensic anthropologist to undertake analyses is fundamentally determined by the preservation of the remains. In turn, the success of identifying an individual based on badly decomposed or skeletonised human remains depends largely on the completeness of the material. It is, therefore, fundamentally important that complete and accurate recovery of skeletal parts and information on their associations with one another and other items are undertaken at a crime/disaster scene. Such recovery relies on controlled excavation employing archaeological techniques. Part II, Forensic Archaeology, thus details current practices in forensic archaeology with a focus on methodologies employed in the search, location, and recovery of various types of evidence associated with crime and disaster scenes.

Thomas Holland and Samuel Connell outline traditional methods, including surveying and testing (probing, coring, and limited excavation), as well as covering remote sensing techniques (including resistivity, magnetometry, and ground-penetrating radar). Paul Cheetham and Ian Hanson discuss the importance of involving archaeologists in the excavation and recovery of human remains, detailing the skills required. They outline the important notion that there is no "normal" way to excavate a site and that the key concept is the ability to be flexible and adapt to each unique scene. The ability to select appropriate field methods and therefore obtain results has important legal implications, which are also considered.

Part III, Forensic Anthropology, includes 15 chapters that provide the reader with information about the fundamental types of analyses undertaken by forensic anthropologists. The contributors provide a background to techniques employed by practitioners and discuss the advantages and limitations of specific methodologies. Dawn Mulhern provides a comprehensive discussion about the initial responsibility of the forensic anthropologist, which is to determine whether the remains are human or nonhuman. Both gross and microscopic approaches are detailed.

Shari Forbes and Kimberly Nugent examine one of the more challenging aspects of forensic anthropology—determination of the postmortem internal. They provide an insight into the history of attempts to determine time since death from the analyses of skeletal remains detailing morphological, chemical, immunological, and radioisotopic analyses. The potentially significant effects of environmental conditions on estimating time since death are also considered.

John Byrd and Bradley Adams examine commingling, a problematic aspect of many anthropological analyses on both a small and large scale. They consider the effects of field recovery techniques in dealing with commingled remains and then detail the techniques used to sort such remains, including visual pair-matching, articulation, size and shape comparison, robusticity, taphonomy, and DNA analysis. Another important aspect of dealing with commingled remains includes quantification. Byrd and Adams outline two main techniques: minimum number of individuals (MNI) and most likely number of individuals (MLNI). Finally, ethical considerations with commingled remains are discussed.

Techniques employed by the forensic anthropologist to establish an individual's biological profile are extensively examined in several chapters. A biological profile includes information concerning the deceased's ancestry, sex, age at death, and stature. Such information provides the parameters of a possible identity (for example, Caucasoid male, aged 20–30 years with a stature of 170–180 cm) and therefore assists in narrowing the search pool.

Norman Sauer and Jane Wankmiller discuss the relationship between race and ancestry determination in forensic anthropology, the methods developed by anthropologists to determine ancestry, and some of the relevant philosophical and ethical issues. Techniques used to determine the sex of an individual are provided by Valeria Braz, followed by Tracy Rogers's in-depth discussion on adult and subadult morphological ageing techniques. Well-established histological methods of age estimation are explored by Christian Crowder, who also looks at the problems associated with the acceptance of these

methods as a conventional tool for the estimation of age at death.

The final aspect of the biological profile, stature, is detailed in Patrick Willey's chapter. The process of estimating adult stature from skeletal remains and comparing that estimation with antemortem height is discussed, as are issues affecting the accuracy of stature comparisons.

Although cause and manner of death are fundamentally the responsibility of the forensic pathologist (cf. Roberts 1996: 101), the forensic anthropologist can make a significant contribution to the recording and interpretation of skeletal trauma. Consequently, considerable attention is given to the forensic anthropologist's role in examining trauma. Eugénia Cunha and João Pinheiro examine all aspects of the analysis of antemortem trauma, and Louise Loe provides a detailed discussion of the principles of perimortem trauma, synthesising the current theoretical and practical issues associated with this analysis of skeletal remains recovered from forensic contexts. This is followed by Stephen Nawrocki's discussion of postmortem alterations.

Forensic anthropologists deal with human remains from a number of different contexts, many of which involve heat-induced transformation. Tim Thompson provides a critical summary of the work undertaken on burnt human remains to date, highlighting specific investigative techniques.

Carl Stephan examines craniofacial identification including techniques of facial approximation and craniofacial superimposition. He details the history of the development of craniofacial identification summarizing the tested and untested guidelines for a range of specific techniques. The role of the forensic odontologist is discussed in detail by John Clement, who outlines the techniques used by odontologists to age and identify individuals.

Part IV, The Crime and Disaster Scene: Case Studies in Forensic Archaeology and Anthropology, provides the reader with a selection of case studies illustrating the ways in which forensic anthropologists and archaeologists contribute to domestic homicide investigations, disaster scenes, and international investigations of atrocities. Dawnie Steadman, William Basler, Michael J. Hochrein, Dennis Klein, and Julia Goodin present a detailed case study illustrating the role of the forensic anthropologist in a North American context. John Hunter discusses the legal setting in which a forensic archaeologist could expect to practise in the United Kingdom and offers 11 short case studies to illustrate the diverse casework of a forensic archaeologist. Paul Sledzik examines the role of the forensic anthropologist in responding to disaster scenes. A series of cases studies are provided that document the history of forensic anthropology in responding to mass disasters in the United States. These case studies highlight the traditional role of the forensic anthropologist as well as newly established contributions.

The range of disaster scenarios to which forensic anthropologists have (or should have!) contributed are highlighted by discussions of the role of forensic anthropology in the investigation of militia violence in the Solomon Islands (Melanie Archer and Malcolm Dodd), the 2004 Boxing Day Tsunami (Sue Black), and the 2002 and 2004 Bali Bombings (Chris Briggs and Alanah Buck). Other chapters examine the contributions that forensic anthropology has made to investigations of genocide and crimes against humanity in the former Yugoslavia (Jon Sterenberg), Guatemala (Ambika Flavel and Caroline Barker), and Iraq (Derek Congram and Jon Sterenberg).

The final section of the volume, Part V, The Professional Forensic Archaeologist and Forensic Anthropologist, examines topics that are essential to the professional practice of forensic anthropology and archaeology. These include a discussion about important ethical considerations associated with training, accreditation, the development of anthropological techniques, limitations of evidence, and research (Soren Blau); working for large organisations such as the United Nations (Richard Wright and Ian Hanson); the use of statistics in forming conclusions and opinions (Ann Ross and Erin Kimmerle); and presenting expert testimony in court (Maciej Henneberg). The final chapter in this section presents a detailed overview of the legal and scientific process of death investigation (David Ranson). Both the practical and personal (community) aspects of the investigation process are discussed.

Conclusion

In assembling this volume, the editors have attempted to augment the traditional and now widely published North American perspective of forensic anthropology. The North American contributions in the volume are fundamental to understanding the origins and development of the discipline; however, we also acknowledge that a lack of publications in the English language does not mean that significant contributions from other parts of the world have not been made.

This volume illustrates the degree to which forensic anthropology and archaeology are disciplines that have the potential to make significant

contributions to the search, location, and recovery of evidence as well as to the analysis of a variety of differential preserved human remains from both crime and disaster scenes; ultimately, the contributions made by forensic anthropology and archaeology assist in investigations undertaken for humanitarian and judicial purposes. Such contributions are achieved through methodological rigour and effective collaboration and communication.

We hope that this volume provides a comprehensive and useful resource for students and emerging practitioners of forensic anthropology and forensic archaeology, as well as other interested professionals. The wide-ranging content of the volume ensures that the book is of interest to both experienced practitioners and those interested in learning more about, the fascinating and rewarding fields of forensic anthropology and forensic archaeology.

Note

1. Spelling used in the volume is in accordance with the author's origin—that is, both American and English versions of words are used (for example,"aging" and "ageing").

References

Black, S. 2000. Forensic osteology in the United Kingdom, in M. Cox and S. Mays (eds.), *Human Osteology in Archaeology and Forensic Science*, pp. 491–503. London: Greenwich Medical Media, Ltd.

———. 2006a. The real world of forensic anthropology. *Nicci French*. www.penguin.co.uk/static/cs/uk/0/minisites/niccifrench/reallife.html (accessed 01/11/06).

———. 2006b. Human identification and forensic anthropology: The role of the forensic anthropologist in forensic science and identification form the living. Paper presented at the 18th International Symposium, The Australian and New Zealand Forensic Science Society, Perth, April 1st.

Cattaneo, C. 2007. Forensic anthropology: Developments of a classical discipline in the new millennium. *Forensic Science International* 165: 185–193.

Cox, M., and Mays, S. (eds.). 2000. *Human Osteology in Archaeology and Forensic Science*. London: Greenwich Medical Media, Ltd.

Fairgrieve, S. I. (ed.). 1999. *Forensic Osteological Analysis: A Book of Case Studies*. Springfield, IL: Charles. C. Thomas.

Hunter, J. R., Roberts, C. A., and Martin, A. 1996. *Studies in Crime: An Introduction to Forensic Archaeology*. London: Batsford.

İşcan, M. Y. 1981. Concepts in teaching forensic anthropology. *Medical Anthropology Newsletter* 13(1): 10–12.

———. 1988. Rise of forensic anthropology. *American Journal of Physical Anthropology* 31: 203–230.

———. 1999. Medicolegal anthropology in France. *Forensic Science International* 100(1–2): 17–35.

———. 2000. Forensic anthropology in Latin America. *Forensic Science International* 109(1): 15–30.

———. 2001. Global forensic anthropology in the 21st century. *Forensic Science International* 117(1–2): 1–6.

Komar, D. R. 2003. Twenty-seven years of forensic anthropology casework in New Mexico. *Journal of Forensic Sciences* 48(3): 521–524.

Krogman, W. M., and İşcan, M. Y. 1986. *The Human Skeleton in Forensic Medicine* (2nd ed.). Springfield, IL: Charles C. Thomas.

Rathburn, A., and Buikstra, J. E. (eds.). 1984. *Human Identification*. Springfield, IL: Charles C. Thomas.

Reichs, K. 1998a. Forensic anthropology: A decade of progress, in K. Reichs (ed.), *Forensic Osteology: Advances in the Identification of Human Remains*, pp. 13–38. Springfield, IL: Charles C. Thomas.

———. (ed.). 1998b. *Forensic Osteology: Advances in the Identification of Human Remains* (2nd ed.). Springfield, IL: Charles C. Thomas.

Roberts, C. A. 1996. Forensic anthropology 1: The contributions of biological anthropology to forensic contexts, in J. Hunter, C. Roberts, and A. Martin (eds.), *Studies in Crime: An Introduction to Forensic Archaeology*, pp. 101–121. London: Batsford.

Rodriguez, J. V. 1994. *Introduction a la Antropologia Forense: Analis e Interpretacion de Restos Oseos Humanos*. Bogotá: C. Anaconda.

Schmitt, A., Cunha, E., and Pinheiro, J. (eds.). 2006. *Forensic Anthropology and Medicine: Complementary Sciences from Recovery to Cause of Death*. Totowa, NJ: Humana Press.

Snow, C. C. 1982. Forensic anthropology. *Annual Review of Anthropology* 11: 97–131.

Steadman, D. W. 2003. *Hard Evidence: Case Studies in Forensic Anthropology*. Upper Saddle River, NJ: Prentice Hall.

Stewart, T. D. 1979. *Essentials of Forensic Anthropology*. Springfield, IL: Charles C. Thomas.

Ubelaker, D. H. 2000. Methodological considerations in the forensic applications of human skeletal biology, in M. A. Katzenburg and R. Shelley (eds.), *Biological Anthropology of the Human Skeleton*, pp. 41–67. New York: Wiley-Liss.

———. 2004. Forensic anthropology. *Encyclopedia of Medical Anthropology* 1, pp. 37–42. New York: Springer Verlag.

———. 2006. Introduction to forensic anthropology, in A. Schmitt, E. Cunha, and J. Pinheiro (eds.), *Forensic Anthropology and Medicine: Complementary Sciences from Recovery to Cause of Death*, pp. 3–12. Totowa, NJ: Humana Press.

PART
ONE

HISTORY OF THE DISCIPLINES

2

FORENSIC ANTHROPOLOGY AND ARCHAEOLOGY: PAST AND PRESENT—A UNITED KINGDOM PERSPECTIVE

Margaret Cox

No man is an island, entire of it; everyman is a piece of the Continent, a part of the main . . . —John Donne 1572–1631: *Devotions upon Emergent Occasions* (Booth 1994)

Forensic anthropologists and archaeologists respectively apply the principles of biological anthropology and archaeology to the process of justice. Although, in purely semantic terms, *forensic* prefixing an area of expertise means use of that science for the "courts of law" (*Oxford English Dictionary* 1990), most forensic practitioners recognise that the term has many facets. These include working for processes of justice, which are not necessarily synonymous with courts of law, and humanitarian work that provides an element of justice for survivors of atrocity crimes and mass disasters seeking to find, bury, and mourn their dead, and to undertake such legal processes as probate. *Justice* is a word with a variety and range of meanings (see Cox 2003; Cox et al. 2008). The term *forensic* is, however, increasingly misused in the United Kingdom (U.K.) in popular culture, television archaeology, and media reporting generally. This chapter concerns the correct application of the term and its humanitarian applications, specifically as they relate to forensic anthropology and archaeology in the U.K. As will become evident in this discussion, the development of forensic anthropology and archaeology within the U.K., as elsewhere, is not an isolated phenomenon. United Kingdom practitioners and the development of the disciplines within the U.K. are part of a larger global response to a range of social, political, economic, and environmental factors; it is within that wider context of engagement and participation that this discussion takes place.

Context: Past and Present

As was articulated in the 17th century by Donne, neither human beings nor facets of their identity, concerns, or responses develop in isolation. Forensic anthropology and archaeology have developed in the U.K. in response to a number of key factors, some obvious and others less so (for a full discussion see Cox 2001; Hunter and Cox 2005). It is generally accepted that most forensic practitioners gain some satisfaction from contributing to the process of justice when crimes are committed and thus perhaps to a safer society. This fact is particularly pertinent in the current professional context for "traditional" anthropologists and archaeologists practicing within the U.K. Here a sanitised planning and development-led professional arena exists, where opportunities for making a significant social or intellectual contribution, or for empowering the present, are few (Hunter and Cox 2005). Contributing to the process of justice is, of course, relevant not only in a domestic context but also in the international arena, where the crimes of genocide, crimes against humanity, war-crimes, and mass murder[1] invite our engagement in their resolution.

The context for the development of these emergent disciplines is in itself extremely complex and sits alongside the role of popular culture and media portrayal in influencing responses. Both of these factors foster and influence belief and value systems, influence responses, and bias and influence perceptions of reality (Cox 2001; Hunter and Cox 2005; McNeely 1995). Such perceptions sit within a world that may be no more dangerous than previously but that is made to appear so by biased and inaccurate global reporting available 24 hours a day, seven days a week. Such reporting increasingly focuses on crime and conflict, and we are presented with an image of life in a threatened society. This picture is also shaped and invoked by politicians and other "leaders" whose vested interests contribute significantly to the context for what some call "global terrorism" and others "wars against repression." The media and power structures, such as governments and religious organisations, also attempt to shape and portray our responses to events and contexts, and they gain, exert, and maintain power through them.

Engagement in such conflicts by forensic practitioners can bring with it a paramilitary association that is, for some, seductive. Equally, the desire to engage in humanitarian work can be compelling for others, and in this context care has to be taken to ensure that such engagement is not tainted with overtones of neocolonialism—in practice, if not intent. Issues arising from differing standards of professional practice for judicial and humanitarian responses clearly demonstrate this. Investigations with solely humanitarian objectives usually have "lower" standards applied to them, and investigations with this constraint on their terms of reference would not be countenanced in the U.K. The question must, therefore, be asked as to why it is thought appropriate or acceptable that wealthy nations should finance and undertake humanitarian programmes that use lower standards in (usually) poorer countries? There is another risk inherent in using lower standards that result in not all of the evidence from graves and human remains being recorded and recovered (whether in a humanitarian or judicial context). It leaves the

door wide open for revisionist histories to be constructed by those with a vested interest in doing so. The Missing and their families and communities deserve the truth. What they do with that truth is up to them, but as scientists it is our responsibility to ensure that all evidence is recovered and has the potential to be appropriately interpreted.

Practicing anthropology and archaeology in a forensic context arguably allows us to be socially relevant, to assist in the resolution of criminal investigations, and to contribute to a safer world. Such engagement is inevitably accompanied by a responsibility to contribute to the debate on the overarching contexts and issues. Perhaps, at an appropriate time, we should debunk some of the myths and expose some of the realities that influence wider perceptions of the social, economic, professional, ethical, and political contexts of serious and atrocity crimes, and the various processes for their resolution. These responsibilities also extend to commenting on the justice and the injustice of, and international responses to, postconflict and mass fatality contexts. We have a moral duty to consider and to comment on these matters and also on our responses as professionals. This duty relates not only to professional, methodological, and technical issues but also to those of motive, intent, and impact. Clearly such responses must fit into frameworks of legal and regulatory process and rules of *sub judice* (before a judge or court of law). Assessment of the broader impact of the involvement of international forensic teams in overseas contexts is generally not undertaken.

Impact assessments are standard practice for development agencies working in international contexts and are also undertaken in the U.K. in police operations (ACPO Centrex 2005) with reference to affected local communities. Consideration of the wider effects of forensic work undertaken should also be standard practice, with assessments including (1) impact on those directly affected by such work by its very nature, (2) impact on those indirectly affected by the work, and (3) incidental impacts on local communities and others caused by the presence of "foreign" nationals with all their trappings and expectations.

Traditional archaeology and biological anthropology (that is, as applied in nonforensic contexts) developed separately in the U.K. and, generally speaking, their forensic applications are considered as separate disciplines and skills. Today, they are increasingly taught together at undergraduate level with archaeology degree programmes including one or more units on biological anthropology. This situation reflects the fact that archaeology is considered the overarching discipline in which anthropology plays a role, in both educational frameworks and in professional practice. Until recent decades, most archaeologists were classics or geography graduates, and most anthropologists were medical practitioners who were interested in palaeopathology. Today, there are a handful of U.K. practitioners who by coincidence fall into the U.S. model, whereby forensic anthropologists generally also have some archaeological skills (although in the U.K. usually the archaeologists have some anthropological skills). Some archaeology graduates in the U.K. subsequently undertake postgraduate study in forensic anthropology, and these individuals may go on to gain experience and expertise in both fields.

Forensic Anthropology in the United Kingdom

Forensic anthropology seeks to employ the science of biological anthropology to contribute toward establishing a presumptive and/or positive identification for a deceased individual(s) and, when possible, to contribute toward determining the cause and manner of death, as well as events leading to death (for example, evidence of torture or starvation).[2]

Forensic anthropologists primarily undertake their analysis on hard tissues but may work with human remains that are not completely skeletonised and may also work closely with pathologists in cases where soft tissues are well preserved. They usually work in a mortuary or anthropology laboratory, often also working closely with radiographers and anatomical pathology technicians. Anthropologists may also play a role in the recovery of remains, working alongside forensic archaeologists, scene-of-crime examiners, and police officers. Such team work is recommended, just as biological anthropologists should work at archaeological sites with traditional archaeologists. Attendance and possibly participation during recovery is particularly important when remains are in friable and fragile condition and may deteriorate further between discovery context and laboratory. In the following discussion, reference is made to forensic archaeology where appropriate to avoid repetition.

History of Forensic Anthropology in the United Kingdom

A detailed history of forensic anthropology in the U.K. is yet to be written, but an overview was provided by Black in 2003. The application of biological anthropology within a forensic context in the U.K. began in 1935 with the case of Dr. Buck Ruxton, who killed and dismembered his wife and a nursemaid (Glaister and Brash 1937; Hunter, Roberts, and Martin 1996; Saukko and Knight 2004). Half a century later, 1988 marked an important step in the history of both forensic anthropology and archaeology in the U.K. The body of a child, Stephen Jennings, was found in a small Pennine town, and both skill sets contributed to the recovery of his remains, his identification, and the reconstruction of the events surrounding his death (Hunter, Roberts, and Martin 1996). Both archaeological and anthropological skills were first requested of this author in 1992 and continue to be requested.

As a profession and as a recognised subject, forensic anthropology in the U.K. has a shorter history than in the U.S. The degree and the extent of involvement of anthropologists in what has historically been the domain of the forensic pathologist have been slow and sporadic, and they vary regionally. Exemplifying this, the most recent edition of a classic and much respected U.K. text in forensic pathology (Saukko and Knight 2004) describes some techniques and references for the analysis of skeletal remains (many of which have been superseded) but does not recommend that an anthropologist applies them. Such an omission is regrettable.

As Black (2003: 188) points out, over the last two decades those entering this arena have backgrounds in either anatomy or osteoarchaeology. I disagree with the view expressed that those previously and primarily practicing within the archaeological arena are unfamiliar with soft tissue. Some anthropologists practicing primarily as osteoarchaeologists have medical backgrounds, and some have experience of working with remains from lead coffins from both intra- and extramural burial contexts, with bog-bodies, with remains found in permafrost, and with mummies. In all cases, soft tissue of some type may survive. In my and many other forensic anthropologists' experience, police and pathologists are happy to work with those without a degree in anatomical sciences or medicine, and they and the courts have confidence in our observations and opinions. The considerable experience that osteoarchaeologists have in working with degraded and fragmented remains provides invaluable expertise for forensic contexts, particularly when severe fragmentation of hard tissue that often characterises cases where explosive forces, or excessive mutilation of remains, is involved. Similarly, many osteoarchaeologists in the U.K. have experience working with skeletal

material that has been subject to heat modification. In this debate, one should acknowledge that
within any discipline it is essential to recognise
and to celebrate the diversity of backgrounds and
areas of specialisation of those practicing within
the broader framework of the subject. Equally valid
and significant contributions are made by those
with relevant experience and expertise, whether
their educational backgrounds and underlying professional experience are in medicine, anatomy, or
osteoarchaeology.

Practicing in the United Kingdom

There are approximately 30 practicing forensic
anthropologists in the U.K. The majority of these
have an archaeological background and have
undertaken only a small number of cases (some of
course have more experience). Level of experience
need not, however, infer level of expertise or the
converse. Most cases do not result in the anthropologist attending court as an expert witness, and, consequently, where work is less than satisfactory, this
fact is unlikely to ever become apparent—which
is why the principle of accreditation is sound and
useful. Equally, some very competent practitioners
cannot undertake large case loads, because their
primary professional responsibilities (for example,
as university lecturers) may prevent this.

As Thompson (2003) points out, the public
and the police have an increasing awareness of
the contributions that forensic anthropology can
make to the resolution of crime and to finding and
identifying the Missing. However, this awareness
is very patchy across the U.K. and also reflects the
level of understanding on the part of the relevant
forensic pathologist of what anthropologists can
contribute to the process. In a recent example,
forensic archaeologists played a key role in the
recovery and the recording of a skeletonised individual for a county police service. Despite the fact
that two of the team were also very experienced
forensic anthropologists, something that was made
very clear during the site-based work, neither was
involved in the analysis of the remains. The reason
for this situation may be that the pathologist did
not consider their involvement to be either necessary or appropriate, or that he considered himself
to be an expert in anthropological analysis. The
degree to which different counties' police services
make use of anthropologists and/or archaeologists
varies enormously, as does the attitude of pathologists to anthropology and anthropologists.

In the U.K., practicing forensic anthropologists work within and from a variety of contexts.
The majority are in universities (for example, the

universities of Birmingham, Cranfield, Dundee,
and Sheffield) where their main roles are education
and research, and from which they may undertake
occasional casework. Some are employed by commercial organisations or charities that are multidisciplinary forensic providers (for instance, LGC
Forensics and the Inforce Foundation, respectively),
where to practice is their principal activity. Some
work for large commercial archaeology organisations (for example, MoLAS, Oxford Archaeology,
and Wessex Archaeology), where a small number
of cases are undertaken annually. The remainder
are freelance consultants working both in the U.K.
and internationally.

Forensic Organisations in the United Kingdom

CIFA. The U.K. is home to one organisation
whose primary function is served through a forensic database (contra Thompson, 2003), the Centre
for International Forensic Assistance (CIFA) (www.
cifa.org.uk), where forensic experts, including
forensic anthropologists and archaeologists, are
registered. Accreditation through the Council for
the Registration of Forensic Practitioners (CRFP)
is not necessary for inclusion in this database, and
competence is not assured by any other means
(Professor Sue Black, Director of CIFA, University
of Dundee, personal communication 2006).

Inforce. The U.K.'s only forensic organisation that is a registered nonprofit organization
is the Inforce Foundation. Inforce is multidisciplinary in its approach, and its core staff in
2006 included two forensic anthropologists, two
archaeologists, and a radiographer. Registration
with the CRFP is not considered essential for
Inforce employees or consultants, and no other
type of formal accreditation is currently in use.
Suitability for employment is based on experience, education, and often personal knowledge
or peer recommendation.[3]

Inforce undertakes work both in the U.K. and
internationally, within a variety of judicial and
humanitarian contexts, including capacity building[4] for those from postconflict regions, and mass
fatality recovery and identification. As yet, Inforce
does not maintain a formal database of practitioners, although it regularly receives *curriculum
vitae* from individuals. Inforce has a core staff and
also offers short-term contracts to experts and
occasionally to interns, as appropriate to the role
and context; it does not employ students. Inforce
has scientific and legal advisors and an Advisor's
Forum that meets at its annual conference. This
group of international experts includes forensic

archaeologists (five) and anthropologists (six), some of whom are U.K.-based (two and four, respectively). Advisors are selected on the basis of their experience and expertise covering the breadth of each discipline (www.inforce.org.uk) and its various applications. Inforce staff (including its anthropologists and archaeologists) deliver and contribute to various education and training activities and to domestic and international casework in serious and atrocity crimes and mass fatalities. All those working for Inforce, whether as full- or part-time employees or on a consultancy basis, have to agree to abide by the Inforce code of conduct (ibid.) and undertake work that meets its protocols and standard operating procedures (Cox et al. 2008).

Applications and Engagement

As Thompson sets out (2003: 185), forensic anthropology in the U.K. is fluid in terms of its professional development as it strives to establish its role within investigative processes; the same is true for forensic archaeology. The contexts in which anthropology is applied are expanding, and the role we play is ever-changing as we face new challenges. Anthropologists and archaeologists practicing within the U.K., or for U.K.-based organisations in the U.K. and/or overseas, can work in a variety of contexts. The scope of work undertaken by anthropologists may range from determining if hard-tissue elements are human or otherwise to potentially playing a key role in triage[5] in mass-fatality incidents. The principal areas of engagement are briefly described:

1. *Domestic police service cases*: The forensic anthropologist's involvement with domestic cases is increasing in the U.K., but as mentioned above, this is by no means universal. Notable cases involving skeletonised remains in which there was no anthropological involvement included the West case in the 1990s: the skeletons of 12 victims of Fred and Rose West were recovered (in February 1994) from three different sites. Despite obvious dismemberment and missing skeletal elements (Cox and Bell 1999), the pathologists involved did not advise the use of anthropologists, and the relevant police service also did not recognise such a need. Archaeological advice (not from a forensic archaeologist) was employed on one site. Despite this, forensic anthropologists and archaeologists increasingly make useful contributions to the investigation of domestic cases (see Hunter and Cox 2005 for numerous case studies) and appear as expert witnesses (see Henneberg this volume).

2. *International investigations of atrocity crimes:* The investigation of atrocity crimes internationally is an arena where U.K.-based and/or U.K.-trained forensic anthropologists and archaeologists have been regularly involved since the mid-1990s—specifically, with such investigations as those conducted by the *ad hoc* International Criminal Tribunal for the Former Yugoslavia and missions in such places as Rwanda, East Timor, the DR Congo, Sierra Leone, and Iraq. (For further discussion of this area see Sterenberg; Flavel and Barker; Congram and Sterenberg this volume).

3. *International humanitarian missions relating to atrocity crimes:* Over the last decade or so, U.K. practitioners have participated in humanitarian missions arising from atrocity crimes in contexts such as Central America (see Flavel and Barker this volume) and Cyprus (Inforce in 2005).

4. *Ministry of Defence/Commonwealth War Graves Commission cases:* Unlike in the U.S., where the repatriation of war dead from the last century is considered essential, in the U.K. that is not the case, particularly with reference to noncurrent conflicts. Although the repatriation of the remains of military personnel from very recent and ongoing conflicts is undertaken, those relating to, for example, WWI and WWII are not. This situation involves tens of thousands of missing service personnel. When remains are recovered, unless they have some form of associated identification (for example, an ID "dog" tag), no anthropological analysis is undertaken, and the remains are interred in a local Commonwealth War Graves Commission cemetery with full-military honours. The headstone states: "Known unto God." The role of the anthropologist in cases in which an indication of the identity of the individual is recovered (the anthropologist is not informed of this detail prior to the analysis) is to provide a biological profile of the individual. Blind assessment is made of ancestry, sex, age, stature, handedness,

and any individuating feature that may be evident in a photograph (for instance, protruding upper anterior dentition, healed fractures, and so on) or in surviving military or medical records. If what is known of the individual concurs with the biological profile, a match is assumed. The individual's relatives are then traced and informed, and invited to the funeral (with full military honours). The name of the recovered individual is then removed from the relevant memorial (for example, the Menin Gate, Ypres, Belgium) of the Missing.

Anthropologists are regularly involved in the analysis of remains from recent and past conflicts, but forensic or traditional archaeologists are only rarely involved in location and recovery in recent and older cases (for instance, the World Wars). In my experience as a forensic anthropologist for the Ministry of Defence (since 2000), working with remains from WWI and WWII usually involves analysis of multiple cases that may vary in completeness and condition and includes many cases exhibiting evidence of explosive or blast injury as well as sharp- and blunt-force trauma and ballistics trauma.

5. *Mass fatality events including anthropogenic (for example, mass transport accidents or terrorist attacks) and natural disasters:* The London bombings atrocity (July 7, 2005) is believed to be the first case in the U.K. in which anthropologists worked in "triage." They also undertook the reconstruction of fragmented remains. In this case, no anthropologist was involved at the outset; it was on the advice of a forensic radiographer that anthropologists were brought into the mortuary team (Mark Viner, Programmes and Operations Director, Inforce Foundation, personal communication 2006). The "London Mass Fatality Plan" (London Resilience Team and Mass Fatalities Working Group 2005) was published weeks before this incident and makes no mention of the involvement of either forensic anthropologists or archaeologists (the latter were not involved in recording or recovery). Although U.K. anthropologists have been involved in mass-fatality responses overseas—for example, the Asian Tsunami (December 26, 2004)

(see Black this volume)—and terrorist attacks in the U.S. (September 11, 2001) (Mackinnon and Mundorff 2007), forensic archaeologists have been involved to a much lesser extent. To date, neither forensic anthropologists nor archaeologists have been involved in the investigation of rail or air crash accidents in the U.K.

6. *Higher education:* Both forensic archaeology and anthropology are taught in U.K. universities, and those with appropriate educational qualifications, research experience, and professional experience undertake the delivery of under- and postgraduate programmes (see below for further discussion).

7. *Professional training for disaster-victim-identification response teams and atrocity-crime respondents and for capacity-building programmes:* Both archaeologists and anthropologists are involved in designing and delivering training for U.K. and other professionals and for those from postconflict and other troubled regions. Relative to the latter context, I consider capacity building to be an ethically sound approach intended to empower those whose human rights have recently been abused. Examples of professional training include a programme that Inforce recently developed and delivered with the Dorset Police Service on mass-fatality response. In this case, a light-airplane crash was simulated (Figures 2.1–2.3) and a temporary mortuary established. Capacity-building programmes have also been delivered in the U.K. and internationally. Inforce delivered three for Iraq in 2004 to 2005[6] (see www.inforce.org.uk for details of these), and two of these included simulated mass graves (Figure 2.4) and a simulated temporary mortuary with a radiography facility (Figures 2.5 and 2.6) as training components to build on theoretical and field/laboratory-based training.

The forensic anthropologist or archaeologist working within some of the contexts described above can ultimately be required to act as an expert witness in the Crown and/or Coroner's Courts, or in an international court. As mentioned above, not all casework involves appearance in court, and U.K. specialists have only rarely acted as expert witnesses in international or special courts. An exception was in 2006, when a U.K. practitioner

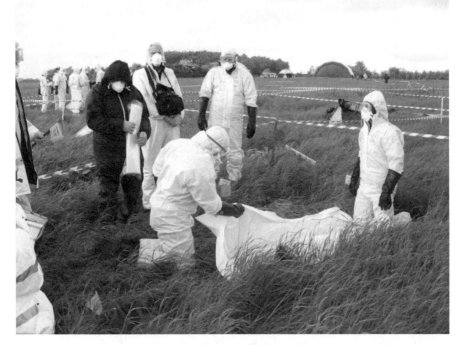

Figure 2.1   Simulated air-crash scene grided for controlled recording and recovery of remains and other evidence. This project was designed and delivered by the Inforce Foundation (2006) in collaboration with the Dorset Police Service (photograph Inforce Foundation).

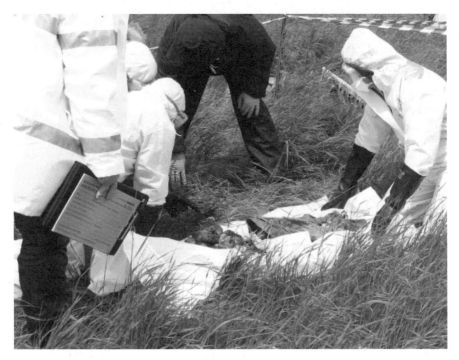

Figure 2.2   Detail of the simulated human remains used in the air-crash simulation (see Figure 2.1) (photograph Inforce Foundation).

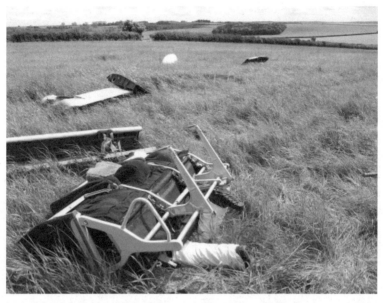

Figure 2.3 Further detail from the simulated air crash (see Figure 2.1) showing seats and remains (photograph Inforce Foundation).

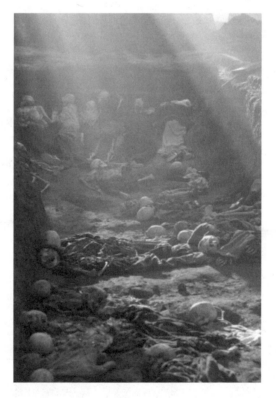

Figure 2.4 A simulated mass grave located and excavated by Iraqi forensic archaeologists and scene-of-crime officers in Dorset, U.K. (2005) as a component of a capacity-building programme (photograph Inforce Foundation).

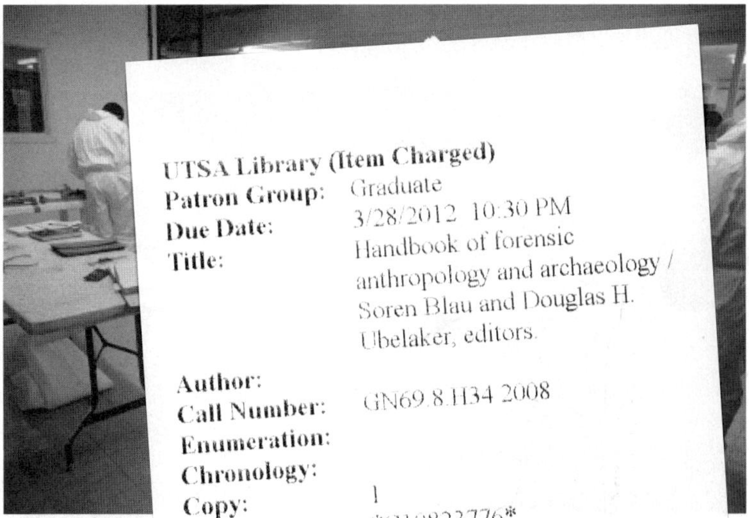

Figure 2.5 Detail from a s[...] ...ortuary snowing trainees examining human remains. Resin skeletons were buried within the grave and recovered by archaeologists. After these mock remains had been taken to the mortuary by scene-of-crime examiners, they were replaced with archaeological human remains prior to examination by fluoroscope and a full anthropological examination (photograph Inforce Foundation).

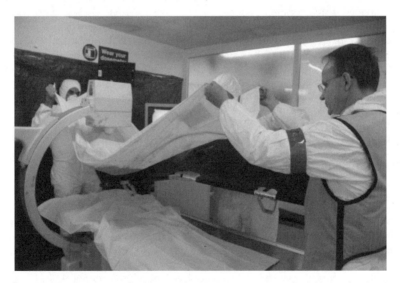

Figure 2.6 Detail from the X-ray facility at Inforce's mortuary site, taken during the training of Iraqi radiologists in forensic radiography (photograph Inforce Foundation).

working for Inforce provided evidence for the Iraq High Tribunal in Baghdad.

Forensic Archaeology

Forensic archaeology in the U.K. is the application of archaeological principles and methods to a forensic context (see Cheetham and Hanson; Hunter this volume). Archaeological skills are applied to the location of sites, site assessment, excavation and recording, recovery of human remains and other evidence, and recording the wider forensic landscape (Hanson 2004). The context of such application (for example, domestic crime, humanitarian recovery, and so on) is briefly discussed above, as are some aspects of the current concerns and challenges facing forensic archaeologists; this section focuses on remaining issues.

One of the first U.K. scientists to recognise the value and the challenges of archaeology in the context of a mass grave was Sir Sydney Smith (Regius Professor of Forensic Medicine at University of Edinburgh from 1928–1953) during his work in Alexandria in 1920 (Smith 1959). Another significant U.K. contributor to forensic archaeology (and anthropology) was A. K. Mant (late Professor of Forensic Medicine, Guy's Hospital, London), whose M.D. thesis (1950) and subsequent contributions (for example, 1987) consider aspects of recovery, taphonomy, and decomposition in respect to recovering bodies from the graves of World War II servicemen. The first U.K. archaeologist to apply archaeological principles to a scene-of-crime was John Hunter (Professor of Archaeology, University of Birmingham) in 1988. The early history and development of forensic archaeology in the U.K. is discussed in depth in Hunter and colleagues (1996) and that of more recent years in Hunter and Cox (2005).

Forensic archaeology is increasingly well integrated into overarching search, location, and recovery strategies within U.K. policing. The vehicle for this integration has, in part, been the Forensic Search Advisory Group (FSAG), which was established in the mid-1990s (ibid.). This group is multidisciplinary and includes all the sciences and police service functions involved in search and location, including archaeologists and geophysical specialists. It provides a 24-hour advisory service for the police in the U.K. and a central contact point through which to access advice and on-site support. The group promotes phased search strategies, instigates research, and discusses case studies in a confidential forum to promote dissemination of the lessons learned from case experience. It works to a code of conduct and does not require CRFP registration of participants, although this is encouraged.

Not all practicing forensic archaeologists work through the FSAG, and some FSAG members are involved in casework through their own links and relationships with local or regional police services. The fact that an increasing number of practicing U.K. police officers and scene-of-crime examiners have completed a B.Sc. in Archaeology or M.Sc. in Forensic Archaeology is helpful in that these individuals can advise their service on whether or not to employ a specialist. Their expertise limits unnecessary call-outs and increases in-house police expertise in search and recovery. As stated in Hunter and Cox (ibid.: 17),

all these factors move the goal posts on issues of accreditation[7] and raise the issue of where the line should be drawn regarding who should be accredited. The role and the development of forensic archaeology must accommodate this fluid context.

Education

Archaeology and anthropology and their forensic counterparts can be studied at U.K. universities at both under- and postgraduate levels, and recent years have seen shifts of emphasis. At an undergraduate level, archaeologists no longer read cultural anthropology (which is a great loss in a forensic context), and few biological anthropology modules and degree programmes include significant training in human anatomy other than skeletal anatomy (regrettable in the context of forensic applications where remains may have associated soft tissues). Formal education in these subjects at the Master of Science level began in the U.K. in 1994 and is now delivered at several universities including Cranfield. There are no undergraduate programmes that focus entirely on forensic archaeology,[8] and only one undergraduate programme exists in forensic anthropology (offered at University of Dundee), with most practitioners reading the subject at Master's level (Bradford, Bournemouth, Central Lancashire, and Cranfield). Postgraduate students on such programmes have a diverse range of academic and professional backgrounds, and although some universities insist on a relevant undergraduate and/or professional background (that is, a relevant science degree for anthropology), some do not. The varying quality of, and subject matter included within, postgraduate provision in the U.K. seems not to deter students (both local and international) interested in these areas of study in England.

The status of university-level education in the U.K. in 2003 was discussed in depth by Black (2003), but that paper omits some key points. The first is that neither under- nor postgraduate educational qualifications are in themselves sufficient to denote professional competence, nor do they purport to. Tertiary or higher education in the U.K. is not professional training.[9] This concept can be difficult for some students to grasp. Some mature students from policing backgrounds, for example, tend to see such a programme of "education" as "training"; the reality of the situation must be made explicit to prospective students. Training suggests the acquisition of competence to practice. Both undergraduate and masters' level "education" is just that; it is primarily designed to take students to a higher level of intellectual competence and engagement—not practice. No one expects a recent graduate of history, law, chemistry, or medicine to be competent to enter professional practice upon graduation. Further, it is my experience that many of those undertaking masters' level education in forensic anthropology and archaeology do not aspire to practice these subjects. Instead, they see such a degree as a part of their educational progression into such areas as policing, scene-of-crime examination, or, for many North American students, undertaking further education and training in law and subsequently entering the legal profession. The same holds true for many other disciplines.

Accreditation

Black (2003) suggests that those teaching in forensic programmes will, in time, be required to register with the Council for the Registration of Forensic Practitioners (CRFP). This is not currently a requirement for an academic post in forensic archaeology or anthropology in a U.K. university, nor should it be. As already stated, neither is higher education professional training, nor does it infer that graduates have any level of professional competence. Many of those teaching in forensic anthropology programmes in the U.K.'s higher education sector are in fact teaching the biological anthropology or anatomy that underpins the forensic application for which they are more than adequately qualified. Those teaching forensic applications in such courses must know their subject, be active in research in that subject, and also have some professional experience. At present, accreditation in the U.K. largely reflects professional experience in casework. Proficient practitioners can be poor academics and teachers (and vice versa)—to conflate the two is misguided.

Practicing forensic scientists are encouraged by some to register with the CRFP, stemming from the problems with expert evidence as highlighted by the Royal Commission of Justice Report (1993). Registered in 1999 and formally opened in 2000, the purpose of the CRFP is to ensure adequacy of professional standards in all aspects of relevant science and crime-scene practice, including forensic archaeology and anthropology. The process of registration is designed to ensure that those asked to contribute to an investigation have relevant skills and experience, although not registering need not infer the converse. At present there are about 30 practicing

forensic anthropologists and the same number of forensic archaeologists in the U.K. (Hunter and Cox 2005: 16). In mid-2006, only eight anthropologists and five archaeologists were registered (www.crfp.org.uk/register_result.asp, accessed 01/06/06); clearly many experienced practitioners have not done so.

Although this subject is not discussed in the literature, informal discussions at meetings and anecdotal comments by practitioners suggest that reluctance to register reflects a variety of factors. These include "not having the time," cost, objections to aspects of the criteria employed, and concerns about the assessment process. Black (2003: 109) is correct when she says that those electing not to register may be asked to explain their reluctance to do so by the courts and police services. However, it should be considered that responses to such queries may raise concerns about aspects of registration as it currently exists. It is appropriate to mention here that similar concerns were evident when U.K. archaeologists attempted to "professionalise" their subject in the 1980s. The establishment of the Institute of Field Archaeologists was resisted for some years by many but has developed and proved to be beneficial to members and the profession as a whole. Today, most archaeologists choose to apply to become members; with time, the same may be true for the CRFP.

Challenges

One of our biggest challenges is to overcome the personal and professional conflicts that are often seen to dominate practice and behaviour in forensic archaeology and anthropology. The reason underlying this situation is difficult to deduce and may reflect one or more factors. For instance, while contributing to the process of justice and humanitarian need, we are working in a marketplace, and although this is without doubt a growth industry with a growing market, full-time posts and freelance opportunities remain few. Consequently, competition for prestige, reputation, positions, and contracts leads to a competitive and often destructive environment that most of those working in "industry" would recognise. We may also have cause to question the motives of some of the individuals that desire to carry out this work. Some may indeed be those taking advantage of the "cash cow" (Black 2003) or alternatively may be attracted by the seductive but superficial and misleading frisson of risk, glamour, and importance (Cox 2001) associated with forensic sciences today.

A more charitable interpretation for the divisions between forensic practitioners and organisations is that expressed by a colleague working toward the prevention of atrocity crimes:

> genocide produces such anger amongst those who see it and want to do something about it, that when they feel powerless they displace their anger onto those people who are also trying to take action against it. They become quite personal and spiteful as a result, just as they would against the perpetrators. What is ironic is that the displacement is most powerful against those who are nearest to them in their goals or ideas.
> (Dr. G. H. Stanton, President, Genocide Watch; Coordinator, International Campaign to End Genocide, personal communication 2006)

Conclusion

Significant steps forward have been taken in the development and the applications of forensic anthropology and archaeology in the U.K. over the last two decades, and much has been achieved within that time frame. There is, however, a very long way to go if we are to do justice to the disciplines and professions that we seek to represent and, more importantly, to contribute effectively to the process of justice in all its diversity. Our role is diverse and includes assisting in the location, recovery, and identification of the Missing and all forms of evidence that have the potential to illuminate our understanding of their deaths and burial or deposition. Improving our approaches to, and methods of recovering, analysing, and reconstructing the past and the identities and causes of death of the deceased must be the focus of our activities and engagement. If we are to continue to move forensic anthropology and archaeology forward, both in the U.K. and internationally, and we must, then there is no room for the seemingly global tendency for internecine disputes and lack of collegial spirit that has somewhat marred the impressive growth and development that the last decade has witnessed.

Acknowledgments

Thanks are due Ian Hanson for providing the reference to Sir Sydney Smith and for reminding me that Mant was a U.K. citizen, and Sue Black for providing information about CIFA and the B.Sc. Forensic Anthropology at University of Dundee. I am grateful to Barrie Fitzgerald and Mark Viner for providing specific unpublished information and to Mary Lewis, Jonathan Forrest, and Derek Congram for commenting usefully on an earlier version of this paper.

Notes

1. David Scheffer (U.S. Ambassador at Large for War Crimes under the Clinton administration, at the 50th Anniversary of the Genocide Convention, 13 June 2001) considered that for the sake of simplicity and to avoid incorrect application of legal terms all such serious crimes should be encompassed within a common phrase—"atrocity crimes."

2. The former may be seen through trauma to bone and the latter from elevated nitrogen isotope levels.

3. The author of this chapter is the Chief Executive of the Inforce Foundation.

4. *Capacity building* is a term much used in the development sector to describe providing training and education that is primarily designed to build in-country capacity in areas where there is little or no previous skills base. As an example, in 2004, Iraq had no osteoarchaeologists or biological or forensic anthropologists. Inforce consequently trained 12 medical doctors in this subject to Master of Science level.

5. Technically, *triage* refers to assigning degrees of urgency to the treatment of wounds in the context of an incident usually involving fatalities. However, in the context of mortuary analysis, its meaning in terms of "sorting" remains has become commonplace.

6. Programme I ran for five months. Thirty-three individuals (whose professional backgrounds included archaeology, dentistry, medicine, policing, and radiology) were trained in forensic archaeology, anthropology, radiography, pathology, logistics, project management, and scene-of-crime examination. This training provided the suite of skills required in a team to locate, excavate, record, and recover all evidence from a mass gravesite and to analyse the remains. All of this training was set within legal and scene-of-crime frameworks. Programme II was for 39 lawyers who were the investigators for the Iraq Special/High Tribunal. Programme III was for 12 of the first group, who were trained in training skills. This programme comprised teacher training, skills enhancement, and a professional placement; it has already borne fruit. The first training courses designed and delivered by these trainees have been delivered in Iraq.

7. And the same principle must apply to anthropology, which is affected by the same trend, particularly in basic issues such as bone/nonbone and human/nonhuman identification, and the use of anthropologists in the field.

8. It may be taught as a specialist third-year option.

9. Exceptions include law, medicine, and dentistry, all of which require subsequent periods of training and mentored practice.

References

ACPO Centrex. 2005. *Practice Advice on Core Investigative Doctrine*. Cambridge: National Centre for Policing Excellence.

Black, S. M. 2003. Forensic anthropology: Regulation in the United Kingdom. *Science and Justice* 43(4): 187–192.

Booth, R. 1994. *The Collected Poems of John Donne*. London: Wordsworth Editions Ltd.

Cox, M. 2001. Forensic archaeology in the U.K.: Questions of socio-intellectual context and socio-political responsibility, in V. Buchli and G. Lucas (eds.), *Archaeologies of the Contemporary Past*, pp. 145–157. Cambridge: Cambridge University Press.

———. 2003. A multidisciplinary approach to the investigation of crimes against humanity, war crimes and genocide: The Inforce Foundation. *Science and Justice* 43(4): 225–229.

Cox, M., and Bell, L. S. 1999. Recovery of human skeletal elements from a recent U.K. murder enquiry: Preservational signatures. *Journal of Forensic Sciences* 44: 945–950.

Cox, M., Flavel, A., Hanson, I., Laver, J., and Wessling, R. (eds.). 2008. *The Scientific Investigation of Mass Graves: Towards the Development of Protocols and Standard Operating Procedures*. Cambridge: Cambridge University Press.

Glaister, J., and Brash, J. 1937. *The Medicolegal Aspects of the Ruxton Case*. Edinburgh: Livingstone.

Hanson, I. D. 2004. The importance of stratigraphic in forensic investigations, in K. Pye and D. J. Croft (eds.), *Forensic Geosciences: Principles, Techniques and Applications*, pp. 39–48. Geological Society Special Publication 232. London: Geological Society.

Hunter, J., and Cox, M. 2005. *Forensic Archaeology: Advances in Theory and Practice*. London: Routledge.

Hunter, J., Roberts, C., and Martin, A. 1996. *Studies in Crime: An Introduction to Forensic Archaeology*. London: Batsford.

London Resilience Team and Mass Fatality Working Group. 2005. *London Mass Fatality Plan*. Restricted document.

Mackinnon, G., and Mundorff, A. Z. 2007. The World Trade Center, September 11th, 2001, in T. J. U. Thompson and S. M. Black (eds.), *An Introduction to Biological Human Identification*, pp. 485–499. Boca Raton, FL: CRC Press.

Mant, A. K. 1950. A Study in Exhumation Data. Unpublished M.D. thesis. University of London.

———. 1987. Knowledge acquired from post-war exhumations, in A. Boddington, A. N. Garland, and R. C. Janaway (eds.), *Death, Decay and Reconstruction*, pp. 65–78. Manchester: Manchester University Press.

McNeely, C. L. 1995. Perceptions of the criminal justice system: Television and popular imagery and public knowledge in the United States. *Journal of Criminal Justice and Popular Culture* 3(1): 1–20.

Oxford English Dictionary. 1990. Oxford: Clarendon Press.

Royal Commission on Criminal Justice. 1993. Report Cm 2263, London: Her Majesty's Stationary Office.

Saukko, P., and Knight, B. 2004. *Knight's Forensic Pathology* (3rd ed.). London: Arnold.

Smith, S. 1959. *Mostly Murder*. London: Companion Book Club.

Thompson, T. J. U. 2003. Supply and demand: The shifting expectations of forensic anthropology in the United Kingdom. *Science and Justice* 43(4): 181–183.

FORENSIC ANTHROPOLOGY AND ARCHAEOLOGY: PERSPECTIVES FROM ITALY

Cristina Cattaneo

Having to give a perspective of forensic anthropology in Italy could be considered a frustrating experience, since there is very little to say from an academic and professional point of view. However, there is a bright side: after approximately ten years of painstaking insistence, pathologists and judges are beginning to understand and to appreciate the discipline and its expertise. The aim of this brief chapter is therefore to give a short history of forensic anthropology in Italy and then to illustrate the status quo with examples of real cases concerning several fields of application.

Forensic Anthropology in Italy: History, Politics, and Academics

Forensic anthropology in Italy was born about a decade ago, with the works of two major Italian universities: Bari in the South and, shortly after that, Milano in the North. These two academic centres started to perform research and to publish in areas concerning sexing, ageing, personal identification, and such and then started to educate judges about the usefulness of the discipline in cases of skeletal remains. The University of Milano went on to create what is now known as LABANOF (Laboratorio di Antropologia ed Odontologia Forense) at the Institute of Legal Medicine, a centre for forensic anthropology research, teaching, and professional activity. Although there are 13 university departments of legal medicine in Italy that offer postgraduate training in forensic pathology and 11 universities that offer undergraduate training in physical anthropology, Milano is currently the only university that offers postgraduate training in forensic anthropology, alternately in the form of a Masters course (M.Sc.) or a "Corso di Perfezionamento" (a taught course of 50 hours of theory and practice). (In the academic year 2008/2009, a Masters Course in Bioarchaeology, Palaeopathology and Forensic Anthropology, organised by the Universities of Bologna, Milano and Pisa, will start.) No undergraduate courses in forensic anthropology are currently offered in Italy. Many forensic pathology and physical anthropology teachers slip in the occasional forensic anthropology lecture in his/her pathology or anthropology course; however, proper training is practically non-existent. This is true for two main reasons: first, forensic anthropology is a relatively new applied discipline; second, nobody really knows who the forensic anthropologist should be—an anthropologist or a pathologist?

This question has been considered in a recently published textbook on forensic anthropology and pathology:

What is a forensic anthropologist? Particularly across Europe, this is a very delicate issue, and it may concern experience and training more so than specific academic qualifications, at least at the moment. In Anglo-Saxon countries, namely, the U.S. and the U.K., the forensic anthropologist at least falls into a defined category, i.e., that of he/she who practices forensic anthropology, this being "the application of physical anthropology to the forensic context." (Cunha and Cattaneo 2006: 40)

Compared to forensic anthropology in the United States, forensic anthropology in Europe is highly disorganised as far as training is concerned.

One of the obstacles to overcome in Europe is cultural. In many European countries, there remains a distinct division between experts who work in a forensic context, namely, forensic pathologists, and those who work in the anthropological context, mainly anthropologists working on archaeological material. Let us take the example of human remains. The scientific and forensic communities have come to realise that there is a void when human remains are found in a forensic scenario: most forensic pathologists do not have anthropological and osteological expertise, and classical anthropologists may not be used to working with human remains still bearing some soft tissue or found in a modern criminal context. In addition to ethnographers, cultural anthropologists, and geneticists who work on human variation, physical anthropologists have always included practitioners considered as experts in human osteology. Thus the anthropologist's contribution to anything coming from the forensic scenario traditionally deals with the determination of ancestry, sexing, ageing, and stature; in other words, similar assessments to those undertaken by the anthropologist when studying skeletal remains of ancient populations.

However, traditional anthropology is not enough for the forensic context. Forensic anthropologists must deal with questions pertaining to identification and manner of death that have legal and social implications. The anthropologist and the pathologist both have to deal with the human body *in toto*: the more soft tissue on it, the more it is the domain of the pathologist; the more skeletonised, decomposed, or burnt, the more it is the domain of the anthropologist.

One could go as far as to say that forensic anthropology is a field that works in parallel with forensic pathology. In other words, just as the pathologist deals with the human cadaver from the scene of crime to establishing time and cause of death, the anthropologist, when nothing remains of a victim but bones, must deal with the search and proper retrieval of the skeleton (using subdisciplines such as forensic archaeology) and with such issues as identification and detection of signs of trauma that may lead to establishing cause and manner of death.

While forensic anthropologists typically deal with the dead, practitioners are increasingly requested to handle the identification and ageing of living individuals. In the past few years, specialists have applied notions of anthropology and associated disciplines to ageing juvenile perpetrators, identifying bank robbers taped on video surveillance systems and establishing whether presumed victims of pedopornography are under age.[1]

Returning to the Italian scenario, a frequent problem is that cases involving human remains are dealt with by forensic pathologists, who have no training in forensic anthropology, with all the imaginable consequences. However, regardless of who should apply forensic anthropology, the main issue is that the discipline be taught, either to pathologists or anthropologists, so that human remains can be examined in the best possible manner. At the moment, in Italy, a pathologist has better chances than an anthropologist does of working as a forensic anthropologist. This is because, by tradition, magistrates give cases to pathologists, who choose a team of experts (including geneticists, experts in ballistics, toxicologists, entomologists, and so on). Frequently, the pathologist feels qualified enough to do the forensic anthropology work. However, properly trained anthropologists may one day enter the expert witness status.

If training and lack of expert pathologists and anthropologists are still issues, research in forensic anthropology in Italy is somewhat present, although sporadic. If we look at books and publications in this discipline on a national basis, we see only one textbook on forensic anthropology, *Lo Studio dei Resti Umani: Testo Atlante di Antropologia ed Odontologia Forense* (Cattaneo and Grandi 2005), and one small booklet on forensic odontology, *Identificazione in Odontologia Forense* (Cameriere 2003). In the last ten years, a few forensic anthropology articles have been published in international journals from Italy, mainly by the teams from Milano (Cattaneo et al. 1999), Bari (Introna et al. 1997; Introna, Di Vella, and Campobasso 1999), Macerata (Cameriere et al. 2005) (strictly odontology), and Rome (Ricci, Marella, and Apostol 2006). The Universities of Milano and Bari, however, remain at the moment the specialists in Italy in this field.

As far as scientific groups and associations are involved, Italy has only one group remotely interested in forensic anthropology, called GIAOF—Gruppo Italiano di Antropologia ed Odontologia Forense. First established in 1996, this group has over the years unfortunately become mainly interested in strictly medico-legal malpractice aspects of forensic odontology and has grown away from forensic anthropology. At this point, the Forensic Anthropology Society of Europe (FASE) is the only society that groups Italian forensic anthropologists and forensic pathologists with an interest in forensic anthropology.

Forensic Anthropology in Practice

However, if we look at the real-world scenario, one can see that in Italy there is a need for forensic anthropology. It is impossible to have a picture of the activity of all Italian medico-legal institutes, but the requests that reach our laboratory every year likely are representative of the enormity of the problem.

Milano is a city with a population of around 1.5 million people. The medico-legal institute performs around 800 autopsies every year, and there are on average 50 cadavers or human remains requiring personal identification. Approximately ten cases every year require the construction of a biological profile through sexing, ageing, stature, ancestry determination, and sometimes facial reconstruction; in these cases, forensic anthropology is crucial. The other cases involving remains that are skeletonised, burnt, or in an advanced stage of decomposition arrive with a suspicion of identity. Identity is confirmed in approximately one-third of cases by DNA analysis and in the other two-thirds by anthropological and/or odontological methods (Cattaneo et al. 2005). Once again, then, forensic anthropology is crucial. Furthermore, in many of these cases, where soft tissue is scarce, forensic anthropology is also critical for verifying the presence of traumatic lesions on bone. In addition, every year there are on average five requests involving scene-of-crime activities that require forensic anthropology and forensic archaeology expertise for the search and recovery of human remains. Increasingly, anthropological expertise is requested for identifying the living from images on video surveillance systems in an average of about eight cases every year. Thus, although forensic anthropology is not needed on a daily basis in the typical Italian medico-legal institute, it is requested quite frequently.

Thus, forensic anthropology in Italy still needs to be developed both professionally and academically. However, the situation is slowly changing, as exemplified by two cases described below. These cases illustrate how crucial forensic anthropology is in cases involving skeletal remains and the extent to which forensic anthropology expertise is beginning to be recognised by judges and pathologists.

Two Emblematic Cases

Case 1

As a preliminary note to Case 1: in 1998, a member of the mafia confessed to a magistrat that ten years before, a man had been murdered and buried in the woods in the outskirts of Milano. The magistrate proceeded to recover the remains, buried about1 m beneath the soil surface, with picks and shovels, using non-expert personnel. The result was that the skeleton was severely damaged and was identified with great difficulty. It was also difficult to distinguish peri- from postmortem lesions on the skeleton (Figure 3.1).

In Italy it used to be quite rare that archaeological methods were used for recovery of skeletal remains or that anthropological analyses of a skeleton were requested in order to create a biological profile to send to newspapers and television for identification. But after the experience of the above-mentioned mafia case, magistrates started to acknowledge the value of expert recovery and anthropological analysis. This was exemplified in a case that occurred five years ago.

On October 5, 2001, in a woody area at the outskirts of a small town near Milano, a group of children saw a boot emerging from the ground and kicked it, uncovering tibia and fibula. Investigating authorities immediately isolated the area and called the Istituto di Medicina Legale in Milan. A team of forensic pathologists, anthropologists, archaeologists, and botanists then arrived at the site, and an archaeological recovery was performed. Over the entire afternoon and night the skeletal remains (Figure 3.2) were uncovered following a stratigraphic method: strict archaeological excavation techniques allowed for the non-destructive recovery of all skeletal elements and associated objects (synthetic clothes, earrings, and so on), their topographic recording and registration, and correct sampling of tree roots crossing the femur and the auditory meati of the cranium, which proved essential for determining the postmortem interval.

Then the skeleton was cleaned and reassembled in the laboratory, where classical anthropological studies were performed (Ubelaker 1998): determination of ancestry (see Sauer and Wankmiller

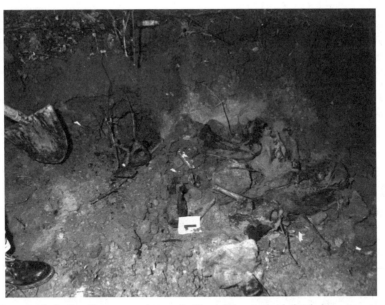

Figure 3.1 Damage, including fractures and commingling of the single skeletal elements, caused by a gross excavation methodology. The lack of a controlled recovery led to loss of information on identity, position of burial, postmortem interval, and trauma.

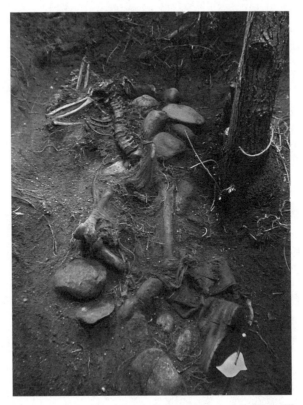

Figure 3.2 Skeleton recovered using archaeological methods. One can note the difference between the case in Figure 3.1 and this case. It was possible to recover every bone and personal effect, to determine PMI, and to interpret skeletal lesions as perimortem trauma.

this volume); sexing (see Braz this volume); ageing (see Rogers and Crowder this volume), height (see Willey this volume); assessment of pathologies and dental status (see Clement this volume) were undertaken leading to a biological profile consistent with a white, young (20–25 year old) female, approximately 1.60 m in height, possibly of Balkan origin. Finally a plaster cast was made from the cranium, on which facial reconstruction was performed. Given the peculiar dentition (a large diastema [space] between the two central upper incisors and the absence of lateral upper incisors), personnel decided to reconstruct the face in a "smiling" attitude, in order to visualize a possibly peculiar smile. A replica of the dentition was made in white resin for the teeth and pink plasticine for the gums. Since tufts of hair of a brownish colour and of medium length were found near the cranial vault, several possible hairdos were also prepared for the final reconstruction. Furthermore, analyses of tree roots and of the clothes allowed personnel to place the time of death between 1995 and 1998; macroscopic and microscopic analysis of the costal margins revealed a cutmark with "green fracture" characteristics on the lower margin of the tenth left rib. Thus biological profile, time of death, and probable cause of death had been achieved. The final image of the victim's face was then passed on to national newspapers and to Italian national television (RAI) (Figure 3.3).

At the end of a popular television programme that deals with missing persons and murder cases, several calls were made to the producers; one in particular seemed interesting for investigating authorities. Information from this call led to the victim being positively identified and to prosecution of members of a prostitution ring accused of her murder.

This case—to our knowledge, the first in Italy in which investigating authorities requested and allowed forensic pathologists, anthropologists, archaeologists, and botanists to deal with the buried skeletal remains from the moment of their discovery—led to determination of postmortem interval, construction of an accurate biological profile, and diagnosis of the possible cause and manner of death. This result stresses how important it is for skeletal remains to be recovered by specialists in order to preserve stratigraphic and botanical evidence for the postmortem interval (PMI) estimate and to properly recover all evidence without fracturing the bones, which would cause difficulty in the interpretation of fractures and manner of death. In conclusion, this case proved to the judges the need for forensic anthropologists and archaeologists at the scene of crime, and also that it is possible, with good collaboration with investigating authorities and the media, to deal adequately with the retrieval of human remains from the start and to solve what may seem, initially, a hopeless case.

Case 2

In the summer of 2001, a skeleton was found within the cellar of an abandoned building in a city near the outskirts of Milano. The body was completely skeletonised, still dressed, and surrounded by garbage, with its feet bound in chains that were attached to the wall. Scene of crime investigators collected most of the bones (although many animal bones, especially chicken, were initially taken for human bones), which underwent full anthropological, odontological, and genetic investigations.

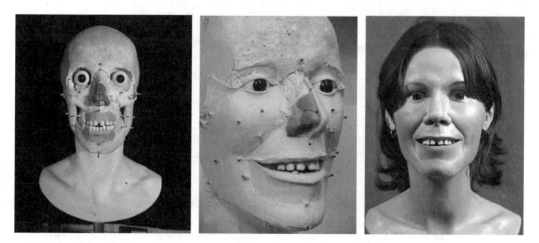

Figure 3.3 Various phases of facial reconstruction that followed anthropological analysis of the skeleton.

Anthropological analyses were performed on two fronts. First of all, a biological profile of the deceased was built according to standard sexing and ageing methods; estimation of ancestry, height, and dental status were also performed (Ubelaker 1998). The biological profile subsequently led to suspicion of identity, so antemortem data related to a young North-African who had gone missing and postmortem data belonging to the skeleton were compared, particularly the dental status. Finally, craniofacial superimposition and genetic analysis were performed (Yoshino et al. 2001). Trauma analysis was also undertaken, because the skeleton presented recent (perimortem) and healed fractures. This was done by macroscopic and stereomicroscopic observation of the bone lesions and by radiological analysis, in order to establish postmortem, perimortem, and antemortem trauma and its manner of production. Ageing of antemortem trauma was also attempted.

Results showed that the skeleton belonged to a 35- to 44-year-old male of Caucasian (Mediterranean) origin, approximately 1.69 m tall, whose two central superior incisors had gone missing long before the time of death. Craniofacial superimposition, along with consistent antemortem and postmortem data concerning the missing incisors (the young man had a removable prosthetic appliance corresponding to the two upper incisors), indicated a high probability of identification

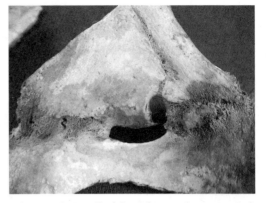

Figure 3.5 Detail of the right scapula, supraspinal portion, showing a recent fracture with initial healing and woven bone.

(Figure 3.4), which was then confirmed by genetic analyses. However, as is frequently the case with illegal immigrants, genetic antemortem or parental material was not available; this case shows the importance therefore of anthropological and odontological identification methods.

Trauma analysis (see Cunha and Pinheiro; Loe; and Nawrocki this volume) showed signs of sharp force perimortem trauma on the blade of the left scapula along with antemortem trauma resulting probably from blunt force injury to the left scapula and the right fibula. The radiographic and macroscopic study of the initial osseous remodelling of the antemortem trauma, still at the stage of "periostitis" (Figure 3.5), indicated that these lesions had probably been produced 15–30 days prior to death. Note that the highly qualified forensic pathologist who had previously studied the skeleton had not noticed the periosteal reaction, which would have led to loss of important information, hence the importance of the forensic anthropologist. Such indications confirmed a witness's report, which stated that the victim had been initially hit with a blunt object and then chained to the wall. Anthropological evidence further showed that the victim survived these blows, but after a period roughly of 15–30 days, he was stabbed and died shortly after. This case report showed the judges the important applications of forensic anthropology not only to problems concerning identification but also to the interpretation of trauma on bone.

Conclusion

Forensic anthropology in Italy is slowly developing both academically and practically. In Milano,

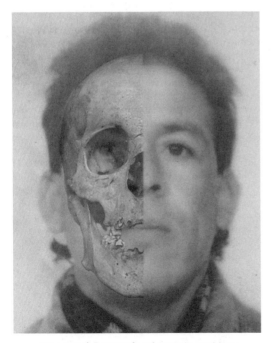

Figure 3.4 Craniofacial superimposition.

where the disciplines of forensic anthropology and archaeology have been strongly publicised in Courts and newspapers and television (thanks to the resolution of the cases mentioned above and others), judges and magistrates are slowly coming to realise the importance of their application. This activity has also had reverberations in other parts of Italy, and skeletal cases are slowly receiving proper attention and treatment. However, much work still needs to be done.

It is not only the judges who need to be "educated" but also, and especially, the forensic pathologists; they are the main characters in the investigation of human remains. When human remains are found, a pathologist is almost certainly called in, and it is he/she who will advise the magistrate on what should be done and which experts to involve. As stated previously, the pathologist is and should necessarily be called in. In fact, by Italian law, the forensic pathologist is the only person who can subsequently certify both death and the cause of death. However he/she is rarely competent in forensic anthropology (and archaeology). Thus, because forensic pathologists may not necessarily be trained in osteology, it is fundamental that a forensic anthropologist be consulted in cases involving skeletonised or partially skeletonised remains. This necessity leads us to the delicate question of the lack of trained personnel (because of the lack of structured training courses—a problem that is slowly reaching a solution) and the inevitable appearance of "self-made" anthropologists on the forensic scene. The problem of unqualified personnel trying to make their way in a new discipline is well known. For this reason, teaching and certification are the next important goals, not only for Italian but also for European anthropology.

Note

1. Thus, only recently has the need arisen—both for issues involving the dead and those involving the living—for the constitution of a European association to discuss and to solve these types of questions. Hence, the main goals of the recently formed FASE (Forensic Anthropology Society of Europe), a subsection of the International Academy of Legal Medicine, are education, harmonisation, and certification, along with the promotion of research (Baccino 2005).

References

Baccino, E. 2005. Forensic Anthropology Society of Europe (FASE), a subsection of IALM, is 1 year old. *International Journal of Legal Medicine* 119(6): N1.

Cameriere, C., Ferrante, L., Mirtella, D., Rollo, R., and Cingolani, M. 2005. Frontal sinuses for identification: Quality of classifications, possible error and potential corrections. *Journal of Forensic Sciences* 50: 770–773.

Cameriere, R. 2003. *Identificazione in Odontologia Forense*. Torino: Edizioni Minerva Medica.

Cattaneo, C., and Baccino, E. 2002. A call for forensic anthropology in Europe. *International Journal of Legal Medicine* 116: N1–N2.

Cattaneo, C. and Grandi, M. 2005. *Lo Studio dei Resti Umani: Testo Atlante di Antropologia ed Odontologia Forense*. Bologna: Monduzzi.

Cattaneo, C., Di Martino, S., Scali, S., Craig, O. E., Grandi, M., and Sokol, R. J. 1999. Determining the human origin of fragments of burnt bone: A comparative study of histological, immunological and DNA techniques. *Forensic Science International* 102: 181–191.

Cattaneo, C., Giovanetti, G., Porta, D., Marinelli, E., D'Agostino, N., and Grandi, M. 2005. Il problema del cadavere sconosciuto visto attraverso uno studio retrospettivo di nove anni (345 casi): Un problema ancora e sempre da risolvere. *Minerva Med Leg*, 125: 9–18.

Cunha, E., and Cattaneo, C. 2006. Forensic pathology and forensic anthropology, in A. Schmitt, E. Cunha, and J. Pinheiro (eds.), *Forensic Anthropology and Medicine*, pp. 39–53. Totowa, NJ: Humana Press.

Introna, F., DiVella, G., and Campobasso, C. P. 1999. Determination of postmortem interval from old skeletal remains by image analysis of luminol test results. *Journal of Forensic Sciences* 44(3): 535–538.

Introna, F., DiVella, G., Campobasso, C., and Dragone, M. 1997. Sex determination by discriminant analysis of calcanei measurements. *Journal of Forensic Sciences* 42: 725–728.

Ricci, A., Marella, G. L., and Apostol, A. M. 2006. A new experimental approach to computer-aided face/skull identification in forensic anthropology. *American Journal of Forensic Medicine and Pathology* 27(1): 46–49.

Ubelaker, D. H. 1998. *Human Skeletal Remains*. Washington, D.C.: Taraxacum Press.

Yoshino, M., Matsuda, H., Kubota, S., Imaitsumi, K., and Myhasaka, S. 2001. Computer-assisted facial image identification system. *Forensic Science Communication* 3(1): 53–59.

4

FORENSIC ANTHROPOLOGY: PERSPECTIVES FROM FRANCE

Eric Baccino

The fact that the writer of this chapter is a medical doctor and a Professor of Legal Medicine is an indicator of the status of forensic anthropology in France, where forensic anthropology is an activity (and not an individualized specialty) undertaken mainly by medico-legal doctors to answer demands from the French judicial system (the organization of which is briefly described below). An historical overview will, however, show that anthropologists played an important role in research and publications in forensic anthropology but were rarely involved in practical cases.

During the past 20 years, forensic anthropology in France has undergone spectacular changes. The number of people trained in forensic anthropology dramatically increased, as did the number of Ph.D.s awarded, conferences attended, and articles published in forensic anthropology. A French disaster victim identification (DVI) team (which acknowledges the role of the forensic anthropologists) was created and became very active at home and abroad. A boost in international collaboration was another characteristic of the last two decades. Since 1990, with the assistance of colleagues from the United States (particularly Dr. Douglas Ubelaker, Smithsonian Institution), several English-speaking workshops in forensic anthropology have been given in France. With

the creation of the Forensic Anthropology Society of Europe (FASE) in 2003, workshops in other European countries have been organized. This chapter aims to explain who the forensic anthropologists in France are and their academic output, as well as field activity. The future of French forensic anthropology within a European context is considered.

In France (similar to many Mediterranean countries), there are two police forces at the national level: "La Police Nationale," under the control of the Minister of the Interior in charge of urban areas, and "La Gendarmerie Nationale," part of the army, for rural areas. Both have local teams trained in forensic sciences, crime laboratories, and DVI teams, but only the National Crime Lab of Gendarmerie has a permanent staff of four (three forensic anthropologists and one odontologist).

Both police forces are under the permanent control of the judges who are present and active from the report of the case and the scene investigation all through the investigation until the trial. Judges also have complete control over the choice of any expert who becomes involved in the case. Although it is not mandatory, the judges choose the experts from an official list established by the courts, which includes (but only since 2005) a section on "Anthropology and Identification." Official experts in forensic anthropology in France are pathologists or odontologists and not anthropologists. The main reason for this situation is that most magistrates know very little about forensic anthropology and think that identification (especially of decomposed bodies) is only a part of the autopsy.

Besides identification, judicial needs include information about the postmortem interval (PMI),[1] the cause of death, and age determination of both deceased and living individuals. Forensic anthropologists in France are often asked to determine the age of living individuals, particularly in cases involving juvenile delinquents or illegal immigrants: below 18 years of age, an immigrant in France cannot be expelled from the country, and individuals younger than 13 years cannot be detained in custody or in jail. A combination of clinical examination and interpretation of wrist and dental X rays is thus necessary.

The complete independence of the judges, especially the "Instruction Judge," explains why judges mainly choose (even in high-profile cases) local experts, that is, experts with whom they are familiar. This is also the case in mass disasters, when the national DVI team will be involved, only at the request of the magistrate in charge and as a complement to the local forensic pathology unit. The fees for forensic anthropology experts are prescribed in a code and, unlike other areas of expertise (for example, DNA and toxicology), forensic anthropology activities are largely undervalued.

The fact that the decision-making process is entirely in the hands of the judges, full-time medico-legal doctors are relatively scarce, and wages are low explain the low number of forensic autopsies (7,000 per year—that is, grossly tenfold less than in the U.K.). The medico-legal field in France is, however, much larger than forensic pathology, because it includes clinical forensic medicine, which comprises, for example, examination of victims of domestic violence and alleged police violence. This very low level of forensic autopsies explains why most medico-legal doctors are part-time "specialists" whose versatility excludes any specialization or experience in forensic anthropology. Moreover, forensic anthropology is just one (small) aspect of medico-legal activity from the judiciary point of view, and one is hardly surprised that there is no admissibility procedure for this information or testimony in the French courts, such as there is in the United States, owing to the Daubert rulings (United States Supreme Court in *Daubert v. Merrell Dow Pharmaceuticals* 1993).

Despite a recent policy on accreditation of judiciary experts, magistrates still, in practice, have the power to do "quality control" for all types of experts (including forensic anthropologists). This cultural prominence of justice is a strong obstacle to accreditation processes and guidelines issued by the scientific community. The overall result is a heterogeneity or unevenness in the quality of medico-legal activity. There are huge differences between cities with well-staffed Medico-Legal Units and remote areas with no 24-hour medico-legal facilities. Thus, forensic anthropology in France is what the magistrates decide it is, since they almost exclusively rely on forensic pathologists to do the job. Thus, here forensic anthropology can be considered as part of forensic pathology rather than an independent discipline.

Historical Overview

Interestingly, the man who is considered the father of physical anthropology in France, Paul Broca (1824–1880), was also a surgeon and a medical doctor. In addition to his research on bone torsion and brain morphology (1875), he played a major role in the foundation of "La Société d'Anthropologie de Paris" (1850), "La Revue d'Anthropologie" (1872), and "L'École d'Anthropologie de Paris" (1875). Despite this "hybrid" paternity, forensic pathologists and physical anthropologists seemed to have followed parallel ways.

The end of the 19th century was also the time of Bertillon, who published anthropometrical methods applied to the identification of criminals (1889) (İşcan and Quatrehomme 1999). Afterward and until relatively recently (the mid 1980s), there was an unofficial task repartition between anthropologists, who were at the origin of most of research articles, and forensic pathologists, who tended to concentrate on producing textbooks (with some forensic anthropology content)—for example, Vibert's *Précis de Médecine Légale* (1896) and, more recently, Dérobert's, *Médecine Légale* (Dérobert 1974), which contained two chapters about "Identification." These two chapters, called "Os" (bones) and "Dents" (teeth), explored most of the topics of interest to forensic anthropology: the determination of human and nonhuman skeletal remains, sex, age, ancestry, stature, postmortem interval, facial reconstruction, photograph superposition, and identification (including from mass disasters). Interestingly, there was no or little mention about

Table 4.1 French forensic anthropology publications concerned with aging methods.

Aging Method	Reference
Suchey Brooks System (SBS system)	Baccino and Schmitt 2006
Three-dimensional CT scan development	Pasquier et al. 1999; Telmon et al. 2005
İşcan's 4th rib-based method evaluation and simplification	Martrille et al. 2003
X rays of laryngeal cartilage	De la Grandmaison, Banasr, and Durigon 2003
Pelvic bone	Rouge-Maillart et al. 2004; Schmitt et al. 2002
The multifactorial approach with the Two Step Procedure (TSP)	Baccino et al. 1999

techniques employed to recover remains or analysis of bone trauma.

Quatrehomme (İşcan and Quatrehomme 1999) provides a complete overview of the contributions of French scientists (anthropologists and medical doctors) to various fields of forensic anthropology. These include contributions by Olivier (1960) to general anthropology; Balthazard and Dervieus (1921) to fetal aging, stature determination, and microscopic aging of adult bones; Fully (1956), Manouvrier (1892), and Rollet (1888 in Dérobert 1974) to adult stature and aging from the ribs end and from the sternum; and Dérobert (1974) to aging from cranial suture closure and for dental charting and aging. In the 1980s, Barres, Durigon, and Paraire (1989) published on histological and "chest plate" X-ray aging.

Since the early 1990s, the dominant theme in French forensic anthropology publications has been a concern with aging methods (Table 4.1). Perhaps the most significant French contribution to aging mature adult cadavers is, however, Lamendin's dental method (Lamendin 1988) (which is also a component of the TSP). Lamendin's technique was further developed by forensic pathologists (Lamendin et al. 1992) and validated at the international level (Prince and Ubelaker 2002), where it became one of the most widely used techniques worldwide, owing to its excellent simplicity/accuracy ratio (Baccino and Schmitt 2006).

Quatrehomme and colleagues (1995) focused on facial reconstruction and restoration techniques. The team from Strasbourg (Mangin, Ludes, and Kintz) developed DNA determination and toxicology methods from bone material and decomposed remains and specialized in the genetic analysis of degraded DNA extracted from human bone, tooth, and hair. New markers and new genotyping technologies have been proposed, the latest one being a snapshot minisequencing-based technology (Keyser-Tracqui, Crubézy, and Ludes 2003; Keyser-Tracqui and Ludes 2005; Ludes et al. 1994; Petkovski et al. 2005). Grevin and colleagues (1998) published several articles about burnt remains and Bruzek about sexing from the pelvis (in İşcan and Quatrehomme 1999). The team from the Crime Laboratory of the French Gendarmerie published several articles about mass disasters and cadaver recovery techniques (Schuliar et al. 1996, 1998, 1999). Articles that would have been published initially in the French medico-legal publication (*Annales de Médecine Légale*, then *Journal de Médecine Légale Droit Médical*) have, since the 1980s, been published in English-language journals.

In 1988, a French medical doctor (the author of this chapter) became, for the first time, a member of the American Academy of Forensic Sciences (AAFS), joined later on by many French colleagues. This membership gave them the opportunity to attend the forensic anthropology section of the annual AAFS meeting, which is one of the most active professional associations, with sometimes more than 100 presentations given in this section.

The same year (1988), the Brest Bone Collection (BBC) was started in Brest (Brittany France) and later continued in Montpellier (France). Made initially from hospital and forensic autopsy cases of known age, sex, ancestry, and stature, it was restricted to forensic cases after 1994, when "bioethics laws" were issued in France, making collection of body parts from cadavers impossible. The BBC has now more than 400 individuals with pubic symphyses, 4th ribs, medial clavicles, iliac crests, and teeth.

The BBC is used for training students attending the European Workshop on forensic anthropology, which has occurred every other year since 1991 in Brest (Baccino, Brooks, and Ubelaker 1995), then in Montpellier (last one in 2002). Colleagues from the U.S., including Douglas Ubelaker, Judy Suchey, Norman Sauer, and others, have played a major role in what is the only training program in forensic anthropology in continental Europe. The BBC is also used for training French students individually or in groups and for research purposes. It is the only Western European modern bone collection dedicated to aging criteria.

In 2002, the International Association of Forensic Sciences (IAFS), which meets every three years, held its meeting in France. During this time, French forensic anthropology was looking vigorous (as the second most publishing nation behind the U.S.), but neither medical doctors nor anthropologists had intended to create a national society or section in forensic anthropology. Fortunately, during the International Academy of Legal Medicine (IALM) meeting in Milan in 2003, the FASE was officially created giving the French, at last, an opportunity to join a group dedicated to forensic anthropology at the European Level. Logically, the organization of the European Workshops on forensic anthropology was transferred to FASE, which organized one in Milan in 2004 and a second in Budapest in 2006.

To date, through these workshops more than 150 people have been trained, mainly from Europe but also from Asia and North America, with a slight majority of them being medical doctors followed by anthropologists and a significant number of odontologists. There were more than 30 French participants trained during these workshops (primarily medical doctors). Some French odontologists preferred to create a national association, Association Française d'Identification Odontologique (AFIO), which has been quite active in the field. Since 2000, Quatrehomme has organized a French-language, one-day meeting on forensic anthropology in Nice, which allows French forensic anthropologists to meet and exchange data at least once a year.

Since the origin of physical anthropology in France, more than one and a half centuries ago, anthropologists and medico-legal doctors (along with odontologists) have all participated actively in the scientific development of forensic anthropology. However, there has always been a distinct division between the medical doctor, who works in a forensic context (for justice), and the anthropologist, who deals with archaeological material. Since 1991, international collaboration with U.S. colleagues resulted in the creation of FASE, through which French forensic anthropologists

(medical doctors more than anthropologists and odontologists) seem to thrive.

The Current Situation of Forensic Anthropology in France

Who Are the Forensic Anthropologists?

There are, at least officially, no forensic anthropologists in France, owing to the absence of board certification. So the question arises, who are those who practice forensic anthropology? Even counting the experts registered on the court list in the subsection "Anthropology and Identification," one has no reliable clue, since the decision to put somebody on this list is made by magistrates only. Moreover, most forensic pathologists who actually do routine forensic anthropology cases did not ask to appear on this official list.

Considering the French practitioners who attend the European workshops and the fact that most of the university-hospital-based medico-legal centers seem autonomous in forensic anthropology, around 50 people (with a large majority of those being medical doctors) do most of the routine work at the national level. Probably fewer would meet the American Board of Forensic Anthropology prerequisites, and these are usually medical doctors working in big-city units; only a handful of them are anthropologists specializing in forensic cases (mainly at the gendarmerie crime laboratory).

Activities

A. Routine Cases. Apart from data from the gendarmerie crime laboratory, which does approximately 90 cases per year, there are no national data on the number of annual routine cases undertaken. From a study made between 1997 and 2001 in the Montpellier area (population approximately 1.5 million) (Baccino and Schmitt 2006; Boismenu et al. 2001), extrapolated to the whole country, one can assume that more than 1,500 bodies admitted in the French medico-legal structures raise some kind of identification issue each year. Among these so-called John Does, 10% are well preserved, approximately one-third are charred bodies, one-third decomposed (to various degrees, but making a visual definite identification impossible), and only 20% skeletonized. As in many countries, the caseload is on the rise. The two main reasons for this are isolation, especially of the elderly, and identification problems associated with the death of illegal immigrants. These immigrants often do not have an identification card, and the situation is worsened by the fact that they are not listed as missing persons by French police.

B. Mass Disasters and Mass Graves. Both the National Gendarmerie and the Police have DVI teams (UGIVC and UPIVC, respectively). Since 1992, the Gendarmerie team (the first to be created) was involved in nine cases in France and eight cases abroad. These include mainly plane crashes but also road tunnel fires, terrorist bombings, and assistance with the 2004 tsunami. A police team also participated in the Balkans identification process.

The DVI teams have the logistics to send their people and equipment to the scene and can be activated at any time. In the absence of a national list of available forensic anthropologists for this type of mission, the gendarmerie and the police have the responsibility to recruit practitioners, on a case-by-case basis, relying on voluntary service. The 2004 Boxing Day tsunami and the relief effort in Thailand showed that there was no lack of good will and competence for this purpose.

Academic Structures

There is still no French university that offers specific graduate or postgraduate courses in forensic anthropology. There are, however, a few institutions (including the Universities of Bordeaux, Toulouse, and Marseille), where it is possible (although not common) to prepare a Ph.D. in anthropology with a forensic focus.

The number and quality of forensic anthropologists in France indisputably increased during the past 20 years, probably in connection with the development of international collaboration and the teaching of workshops in forensic anthropology. Unfortunately, there is still no official national recognition of forensic anthropology as an academic specialty in France. This is a major weakness when it comes to funding research projects and to quality control of self-proclaimed forensic anthropology specialists. In a country where neither legal medicine nor forensic sciences has an official Ph.D. program, there is little hope that forensic anthropology will obtain academic recognition as an individualized specialty. There is also little hope that the judicial branch will abandon its complete control over the selection and appointment of experts. In addition, the present national economic mood is far from favorable to increasing expenses in the Health and Judicial system. The only solution might come at the European level.

Although difficult, obtaining funds for possible development of forensic anthropology from the European Council (E.C.) is possible. The E.C. is a big enough market to justify the publication of a book about forensic anthropology as well as an online teaching module, and creating a course on forensic anthropology at the E.C. level that would involve several universities as theoretical teaching and training laboratories makes sense. This would be even more practical if the definition of forensic anthropology were extended to include recovery, biological profile, and identification as well as PMI, cause and manner of death, and identification of the living along with age determination from clinical examination and photographic material (Cunha and Cattaneo 2006). An accreditation process at the Continental level (one of the main aims of the creation of the FASE) (Cattaneo and Baccino 2002) would also be beneficial to achieve an independent specialty (with subsections such as imaging, DNA, toxicology, and so on). The FASE supports this by organizing workshops and advanced courses, guidelines, coordinated research, and publication. There is, however, yet another paradox in viewing the development of forensic anthropology in France: the future of French forensic anthropology might be grim unless we agree to write it in English.

Note

1. If the PMI is over 10 years the case can no longer be prosecuted.

References

Baccino, E., Brooks, S. T., and Ubelaker, D. 1995. Forensic Anthropology workshops in Brest, France, *Proceedings of the American Academy of Forensic Sciences,* pp. 173–174.

Baccino, E., and Schmitt, A. 2006. Determination of adult age at death in the forensic context, in A. Schmitt, E. Cunha, and J. Pinheiro (eds.). *Forensic Anthropology and Medicine: Complementary Sciences. From Recovery to Cause of Death,* pp. 259–280. Totowa, NJ: Humana Press.

Baccino, E., Ubelaker, D. H., Hayek, L., and Zerilli, A. 1999. Evaluation of seven methods of estimating age at death from mature human skeletal remains. *Journal of Forensic Sciences* 44: 39–44.

Balthazard, V., and Dervieux, F. 1921. Etudes anthropologiques sur le foetus humain. *Annales de Médecine Légales* 1: 37–43.

Barres, D. R., Durigon, M., and Paraire, F. 1989. Age estimation from quantification of features of

"Chest Plate" X Rays. *Journal of Forensic Sciences* 34: 228–233.

Boismenu, L., Bertolotti, C., Salerio, G., and Baccino, E. 2001. L'identification Médico légale anthropologique, bilan d'activité autopsique du service de médecine légale de Montpellier au cours des années 1997–2001, presented at the *3rd Congress of Medico-legal Anthropology, Nice, France, November.*

Cattaneo, C., and Baccino, E. 2002. A call for forensic anthropology in Europe. *International Journal of Legal Medicine* 116: N1–N2.

Cunha, E., and Cattaneo, C. 2006. Forensic anthropology and forensic pathology: The state of Art, in A. Schmitt, E. Cunha, and J. Pinheiro (eds.). *Forensic Anthropology and Medicine: Complementary Sciences. From Recovery to Cause of Death*, pp. 13–38. Totowa, NJ: Humana Press.

De la Grandmaison, G. L., Banasr, A., and Durigon, M. 2003. Age estimation using radiographic analysis of laryngeal cartilage. *American Journal of Forensic Medicine and Pathology* 24(1): 96–99.

Dérobert, L. 1974. *Médecine Légale*. Paris: Flammarion Médecine-Sciences.

Fully, G. 1956. Une nouvelle méthode de détermination de la Taille. *Annales de Médecine Légales* 36: 266–273.

Grévin, G., Bailet, P., Quatrehomme, G., and Ollier, A. 1998. Anatomical reconstruction of fragments of burned human bones: A necessary means for forensic identifications, *Forensic Science International* 96: 129–134.

İşcan, M. Y., and Quatrehomme, G. 1999. Medico legal anthropology in France. *Forensic Science International* 100: 17–35.

Keyser-Tracqui, C., Crubézy, E., and Ludes, B. 2003. Nuclear and mitochondrial DNA analysis of a 2,000-year-old necropolis in the Egyin Gol valley of Mongolia. *American Journal of Human Genetics* 73(2): 247–260.

Keyser-Tracqui, C., and Ludes, B. 2005. Methods for the study of ancient DNA, *Methods in Molecular Biology* 297: 253–264.

Lamendin, H. 1988. Determination de l'age avec la méthode de Guftason "simplifiée." *Le Chirurgien Dentiste de France* 58: 43–47.

Lamendin, H., Baccino, E., Humbert, J. F., Tavernier, J. C., Nossintchouk, R., and Zerilli, A. 1992. A simple technique for age estimation in adult corpses: The two criteria dental method. *Journal of Forensic Sciences* 37: 1373–1379.

Ludes, B., Tracqui, A., Pfitzinger, H., Kintz, P., Levy, F., Disteldorf, M., Hutt, J. M., Kaess, B., Haag, R., Memheld, B., Kaempf, C., Friederich, F., Evenot, E., and Mangin, P. 1994. Medico-legal investigations of the Airbus A320 crash upon Mount Ste-Odile, France. *Journal of Forensic Sciences* 39: 1147–1152.

Manouvrier, L. 1892. Détermination de la Taille d'après les Grands Os des Membres. *Revue l'Ecole d'Anthropologie*. 2: 227–233.

Martrille, L., and Baccino, E. 2005. Professional bodies: France—Forensic, medical and scientific training. *Encyclopedia of Forensic and Legal Medicine*. Vol. 3: 499. New York: Elsevier, Academic Press.

Martrille, L., Mbghirbi, T., Zerilli, A., and Baccino, E. 2003. A strategy for age determination combining a dental method (Lamendin) and an anthropological method (Iscan). *Proceedings of the American Academy of Forensic Sciences*.

Olivier, G. 1960. *Pratique Anthropologique*. Paris: Vigot frères.

Pasquier, E., De Saint Martin Pernot, L., Burdin, V., Mounayer, C., Le Rest, C., Colin, D., Mottier, D., Rouxan, C., and Baccino, E. 1999. Determination of age at death: Assessment of an algorithm of age prediction using numerical three-dimensional CT data from pubic bones. *American Journal of Physical Anthropology* 108(3): 261–268.

Petkovski, E., Keyser-Tracqui, C., Hienne, R., and Ludes, B. 2005. SNPs and MALDI-TOF MS: Tools for DNA typing in forensic paternity testing and anthropology. *Journal of Forensic Sciences* 50(3): 535–541.

Prince, D. A., and Ubelaker, D. H. 2002. Application of Lamendin's adult dental aging technique to a diverse skeletal sample. *Journal of Forensic Sciences* 47: 107–116.

Quatrehomme, G., Garidel, Y., Grévin, G., Liao, Z. G., Bailet, P., and Ollier, A. 1995. Method for identifying putrefied corpses by facial casting. *Forensic Science International* 74: 115–124.

Rouge-Maillart, C., Telmon, N., Rissech, C., Malgosa, A., and Rouge, D. 2004. The determination of male adult age at death by central and posterior coxal analysis: A preliminary study. *Journal of Forensic Sciences* 49(2): 208–214.

Schmitt, A., Murail, P., Cunha, E., and Rougé, D. 2002. Variability of the pattern of aging on the human skeleton: Evidence from bone indicators and implications on age at death estimation. *Journal of Forensic Sciences* 47: 1203–1209.

Schuliar, Y., Ceccaldi, B., Salon, J., Chilliard, P., and Vian, J. M. 1999. Catastrophe aérienne à Haïti, 7 décembre 1995, intervention de la cellule d'identification de victimes de catastrophes de la Gendarmerie Nationale (CIVC), *Journal de Médecine Légale Droit Médical* 42: 5.

Schuliar, Y., Corvisier, J. M., Masselin, P., Ceccaldi, B., and Crispino, F. 1996. Identification des victimes de la catastrophe aérienne du Bourget le 20 Janvier 1995. Participation de la Cellule d'identification de Victimes de Catastrophes de la Gendarmerie Nationale. *Journal de Médecine Légale Droit Médical* 39(7–8): 499–500.

Schuliar, Y., Richebe, J., Crispino, F., and Delemmme, E. 1998. Méthodes de recherches de cadavers. *Journal de Médecine Légale Droit Médical* 41 (3–4): 253–260.

Telmon, N., Gaston, A., Chemla, P., Blanc, A., Joffre, F., and Rougé, D. 2005. Application of the Suchey-Brooks Method to three-dimensional in aging of the pubic symphysis. *Journal of Forensic Sciences* 50(3): 507–512.

United States Supreme Court in *Daubert v. Merrell Dow Pharmaceuticals, Inc.*, 509 U.S. 579 (1993).

5

A HISTORY OF FORENSIC ANTHROPOLOGY IN SPAIN

José L. Prieto

Forensic anthropology has developed in different ways across the world in response to country-specific criteria in approaches to forensic investigations, the role that the forensic anthropologist plays in these investigations, and the level of experience and/or the type of training system implemented.[1] In some countries, particularly in the United States, forensic anthropology has developed under the concept of *forensic science* as a subdiscipline of physical anthropology for the purpose of resolving criminal cases and is practiced by physical or biological anthropologists who specialize in the forensic field. Their research and techniques are applied to the identification of human remains in the legal sphere, where assessing sex, age, ancestry, and stature is essential to arrive at a biological profile of the individual in question (Hunter 1996; Krogman and İşcan 1986; Stewart 1979; Ubelaker 1999).

In some European countries, however, what we would now describe as forensic anthropology has been linked to forensic medicine, the specialized branch of medicine at the service of the law, which incorporates the study of living and dead individuals, taking knowledge from scientific disciplines other than medicine itself. Here, forensic anthropology has developed, in practice, as a subdiscipline of legal and forensic medicine, and for this reason forensic doctors with training in physical anthropology frequently carry out forensic anthropological examinations (Baccino et al. 2004; Gulec and İşcan 1994; İşcan and Quatrehomme 1999; Prieto 2007).

Following this introduction, I explain the historic and current roles played by forensic anthropology within the Spanish medical legal system, in organizational, teaching, and research terms.

Historical Roots: Anthropology and Legal Medicine in Spain

Classical Period

Traditionally, forensic anthropology has focused on the identification both of living persons and of human remains based on reconstruction and/or comparison of the biological features observed in the skeleton. In Spain, the problems of identification encountered in the legal sphere when dealing with living subjects and the deceased have always been associated with legal and forensic medicine (Etxeberría 2004; Prieto 2001; Reverte 1991; Sánchez Sánchez 1996), as one of the topics in texts written by leading classic Spanish authors.[2] Historical roots of Spanish forensic anthropology date back to the mid-19th century under the influence of two principal events: (1) the constitution of the *Société d'anthropologie du Paris* by Professor Paul Broca and (2) the development of modern Legal Medicine, which was greatly influenced by anthropology. Doctors and naturalists have had a significant impact on development of anthropology in Spain. One outstanding figure is Dr. Pedro González de Velasco, an anatomist, founder of the Spanish Anthropological Society in 1865 and the Anthropological Museum of Madrid in 1875. It was at this time that the first magazines of anthropology, such as *Anthropological Magazine* (1874) and *Modern Anthropology* (1883), appeared (Reverte 1991).

In 1883, the Anthropology and Ethnography sections of the Anthropological Museum were created. This was followed in 1892 by the appointment of Professor Manuel Antón y Ferrándiz as the first Chair of Anthropology in the Faculty of Sciences at the Central University of Madrid. In 1910, Ferrándiz was named first director of the Museum of Anthropology, Ethnography, and Prehistory. Other significant events include the publication in 1883 of the Cephalic Index of Spain by Dr. Federico Olóriz Aguilera, Chair of Anatomy at the University of Madrid (Olóriz Aguilera 1894), and the creation of the Craniological Museum, which amassed a total of 2,500 skulls, 2,220 of which were identified individuals and came from donated bodies for research to the Department of Anatomy while Olóriz was chair (Gómez Ocaña 1913). Significant research undertaken by Olóriz includes his publication on stature in Spain (Olóriz Aguilera 1896). Unfortunately, the lack of collaboration in collecting data from certain Spanish regions resulted in Olóriz giving up this project. His interest in identification techniques turned to fingerprinting, as one of the founders in developing the so-called monodigital system, or Spanish system (Olóriz 1908, 1909, 1910, 1911).

At the end of the 19th and the beginning of the 20th centuries, publications of other illustrious founders of Spanish anthropology, such as Telesforo de Aranzadi, Chair of Anthropology at the University of Barcelona, and Luis de Hoyos Sáinz (Professor of Physiology at the Teacher Training College), and their texts on anthropometry and ethnography stand out (Aranzadi and Hoyos Sáinz 1917; Hoyos Sáinz and Aranzadi 1913; Hoyos Sáinz 1899, 1939). In the same period, anthropology played a leading role in three fields of Legal Medicine: (1) analyzing the relationship between human physical features and criminal conduct (so-called Criminal Anthropology); (2) establishing the identity of the living, in particular

that of delinquents, with the purpose of augmenting police identification through somatometry or Judicial Anthropometry; and (3) establishing the identity of a corpse, particularly from decayed, mutilated, burnt, and/or skeletonized bodies, on which it is necessary to establish a biological profile (sex, age, stature, and so on).

Criminal anthropology was made famous by the work of Cesare Lombroso, who considered the delinquent to be an abnormal subspecies of the human race. For Lombroso, the criminal develops an innate conduct that represents a regression to previous evolutionary states and that can be recognized owing to a physical series of stigmas or anomalies, such as cranial and face asymmetry, small brow, protruding superciliary arcs, mandibular prognathism, an irregular implantation of the hair and teeth, and—what he considered the most atavistic characteristic of criminals—a pit in the middle of the occipital. From the psychological point of view, the primitive instincts with congenital incapacity to resist the forces of evil are predominant (Lombroso 1897).[3] In Spain, one of this perspective's more outstanding representatives was Rafael Salillas (Salillas 1888, 1908). Other famous psychiatrists of the time also incorporated anthropological theories in their interventions in the courts. Doctors Ángel Pulido Fernandez, Jose Maria Esquerdo Zaragoza, Luis Simarro Lacabra, and Jaime Vera Lopez often took part in judicial processes by contributing scientific valuations of criminal behaviors to the courts (Fernández 1991).

The anthropometric method, presented by Alphonse Bertillon in the medical Congress of Rome of 1882 (Barahona Holgado 1908), aimed at identifying criminal recidivists using the almost absolute fixedness of the human skeleton in adult individuals, the interindividual variability of the skeleton measurements, and their simplicity and precision in the living. This method resulted in a practical, simple, and exact classification and was adopted quickly by Spain, contributing to the diffusion works of such Spanish physical anthropologists as Alvarez Taladriz, García Plaza, Alonso, and Aranzadi (Lecha Martínez 1912). The later development of fingerprinting, following the works of Vucetich and especially Olóriz in Spain, suggested the end of the anthropometric Bertillon's identification techniques. However, somatometric techniques have again returned in the identification of offenders through images caught by video cameras (Porter and Doran 2000; Ventura et al. 2004).

A significant figure in the history of Legal Medicine in Spain is Dr. Pedro Mata Fontanet. In

1843, the first Chair in Legal Medicine was created at the University of Madrid, headed by Dr. Mata. To Dr. Mata we owe the creation in 1862 of a body of state doctors reporting to the Ministry of Justice, at the service of courts and tribunals, named the National Forensic Physicians Corps. Following the introduction of the Criminal Indictment Act in 1882, the title and functions of forensic doctors were officially recognized: "each court of first instance will have a doctor in charge of assisting the legal authorities in all cases or actions where their participation is necessary or advisable throughout the judicial district" (Criminal Indictment Act 1997: 249). Summing up, we can say that forensic doctors are the official advisors or experts in medical and biology matters for the Spanish courts and tribunals. However, the legal authorities have other official institutions that act as advisors in legal medical matters, including the National Institute of Toxicology and Forensic Sciences, governed by the Ministry of Justice, and other independent bodies, such as the University Legal Medicine schools, professional medical associations, and the Royal Academy of Medicine. Within this context, anthropology is recognized as one of the main subjects of forensic medicine. On the 1915 list of official exam questions for access to the Forensic Physician Corp, 28 subjects were anthropology related, referring to anthropometry, craniometry, and skeletal characteristics of sex and age, or dental evolution (Vibert 1916).

The work of such Spanish anthropologists as Olóriz, Salillas, and Aranzadi are referred to in legal medicine texts of the time (Barahona Holgado 1908; Lecha Marzo 1917; Piga y Pascual 1928), and the anthropological techniques are described in those same texts with respect to cadaver identification. In them are anthropometric references and descriptions on the estimation of stature (tables of Orfila, Rollet, and Manouvrier); sex; age (ossification points, obliteration of the sutures, laryngeal ossification, state of the teeth) (Barahona Holgado 1908; Lecha Martínez 1912; Peiró and Rodrigo 1844; Piga y Pascual 1928); particular signs of identity (old fractures, occupational malformations, stigmas, and skeletal X rays) (Barahona Holgado 1908); and dental analysis (Piga y Pascual 1928). Some authors, such as Lecha Marzo (1917), warn of the importance of microscopic bone analysis in time-since-death estimation and the age of death from the studies developed by Tirelli. The teachings of Maestre (Ballesteros 1913), first director of the Institute of Legal Medicine, Toxicology, and Psychiatry of Spain, created in 1914, and Piga y Pascual (1928, 1935), successor of Maestre in the Legal Medicine Chair of Madrid, are particularly complete with respect to aspects of corpse identification and, although for the most part they present data from works elaborated by other authors, contribute valuable elements of their own personal experience.

The period between the second half of the 19th century and the Spanish Civil War (1936–1939) is known as the "Silver Age" of Spanish culture and science. During this time, institutions such as the Ateneo de Madrid and particularly the Institución Libre de Enseñanza, enjoyed great influence on scientific and cultural environments. The Institución Libre de Enseñanza was founded in 1876 by a group of university professors (including Francisco Giner de los Ríos, Gumersindo de Azcárate, and Nicolás Salmerón), who separated from the University to defend academic freedom. The Institución, with which the majority of the best Spanish scientists of the moment collaborated, marked a significant time in the development of Spanish scientific culture. One of its main outcomes was the creation of the Junta para la Ampliación de Estudios, in charge of the creation of the National Institute of Physical-Natural Sciences, to which was added, among other institutions, the Museum of Anthropology. The main purpose of this museum was to introduce to Spain pedagogical and scientific theories that were being developed internationally. Unfortunately, the civil war resulted in the destruction of this institution and with it, the incipient scientific system that had begun to develop in Spain (Otero Carvajal 2001).

Forensic Anthropology in the Present: Spanish Medical Legal Structure

Modern Period

While the field of forensic anthropology was rapidly developing outside Spain, especially in post-World War II United States under the direction of Drs. Aleš Hrdlička, Wilton Marion Krogman, Ellis R. Kerley, and T. D. Stewart, relatively little progress was made in this field in Spain. Although some investigations involving the study of skeletal remains with forensic aims were undertaken by people such as Drs. Blas Aznar, who was a driving force in criminology in Spain (Aznar 1931), and the already mentioned Tomás Maestre (Aznar and Maestre 1945), the texts of renowned authors such as Drs. Royo-Villanova (Royo-Villanova Morales 1952), López Gómez (1967), and Gisbert Calabuig (1985), along with other scientific publications related to the study of human remains, continued making exclusive reference to the most classic authors of the discipline and to outdated knowledge.[4]

It was not until the early 1980s that a new "modern period" began for Spanish forensic anthropology. The point of reference can be located in the creation of the Laboratory of Anthropology Forense and Paleopatología at the Legal Medicine School of Madrid by Dr. Jose M. Reverte Coma (Reverte Coma 1997).

Through Dr. Reverte and the publication of his book *Forensic Anthropology* (Reverte Coma 1991)—the first book published in Spain on forensic anthropology—the techniques and knowledge developed by the American forensic anthropologists spread into Spanish legal medicine at a time when the structure of legal medicine in Spain was being modernized. Forensic anthropology was added to the curriculum of legal medicine and employed successively in daily forensic medical practice.

In 1984, legal and forensic medicine was officially recognized as a medical speciality in Spain. Today, through a system called M. I. R. (Resident Intern Doctor), a single exam gives access to any of the state posts offered for all medical specialities. For legal and forensic medicine, training is carried out at the Legal Medicine schools governed by University Medicine faculties. At present, the legal and forensic medicine speciality is offered in Madrid (Complutense University) and in Granada. Successful students can opt for one of three paths: (1) taking the state exam for the Forensic Physician Corps (FPC), for which the speciality is not an indispensable requirement; (2) University professorship, which is separate from normal forensic practice; or (3) entering the private advisory sector.

The official organizational structure of forensic medicine in Spain has led to a general isolation of forensic doctors in professional and scientific terms and a complete separation (save in exceptional cases) of official forensic practice (governed by the FPC) from the university mandate in legal and forensic medicine teaching (and theoretically in research). Forensic medical work until now had been performed directly in legal spheres, in court buildings lacking adequate medical or scientific infrastructure and equipment, with scant means, and in an individualistic and personal manner, without any specialization. Only the leading regional capitals, such as Madrid and Barcelona, boast forensic medical clinics and forensic institutes. At the clinics, specialist forensic doctors perform examinations of live subjects in areas such as forensic psychiatry, traumatology (body damage evaluation), gynaecology, and others. The forensic

institutes meanwhile deal with legal autopsy of corpses in their judicial district and are simply official mortuaries. In Madrid, since the late 1980s, the Forensic Institute (FI) has gradually developed diverse services related to corpse investigation. Thus forensic pathology, toxicology, anthropology, dentistry, and radiology services have been introduced, being the first in their respective specialities to be implemented among the collective of Spanish forensic doctors.

In 1985, Spanish legislation, through the Organic Judicial Powers Act, recognized the need to transform the organizational system of forensic medicine by proposing the creation of so-called Legal Medicine Institutes. The aim of these institutes is to promote the modernization of forensic medicine and to foster teamwork and specialization in adequately equipped centres. This reform is currently at the stage of introducing nationwide Legal Medicine Institutes. The Spanish state is divided into autonomous regions, the majority of which, following devolution by the central authorities, hold legal justice powers, making the regions responsible for innovating the Institutes. The Legal Medicine Institutes, therefore, are being founded as technical bodies that centralize forensic medical expertise to tap its legal advisory capacity.

The Institutes are structured into services and departments, which include all the forensic doctors of a given autonomous region. Their mission is the same as the mandate held until now in a personal and individual manner by all forensic practitioners—namely, to assist the courts and tribunals through expert medical tests. This mandate has increased to include other responsibilities, such as forensic medicine teaching and research, the latter in coordination with the Universities and the National Toxicology Institute. The Madrid Forensic Institute has attempted, over the last 15 years, to create the embryo of what would become the Madrid Legal Medicine Institute.

Forensic anthropology forms part of the Institutes' Forensic Pathology service, charged with "legal medical investigation in all cases of violent or suspected criminal death occurring in their judicial district, as well as corpse and human remains identification." The future Madrid LMI will have a forensic anthropology department inside the Forensic Pathology Service. Its mission will be the identification of living and deceased subjects, as well as the forensic study of remains to identify the cause and circumstances of death.

Although the Spanish Ministry of Education and Science follows the international UNESCO definition and considers Forensic Anthropology as a subdiscipline (2402.03) of Physical Anthropology (2402) in the Life Sciences field (24), as it has been stated earlier, legal case resolution in medical and biology matters in Spain has always been the remit of forensic medicine. The problems of identification when dealing with living subjects and that of the deceased in the legal sphere have always been associated with legal and forensic medicine (Etxeberría 2004; Prieto 2001; Reverte Coma 1991; Sánchez Sánchez 1996). Inside the Spanish legal medicine system, forensic anthropology is considered a "special branch of forensic medicine whose purpose is legal medical study of badly preserved corpses with the aim of identifying them and establishing the cause and circumstances of death."

At present, forensic anthropology is practiced mainly by forensic doctors with specialized knowledge in physical anthropology who are based in legal medicine centers (Forensic Institutes and University departments). They are considered specialists able to carry out forensic medical consultation in diverse cases of legal interest relating to both living subjects (identification, age estimation in undocumented youths, and so on) and cadavers. In the examination of human remains, the objectives are to establish the physical features and personal characteristics that enable identification, as well as the possible cause and circumstances of death (Prieto 2001). These two elements are fundamental in resolving any death case within a legal context and constitute indisputable objectives of any medico-legal autopsy (as stipulated by Spanish criminal law), whatever the condition of the corpse. The European Union (EU) recognizes the same fundamental elements in Recommendation number 99 (3) of the Council of Ministers of Member States for Harmonisation of Medico-legal Autopsies (1999), which states in its Principles and Rules relating to medico-legal autopsy procedures: "Autopsies should be carried out in all obvious or suspected unnatural death, even where there is a delay between causative events and death, in particular: . . ., unidentified or skeletonized bodies" (Council of Europe Committee Ministers 1999: 3).

Forensic anthropologists are being incorporated in many cases routinely undertaken in forensic institutes.[5] They contribute to diagnosis of cause and circumstances of death and complement the work of the forensic pathologist when dealing with fresh corpses on which a conventional autopsy is practiced. The forensic anthropologist is particularly useful in providing complementary analyses of perimortem injuries to skeletonized remains (see Loe this volume) and in supplying valuable additional data on the characteristics of wounds and the objects or weapons responsible for them (blunt trauma, sharp force, or gunshot wounds). The fact that forensic anthropological assessments are performed in these centers, where conventional autopsies are carried out daily, serves to provide unequaled experience in the diagnosis of trauma when one is studying skeletonized remains and provides a personal perspective different from that of forensic pathologists, who are not trained in the analysis of skeletal structures and their interpretation. Meanwhile, the links between these forensic centers and the universities have enabled practice, teaching, and analysis to develop unavoidably hand in hand.

There are a total of nine laboratories: four in Madrid, two in Valencia, and one each in Catalonia, the Basque Country, and Andalucía. The total annual number of forensic anthropology cases studied at the nine Spanish labs is about 200. This figure is probably far smaller than the number of cases objectively requiring study, as observed in other countries (Cattaneo and Baccino 2002). To give an example, at the Madrid FI, approximately 2,500 corpses are received annually, with only 40 requiring the services of a forensic anthropologist. Installation of the Legal Medicine Institutes will enable objective and homogeneous study criteria to be introduced. This will eliminate the current purely personal criteria, whereby the forensic practitioner in charge of the case is the person who decides if examination is necessary—whether complete, in which case it is remitted to the anthropology department, or partial, as support for the conventional autopsy in the evaluation of skeletal injuries.

Teaching

Forensic anthropology teaching in Spain largely forms part of forensic medicine programs, in some cases under the criminology and biology programs that govern physical anthropology. Over recent years, forensic anthropology has raised its profile, thanks to the boost given to training in both the university and the legal spheres. University training is offered at both undergraduate and postgraduate levels.

University Training

Undergraduate Studies. Some topics included in legal medicine undergraduate study incorporate concepts related to forensic anthropology, such as the study of burnt corpses, identification techniques, decomposition and preservation techniques, and responses to mass disasters. The Basque Country University in its undergraduate program includes an optional subject called Anthropological Identity and Identification, lasting four quarters and covering 20 topics worth 5 credits (2 theory, 3 practical). Only the University of Navarra specifically includes forensic anthropology as part of its subject list.

Postgraduate Studies

Legal and Forensic Medicine Specialist Subject. The subject of forensic anthropology is covered under the topic Criminology (rather than Legal and Forensic Medicine), specifically in relation to issues of identification.

Doctorate. The only specific legal and forensic medicine course is offered by the Madrid Complutense University (Toxicology and Health Legislation Department). The course includes forensic anthropology (5 credits), with forensic anthropology as a research subject worth 12 credits in the doctoral thesis. The University Miguel Hernández (Alicante) includes forensic anthropology, forensic police work, and fingerprint analysis as obligatory subjects in its Legal Medicine doctorate program, worth a total 3 credits. Other legal medicine and some biology faculties offer doctorate courses that include topics more or less specifically related to forensic anthropology. Over the last decade, about 10 theses with a focus on forensic anthropology have been produced.

Specific Forensic Anthropology University Qualifications

Basic Forensic Anthropology Courses. There are numerous basic courses in forensic anthropology available at Spanish universities. The Complutense University offers a "basic course" for graduates of medicine, law, journalism, history and archaeology, biology, health sciences, criminology, and those interested in physical and forensic anthropology in general. The course is 60 hours of classes, worth 6 academic credits. The Complutense also offers a "practical course" for students completing the basic forensic anthropology course or having basic knowledge on the subject. The course is 80 hours long, worth 8 credits, and limited to a total 8 students. The two courses (basic and practical) are given once a year.

Other universities, such as the Barcelona Autonomous University, the Canary Palaeopathology and Bioanthropology Institute, and the University of La Laguna organize sporadic basic courses in forensic anthropology or include related topics in their palaeopathology courses.

Specialist and Master Courses. Since 1997, the Medicine Faculty of the Madrid Complutense University has offered a specialist qualification in forensic anthropology. The course comprises 300 teaching hours: 150 theory and 150 practical, worth 30 credits. The requirements to apply are graduate status and at least 4 years experience in the field of forensic anthropology. The maximum number of students is 16. In 2003, the University of Granada inaugurated two internet-based courses organized by the Centre for Internet Education. The first is a course in Specialisation in Anthropological Techniques for Human Identification and is worth an optional 7 credits for medicine students. The second course is the Virtual Masters in Forensic Anthropology and Genetics, including 2 blocks on forensic anthropology, over 260 teaching hours and worth 26 credits.

Masters in Forensic Medicine, organized by the Business Foundation University in Valencia for medicine, biology and dentistry graduates, includes a unit on forensic anthropology worth a total 3 credits.

Training in the Forensic Field

The program for entry to the FPC includes 6 topics on identification process, 3 of them on forensic anthropology. Furthermore, the course program of initial training for forensic doctors offered at the Law Study Centre, once the entrance exam has been passed, offers a basic list of 10 hours of theory and practical seminars in forensic anthropology.

Meanwhile, a training program for forensic doctors has been offered by the Justice Administration Law Study Centre since 1997. The Basic Course in Forensic Anthropology has been offered biennially, under my coordination with assistance from Douglas Ubelaker. This course aroused great interest in other regions independent of the Legal Studies Centre and was offered in Galicia in 2000 and Andalucia in 2001 with the collaboration of these regions´ forensic doctors' associations.

Apart from the regular courses offered by the Complutense, Granada and Valencia Universities, and those organized by the FDC, the other courses available are sporadic and aimed at a wide range of students proceeding from any scientific field.

Research

Relatively little research in forensic anthropology has been undertaken in Spain. The lack of contemporary skeletal collections has greatly limited research, with most work being undertaken on archaeological collections in the physical anthropology field and subsequently applied to questions relating to forensic anthropology. The majority of research projects are carried out in university departments linked to the legal and forensic medicine field of learning, inside doctorate courses. The leading centers doing research in this field are those that perform forensic case studies for the legal authorities: Madrid Complutense, Granada, Basque Country, Valencia, Barcelona Autonomous, Alicante, and Zaragoza universities.

State grants and aid for research in the biomedical area do not include forensic medicine and, even less often, forensic anthropology. This is due to the fact that forensic anthropology is considered a subdiscipline of physical anthropology, and most grants in physical anthropology are aimed at research in archaeological fields (for example, population dynamics, demography, and so on). Further, there is a lack of grants in forensic sciences in general, and forensic anthropology is therefore in competition with basic science projects (mainly physiology). This background makes project development extremely difficult, because projects in the main must be financed by the researchers themselves.

In contrast, there is an increase in research being undertaken at the recently established Legal Medicine Institutes, as reflected in the number of scientific magazine texts and publications in national and international journals.

Forensic Anthropology Texts in Spain

Following the first work on forensic anthropology in Spain by Dr. J. M. Reverte entitled *Forensic Anthropology* (1991 and 1999), there have been several monographs focusing on this area, such as *Police and Forensic Anthropological Identification* (Villalaín and Puchalt 2000); *Criminological Anthropology* (Rodes and Martí 2001), and *Forensic Anthropology* (Prieto et al. 2001), constituting the texts for the basic forensic anthropology course held in Galicia.

Other important contributions to the field of physical archaeological anthropology include the work by Trancho and colleagues (1997) and the bibliographical database on pathology of skeletal remains (Etxeberría 2001). Forensic anthropology related articles published by Spanish authors are also hard to find in national and international magazines (see below).

National Publications

There are currently four Spanish publications related to forensic medicine: Revista Española de Medicina Legal (www.arrakis.es/~anmf/), Cuadernos de Medicina Forense (www.cica.es/~aamefo/es_index.html), Boletín Galego de Medicina Legal e Forense, and Revista Aragonesa de Ciencias Forenses. Over the last 15 years (1992–2006), a total of 17 articles related to forensic anthropology have been published.[6]

International Publications

There have been relatively few published articles on forensic anthropology by Spanish authors. Over the last 15 years, practitioners have published around nine articles in leading forensic science reviews.[7]

It seems clear that forensic anthropological expertise is needed. With the purpose of obtaining properly trained forensic anthropologists and qualified forensic anthropology laboratories across Europe, the Forensic Anthropology Society of Europe (FASE) was created in Milan in 2003, under the umbrella of the International Academy of Legal Medicine (IALM). Without doubt, FASE has a major role to play in the evolution of modern forensic anthropology in Europe. Among others, one important role is the necessary development of a European certification in forensic anthropology, similar to that available in the U.S., offered by the American Academy of Forensic Sciences.

Conclusion

In summary, in Spain, forensic anthropology is an activity clearly linked to legal and forensic medicine, practiced inside the organizational system of forensic medicine. Forensic anthropology is a growing scientific discipline in Spain, as evidenced by the increase in specific courses (some of the specialist courses consisting of up to 300 teaching hours) and the increase in specific texts and articles published in national and international magazines.

Although a boost to forensic anthropology research is undoubtedly needed, we can expect that the future organizational model of forensic medicine inside the new Legal Medicine Institutes, with stronger links to universities and centers of training and research, will enable forensic anthropology to develop to its maximum potential in Spain. In this process, FASE should play a major role in promoting and developing forensic anthropology across Europe.

Notes

1. Baccino et al. 2004; Brickley and Ferlini 2007; Gulec and İşcan 1994; İşcan 1998, 2001; İşcan and Olivera 2000; İşcan and Quatrehomme 1999; Rodríguez 2004; Sanabria 2004; Schiwy-Bochat, Riepert, and Rothschild 2004; Ubelaker 1996.

2. Aznar and Maestre 1945; Ballesteros 1913; Barahona Holgado 1908; Gisbert Calabuig 1985; Lecha Martínez 1894; López Gómez and Gisbert Calabuig 1967; Mata Fontanet 1874; Peiró and Rodrigo 1844; Piga y Pascual 1928; Royo-Villanova Morales 1952.

3. Lombroso's theories are no longer well accepted (Gould 1981).

4. Martínez Estrada 1951, 1952; Muñoz Tuero and De Portugal Álvarez 1966; Muñoz Tuero, Moya Pueyo, and Villalaín 1972; Muñoz Tuero and Díaz Domínguez 1981; Pérez de Petinto Bertomeu 1952, 1980; Romero Palanco 1980; Serrano Cepedano 1982; Villalaín Blanco and Buján Varela 1981; Villalaín Blanco and Ramos Almazán 1981.

5. A number of laboratories have been promoted by different institutions. These include from the Ministry of Justice (FDC): Madrid Forensic Institute, National Toxicology Institute, Catalonia Legal Medicine Institute; from universities (Legal Medicine faculties): Complutense (Legal Medicine School), Basque Country, Valencia, Alicante, Granada (Anthropology Chair at the Medicine faculty); from the Home Office (Forensic Police): National Police.

6. Agudo, Sancho Ruiz, and del Muñoz 1998; Chiarri, Rodes, and Martí 2003; del Río Muñoz and Sánchez Sánchez 1997; del Río, Sánchez Sánchez, and Prieto Carrero 2000, 2001; Etxeberría 1992; Etxeberría and Carnicero 1998; Miquel Feucht and Villalaín Blanco 1996; Prieto 1996; Prieto and Abenza 1998; Prieto et al. 2005a, 2005b; Ramírez Álava et al. 2000; Reverte 1997; Rodes 2004; Rodes et al. 2004; Sánchez Sánchez 1996, 1997.

7. Bolaños et al. 2003; Garamendi et al. 2005; Lorente et al. 2001; Martín de las Heras et al. 1999; Muñoz et al. 2001; Prieto, Magaña, and Ubelaker 2004; Prieto et al. 2005a; Trancho et al. 1997; Valenzuela et al. 2000.

References

Agudo Ordóñez, J., Sancho Ruiz, M., and del Muñoz, P. A. 1998. Identificación positiva mediante la radiografía de los senos frontales. *Revista Española de Medicina Legal* 82: 45–47.

Aranzadi, T., and Hoyos Sáinz, L. 1917. *Etnografía: Sus Bases, Sus Métodos y Aplicaciones a España.* Madrid: Biblioteca Corona.

Aznar, B. 1931. *Contribución a la Identificación de restos óseos Fetales.* Madrid: Gráficas Gutenberg.

Aznar, B., and Maestre, T. 1945. Identificación de restos cadavéricos oseos. *Investigación* 211: 79–81.

Baccino, E., Cattaneo, C., Cunha, E., Prieto, J. L., and Penning, R. 2004. *Organization, Teaching and Research in Forensic Anthropology across Europe.* Plenary Session. 1st FASE Meeting. Frankfurt.

Ballesteros, S. 1913. *Apuntes de Medicina Legal y Toxicología Ajustados a las Explicaciones del Dr. D. Tomás Maestre Pérez.* Madrid: Librería Médica de Vidal.

Barahona Holgado, I. 1908. *Lecciones de Medicina Legal.* Salamanca: Marcelino Rodríguez.

Bolaños, M. V., Moussa, H., Manrique, M. C., and Bolaños, M. J. 2003. Radiographic evaluation of third molar development in Spanish children and young people. *Forensic Science International* 133(3): 212–219.

Brickley, M. B., and Ferlini, R. 2007. Forensic anthropology: Developments in two continents, in M. B. Brickley and R. Ferlini (eds.), *Forensic Anthropology: Case Studies from Europe,* pp. 3–18. Springfield, IL: Charles C. Thomas.

Cattaneo, C., and Baccino, E. 2002. A call for forensic anthropology in Europe. *International Journal of Legal Medicine* 116: N1–N2.

Cattaneo, C., Gigli, F., Lodi, F., and Grandi, M. 2003. The detection of morphine and codeine in human teeth: An aid in the identification and study of human skeletal remains. *Journal of Forensic Odontostomatology* 21(1): 1–5.

Chiarri, M., Rodes, F., and Martí, J. B. 2003. Identificación positiva a partir del estudio de restos óseos en un caso de desaparecido. *Boletín Galego de Medicina Legal e Forense* 11: 35–40.

Council of Europe Committee of Ministers. Recommendation No. R (99) 3 of the Committee of Ministers to Member States on the Harmonisation of Medico-Legal Autopsy Rules (adopted by the Committee of Ministers on February 2nd). 1999. 658th meeting of the Ministers' Deputies, pp. 2–3.

Criminal Indictment Act (Ley de Enjuiciamiento Criminal). 1997. Madrid: Colex ed.

del Río Muñoz, P. A., and Sánchez Sánchez, J. A. 1997. Discriminación sexual en la séptima vértebra cervical mediante el análisis de imagen. *Revista Española de Medicina Legal* 80-81: 49–54.

del Río Muñoz, P. A., Sánchez Sánchez, J. A., and Prieto Carrero, J. L. 2000. Determinación del sexo mediante el análisis de imagen en el atlas. *Cuadernos de Medicina Forense* 22: 45–52.

———. 2001. Estimación del sexo en la mandíbula mediante funciones discriminantes. *Cuadernos de Medicina Forense* 26: 21–28.

Etxeberría, F. 1992. Aspectos macroscópicos del tejido óseo sometido al efecto de las altas temperaturas. Aportación al estudio de las cremaciones. *Revista Española de Medicina Legal* 72-73: 159–163.

———. 2001. Bibliografía de las investigaciones sobre paleopatología en España. www.aranzadi-zientziak.org/old/antropologia/01t.htm

———. 2004. Panorama Organizativo Sobre Antropología y Patología Forense en España. Algunas Propuestas para el Estudio de Fosas con Restos Humanos de la Guerra Civil Española de 1936, in E. Silva, A. Esteban, J. Castan, and P. Salvador (eds.), *La Memoria de los Olvidados: Un Debate sobre el Silencio de la Represión Franquista*, pp. 183–219. Valladolid: Ámbito Ediciones.

Etxeberría, F., and Carnicero, M. A. 1998. Estudio macroscópico de las fracturas del perimortem en Antropología Forense *Revista Española de Medicina Legal* 84-85: 36–44.

Fernández, P. T. 1991. *La defensa de la sociedad: Cárcel y delincuencia en la España de los siglos XVIII–XIX*, p. 268. Madrid: Alliance.

Garamendi, P. M., Landa, M. I., Ballesteros, J., and Solano, M. A. 2005. Reliability of the methods applied to assess age minority in living subjects around 18 years old: A survey on a Moroccan origin population. *Forensic Science International* 154(1): 3–12.

Gisbert Calabuig, J. A. 1985. *Medicina Legal y Toxicología*, pp. 675–682. Valencia: Fundación García Muñoz.

Gómez Ocaña. 1913. *Memorias de la Real Sociedad Española de Medicina Natural* 7(5): 343–454.

Gould, S. J. 1981. *The Mismeasure of Man*. New York: Norton.

Gulec, E. S., and İşcan, M.Y. 1994. Forensic anthropology in Turkey. *Forensic Science International* 66(1): 61–68.

Hoyos Sáinz, L. 1899. *Técnica Antropológica y Antropología Física*. Madrid: Romo y Fussel (Imp. del Asilo de Huérfanos del S.C. de Jesús).

———. 1929. *Una Hoja para el Estudio de la Herencia en el Hombre: Grupos Sanguíneos y Caracteres Antropológicos*. Madrid: Laboratorio de Antropología Fisiológica.

———. 1939. *Ficha Antropológica para la Investigación de Herencia*. Madrid: [s.n.].

Hoyos Sáinz, L., and Aranzadi, T. 1913. *Unidades y Constantes de la Crania Hispanica*. Madrid: Asociación Española para el Progreso de las Ciencias.

Hunter, J. R. 1996. A background to forensic archaeology, in J. Hunter, C. Roberts, and A. Martin (eds.), *Studies in Crime: An Introduction to Forensic Archaeology*, pp. 7–23. London: Batsford Ltd.

İşcan, M. Y. 1998. Progress in Forensic Anthropology: The 20th Century. *Forensic Science International* 98(1-2): 1–8.

———. 2001. Global forensic anthropology in the 21st Century. Editorial. *Forensic Science International* 117: 1–6.

İşcan, M. Y., and Olivera, H. E. 2000. Forensic anthropology in Latin America. *Forensic Science International* 109(1): 15–30.

İşcan, M. Y., and Quatrehomme, G. 1999. Medicolegal anthropology in France. *Forensic Science International* 100(1-2): 17–35.

Krogman, W. M., and İşcan, M. Y. 1986. *The Human Skeleton in Forensic Medicine*. Springfield, IL: Charles C. Thomas.

Lecha-Martínez, L. 1894. *Elementos de Medicina Legal Complementarios a la Obra de Hofmann*. Valladolid: Hijos de Rodríguez.

———. 1912. *Manual de Medicina Legal*. Madrid: Imprenta y Librería de Nicolás Moya.

Lecha Marzo A. 1917. *Tratado de Autopsias y Embalsamamientos. El Diagnóstico Médico Legal en el Cadáver*. Barcelona: Manuel Marín.

Lombroso, C. 1897. *L'uomo Delinquente: In Rapporto all'Antropologia, alla Giurisprudenza ed alle Discipline Carcerarie*. Torino: Fratelli Bocca.

López Gómez, L., and Gisbert Calabuig, J. A. 1967. *Tratado de Medicina Legal*. Valencia: Saber.

Lorente, J. A., Entrala, C., Alvarez, J. C., Arce, B., Heinrichs, B., Lorente, M., Carrasco, F., Budowle, B., and Villanueva, E. 2001. Identification of missing persons: The Spanish "Phoenix" program. *Croatian Medical Journal* 42(3): 267–270.

Martin de las Heras, S., Valenzuela, A., Villanueva, E., Marques, T., Exposito, N., and Bohoyo, J. M. 1999. Methods for identification of 28 burn victims following a 1996 bus accident in Spain. *Journal of Forensic Sciences* 44(2): 428–431.

Martínez Estrada, J. M. 1951. La Sinóstosis de los huesos del cráneo. *Revista Española de Medicina Legal* 64-65: 291–303.

———. 1952. Determinación de la edad en el cráneo en el niño. *Revista Española de Medicina Legal* 70-71: 31–47.

Mata Fontanet, P. 1874. *Tratado de Medicina y Cirugía Legal*. Madrid: Bailly-Bailliere.

Miquel Feucht, M. J., and Villalaín Blanco, J. D. 1996. El primer tiro de gracia: Estudio criminológico de un cráneo morisco. *Revista Española de Medicina Legal* 76-77: 47–62.

Muñoz, J. I., Linares-Iglesias, M., Suarez-Penaranda, J. M., Mayo, M., Miguens, X., Rodriguez-Calvo, M. S., and Concheiro, L. 2001. Stature estimation from radiographically determined long bone length in a Spanish population sample. *Journal of Forensic Sciences* 46(2): 363–366.

Muñoz Tuero, L. M., and De Portugal Álvarez, J. 1966. Aportación a la determinación de la edad en un cráneo. *Anales de Medicina Forense de la Asociación Española de Médicos Forenses*, VIII. Zaragoza: Jornadas Médico Forenses.

Muñoz Tuero, L. M., and Díaz Domínguez, J. 1981. Aportación a las lesiones en restos óseos. *Revista Española de Medicina Legal* 26-27: 102–105.

Muñoz Tuero, L. M., Moya Pueyo, V., and Villalaín Blanco, J. D. 1972. Aportación a las muertes por proyectiles de arma corta de fuego: Estudio de restos óseos. *Anales de Medicina Forense*, pp. 179–184. Pittsburg-Madrid: Primera Reunión Hispanonorteamericana de Medicina Forense.

Olóriz Aguilera, F. 1884. *Recolección de Cráneos para Estudios Antropológicos*. Granada: Librería de Paulino Ventura Sabatel.

———. 1894. *Distribución geográfica del índice cefálico en España deducida del examen de 8.368 varones adultos*. Memoria presentada al Congreso Geográfico Hispano-Portugués-Americano en sesión de 19 de octubre de 1892. Madrid: Imp. del Memorial de Ingenieros.

———. 1896. *La Talla Humana en España: Discursos Leídos en la Real Academia de Medicina el día 24 de mayo de 1896 para la Recepción Pública del Académico Electo*. Madrid: Imp. y Libr. de Nicolás Moya.

———. 1908. *Dactiloscopia*. Madrid: Imprenta de Eduardo Arias.

———. 1909. *Guía para Extender la Tarjeta de Identidad Según las Lecciones Dadas en la Escuela de Policia de Madrid*. Madrid: Imprenta de los Hijos de M. G. Hernández.

———. 1910. *Experimentos de Identificación Monodactilar en la Universidad de Madrid*. Madrid: Hijos de Reus.

———. 1911. *Manuel pour l'identification des délinquants de Madrid*. Bruxelles: Ferdinand Larcier.

Otero Carvajal, L. E. 2001. La destrucción de la Ciencia en España. Las consecuencias del triunfo militar de la España franquista. *Historia y Comunicación Social* 6: 149–186.

Peiró P. M., and Rodrigo, J. 1844. *Elementos de Medicina y Cirugía Legal Arreglados a la Legislación Española*. Zaragoza: Imprenta de Mariano Peiró.

Pérez de Petinto Bertomeu, M. 1952. Valor jurídico de la identificación de reliquias. *Revista Española de Medicina Legal* 72-73: 122–158.

———. 1980. La estatura de una persona en vida deducida por la proporcionalidad ósea de sus restos esqueletizados. *Revista Española de Medicina Legal* 24-25: 64–71.

Piga y Pascual, A. 1928. *Medicina Legal de Urgencia. (La Autopsia Judicial)*. Madrid: Mercurio.

———. 1935. *Manual Teorico-práctico de Medicina Legal*. Madrid: Instituto Reus.

Porter, G., and Doran, G. 2000. An anatomical and photographic technique for forensic facial identification. *Forensic Science International* 114(2): 97–105.

Prieto, J. L. 1996. Identificación dental: Técnicas radiológicas. *Revista Española de Medicina Legal* 76-77: 71–83.

———. 2001. Sistemática de la recuperación de restos cadavéricos. *Boletín Galego de Medicina Legal e Forense* 10: 5.

———. 2007. Stab wounds. The contribution of forensic anthropology: A case study, in M. B. Brickley and R. Ferlini (eds.), *Forensic Anthropology: Case Studies from Europe*, pp. 19–37. Springfield, IL: Charles C. Thomas.

Prieto, J. L., and Abenza, J. M. 1998. Métodos para valorar la edad en el adolescente. *Revista Española de Medicina Legal* 84-85: 45–50.

Prieto, J. L., Barberia, E., Ortega, R., and Magaña, C. 2005a. Evaluation of chronological age based on third molar development in the Spanish population. *International Journal of Legal Medicine* 119(6): 349–354.

Prieto J. L, Magaña, C., Bedate, A., Segura, L., Tortosa, C., Conejero, J., Abenza, J. M., Mariscal de Gante, M. C., and Perea, B. 2005b. Los atentados de Madrid del 11 de Marzo de 2004. Organización de las tareas médico-forenses en el pabellón No. 6 de IFEMA. *Boletín Galego de Medicina Legal e Forense* 14: 19–26.

Prieto, J. L., Magaña, C., and Ubelaker, D. H. 2004. Interpretation of postmortem change in cadavers in Spain. *Journal of Forensic Sciences* 49(5): 918–923.

Prieto, J. L., Sánchez, J. A., Magaña, C., Roselló, J., and Gremo, A. 2001. Curso Básico de Antropología Forense. *Boletín Galego de Medicina Legal e Forense*. Ponencias del curso organizado por la Asociación Gallega de Médicos Forenses 10.

Ramírez Álava, M. A., Carnicero Giménez de Azcárate, M. A., Baigorri Soler, M. C., and Etxeberría Gabilondo, F. 2000. El valor de la patología ósea en la identificación personal, a propósito de un caso con espondilitis anquilosante. *Cuadernos de Medicina Forense* 22: 53–58.

Reverte, J. M. 1991. *Antropología Forense*. Madrid: Ministerio de Justicia.

———. 1997. Historia del Museo de Antropología Forense, Paleopatología y Criminología de la Escuela de Medicina Legal de la Universidad Complutense. *Anales de la Real Academia Nacional de Medicina* 114(4): 865–882.

Rodes Lloret, F. 2004. Foramen esternal vs orificio por proyectil de arma de fuego. *Cuadernos de Medicina Forense* 35: 71–74.

Rodes Lloret, F., Giner Alberola, S., Pastor Bravo, M., Martí Lloret, J. B., and Dorado Fernández, E. 2004. Herida craneal por arma de fuego en forma de "orificio en herradura": A propósito de un caso. *Boletín Galego de Medicina Legal e Forense* 13: 59–61.

Rodes Lloret, F., and Martí Lloret, J. B. 2001. *Antropología Criminológica*. Alicante: Universidad Miguel Hernández.

Rodríguez, J. V. 2004. *La Antropología Forense en la Identificación Humana*. Bogotá: Universidad Nacional de Colombia.

Romero Palanco, J. L., Torres Ortiz, M. A., and Vila Lopez, E. 1980. Estudio de la flora en cadáveres momificados. *Revista Española de Medicina Legal* 24-25: 199–202.

Royo-Villanova Morales, R. 1952. *Lecciones de Medicina Legal*. Madrid: Marbán.

Salillas, R. 1888. *La Antropología en el Derecho Penal: Tema de Discusión en la Sección de Ciencias Exactas, Físicas y Naturales del Ateneo Científico, Literario y Artístico de Madrid para el curso de 1888–1889*. Madrid: Imprenta de la Revista de Legislación y Jurisprudencia.

———. 1908. *Sentido y Tendencia de las Ultimas Reformas en Criminología*. Madrid: Asociación Española para el Progreso de las Ciencias. Imprenta de Eduardo Arias.

Sanabria, C. 2004. *Antropología Forense y la Investigación Médico-Legal de las Muertes*. Bogotá: Facultad de Investigación Criminal.

Sánchez Sánchez, J. A. 1996. Antropología forense: Revisión histórica y perspectivas actuales. *Revista Española de Medicina Legal* 76-77: 63–70.

———. 1997. Desastres de masas: Legislación y tipo de accidentes. *Revista Española de Medicina Legal* 78-79: 51–56.

Schiwy-Bochat, K. H., Riepert, T., and Rothschild, M. A. 2004. The contribution of forensic medicine to forensic anthropology in German-speaking countries. *Forensic Science International* 144: 255–258.

Serrano Cepedano, F. 1982. Acción del tiempo y la naturaleza sobre restos humanos. *Revista Española de Medicina Legal* 30-31: 79–82.

Stewart, T. D. 1979. *Essentials of Forensic Anthropology: Especially as Developed in the United States*. Springfield, IL: Charles C. Thomas.

Trancho, G. J, Robledo, B., and López Bueis, I. 1997. *Anthropological Investigations in Spain*. Madrid: University of Complutense.

Trancho, G. J., Robledo, B., López Bueis, I., and Sánchez Sánchez, J. A. 1997. Sexual determination of the femur using discriminant functions: Analysis of a Spanish population of known sex and age. *Journal of Forensic Sciences* 42(2): 181–185.

Ubelaker, D. H. 1996. Skeletons testify: Anthropology in forensic science. *Yearbook of Physical Anthropology* 39: 229–244.

———. 1999. *Human Skeletal Remains: Excavation, Analysis, Interpretation*. Washington, D. C.: Taraxacum.

Valenzuela, A., Martin-de las Heras, S., Marques, T., Exposito, N., and Bohoyo, J. M. 2000. The application of dental methods of identification to human burn victims in a mass disaster. *International Journal of Legal Medicine* 113(4): 236–239.

Ventura, F., Zacheo, To, Luck, To, and Shovel, A. 2004. Computerised anthropomorphometric analysis of images: Case report. *Forensic Science International* 146 Suppl: S211–213.

Vibert, Ch. 1916. *Manual de Medicina Legal y Toxicología Clínica y Médico-Legal*. Traducción castellana enriquecida con notas y referencias a la legislación española vigente por Manuel Saforcada. Barcelona: Hijos de J. Espasa.

Villalaín Blanco, J. D., and Buján Varela, J. 1981. Estudio de un cuerpo momificado hallado en Colmenar Viejo (Madrid). *Revista Española de Medicina Legal* 26-27: 56–58.

Villalaín Blanco, J. D., and Puchalt Fortea, F. J. 2000. *Identificación Antropológica Policial y Forense*. Valencia: Tirant Lo Blanch.

Villalaín Blanco, J. D., and Ramos Almazán, M. T. 1981. Consideraciones médico legales en relación al cuerpo momificado de Colmenar Viejo. *Revista Española de Medicina Legal* 26-27: 68–80.

The Application of Forensic Anthropology to the Investigation of Cases of Political Violence: Perspectives from South America

6

Luis Fondebrider

This chapter reflects on the development of forensic anthropology in investigating cases of political violence. It seeks to contextualize the boom that has been taking place since 1996,[1] following the beginning of extensive forensic investigations in the Balkans. In addition, this chapter intends to confront the apparent novelty of this application of the discipline with reference to its significant development in the Latin American context, where the Argentine Forensic Anthropology Team (EAAF) has been one of the pioneers in the field through its activities since 1984.[2]

Although the literature on the origins and the current status of this particular application of forensic anthropology[3] has substantially increased in the last five years (Doretti and Fondebrider 2001; Fondebrider 2004; Haglund 2001, 2002; Haglund, Connor, and Scott 2001; Hunter et al. 2001; Simmons and Haglund 2005; Skinner, Alempijevic, and Djuric-Srejic 2003; Skinner and Sterenberg 2005; Steadman and Haglund 2005), there is a still a lack of understanding about the nature of the work and the contribution made by organizations and individual anthropologists outside the Anglo-Saxon world. As an example, work carried out by the two largest organizations in Latin America, EAAF and Fundación de Antropología Forense de Guatemala, or FAFG (the Guatemalan Forensic Anthropology Foundation), are mentioned as

merely early and local developments (Simmons and Haglund 2005) (which in the case of EAAF is not true, since they have been working outside Argentina since 1986), incorrectly described (Klonowski et al. 2004), or ignored (Hunter 2002). This situation could have resulted from a number of factors: a lack of knowledge regarding the activities of the discipline in other parts of the world or an almost non-existent bibliography that ignores other experiences and mostly concentrates on Anglo-Saxon activities in the Balkans. Because the Balkans is the only region where the majority of Anglo-Saxon forensic anthropologists have worked, this experience is taken as paramount and as a model to apply—for example, in Iraq, the new popular destination for forensic anthropologists (Bernardi and Fondebrider 2007).

Additionally, there is no single criterion for the type of contribution made by forensic anthropology to "contexts of political violence," which are therefore designated as "humanitarian," "human rights," "war crimes," or "genocide" investigations, all of which are but partial and incomplete names that simplify the complexity of the problem. This situation may be due to the fact that most of the practitioners of such name applications do not have a profound and comprehensive insight into what political violence entails, the different local contexts, or the judicial and humanitarian dimensions of the investigations. Finally, it is worth mentioning that such applications of forensic anthropology are new for many professionals, who until 1996 had excavated only individual graves in their own countries. Many such professionals have very little to no knowledge of the human rights situations in the places where have worked—for example, the importance of the relatives of the victims in the process.

Facts and Aspirations

In the last ten years, a great number of forensic anthropologists of different nationalities have worked in the Balkans, acquiring expertise in exhumation and analysis of skeletal remains, as well as an understanding of how significant it is to interact with the victims' relatives. In most cases, these scientists have worked daily throughout several months excavating graves and analyzing skeletons. There are others, however, who instead have made only short visits to Bosnia, Croatia, or Kosovo and have subsequently published methodological guidelines on these issues. Unfortunately, some colleagues, reputed as international experts in mass grave excavations, analysis of large collections of skeletons, and communication with victims' relatives have failed to consider the experiences gained by those who have actively participated in the worldwide development of these applications of forensic anthropology.

The progress made since 1996, when the International Criminal Tribunal for the Former Yugoslavia (ICTY) started its intensive investigations of mass graves in Bosnia, has been enormous from all standpoints.[4] The collective nature of these contributions is highlighted here: hundreds of archaeologists and anthropologists have worked long hours excavating graves and analyzing remains. A great number of these professionals, particularly those from countries lacking experience in this kind of massive investigation, had to start from the basics. They had never seen a real mass grave before or, in the best of cases, had exhumed only individual graves associated with domestic crimes. Some had a Master's Degree in Forensic Archaeology but were not prepared for fieldwork. Very seldom had they worked with contemporary skeletons or were used to perimortem injuries caused by gunshot or accustomed to interacting with forensic pathologists. However, there were other professionals who arrived in Bosnia, and later in Croatia and Kosovo, with experience in cases of this kind. These were professionals (particularly those from the United States) who had worked in criminal contexts or in the recovery of

missing American citizens in wars and professionals (from Argentina, Guatemala, and Colombia) for whom working in mass graves and analyzing remains were ordinary rather than exceptional cases.

A good example of the lack of acknowledgement of the origins of this application of forensic anthropology to the investigation of political cases and the nature of the collective contributions is the subject of the protocols used for field and laboratory work and the collection of antemortem data. The majority of organizations mentioned in this chapter have been involved in the development of protocols and have always clearly attributed such protocols to a specific organization. The protocol documents are the result of collective contributions from many anthropologists involved in this work over the last 20 years. In developing protocols, practitioners rely on models *already created* that are modified and adapted for particular contexts.

It is important to present a fair and balanced description of how forensic anthropology started to be applied to investigations of political violence and what the contribution made by each organization has been. The fact that there are almost no scientific papers published by researchers outside the United States and the United Kingdom does not mean that there are no such researchers or that they should be ignored or mentioned only casually when discussing this issue.[5] For example, to disregard the fact that the EAAF has worked in 35 countries, that it has its own laboratory where dozens of remains are analyzed every year, that since 1992 it has been one of the points of reference for the United Nations in these kinds of investigations, that it has contributed to the training of other teams and professionals in no less than seven countries, and that it has kept almost daily contact with the victims' relatives for 23 years does not help to ensure an evenly balanced exchange among the parties involved. Furthermore, to ignore the fact that the FAFG is an organization staffed by a large number of full-time anthropologists, equipped with their own laboratory and 14 years of experience in excavating highly complicated mass graves and analyzing hundreds of skeletons per year (Steadman and Haglund 2005; www. eaaf.org; www.fafg.org.), does not help advance our discipline. It also denies the significant contributions made to acknowledging the role of the victim's families as true protagonists rather than as mere secondary actors.

At the same time, one should mention that the two major organizations in Latin America, as well as other individual anthropologists, do not publish enough papers describing all the experiences accumulated. This is a weakness that has to be challenged. It is not a question of drawing attention to personalities, or of drawing a dividing line between Europeans and Americans, on the one hand, and Latin American professionals, on the other, but of joining efforts, acknowledging professional weaknesses or deficiencies, enhancing capabilities, and ultimately contributing to the development and improvement of this specific application of forensic anthropology.

A Briefing on History: The Latin American Context

Figures are tangible evidence and also hard to dispute. To mention only the best-known cases: more than 200,000 people disappeared and/or were murdered in Guatemala between 1960 and 1996; 15,000 in Argentina between 1976 and 1983; 70,000 in El Salvador between 1981 and 1991; 70,000 in Peru between 1980 and 2000; 3,000 in Chile between 1973 and 1989; and thousands in Colombia, an estimate that increases daily. One should keep in mind that these figures refer to real human beings with first and last names, with families and friends still longing to know what has happened to them and, if applicable, demanding to know where their remains are, who killed them, and that justice be brought to those responsible for the crimes.

What was the prevailing modus operandi? It mainly involved: (1) the victim's illegal detention, immediate extrajudicial killing, and disappearance of his/her body; (2) the victim's kidnapping, transfer to a legal or clandestine detention centre, torture, extrajudicial killing, and disappearance of his/her body; or (3) a confrontation between State security forces and a guerrilla group, resulting in the robbery and disappearance of dead guerrillas' remains.

What happened to the remains? The bodies were either buried in official cemeteries as John Does; buried in clandestine cemeteries without any identification on the grave, or on crop lands, in military compounds, ravines, and so on; thrown into dried-up water wells; thrown into the sea or volcanoes from airplanes; burnt; or destroyed with explosives or chemicals.

More often than not, the State was the main perpetrator (with the exception of Colombia and Peru). This fact resulted in families and the community as a whole being terrorized: families were unable to ascertain the fate of their loved ones and failed to obtain a response from the State to their claims for truth, justice, and reparation.

When Dr. Clyde Snow arrived in Argentina in 1984 as part of a scientific delegation organized by the American Association for the Advancement of Science (AAAS), he knew nothing of this situation. He disinterestedly traveled to Argentina to help victims' family members to look for and identify their loved ones' remains and consequently became the pioneer of the application of forensic anthropology to the investigation of cases of political violence. From this initial trip onward, Dr. Snow, imbued with the same spirit, repeatedly visited several countries, training young scientists, building a bridge between scientists and the victims' relatives and raising awareness among public authorities that there should not be any gap between these parties (Joyce and Stover 1991; Snow 1984a, 1984b).

At that time, it was most unusual to talk about forensic anthropology in Latin America; indeed, the discipline was unknown to judges and prosecutors. Forensic physicians were acquainted with some general notions from legal medicine publications, which used to include a small section with tables from European publications from the end of the 19th century. Physical anthropologists, instead, were better positioned to make anthropological analyses of skeletons but were only seldom consulted by authorities, and there was little interest in incorporating them into forensic circles.[6] The picture for remains recovery was even worse, since this task was left in the hands of the police, fire fighters, or gravediggers.

To draw a complete picture of this time, one must describe the political context. The same countries that had undergone political violence, causing massive human rights violations, were gradually returning to democracy. Transition to democracy was a complex process, during which those responsible for "the disappearances" were free or, in some cases, occupying political positions in the new governments. This was the reason why investigations, from their very beginnings, were strongly conditioned by several factors, namely: (1) a strong presence of human rights organizations, particularly those involving victims' relatives; (2) little or no independence of forensic institutions, very often complicit in the crimes[7]; (3) lack of information on burial sites; (4) an almost complete lack of interest from the academic world to participate in investigations; (5) after an initial period, a decline of the State's interest in continuing with the investigations; and (6) ensuing decline in the support given by the international community.

This was the situation encountered by Dr. Snow at the time of his arrival in Argentina, with the exception of (5) and (6) (see above). Consequently, he decided to work with a group of anthropology and medical students, who later on were to found EAAF (Joyce and Stover 1991). Snow's pioneering work extended to Chile in 1989 and to Guatemala in 1992, thus contributing to beginning the training process of independent forensic anthropologists in these two countries.

The fact that forensic anthropology in Latin American countries was born out of a dire need to meet the demands of the social sectors hardest hit by violence is one of the most striking differences between the development of forensic anthropology in Latin America and in the United States and Europe. It was not the result of an academic decision or a decision from an anthropology department eager to fulfill its civic responsibility to undertake this task; indeed, the academic community was not interested in the process. Therefore, forensic anthropology in Argentina, Chile, Guatemala, and later in Peru was initially pushed to broaden its traditional role of determining the biological profile of a skeleton for identification purposes; but this was not good enough. There was a need not only to recover bodies following correct procedures but also to respond to issues associated with the political and legal contexts in the places where the work was being performed, to ensure the logistics and security required for each intervention, and, most especially, to establish a relationship with the victims' relatives and their communities. That the victim's relatives, rather than the judge or the forensic anthropologists, are the true protagonists is still hard for most scientists to understand. Given all these considerations, anthropologists had to interact with other actors in the process and broaden their scope of action; for example, establishing ties with the victims' relatives, a task that goes well beyond collecting antemortem data, is a long, slow process that requires a relationship built on mutual trust.

Building an atmosphere of trust is, of course, not a smooth or simple process for the teams involved. We had to learn how to interact with relatives, to understand their doubts, uncertainties, to respect their need for time. For example, not all family members are always willing to start an investigation; sometimes some of them are afraid of the political consequences. On other occasions, the perpetrators still live in the same village, and to ask a relative or a witness to point out the gravesite might put the person in danger. For all these reasons, we think that it is a mistake to see the relatives as simple providers of antemortem data or blood samples for DNA analysis. It is much a more complex procedure entailing hours with the relatives, explaining the process of exhumation, the realistic probability of finding remains, the difficulties of identification, but also to hear their histories, to try to understand, for example, how the disappearance of their loved one has affected the family and changed their lives. All these things are unrelated to the traditional field of forensic anthropology but were important skills we had to learn along the way (Doretti and Fondebrider 2004; Doretti and Snow 2003; Stover and Shigekane 2002).

The other main difference between Latin American and North American and European forensic anthropology organizations is that for the EAAF, and in certain respects also for other Latin American teams, the preliminary investigation of each case is an essential part of the work. The lack of interest of the judiciary to investigate properly, the lack of support from the state, and the reluctance of the perpetrators to provide information require that from the very beginning we construct our own hypotheses about the location of the remains of the disappeared people. We cannot ask the police or criminal investigators for help. They were in many cases part of the same system. Based on the idea that perpetrators, especially when they are the State, leave traces of their actions in various media, we started searching cemetery records, death certificate archives, court records, intelligence reports produced by the army or the police, and press information, and we interviewed not only relatives of the victims but also witnesses that participated in or saw the killings and burials of the bodies (Bernardi and Fondebrider 2007; Doretti and Snow 2003, Snow and Bihurriet 1992).

It is worth mentioning, therefore, that when extensive investigations started in Bosnia in 1996, under the ICTY, the processes of investigating cases of political violence (including the relationship with the victims' relatives, the exhumation of graves, and the analysis of skeletal remains) were firmly rooted in the work of EAAF, in Argentina. In Guatemala, many useful experiences were also gained during four years of exhumations of mass graves and analysis of remains. In Colombia, individual anthropologists were engaged in the investigation of political cases as well as in ordinary crimes.

The International Context: The Balkans and the Rest of the World

Dr. Snow worked in isolation for several years, since very few colleagues from the United States joined his efforts. In Europe, only a few forensic pathologists lent their support following requests from Amnesty International to investigate cases of torture or death in custody in the countries where such crimes were reported. It was not until the ICTY's investigations that anthropologists became more interested in the forensic application of their field.

Thus, one must begin the history of the application of forensic anthropology to the investigation of political violence by mentioning the work of the American Association for the Advancement of Science (AAAS) that in 1984 engaged a group of American scientists, among them Dr. Clyde Snow, to go to Argentina, after which the AAAS helped to start the process in Guatemala. Before 1996, when the work in Bosnia started, there were two organizations working at the international level: the EAAF and the PHR. The EAAF,[8] created in 1984 after Snow's visit, began in 1986 to participate in forensic investigations in other countries that, after periods of violence, were starting to analyze their past. So, in those 12 years before the work in Bosnia, EAAF had been working already in Argentina, Bolivia, Brazil, Colombia, Croatia, Chile, El Salvador, Ethiopia, Guatemala, Iraq, the Philippines, Romania, and South Africa.

PHR, founded in 1986 with a wider objective, also developed forensic anthropology through its forensic program, directed initially by Dr. Robert Kirshner and later by Dr. William Haglund. Mr. Eric Stover participated in the original delegation of the AAAS to Argentina and played a major role in this process as executive director of PHR until his retirement in 1995. Until 1996, PHR conducted forensic missions to Croatia, Mexico, Guatemala, Honduras, and Rwanda. Instead of counting on its own team of forensic anthropologists, the forensic program of PHR is presided over by a forensic specialist (until recently, Dr. W. Haglund), who recruits anthropologists and other professionals from different countries whenever they are assigned a specific mission. Once the mission is finished, each specialist returns to his/her country of residence. The longest and most significant project for PHR was in the Balkans, beginning in 1996, and then in Cyprus, beginning in 1999 (www. phrusa.org). For specific missions, such as those in Iraq (1992) and Croatia (1993 and 1996), EAAF as well as colleagues from the Guatemalan and Chilean teams were invited to participate by PHR, the coordinating organization.

In 1996, PHR was commissioned by the ICTY for the Balkans mission to conduct the first mass exhumations in Bosnia. Again, it recruited a large group of experts from different countries giving many international anthropologists the opportunity to participate in this kind of work for first time. For most of the anthropologists who traveled to Croatia and Bosnia in those years (1996 and 1997), this was their first experience with a mass grave and with analyzing the skeletal remains of different populations. Many of the pathologists, radiologists, and crime-scene investigators who were part of the teams in those years had never investigated the kinds of cases in which the state was responsible for the killing of large numbers of people. It was not a typical mass disaster, such as an airplane crash. In this case, the perpetrators went free, the bodies hidden in mass graves, and thousands of families were involved. Very few of those scientists recognized that they were not prepared for such a different task. In contrast to the experience in Latin America, these first years had a very technical profile, almost without contact between forensic specialists and families, quite the opposite from what Snow had promoted since 1984.

Some time later, the Tribunal decided to hire its own forensic specialist, José Pablo Baraybar from Peru, who opened up the path for another important group of anthropologists, mainly from Latin America, the United States, and the United Kingdom, to work in this field. Also in the Balkans, in 1996, the International Commission on Missing Persons (ICMP) was created, with a strong emphasis on the use of DNA analysis to identify remains. A few years later, ICMP also began to hire anthropologists for the recovery of remains from mass graves and their analysis. During some periods, the ICTY, PHR, and ICMP worked at the same time in Bosnia. Some of the most interesting articles about the exhumation of mass graves and anthropological analyses were produced by anthropologists who worked for ICTY and later for ICMP (e.g., Baraybar and Maraek 2006; Haglund 2002; Komar 2003; Skinner, Alempijevic, and Djuric-Srejic 2003, Skinner and Sterenberg 2005; Tuller and Duric 2006; Tuller, Hofmeister, and Daley 2008). In 2002, the United Nations Mission in Kosovo (UNMIK) created the Office on Missing Persons and Forensics (OMPF) within the Department of Justice, with the objective of determining the whereabouts of missing persons, identifying their remains, and returning them to the families. The OMPF was also assigned to establish a medical examiner's office to provide medico-legal forensic examinations according to international standards and to build local institutional capacity to carry out this work.[9]

Finally, in 2001, INFORCE was created. This organization is staffed mostly by English scientists who have been trained in forensic anthropology and archaeology and who gained practical experience in the Balkans between 1996 and 2001 working for PHR, ICTY, or ICMP. To date, INFORCE as an institution has worked in the Balkans, Cyprus, and Iraq, and one of its members participated in a mission to the Democratic Republic of Congo in 2003, under the coordination of EAAF. In addition, many anthropologists, although not members of any of the above-mentioned organizations, have worked for them in the Balkans, providing input from their countries of origin.

The Joint POW/MIA Accounting Command from the U.S.A. deserves a special mention. Even though it cannot be regarded as a typical organization engaged in the kinds of cases discussed here, it has gained broad experience in the recovery and analysis of remains of American citizens disappeared in war, particularly in Southeast Asia.

This brief description illustrates that, with the exception of the EAAF and PHR, the other organizations outlined above have focused their activities in the Balkans. Consequently, the great majority of forensic anthropologists who have been working for the last ten years in applying their disciplines to cases of political violence have done so almost exclusively in this region of the world. Only in exceptional cases have these scientists been faced with circumstances in other countries.[10] Consequently, many publications on the application of forensic anthropology to political violence are biased owing to the fact that the authors' experience in this area is an exception rather than a rule.

There were several negative experiences in the Balkans, including a profusion of local and international agencies involved in the task that disagreed about methodologies and that applied different work protocols. The lack of coordination resulted, in many occasions, in problems with the identification of the remains and the re-analysis of bodies. This, in turn, created uncertainty among the relatives about the process. As a consequence, the International Committee of the Red Cross (ICRC) launched The Missing project (www.icrc.org/TheMissing). This important initiative promotes *the right to know* of the relatives of the missing around the world, as well as raising the profile of legal, humanitarian, psychological, and scientific aspects of the work. This initiative involved an important effort to draw lessons from experiences gained in the Balkans and other parts of the world, such as Latin America, where science has been used to investigate cases of missing people.

The Current Situation in Latin America

In Latin America, forensic anthropology may be applied to three types of cases: (1) domestic crimes; (2) mass disasters (aircraft accidents, earthquakes, car bombs, and so on); and (3) political violence (kidnapping/disappearance of persons and executions). The first two scenarios involve forensic anthropologists working for an official institution (for example, medico-legal services, judicial police, offices of prosecutors, and/or scientific police). Argentina, Colombia, Costa Rica, Cuba, Chile, Mexico, Peru, Puerto Rico, Uruguay, and Venezuela are some of the Latin American countries that have incorporated forensic anthropologists in at least one of the services mentioned above. In general, they focus on the analysis of remains rather than on their recovery, but they have undoubtedly acquired important case-based knowledge.

The third type of case has been largely left in the hands of nongovernment organizations, with a few executions, such as Peru very recently. In addition to the EAAF and FAFG, there are other organizations that investigate political violence in Latin America, including the Guatemalan organization Centro de Antropología Forense y Ciencias Aplicadas or CAFCA (Center for Forensic Anthropology and Applied Sciences), the Equipo Peruano de Antropologia Forense or EPAF (Peruvian Forensic Anthropology Team), and the Centro Andino de Investigaciones Antropológico Forenses or CENIA (Andean Center for Forensic Anthropology Research). Similar activities are undertaken by the Equipo Forense Especializado (Specialized Forensic Team) in the Legal Medicine Institute in Peru, also under the purview of the Public Ministry. In Colombia, these activities are performed by the Legal Medicine Institute and the Prosecutor's office, with their own anthropologists, and recently an independent organization was formed called Equipo Colombiano Interdisciplinario de Trabajo Forense y Asistencia Psicosocial, or EQUITAS (Colombian Interdisciplinary Team for Forensic Work and Psychosocial Services).

Why are most of the initiatives from private and not State-run organizations? There are countless reasons to account for this peculiar feature, but two stand out: first, there is the relatives' lack of trust in public agencies to conduct this kind of investigation, despite the new democratic wind blowing in the region; and, second, there is the State's lack of interest in digging deep into the past.

Conclusion

This chapter has briefly described how forensic anthropology first began to be applied in 1984 to investigations into political violence in Latin America and has highlighted differences between investigations undertaken in Latin America and those conducted in the Balkans from 1996 onward. Differences in development and experience between Latin American and European and U.S. scientists result from a series of the above-mentioned factors:

1. There are disappeared people and mass graves containing their remains throughout Latin America, Africa, the Middle East, and Asia. Also, the rate of criminal cases (including those requiring analysis of skeletal remains) is high in several countries. This means that forensic anthropologies have the possibility to have a permanent and full-time job in official and non-official organizations, to obtain experience with domestic cases, and to develop new field and laboratory population standards.

2. There are practically no mass graves or large numbers of remains to be identified in the United States or Europe (with the exception of Spain and countries in the east, and WWII graves, particularly in Germany and Austria). The U.S., in turn, has a high rate of domestic crimes and, since September 2001, cases related to terrorism, many of which require the analysis of remains. In Europe, particularly in the northern countries, the rate is very low. Consequently, there are limited jobs for forensic anthropologists in Europe. Most of the cases involving skeletal remains are analyzed by forensic pathologists, and the exhumations are done by the police or personnel from a criminalistic field.

3. Latin American forensic anthropology organizations specializing in political cases have focused closely on their relationship with the victims' relatives. For European and U.S. organizations and anthropologists, this aspect has been just one among many others, often left to the responsibility of the United Nations or other organizations, so as to focus exclusively on technical issues.

4. Compared to the U.S., the U.K. offers relatively few training courses in forensic anthropology. There are even fewer training courses available in Latin America.

5. Forensic anthropologists in Latin America have a strong empirical knowledge, based on vast experience, but only a few have a Ph.D. In developed countries, the situation is just the opposite.

Cooperation under equal conditions is absolutely desirable. In fact, the differences listed above should not divide forensic anthropologists working in this field of application but on the contrary should enrich our task, by fostering a balanced and open dialogue with a view to rendering a better service to the victims' relatives, doing justice and preventing impunity.

Notes

1. In spite of the fact that specific forensic investigations began in the Balkans in 1992 with the United Nations appointed Commission of Experts, assisted by Physicians for Human Rights (PHR), extensive investigations did not start until 1996, when the International Criminal Tribunal for the Former Yugoslavia (ICTY) commissioned PHR to conduct the forensic exhumations resulting in the contracting of large numbers of scientists.

2. EAAF is a nongovernment, independent organization created in 1984. To date, the EAAF has carried out forensic missions in Angola, Argentina, Bolivia, Brazil, Colombia, Côte d'Ivoire, Cyprus, Chile, Democratic Republic of the Congo, El Salvador, Ethiopia, Guatemala, Honduras, Indonesia, Kenya, Mexico, Morocco, Namibia, Panama, Paraguay, Philippines, Romania, Sierra Leone, South Africa, Sudan, Togo, Uruguay, Venezuela, and Zimbabwe. In addition, the EAAF has participated as a member of international teams in missions in Bosnia, Croatia, Georgia/Abkazia, Haiti, Iraq, Kosovo, Peru, Philippines, and Timor-Leste.

3. The term *forensic anthropology* is used in its widest sense, comprising the activities of both archaeologists and anthropologists who are concerned with the investigation of cases of criminal and political violence.

4. The author, as a member of EAAF, participated in some of its investigation stages from 1993 through 2000.

5. The group of forensic anthropologists engaged in investigations of this kind is a small one, and we all know one another very well. Therefore, we know what other colleagues have done, where they work, and for whom they have worked. The volume and extent of the experience gathered can be very simply evaluated by looking at the reports issued by each organization, at least those who produce a report every year.

6. In this brief summary I should mention the pioneering work of Dr. José Vicente Rodríguez from Colombia in the training of young generations of forensic anthropologists in his country.

7. In most Latin American countries, forensic experts form part of (1) the judicial system, (2) the prosecutor's office, and (3) the security forces.

8. The EAAF is based in Argentina, and despite the fact that the organization has a branch office in New York, it is still, on some occasions, denied a status as an international organization. It appears as if only those based in the U.S.A. or Western Europe may be called "international."

9. Also it should be mentioned that apart from the organizations mentioned above, local governments in Bosnia, Croatia, and Republica Srpksa exhumed graves, in some cases, with advice or participation from foreign scientists.

10. One of the exceptions is the participation of several forensic anthropologists since 2001 in investigations in East Timor, under the direction of the United Nations Serious Crimes Investigation Unit (SCIU).

References

Baraybar, J. P., and Marek, G. 2006. Forensic anthropology and the most probable cause of death in cases of violations against international humanitarian law: An example from Bosnia and Herzegovina. *Journal of Forensic Sciences* 51(6): 103–108.

Bernardi, P., and Fondebrider, L. 2007. Forensic archaeology and the scientific documentation of human rights violations: An Argentinean example from the early 1980s, in R. Ferllini (ed.), *Forensic Archaeology and the Investigation of Human Rights Abuses*, pp. 205–232. Springfield, IL: Charles C. Thomas.

Doretti, M., and Fondebrider, L. 2001. Science and human rights: Truth, justice, reparation and reconciliation: A long way in Third World countries, in V. Buchli and L. Gavin (eds.), *Archaeologies of the Contemporary Past*, pp. 138–144. London: Routledge.

———. 2004. Perspectives and recommendations from the field: Forensic anthropology and human rights in Argentina. *Proceedings of the 56th of the Academy of Forensic Sciences*, February 16–21, Dallas, Texas. Annual Meeting of the American Academy of Forensic Sciences, Dallas.

Doretti, M., and Snow, C. 2003. Forensic anthropology and human rights: The Argentine experience, in D. W. Steadman (ed.), *Hard Evidence: Case Studies in Forensic Anthropology*, pp. 290–310. Upper Saddle River, NJ: Prentice Hall.

Fondebrider, L. 2004. *Uncovering Evidence: The Forensic Sciences in Human Rights*. Project of the Center for Victims of Torture (CVT; US).

Haglund, W. 2001. Archaeology and forensic death investigations. *Historical Archaeology* 35: 26–34.

———. 2002. Recent mass graves, an introduction, in W. D. Haglund and M. H. Sorg (eds.), *Advances in Forensic Taphonomy: Method, Theory and Archaeological Perspectives*, pp. 243–262. Boca Raton, FL: CRC Press.

Haglund, W., Connor, M., and Scott, D. 2001. The archaeology of contemporary mass graves. *Historical Archaeology* 35: 57–69.

Hunter, J. 2002. Foreword: A pilgrim in forensic archaeology—A personal view, in W. D. Haglund and M. H. Sorg (eds.), *Advances in Forensic Taphonomy: Method, Theory and Archaeological Perspectives*, p. xxix. Boca Raton, FL: CRC Press.

Hunter, J., Brickley, M. G., Bourgeois, J., Bouts, W., Bourguignon, L., Hubrecht, F., DeWinne, J., Van Haaster, H., Hakbul, T., De Jong, H., Smits, L., Van Wijngaarden, L. H., and Luschen, M. 2001. Forensic archaeology, forensic anthropology and human rights in Europe. *Science and Justice* 4: 173–178.

Joyce, C., and Sover, E. 1991. *Witnesses from the Grave*. Boston: Little Brown.

Klonowski, E. 2004. Piotr Drukler and Nermin Sarajilic. The American Academy of Forensic Sciences, Vol. 10. Annual meeting, Dallas, Texas, February 16–21. Abstracts.

Komar, D. 2003. Lessons from Srebrenica: The contributions and limitations of physical anthropology in identifying victims of war crimes. *Journal of Forensic Science* 48(4): 713–716.

Simmons, T., and Haglund, W. D. 2005. Anthropology in a forensic context, in J. R. Hunter and M. Cox (eds.), *Advances in Forensic Archaeology*, pp. 159–176. New York: Routledge.

Skinner, M. F., Alempijevic, D., and Djuric-Srejic, M. 2003. Guidelines for international forensic bio-archaeology monitors of mass grave exhumations. *Forensic Science International* 134: 81–92.

Skinner, M. F., and Sterenberg, J. 2005. Turf wars: Authority and responsibility for the investigation of mass graves. *Forensic Science International* 151: 221–232.

Snow, C. 1984a. The investigation of the human remains of the disappeared in Argentina. *American Journal of Medicine and Pathology* 5: 297–300.

———. 1984b. Forensic anthropology in the documentation of human rights abuses. *American Journal of Forensic Medicine and Pathology* 5: 297–299.

Snow, C., and Bihurriet, M. J. 1992. An epidemiology of homicide: Ningun Nombre burials in the Province of Buenos Aires 1970 to 1984, in T. B. Jabine and C. P. Claude (eds.), *Human Rights and Statistics: Getting the Record Straight*, pp. 328–363. Philadelphia: University of Philadelphia Press.

Steadman, D.W., and Haglund, W. D. 2005. The scope of anthropological contributions to human rights investigations. *Journal of Forensic Sciences* 50(1): 1–8.

Stover, E., and Shigekane, R. 2002. The Missing in the aftermath of war: When do the need of victims' families and international war crimes tribunals clash? *International Review of the Red Cross* 848(84): 845–866.

Tuller, H., and Duric, M. 2006. Keeping the pieces together: A comparison of mass grave excavation methodology. *Forensic Science International* 156: 192–200.

Tuller, H., Hofmeister, U., and Daley, S. 2008. Spatial analysis of mass grave mapping data to assist in the re-association of disarticulated and commingled human remains, in B. Adams and Byrd, J. (eds.), *Recovery, Analysis, and Identification of Commingled Human Remains*, pp. 7–30. Totowa, NJ: Humana Press.

7

HISTORICAL DEVELOPMENT OF FORENSIC ANTHROPOLOGY: PERSPECTIVE FROM THE UNITED STATES

Douglas H. Ubelaker

Much of the intellectual growth of forensic anthropology in the past several decades can be traced to initiatives within the United States. Key themes in this development are significant early involvement of anthropologists in high profile cases, a research focus on problems centered in forensic anthropology, organizational developments, and the formation of relevant graduate programs. This chapter reviews that history with an emphasis on these themes.

Although the academic roots of forensic anthropology in the United States extend into Europe, within the country they originate with early anatomists and physicians who applied their knowledge to medico-legal issues. Some of these applications were serendipitous, as when major crimes and court trials happened to occur in the vicinity where the experts worked. In other cases, research interests in skeletal anatomy and human variation led them into the forensic arena.

The Parkman Trial

The Boston Parkman trial stands out as an early benchmark (Snow 1973; Stewart 1979a, 1979b). In 1849, Dr. George Parkman, a prominent local physician, was killed by Harvard professor and chemist John W. Webster. The murder took place at Harvard Medical School in a building constructed on land that Parkman had donated to the university. In addition to his philanthropy, Parkman had made loans to faculty members, including Webster. When Webster failed to make proper payment on his loan, Parkman began to apply pressure. Ultimately, Webster invited Parkman to his university laboratory, allegedly to make a payment, but instead Webster killed Parkman. In an effort to conceal the crime, Webster dismembered the body, attempted to burn the dismembered parts in the building furnace, and dispatched the bulk of the remains in the sewage system associated with his laboratory. Thanks to the efforts of a suspicious janitor and the local authorities, the remains were discovered.

In the trial, Harvard professors Oliver Wendell Holmes (1809–1894) and Jeffries Wyman (1814–1874) testified on anatomical issues of the recovered remains, bringing local public attention to the applied aspects of anatomy studies. At the time, Holmes was the initial appointee to the Parkman Professorship of Anatomy at Harvard, a position established by the university to recognize Parkman for his generous donation.

Wyman had graduated from medical school at Harvard and subsequently (1843) held the Harvard position of Hersey Professor of Anatomy. After the Parkman trial in 1866, Wyman became the first curator of Harvard's Peabody Museum of American

Archaeology and Ethnology and was recognized as a leading physical anthropologist of the time for his research on the skeletal anatomy of gorillas and humans, as well as on human remains recovered archaeologically from shell mounds in Florida (Hrdlička 1919). At the Webster trial, Wyman testified that cremated fragments found within the furnace were consistent with an origin from the same individual as the remains recovered from the laboratory sewage system. The verdict was guilty, and Webster was put to death by hanging.

Thomas Dwight (1843–1911)

At the time of the high-profile Parkman trial, Thomas Dwight was a child living in Boston. Likely influenced by discussions of the trial testimony and anatomical topics, Dwight developed an interest in medico-legal applications of anatomy and 29 years after the trial (1878) published a historically important essay, "The Identification of the Human Skeleton: A Medico-Legal Study." The essay won an award from the Massachusetts Medical Society and launched Dwight's career focusing on these issues. Dwight succeeded Holmes in holding the Parkman Professorship of Anatomy at Harvard. He followed up his landmark 1878 study with separate investigations of sex and age variation of the sternum (1881, 1890a), age changes in cranial suture closure (1890b), stature estimation from skeletal elements (1894a), the role of variation in skeletal interpretation (1894b), and sex differences in the size of bone articular surfaces (1905). Along the way, he also apparently participated in forensic cases (Stewart 1979a; Warren 1911). Dwight's early contributions were sufficiently important for T. D. Stewart (1979a: xii) to designate him "the father of forensic anthropology in the United States."

George A. Dorsey (1868–1931)

As an anthropology student at Harvard, George Dorsey was influenced by Dwight's research on skeletal variation and forensic applications (Stewart 1979a). While still a graduate student, he conducted archaeological excavations at Ancon, Peru, and assembled an archaeological exhibit for the 1893 World's Columbian Exposition in Chicago. In 1894, he received Harvard's first Ph.D. in anthropology, with a dissertation focusing on the Ancon material. From 1895–1896, Dorsey was an instructor at Harvard University. He subsequently (1898) became Curator at the Field Columbian Museum in Chicago and conducted his own research on sex variation of the heads of the femur and humerus (Dorsey 1897) and general bone identification, age, sex, and ancestry determination (Dorsey 1899). During his career Dorsey held professorships in comparative anatomy at Northwestern University Dental School and in anthropology at the University of Chicago, and he was also a founding member of the American Association of Physical Anthropologists.

Dorsey offered testimony in the high-profile Chicago trial of a local sausage maker, Adolph Luetgert, accused of murdering his wife Louisa and disposing of her remains in a vat at the sausage factory. Dorsey opined on small bone fragments that had been recovered at the scene. Although challenged by other experts, his testimony received extensive favorable media coverage in this high-profile trial. Subsequently, however, he shifted his interests toward ethnology, travel, and government service.

H. H. Wilder (1864–1928) and Paul Stevenson (1890–1971)

Harris Hawthorne Wilder began his career as a European-trained zoologist but developed a research interest in forensic anthropology while a professor at Smith College in Massachusetts (Stewart 1982a, 1982b). After graduating from Amherst College in Massachusetts in 1886, he studied zoology in Germany, receiving his doctorate there. He began his long career at Smith College in 1892. Wilder's interests included forensic aspects of dermatoglyphics and techniques of facial reproduction, improving on methodology he had been exposed to in Germany. In 1918, he coauthored a book on personal identification (Wilder and Wentworth 1918).

Wilder's career overlapped that of Paul Stevenson, an American anatomist who spent much of his career outside the United States. His one major publication from the United States offered detailed information on the age progression of epiphyseal union (Stevenson 1924). Although this information is of limited use today, because his study did not separate the sexes, historically the publication represents a key development in demonstrating the variation in the timing of union with detailed data.

Earnest A. Hooton (1887–1954) and Aleš Hrdlička (1869–1943)

Hooton and Hrdlička are widely recognized as key figures in the development of American physical anthropology. Earnest Hooton was a faculty member at Harvard University from 1913 to 1954. His major research interests included the skeletal biology of past peoples, race and human variation, and the relationship between body form and behavior—particularly that of criminals. Through his position at Harvard, Hooton trained many physical anthropologists who went on to make major contributions to forensic anthropology (including W. W. Howells, C. E. Snow, S. L. Washburn, and J. L. Angel, among others). Although active in forensic applications (Stewart 1979a), Hooton published relatively little on the subject (Hooton 1943).

Aleš Hrdlička immigrated to the United States with his family from Bohemia (now the Czech Republic) in 1881. He later acquired a medical degree and became interested in legal medicine, including the possible biological basis of insanity and criminal behavior. His research included anthropometry and its application to medicine and prehistoric populations. In 1902, Hrdlička began his 40-year career at the Smithsonian Institution in Washington, D.C.; during this time he assembled large collections of human remains that enabled much research in skeletal biology and forensic anthropology.

After founding the *American Journal of Physical Anthropology* in 1918 and the American Association of Physical Anthropologists, Hrdlička investigated a variety of anthropological topics, such as the peopling of the New World, human origins, and forensic anthropology. His many publications included forensic topics (see all Hrdlička references in Ubelaker 1999) and the 1939 edition of *Practical Anthropometry*, which presented a major section for forensic anthropology topics.

As early as 1896, Hrdlička presented court testimony on issues of epilepsy and insanity in a jury trial (Ubelaker 1999). Subsequently, forensic activities included analyses of human remains in Argentina and Peru (1910), studies of ancestry issues in litigation involving Chippewa Indian status in Minnesota (1915 to 1920), and a comparison of a skull recovered in Arizona with photographs and stereoscopic photographs of a missing person (1932). By 1936, his expertise was recognized by the Federal Bureau of Investigation (FBI), and he subsequently reported on evidence submitted by them. The record indicates he reported on at least nine cases over his career, but the actual number was probably much greater.

The Modern Era

In 1939, Wilton M. Krogman (1903–1987) published his *Guide to the Identification of Human Skeletal Material,* launching what many consider to be the modern era of forensic anthropology in the United States. During a seven-year academic appointment at (Case) Western Reserve Medical School, Krogman had worked closely with T. Wingate Todd (1885–1938), who had published key articles on age changes in the pubic bone (1920–1921), the clavicular epiphysis (Todd and D'Errico 1928), and the cranial sutures (Todd and Lyon 1924–1925). Krogman's book was published the same year as a revised edition of Hrdlička's *Practical Anthropometry*, but the guide's enhanced importance relates to its stand-alone emphasis on forensic applications and its publication in the FBI's law-enforcement-oriented publication. It rapidly became the authoritative work in forensic anthropology and was widely utilized (Stewart 1979a).

Although much of Krogman's research focused on growth and development, he went on to publish other important forensic contributions (1943, 1946, 1949) including his key text, *The Human Skeleton in Forensic Medicine* (1962). Krogman's book was widely utilized by those involved in identifying remains for the military, such as H. L. Shapiro (1902–1990) in Europe and Charles E. Snow (1910–1967), Mildred Trotter (1899–1991), and T. Dale Stewart (1901–1997) in Hawaii. The extensive identification effort by these individuals and others elucidated the shortcomings of Krogman's book and led to important research aimed at improving such methodology as Trotter's work on stature (Trotter and Gleser 1952) and Stewart's approach to age changes (McKern and Stewart 1957). The military identification effort not only provided those involved with extensive experience in identification but also led to key publications, such as Stewart's edited volume on mass disaster investigation (1970).

Smithsonian Collaboration with the FBI

Following Hrdlička's retirement in 1942, consultation with the FBI continued at the Smithsonian Institution with Hrdlička's successor, T. Dale Stewart. Like Hrdlička, Stewart had a medical degree. He served as an assistant to Hrdlička for many years but seemingly remained unaware of most of Hrdlička's forensic consultation (Stewart 1979a; Ubelaker 1999, 2000a, 2000b). Stewart immediately began working on FBI cases when he became curator in 1942. By 1969 he had reported on at least 254 cases, including 169 at the request of the FBI, and he had testified in court at least seven times.

With this casework experience, Stewart recognized the need for research aimed specifically at improving methodology in forensic applications. His classic 1957 publication with Thomas McKern (1920–1974), *Skeletal Age Changes in Young American Males*, resulted directly from his experience identifying remains for the military in Hawaii. Stewart recognized that methodology at the time, including that summarized in Krogman's book, was primarily based on anatomical collections such as those developed by Todd in Ohio. These collections represented primarily the elderly, and thus methodology was limited for age changes and other factors in the young. Working with the remains of young men killed in the Korean Conflict, Stewart and his colleagues assembled data from this important age group and revisited existing methodology.

Stewart also became a champion of problem-oriented research aimed at improving methodology. Examples include his research on issues relating to race (Stewart 1944, 1962), identification of cultural attributes on the skeleton (Stewart 1937, 1939, 1941, 1950; Stewart and Titterington 1944, 1946), age changes (McKern and Stewart 1957; Stewart 1953a, 1954a, 1957, 1958), sex estimation (Stewart 1954b), distinguishing human from nonhuman remains (Stewart 1959, 1961), historical issues (Stewart 1978, 1979c, 1982a, 1982b), anatomical aspects of facial reproduction (Stewart 1983), and objectivity in casework (Stewart 1984). Much of this is summarized in synthetic works (Stewart 1948, 1951, 1953b, 1954c, 1968, 1970, 1972, 1973, 1979a, 1979b, 1980; Stewart and Trotter 1954, 1955), including his own classic 1979 text *Essentials of Forensic Anthropology*.

In 1962, Stewart accepted an appointment as Director of the United States National Museum, and J. Lawrence Angel (1915–1986) assumed casework responsibility for the FBI and others. British-born Angel had received his Ph.D. at Harvard working closely with Hooton and Clyde Kluckhohn (1905–1960). Although his dissertation and major research had focused on anatomical issues and human remains from the Near East, his interests shifted toward forensic applications when he left Jefferson Medical College in Philadelphia and joined the Smithsonian Institution in 1962. Assuming the forensic caseload from Stewart, he reported on approximately 565 cases for the FBI and others before his death in 1986. In about 1977, Angel took sabbatical leave, and Douglas H. Ubelaker assumed the Smithsonian Institution forensic consultation for the FBI, and he has continued in that role until 2006, having reported on over 760 cases.

Organizational Advances

In 1972, physical anthropologists launched their own section of the American Academy of Forensic Sciences. Prior to that time, participating anthropologists held membership in the Pathology-Biology or General sections, but formation of the new section galvanized the participation of physical anthropologists at such meetings. The initial formation of 14 founding members grew steadily to a 2006 membership of 334. The annual meeting is well-attended, usually with over two days of scientific papers and posters on a variety of subjects relating to the field. The meeting also has stimulated interaction of anthropologists with others in forensic science through Academy-wide committee appointments and attendance at simultaneous and joint academic sessions.

Ellis R. Kerley (1924–1998) provided leadership in the formation of the section and also in the establishment of the American Board of Forensic Anthropology (ABFA) in 1977/1978. The ABFA provides certification for forensic anthropologists and has grown from an initial enrollment of 22; 74 diplomates have been certified by 2006. The AFBA is important historically in providing recognition to its diplomates and offering the legal system a list of professionals deemed to be qualified by their peers.

Educational Advances

Historically, training in forensic anthropology in the United States has shifted from medical schools to departments of anthropology. Whereas the pioneers in the field largely held medical degrees with specialties in anatomy, all current forensic anthropologists hold degrees from academic departments of anthropology and related disciplines. This development reflects the increasing complexity and specialization of American science, as well as the nature of the development of forensic anthropology. Forensic anthropologists uniquely bring knowledge of archaeological techniques, taphonomic changes, and human variation to their casework—knowledge acquired in graduate school rather than medical school. Historically, several learning institutions have been particularly instrumental in training forensic anthropologists. In the early days, Harvard played a key role, although forensic anthropology assumed a role secondary to the more general field of physical anthropology. Hooton trained many students, and many of them later became involved in forensic applications (for example, Angel).

In more recent years, a variety of universities have trained forensic anthropologists, but special mention is due the University of Kansas in the 1960s and 1970s. William M. Bass III joined the faculty there in 1960, soon to be joined by Ellis R. Kerley and Thomas McKern. Bass brought extensive experience working with archaeologically recovered remains, as well as having completed a dissertation at the University of Pennsylvania under the direction of Wilton Krogman and T. D. Stewart, among others. As noted above, Kerley was especially active in the American Academy of Forensic Sciences and had pioneered research in microscopic approaches to the estimation of age at death in adults. Thomas McKern had worked closely with T. D. Stewart of the Smithsonian Institution on the analysis of the age at death data from the Korean War dead (McKern and Stewart 1957). Until the trio departed the university in the early 1970s for other positions, they had assembled a formidable teaching team that trained many of the forensic anthropologists active today. Bass left Kansas for the University of Tennessee, where he founded another major training program in forensic anthropology and organized a long-term research project to study human postmortem change.

Currently, training for forensic anthropologists in the United States is available at a variety of levels in graduate programs within universities. The nucleus of this activity continues to be the department of anthropology or its equivalent, but, increasingly, training incorporates coursework in related areas of forensic science, law, statistics, anatomy, and other key areas. Workshops and internships supplement this formal training in important ways by providing practical experience.

Recent years have witnessed a quantum leap in student interest in forensic anthropology within the United States. Likely fueled by media presentations of forensic themes, growing numbers of new students are attracted to the field allowing graduate admissions committees to be increasingly selective. The result seems to be a cohort of young forensic anthropologists who are ever more intelligent, focused, well-trained, and capable.

Research Advances

Stimulated by the growing focus on forensic anthropology in graduate programs, increased experience in casework and enhanced communication and publication outlets, forensic anthropologists are undertaking research in a range of key areas. Parts of these advances are fueled by new technology or awareness of the applications of existing technology to problems in forensic anthropology. Molecular analysis (see Baker this volume), radiocarbon analysis (see Forbes and Nugent this volume), sophisticated computer technology, analysis using the scanning electron microscope and mass spectrometer, and a variety of other approaches are finding their way into anthropological research. Much of this research is problem driven; work on forensic cases encounters previously unrecognized problems that require resolution. Research answers can be found in the chemistry department in another building on campus or with the colleague at another institution who is doing work in a relevant area.

Significant research advances are enabled by computer technology and the enlarged databases that are now possible to assemble. Work in forensic research laboratories in the United States currently takes full advantage of this and other technologies to address a variety of research problems. Although large databases have been constructed using samples from the United States, growing awareness of the importance of human variation has stimulated the inclusion of worldwide perspective on such important issues as ancestry, sexual dimorphism, and the timing of age changes. Greater awareness of secular change in the United States populations has tempered interpretation of older databases and led to the formation of more contemporary ones as exemplified by the computerized FORDISC system for the assessment of ancestry, sex, and living stature (Jantz and Moore-Jansen 1988; Jantz and Ousley 1993).

Collections of well-documented human remains play key roles in the development of the scientific methodology of forensic anthropology. Permanent collections not only allow new research but also permit previously published techniques to be reexamined with fresh perspective. On the positive side, global interest in forensic anthropology has stimulated the formation of new collections, many originating from parts of the world and populations previously not well represented.

On the other hand, in the United States, concerns expressed by Aboriginal peoples, political developments, and legislation have limited access to remains relating to American Indians. Although state laws and policies vary considerably (Ubelaker and Grant 1989), two federal laws (the National Museum of the American Indian Act passed in 1989 and the Native American Graves Protection and Repatriation Act passed in 1990) specifically target collections of human remains and call for research to determine if those being curated can be linked to existing American Indian groups (Buikstra 2006). While these laws and associated policy have resulted in reduced access to some collections, they have also stimulated considerable research.

The recent presentations in the Physical Anthropology Section of the American Academy of Forensic Sciences annual meeting in Seattle, Washington (February 2006), provide a sampler of the diversity of research being conducted. In addition to case studies, research topics presented there included new methodologies for identification and individuation; search techniques, taphonomy and dating; microscopic and radiological analyses; and trauma interpretation in individual or mass disaster scenarios.

Individuation and identification are major goals of forensic anthropology. Individuation techniques introduced at the 2006 AAFS meeting include new approaches to stature estimation (Adams and Herrmann 2006; Giroux and Wescott 2006), determination of adult sex (Allbright 2006; Brown, Ubelaker, and Schanfield 2006; Cornelison, Lackey-Cornelison, and Hunter 2006) and subadult sex (Franklin et al. 2006), age estimation of adults (DiGangi et al. 2006; Park et al. 2006; Prodhan, Ubelaker, and Prince 2006) and subadults (El-Sheikh and Ramadan 2006; Schaefer 2006), identifying ancestry (Berg 2006; Hefner and Ousley 2006; Kolatorowicz 2006; Loichinger and Wilczak 2006; Parr 2006; Regan and Falsetti 2006; Wescott 2006), pathology (Child and Austin 2006; Falsetti and Freas 2006; Grivas 2006; Wilson, Bethard, and DiGangi 2006), and distinguishing human from nonhuman bone (Gray and Suchey 2006; Leney 2006; Pope et al. 2006). Advances in photo and video identification in forensic anthropology were also introduced (De Angelis et al. 2006; Fenton and Sauer 2006; Meehan and Mann 2006).

Interpreting traumatic injuries continues to be a key research topic (e.g., Cattaneo et al. 2006; Daegling et al. 2006; Freas 2006; Fulginiti et al. 2006; Hufnagl 2006; Kennedy 2006; Marks, Tersigni, and Mileusnic 2006; Murad 2006; Pope et al. 2006; Potter and Alexander 2006; Symes et al. 2006; see also Cunha and Pinheiro and see Loe this volume). Recent research also focuses on such issues as commingling (O'Callaghan et al. 2006; see also Byrd and Adams this volume), burning (Bodkin et al. 2006; Delvin et al. 2006; Pope et al. 2006; see also Thompson this volume), identification in mass disaster situations (Fulginiti et al. 2006; Martrille et al. 2006; Regan and Falsetti 2006; Simmons and Skinner 2006; see also Sledzik this volume), the use of archaeological techniques to aid in the search and recovery of human remains (Dirkmaat and Cabo 2006; Schultz 2006; see also Holland and Connell this volume), complexities

in the interpretation of decomposition (Albert, Tomberlin, and Johnson 2006; Bunch 2006; Seet 2006) and taphonomy (Cope and Dupras 2006; O'Brien et al. 2006; see also Nawrocki this volume), new approaches to determining the postmortem interval (Ubelaker, Buchholz, and Stewart 2006; Wedel and Bowman 2006; Weitzel 2006; see also Forbes and Nugent this volume), new applications of microscopic and computerized technology (Crowder 2006; Leney 2006; Marks, Tersigni, and Mileusnic 2006; Rodriguez 2006), and the potential of the petrous portion of the temporal in individuation (Wiersema 2006). Although not all these methods will stand the test of time, they indicate the viability and maturity of the field.

The diversity of these research topics and the new concepts and methodology they represent reflect the growth and intensity of forensic anthropology in the United States. The field has changed immensely since its foundation in the 19th century, but it continues to evolve.

References

Adams, B. J., and Herrmann, N. P. 2006. Estimation of living stature from selected anthropometric (soft tissue) measurements: How do these compare with osteometric (skeletal) measurements? *Proceedings of the American Academy of Forensic Sciences, 20–25 February, Seattle.* Denver, CO: American Academy of Forensic Sciences, 279–280.

Albert, A., Tomberlin, J. K., and Johnson, C. 2006. Observations of decomposition in Southern coastal North Carolina. *Proceedings of the American Academy of Forensic Sciences, 20–25 February, Seattle.* Denver, CO: American Academy of Forensic Sciences: 309.

Allbright, A. S. 2006. Sexual dimorphism in the vertebral column. *Proceedings of the American Academy of Forensic Sciences, 20-25 February, Seattle.* Denver, CO: American Academy of Forensic Sciences: 310.

Berg, G. E. 2006. Discriminant function analysis as applied to mandibular morphology to assess population affinity. *Proceedings of the American Academy of Forensic Sciences, 20–25 February, Seattle.* Denver, CO: American Academy of Forensic Sciences: 282.

Bodkin, T. E., Brooks, T., Potts, G. E., and Smullen, S. 2006. Trace element analysis of medical school cadaver cremains. *Proceedings of the American Academy of Forensic Sciences, 20–25 February, Seattle.* Denver, CO: American Academy of Forensic Sciences: 315.

Brown, R. P., Ubelaker, D. H., and Schanfield, M. S. 2006. Evaluation of Purkait's Triangle Method for determining sexual dimorphism. *Proceedings of the American Academy of Forensic Sciences, 20–25 February, Seattle.* Denver, CO: American Academy of Forensic Sciences: 285–286.

Buikstra, J. 2006. History of research in skeletal biology, in D. H. Ubelaker (ed.), *Environment, Origins and Population*, Vol. 3, pp. 504–523. Handbook of North American Indians. Washington, D.C.: Smithsonian Institution.

Bunch, A. W. 2006. A preliminary investigation of decomposition in cold climate. *Proceedings of the American Academy of Forensic Sciences, 20–25 February, Seattle.* Denver, CO: American Academy of Forensic Sciences: 297–298.

Cattaneo, C., Marinelli, E., Andreola, S., Poppa, P., and Grandi, M. 2006. The detection of microscopic markers of haemorrhaging and wound age on dry bone: Beating the barriers between forensic anthropology and forensic pathology. *Proceedings of the American Academy of Forensic Sciences, 20–25 February, Seattle.* Denver, CO: American Academy of Forensic Sciences: 293–294.

Child, S. L., and Austin, D. E. 2006. The differential diagnosis of skullbase osteomyelitis secondary to necrotizing ostitis externa. *Proceedings of the American Academy of Forensic Sciences, 20–25 February, Seattle.* Denver, CO: American Academy of Forensic Sciences: 309–310.

Cope, D. J., and Dupras, T. L. 2006. The effects of household corrosive substances on human bone and teeth. *Proceedings of the American Academy of Forensic Sciences, 20–25 February, Seattle.* Denver, CO: American Academy of Forensic Sciences: 290.

Cornelison, J. B., Lackey-Cornelison, W. L., and Hunter, B. C. 2006. Sex determination from the hyoid body. *Proceedings of the American Academy of Forensic Sciences, 20–25 February, Seattle.* Denver, CO: American Academy of Forensic Sciences: 286.

Crowder, C. M. 2006. Reducing observer error through choice of histological evaluation technique. *Proceedings of the American Academy of Forensic Sciences, 20–25 February, Seattle.* Denver, CO: American Academy of Forensic Sciences: 319.

Daegling, D. J., Hortzman, J., Self, C. J., and Warren, M. W. 2006. Bone fracture mechanics: *In Vitro* strain gauge analysis of the ribs and mandible during failure. *Proceedings of the American Academy of Forensic Sciences, 20–25 February, Seattle.* Denver, CO: American Academy of Forensic Sciences: 315–316.

De Angelis, D., Poppa, P., Sala, R., and Cattaneo, C. 2006. Identification of the living on video surveillance systems: A novel approach. *Proceedings of the American Academy of Forensic Sciences, 20–25 February, Seattle.* Denver, CO: American Academy of Forensic Sciences: 317.

Delvin, J. B., Kroman, A., Symes, S., and Herrmann, N. P. 2006. Heat intensity versus exposure duration,

Part I: Macroscopic influence on burned bone. *Proceedings of the American Academy of Forensic Sciences, 20–25 February, Seattle.* Denver, CO: American Academy of Forensic Sciences: 310–311.

DiGangi, E. A., Bethard, J. D., Kimmerle, E. H., and Konigsberg, L. W. 2006. A new method for estimating age-at-death from the first rib. *Proceedings of the American Academy of Forensic Sciences, 20–25 February, Seattle.* Denver, CO: American Academy of Forensic Sciences: 283–284.

Dirkmaat, D. C., and Cabo, L. L. 2006. The shallow grave as an option for disposing of the recently deceased: Goals and consequences. *Proceedings of the American Academy of Forensic Sciences, 20–25 February, Seattle.* Denver, CO: American Academy of Forensic Sciences: 299–300.

Dorsey, G. A. 1897. A sexual study of the size of the articular surfaces of the long bones in Aboriginal American skeletons. *Boston Medical and Surgical Journal* 137: 82–89.

———. 1899. The skeleton in medico-legal anatomy. *Chicago Medical Recorder* 16: 172–179.

Dwight, T. 1878. *The Identification of the Human Skeleton: A Medico-Legal Study.* Boston.

———. 1881. The sternum as an index of sex and age. *Journal of Anatomy and Physiology (London)* 15: 327–330.

———. 1890a. The sternum as an index of sex, height and age. *Journal of Anatomy and Physiology (London)* 24: 527–535.

———. 1890b. The closure of the cranial sutures as a sign of age. *Boston Medical and Surgical Journal* 122: 389–392.

———. 1894a. Methods of estimating the height from parts of the skeleton. *Medical Record* 46: 293–296.

———. 1894b. The range and significance of variations in the human skeleton. *Boston Medical and Surgical Journal* 13: 361–389.

———. 1905. The size of the articular surfaces of the long bones as characteristic of sex. An anthropological study. *American Journal of Anatomy* 4: 19–32.

El-Sheikh, M. E. E., and Ramadan, S. 2006. Age of closure of the spheno-occipital synchondrosis in the Arabian Gulf Region. *Proceedings of the American Academy of Forensic Sciences, 20–25 February, Seattle.* Denver, CO: American Academy of Forensic Sciences: 277.

Falsetti, A. B., and Freas, L. E. 2006. Lumbosacral transitional vertebrae, spondylolysis and spondylolisthesis: Prevalence in a modern forensic skeletal population. *Proceedings of the American Academy of Forensic Sciences, 20–25 February, Seattle.* Denver, CO: American Academy of Forensic Sciences: 318.

Fenton, T. W., and Sauer, N. J. 2006. Identification of the living from video tape and photographs: The dynamic orientation technique. *Proceedings of the American Academy of Forensic Sciences, 20–25 February, Seattle*. Denver, CO: American Academy of Forensic Sciences: 314–315.

Franklin, D., Oxnard, C. E., O'Higgins, P., Dadour, I., and Napper, R. 2006. Sexual dimorphism in the subadult mandible: Quantification using geometric morphometrics. *Proceedings of the American Academy of Forensic Sciences, 20–25 February, Seattle*. Denver, CO: American Academy of Forensic Sciences: 277.

Freas, L. 2006. Scanning electron microscopy of saw marks in bone: Assessment of wear-related features of the Kerf Wall. *Proceedings of the American Academy of Forensic Sciences, 20–25 February, Seattle*. Denver, CO: American Academy of Forensic Sciences: 296.

Fulginiti, L. C., Hartnett, K. M., Horn, K. D., and Kohlmeier, R. E. 2006. Of butterflies and spirals: Interpretation of fractures in motor vehicle vs. pedestrian accidents. *Proceedings of the American Academy of Forensic Sciences, 20–25 February, Seattle*. Denver, CO: American Academy of Forensic Sciences: 289.

Fulginiti, L. C., Warren, M. W., Hefner, J. T., Bedore, L. R., Byrd, J. H., Stefan, V., and Dirkmaat, D. C. 2006. Anthropology responds to Hurricane Katrina. *Proceedings of the American Academy of Forensic Sciences, 20–25 February, Seattle*. Denver, CO: American Academy of Forensic Sciences: 305.

Giroux, C. L., and Wescott, D. J. 2006. Stature estimation based on dimensions of the bony pelvis and proximal femur. *Proceedings of the American Academy of Forensic Sciences, 20–25 February, Seattle*. Denver, CO: American Academy of Forensic Sciences: 284.

Gray, D. W., and Suchey, J. M. 2006. Mass disasters and non-human remains. *Proceedings of the American Academy of Forensic Sciences, 20–25 February, Seattle*. Denver, CO: American Academy of Forensic Sciences: 306.

Grivas, C.R. 2006. Differential diagnosis of gout in skeletal remains. *Proceedings of the American Academy of Forensic Sciences, 20–25 February, Seattle*. Denver, CO: American Academy of Forensic Sciences: 294.

Hefner, J. T., and Ousley, S. D. 2006. Morphoscopic traits and the statistical determination of ancestry II. *Proceedings of the American Academy of Forensic Sciences, 20–25 February, Seattle*. Denver, CO: American Academy of Forensic Sciences: 282.

Hooton, E. A. 1943. Medico-legal aspects of physical anthropology. *Clinics* 1: 1612–1624.

Hrdlička, A. 1919. *Physical Anthropology: Its Scope and Aims; Its History and Present Status in the United States*. Philadelphia: The Wistar Institute of Anatomy and Biology.

———. 1939. *Practical Anthropometry*. Philadelphia: The Wistar Institute of Anatomy and Biology.

Hufnagl, K. B. 2006. Estimating time since injury from healing stages observed in radiographs. *Proceedings of the American Academy of Forensic Sciences, 20–25 February, Seattle*. Denver, CO: American Academy of Forensic Sciences: 274.

Jantz, R. L., and Moore-Jansen, P. H. 1988. *A Database for Forensic Anthropology: Structure, Content and Analysis*. Report of Investigations 47. Knoxville: The University of Tennessee.

Jantz, R. L., and Ousley, S. D. 1993. *FORDISC 1.0: Computerized Forensic Discriminant Functions*. Knoxville: The University of Tennessee.

Kennedy, K. A. R. 2006. Traumatic modifications of human remains of victims of mass disasters and long-term abuse. *Proceedings of the American Academy of Forensic Sciences, 20–25 February, Seattle*. Denver, CO: American Academy of Forensic Sciences: 304.

Kolatorowicz, A. 2006. Selection of variables for discriminant analysis of human crania for determining ancestry. *Proceedings of the American Academy of Forensic Sciences, 20–25 February, Seattle*. Denver, CO: American Academy of Forensic Sciences: 276–277.

Krogman, W. M. 1939. A guide to the identification of human skeletal material. *FBI Law Enforcement Bulletin* 8: 3–31.

———. 1943. Role of the physical anthropologist in the identification of human skeletal remains. *FBI Law Enforcement Bulletin* 12(4): 17–40; 12(5): 12–28.

———. 1946. The reconstruction of the living head from the skull. *FBI Law Enforcement Bulletin* 15: 11–18.

———. 1949. The human skeleton in legal medicine: Medical aspects, in S. D. Levinson (ed.), *Symposium on Medicolegal Problems* 2: 1–90. Philadelphia: Lippincott.

———. 1962. *The Human Skeleton in Forensic Medicine*. Springfield, IL: Thomas.

Leney, M. D. 2006. Is this bone human or what? In pursuit of human vs. non human determinations in small osseous fragments. *Proceedings of the American Academy of Forensic Sciences, 20–25 February, Seattle*. Denver, CO: American Academy of Forensic Sciences: 321.

Loichinger, J. L., and Wilczak, C. A. 2006. Population variation in the sacrum. *Proceedings of the American Academy of Forensic Sciences, 20–25 February, Seattle*. Denver, CO: American Academy of Forensic Sciences: 275–276.

Marks, M. K., Tersigni, M. A., and Mileusnic, D. 2006. Antemortem vs. perimortem infant rib fracture: The histological evidence. *Proceedings of the American Academy of Forensic Sciences, 20–25*

February, Seattle. Denver, CO: American Academy of Forensic Sciences: 307.

Martrille, L., Cattaneo, C., Schuliar, Y., and Baccino, E. 2006. Anthropological aspects of mass disasters. *Proceedings of the American Academy of Forensic Sciences, 20–25 February, Seattle.* Denver, CO: American Academy of Forensic Sciences: 304.

McKern, T. W., and Stewart, T. D. 1957. *Skeletal Age Changes in Young American Males.* Natick, MA: Quartermaster Research and Development Center, Environmental Protection Research Division; Report No. EP-45.

Meehan, A. L., and Mann, R. W. 2006. Skull and photo superimposition technique used to aid in the identification process. *Proceedings of the American Academy of Forensic Sciences, 20–25 February, Seattle.* Denver, CO: American Academy of Forensic Sciences: 276.

Murad, T. A. 2006. The difference between "Pala" and "Palo" is the instrument of death. *Proceedings of the American Academy of Forensic Sciences, 20–25 February, Seattle.* Denver, CO: American Academy of Forensic Sciences: 295–296.

O'Brien, R. C., Forbes, S. L., Meyer, J., and Dadour, I. 2006. Seasonal variation of scavenging and associated faunal activity on pig carcasses in South Western Australia. *Proceedings of the American Academy of Forensic Sciences, 20–25 February, Seattle.* Denver, CO: American Academy of Forensic Sciences: 297.

O'Callaghan, J., Raskin-Burns, J., Christensen, A. F., Meehan, A., Leney, M., Barritt, S. M., and Smith, B. C. 2006. Resolving extremely commingled skeletal remains from the Korean War through mitochondrial DNA (mtDNA) testing. *Proceedings of the American Academy of Forensic Sciences, 20–25 February, Seattle.* Denver, CO: American Academy of Forensic Sciences: 320.

Park, D., Ko, J., Kim, D., and Han, S. 2006. Morphometrics using radiographic study of thyroid cartilage for age-estimation in Korean males. *Proceedings of the American Academy of Forensic Sciences, 20–25 February, Seattle.* Denver, CO: American Academy of Forensic Sciences: 291–292.

Parr, N. M. 2006. An assessment of non-metric traits of the mandible used in the determination of ancestry. *Proceedings of the American Academy of Forensic Sciences, 20–25 February, Seattle.* Denver, CO: American Academy of Forensic Sciences: 281.

Pope, E. J., Batey, T., and Rose, J. C. 2006. Non-destructive microscopic differentiation of human from non-human fragmentary burned bone. *Proceedings of the American Academy of Forensic Sciences, 20–25 February, Seattle.* Denver, CO: American Academy of Forensic Sciences: 293.

Pope, E. J., Smith, O. C., and Spradly, K. M. 2006. Bevel, bevel in my bone, be it bullet or be it stone? Misidentification of blunt force trauma as ballistic entrance wounds in burned Cranial Bone. *Proceedings of the American Academy of Forensic Sciences, 20–25 February, Seattle.* Denver, CO: American Academy of Forensic Sciences: 295.

Potter, W. E., and Alexander, R. T. 2006. Nail or bullet? A comparison of typical cranial gunshot wounds to a defect resulting from a nail gun. *Proceedings of the American Academy of Forensic Sciences, 20–25 February, Seattle.* Denver, CO: American Academy of Forensic Sciences: 308–309.

Prodhan, R., Ubelaker, D. H., and Prince, D. A. 2006. Evaluation of three methods of age estimation from human skeletal remains (Suchey-Brooks, Lamendin, and Two-Step Strategy). *Proceedings of the American Academy of Forensic Sciences, 20–25 February, Seattle.* Denver, CO: American Academy of Forensic Sciences: 284–285.

Regan, L. A., and Falsetti, A. B. 2006. Isotopic determination of region of origin in modern peoples: Applications for identification of U.S. war-dead from the Vietnam Conflict. *Proceedings of the American Academy of Forensic Sciences, 20–25 February, Seattle.* Denver, CO: American Academy of Forensic Sciences: 292.

Rodriguez, W. C., III. 2006. The impact of high speed-high resolution three dimensional CT scans on forensic anthropology. *Proceedings of the American Academy of Forensic Sciences, 20–25 February, Seattle.* Denver, CO: American Academy of Forensic Sciences: 316–317.

Schaefer, M. C. 2006. Forensic application of epiphyseal sequencing. *Proceedings of the American Academy of Forensic Sciences, 20–25 February, Seattle.* Denver, CO: American Academy of Forensic Sciences: 286.

Schultz, J. J. 2006. Forensic GPR: Using ground-penetrating radar to search for buried bodies. *Proceedings of the American Academy of Forensic Sciences, 20–25 February, Seattle.* Denver, CO: American Academy of Forensic Sciences: 278.

Seet, B. L. 2006. Estimating the postmortem interval in freshwater environments. *Proceedings of the American Academy of Forensic Sciences, 20–25 February, Seattle.* Denver, CO: American Academy of Forensic Sciences: 287.

Simmons, T., and Skinner, M. 2006. The accuracy of ante-mortem data and presumptive identification: Appropriate procedures, applications and ethics. *Proceedings of the American Academy of Forensic Sciences, 20–25 February, Seattle.* Denver, CO: American Academy of Forensic Sciences: 303.

Snow, C. C. 1973. Forensic anthropology, in A. Redfield (ed.), *Anthropology Beyond the University*, pp. 4–17. Athens, GA: Southern Anthropological Society Proceedings, No. 7.

Stevenson, P. H. 1924. Age order of epiphyseal union in Man. *American Journal of Physical Anthropology* 7: 53–93.

Stewart, T. D. 1937. Different types of cranial deformity in the pueblo area. *American Anthropologist* 39: 169–171.

———. 1939. A new type of artificial cranial deformation from Florida. *Journal of the Washington Academy of Sciences* 29: 460–465.

———. 1941. The circular type of cranial deformity in the United States. *American Journal of Physical Anthropology* 28: 343–351.

———. 1944. Reviews of Man's most dangerous myth: The fallacy of Race, M. F. A. Montagu; Race: Science and politics, R. Benedict; The races of mankind, R. Benedict and G. Weltfish; and Race, reason, and rubbish, G. Dahlberg. *American Journal of Physical Anthropology* 2: 321–322.

———. 1948. Medico-legal aspects of the skeleton. I. Sex, age, race and stature. *American Journal of Physical Anthropology* 6: 315–321.

———. 1950. Early description of lambdoid cranial deformity incorrectly attributed to the Navaho: Historical note on R.W. Shufeldt, M.D. (1850–1934). *Journal of the Washington Academy of Sciences* 40: 33–37.

———. 1951. What the bones tell. *FBI Law Enforcement Bulletin* 20: 1–5.

———. 1953a. The age incidence of neural-arch defects in Alaskan natives, considered from the standpoint of etiology. *Journal of Bone Joint Surgery* 35-A: 937–950.

———. 1953b. Research in human identification. *Science* 118: 3.

———. 1954a. Metamorphosis of the joints of the sternum in relation to age changes in other bones. *American Journal of Physical Anthropology* 12: 519–535.

———. 1954b. Sex determination of the skeleton by guess and by measurement. *American Journal of Physical Anthropology* 12: 385–392.

———. 1954c. Evaluation of evidence from the skeleton, in R. B. H. Gradwohl (ed.), *Legal Medicine*, pp. 407–450. St. Louis, MO: Mosby.

———. 1957. Distortion of the pubic symphyseal surface in females and its effect on age determination. *American Journal of Physical Anthropology* 15: 9–18.

———. 1958. Rate of development of vertebral osteoarthritis in American whites and its significance in skeletal age identification. *The Leech* 28: 144–151.

———. 1959. Bear paw remains closely resemble human bones. *FBI Law Enforcement Bulletin* 28: 18–21.

———. 1961. Sternal ribs are aid in identifying animal remains. *FBI Law Enforcement Bulletin* 30: 9–11.

———. 1962. Anterior femoral curvature: Its utility for race identification. *Human Biology* 34: 49–62.

———. 1968. Identification by the skeletal structures, in F. E. Camps (ed.), *Gradwohl's Legal Medicine* (3rd ed.), pp. 123–154. Bristol: J Wright.

———. 1970. *Personal Identification in Mass Disasters*. Washington, D.C.: Smithsonian Institution.

———. 1972. What the bones tell today. *FBI Law Enforcement Bulletin* 41: 16–20, 30–31.

———. 1973. Recent improvements in estimating stature, sex, age and race from skeletal remains, in A. K. Mant (ed.), *Modern Trends in Forensic Medicine*, pp. 193–211. London: Butterworths.

———. 1978. George A. Dorsey's role in the Luetgert Case: A significant episode in the history of forensic anthropology. *Journal of Forensic Sciences* 23: 786–791.

———. 1979a. *Essentials of Forensic Anthropology, Especially as Developed in the United States*. Springfield, IL: Charles C. Thomas.

———. 1979b. Forensic anthropology, in W. Goldschmidt (ed.), *The Uses of Anthropology*: 169–183. Special publication No 11. Washington, D.C.: American Anthropological Association.

———. 1979c. A tribute to the French forensic anthropologist, Georges Fully (1926–1973). *Journal of Forensic Sciences* 24: 916–924.

———. 1980. Responses of the human skeleton to changes in the quality of life. *Journal of Forensic Sciences* 25: 912–921.

———. 1982a. Background of American forensic anthropology. *Criminal Justice Review* 7: 4–7.

———. 1982b. Pioneer contributions of Harris Hawthorne Wilder, Ph.D., to forensic sciences. *Journal of Forensic Sciences* 27: 754–762.

———. 1983. The points of attachment of the palpebral ligaments: Their use in facial reconstructions on the skull. *Journal of Forensic Sciences* 28: 858–863.

———. 1984. Perspective on the reporting of forensic cases, in T. A. Rathbun and J. E. Buikstra (eds.), *Human Identification: Case Studies in Forensic Anthropology*, pp. 15–18. Springfield, IL: Charles C. Thomas.

Stewart, T. D., and Titterington, P. F. 1944. Filed Indian teeth from Illinois. *Journal of the Washington Academy of Sciences* 34: 317–321.

———. 1946. More filed Indian teeth from the United States. *Journal of the Washington Academy of Sciences* 36: 259–261.

Stewart, T. D., and Trotter, M. 1954. *Basic Readings on the Identification of Human Skeletons: Estimation of Age*. New York: Wenner-Gren Foundation for Anthropological Research, Inc.

———. 1955. Role of physical anthropology in the field of human identification. *Science* 122: 883–884.

Symes, S. A., Kroman, A. M., Myster, S. M. T., Rainwater, C. W, and Matia, J. J. 2006. Anthropological saw mark analysis on bone: What is the potential dismemberment interpretation? *Proceedings of the*

American Academy of Forensic Sciences, 20–25 February, Seattle. Denver, CO: American Academy of Forensic Sciences: 301.

Todd, T. W. 1920–1921. Age changes in the pubic bone. *American Journal of Physical Anthropology* 3: 285–334; 4: 1–70, 333–424.

Todd, T. W., and D'Errico, J., Jr. 1928. The clavicular epiphyses. *American Journal of Anatomy* 41: 25–50.

Todd, T. W., and Lyon, D. W., Jr. 1924–1925. Cranial suture closure: Its progress and age relationship. *American Journal of Physical Anthropology* 7: 325–384; 8: 23–71, 149–168.

Trotter, M., and Gleser, G. C. 1952. Estimation of stature from long bones of American Whites and Negroes. *American Journal of Physical Anthropology* 10: 463–514.

Ubelaker, D. H. 1999. Aleš Hrdlička's role in the history of physical anthropology. *Journal of Forensic Sciences* 44: 708–714.

———. 2000a. T. Dale Stewart's perspective on his career as a forensic anthropologist at the Smithsonian. *Journal of Forensic Sciences* 45: 269–278.

———. 2000b. The forensic anthropology legacy of T. Dale Stewart (1901–1997). *Journal of Forensic Sciences* 45: 245–252.

Ubelaker, D. H., Buchholz, B. A., and Stewart, J. 2006. Evaluation of date of death through artificial radiocarbon in distinct human skeletal and dental tissues. *Proceedings of the American Academy of Forensic Sciences, 20–25 February, Seattle*. Denver, CO: American Academy of Forensic Sciences: 316.

Ubelaker, D. H., and Grant, L. G. 1989. Human skeletal remains: Preservation or reburial? *Yearbook of Physical Anthropology* 32: 249–287.

Warren, J. 1911. Thomas Dwight, M.D., LL.D. *Anatomical Record* 5: 439–531.

Wedel, V. L., and Bowman, S. 2006. How to look a gift corpse in the mouth: Season at death determined by cementum increment analysis. *Proceedings of the American Academy of Forensic Sciences, 20–25 February, Seattle*. Denver, CO: American Academy of Forensic Sciences: 300.

Weitzel, M. A. 2006. Temperature variability in the burial environment. *Proceedings of the American Academy of Forensic Sciences, 20–25 February, Seattle*. Denver, CO: American Academy of Forensic Sciences: 299.

Wescott, D. J. 2006. Ontogeny of femur subtrochanteric shape: Implications for determining ancestry using the platymeric index. *Proceedings of the American Academy of Forensic Sciences, 20–25 February, Seattle*. Denver, CO: American Academy of Forensic Sciences: 283.

Wiersema, J. M. 2006. The human petrous temporal bone: Potential for forensic individuation. *Proceedings of the American Academy of Forensic Sciences, 20–25 February, Seattle*. Denver, CO: American Academy of Forensic Sciences, 274–275.

Wilder, H. H., and Wentworth, B. 1918. *Personal Identification: Methods for the Identification of Individuals, Living or Dead*. Boston: R. G. Badger.

Wilson, R. J., Bethard, J. D., and DiGangi, E. A. 2006. Orthopedic devices and the William M. Bass donated skeletal collection: Implications for forensic anthropological identification. *Proceedings of the American Academy of Forensic Sciences, 20–25 February, Seattle*. Denver, CO: American Academy of Forensic Sciences: 289–290.

FORENSIC ANTHROPOLOGY: CANADIAN CONTENT AND CONTRIBUTIONS

Mark Skinner and Kristina Bowie

"The downside is you cannot make a living in Canada in the ultra specialized field of forensic anthropology," he adds. "There just aren't enough homicides," says Dr. Melbye. . . . (Belford 2003: B11)

Despite Dr. Melbye's assertion, forensic anthropology has emerged in Canada as an increasingly important applied science at the core of societal concerns with public safety. Canadian citizens express dismay at horrendous homicides in Montreal, Toronto, and Vancouver that erode the confidence with which we can turn our children out to play. Our job as forensic anthropologists is to try to restore harmony to our society by improving the ability to prosecute criminals and to identify their victims. The point of reviewing the historical trajectory of our discipline must surely be to determine if we are doing the job.

The focus of this chapter is deliberately parochial: an evaluation of the contribution that individual Canadian forensic anthropologists have made and are currently making to death investigation. We are still a small community of scholars with local concerns but who conduct their business within an intellectual nexus shared internationally with forensic scientists facing a common problem.

In this chapter, we first define Canadian content with an emphasis on our contributions to forensic osteology and fieldwork locally and internationally. Then we identify the intellectual lineages of anatomists and biological anthropologists who chose in their careers to engage themselves and their students in specific forensic anthropological concerns with victim identification, elapsed time since death, circumstances of recent deaths, and recovering physical evidence of perpetrator behaviors. Next we examine how and to what extent legal jurisdictions have reached out to academic expertise in our communities in death investigation. We critically evaluate the content of publications by Canadians in forensic anthropology and archaeology over a span of several decades. Finally, we review centers of training in forensic anthropology as they have proliferated recently across Canada. The results of our review are mixed; Canadian contributions to forensic osteology, to the investigation of mass graves internationally, and to forensic taphonomy have been considerable and yet remain insufficiently focused on research initiatives and ongoing, core involvement at crime scenes and in the analysis of human tissues and associated evidence.

For the purposes of this chapter,[1] forensic anthropology embraces the following concerns:

1. archaeology (landscape assessment, GIS, search and recovery techniques, evidence continuity, and conservation)

2. biological anthropology, including osteology (age at death, sex, ancestry, stature, individualization), circumstances of death (tool marks, peri- and postmortem trauma, body disposal), taphonomy, time since death, archaeometry (including bone biology)

3. social anthropology: material culture and practices, human rights, law

4. molecular forensic DNA

As the discipline of forensic anthropology has matured in Canada, collaboration has increased among specialists such that reports and published articles are multiauthored and combine disciplines, making it more difficult to isolate forensic anthropology from closely allied sciences that address identification of historic individuals. For example, John Mayhall, a dental anthropologist, assisted with the DNA-based identification of a 13-month-old infant from the Titanic disaster (1912) buried in Nova Scotia, by identifying dental fragments (Titley et al. 2004). Tanya Peckmann (1998) has termed the positive identification of historical personages using customary forensic techniques "*applied* forensic osteology." Elliott Leyton's enormously influential and reissued study (2003) of the cultural settings of serial homicide, *Hunting Humans,* should remind us that there is such a thing as "cultural forensic anthropology" and that discovering new ways to find and to understand perpetrators may be more of a contribution to society than a discovery of a new way to locate buried bodies or sex the radius. However, in our opinion, such important contributions do not qualify as forensic anthropology, *sensu stricto.*

Canadian Content

To a significant degree, forensic anthropology in Canada differs from that in the United States. Fundamentally, the demand is less due to our lower crime rates. The historical emphasis in America on the determination of ancestry of victim (Ousley and Jantz 1998) and perpetrator has been less frequently relevant in our experience both in Canada and internationally, although this may change with increasing immigration. Similarly, the frequency of gunshot wounds in American forensic cases is not observed in Canada; alarmingly, this is changing with the recent flow of handguns across

our common border. Other distinctions are due to the fact that decay rates slow with higher latitudes and prolonged winters such that we observe soft-tissue tags on some bodies even after many years. Many parts of rural Canada are heavily forested with significant predators, such as coyote, cougar, and bear, who prey on and scavenge remains. Therefore, for a variety of reasons, the demands of Canadian forensic casework are somewhat different from those in the United States.

We have chosen to emphasize Canadian content rather than simply requiring that the practitioners be Canadian. Consequently, this review includes high-profile Canadian cases to which American forensic anthropologists, some of them trained in Canada, contribute their expertise. Similarly, there are several young Canadians whose first-class training in osteology has enabled them to find employment and conduct forensic casework elsewhere in the world.

To discuss forensic anthropology as solely Canadian is parochial; forensic science has no such political boundaries. Expertise is what counts, which is why some of Canada's high-profile cases have had significant input from Americans. For example, Steven Symes (Mercyhurst Archaeological Institute, Pennsylvania) was involved in the Paul Bernardo Case (1995) and in the Reynolds Case (1997), both of which required his expertise in tool-mark analysis (Steven Symes, personal communication 2001). Likewise, Jon Nordby from Final Analysis Forensics (Washington State) worked on the "parking garage homicide" for the Hamilton-Wentworth Police (Jon Nordby, personal communication 2006).

Constructing a "History" of Forensic Anthropology in Canada

The history of Canadian forensic anthropology is best addressed by identifying the intellectual lineages of teachers and students who have conducted casework and advanced the discipline through teaching, research, and publications. Finding the links to scholars in nations other than Canada is part of this enquiry. Another factor is to define which casework is relevant to the history of the discipline in Canada: casework may involve determining whether recovered bones are animal or of heritage significance (as required by law in Canada); a World War II unidentified death may now be considered merely of historical interest but most certainly was considered of immediate forensic interest by earlier generations of forensic anthropologists and still is to the Nation and victim's relatives. A current problem in Canada is the investigation of bodies of persons killed in airplane accidents up to half a century ago, whose skeletal remains are now exposed by melting snow cover, subjecting them to potential theft and disturbance. The bottom line is that, if there are people who are concerned with the personal identification of deceased individuals and the determination of how they died, no matter how long ago, and if this determination draws on forensic science, then this is forensic casework. Evaluation of ancient remains, which are protected by law in Canada, may involve "forensic" techniques, including archaeology, anthropology, and DNA analysis (Dudar, Waye, and Saunders 2003). That said, this chapter does not include discussions of routine examination of unknown ancient remains for repatriation.

Historical Foundations of Forensic Anthropology in Canada

Canada inherited the legal and scientific traditions of Europe, particularly France and the United Kingdom. Consequently, there are many cases of human remains recovered in the 19th and 20th centuries in Canada that relied on familiar techniques of identification performed by anatomists, many of whom shared the contemporary concerns of anthropology with understanding skeletal variation and ancestry. Thus, Dr. William Dunlop, educated in Edinburgh in the 1820s, provided the first identifications in forensic medicine in Ontario (Lucas 1996). Just as medically trained experts dealt with bones, police investigators—not archaeologists—dealt with graves and their contents. In another Ontario case from 1897, Detective Murray delicately re-exhumed an abortive grave intended for Emma Orr, whose remains were found interred elsewhere, and was able to find a well-preserved boot print in the compressed earth. The body in the actual grave was detected by "touch-probing" with a gentleman's walking stick (Campbell 1970). Even our modern concerns with taphonomy (see Nawrocki this volume) and scavenging are clearly nothing new. In the first years of the 20th century, wolf-scavenged remains and fragments of clothing of several children from a Native family in Saskatchewan were collected by a police officer and transported over 1,000 miles to Edmonton, where the children's father was charged with desertion (Young 1968: 75).

Alphonse Bertillon is considered the father of criminal identification. In the final decades of the 19th century, he developed an anthropometric system for recording the body segments of criminals in Paris as a remarkably successful means of identifying repeat offenders. The year 1896 saw the heyday of "Bertillonage" and the zenith of the contribution that anthropology was to make to forensic science for nearly a century. However, Bertillon's system for measuring body segments was flawed, because of lack of independence between measured body parts. This prevented the accurate multiplication of separate probabilities, a realization that prompted reliance on the newly discovered uniqueness of fingerprints as a means of identifying victims and perpetrators. Canada moved in 1897 to introduce Bertillonage into its prison systems, just as it was being abandoned elsewhere (Campbell 1970). British police introduced Bertillonage only in 1895 in a deliberately abbreviated form, substituting dactyloscopy of all ten digits. As is sadly typical of many, even recent, forensic investigations in Canada, police in the late 19th century took upon themselves the technical role of the anthropologist:

> Inspector Stark, of the local detective Department, yesterday received from Chicago a complete set of instruments to be used in the Bertillon system of recording criminals. Instruments finely made [in Paris] consist of large and small calipers for measurement of the body, head, fingers, feet, arms and ears. Inspector Stark gave a brief explanation of the workings of the system yesterday using Crown Attorney Curry as an object lesson. Mr. Curry's measurements, however, were not recorded. (Campbell 1970: 126)

Fingerprinting was adopted in Canada only in 1908 (ibid.).

The first city in North America to establish a criminalistics laboratory was Montreal in 1914. It was run by a physician, while medically trained individuals analyzed human remains (Nafte 2000). Anthropology as a distinct discipline concerned, in part, with human remains identification did not emerge in North America until the 1930s with the founding of the American Association of Physical Anthropologists (AAPA) in alliance with the American Association of Anatomists (Boaz and Spencer 1981). A charter member of AAPA was J. C. Boileau Grant from the University of Toronto, where the Grant Anatomy Collection now serves as a valuable resource in current use for osteological research with forensic relevance (Bedford et al. 1993; Kurki 2005). A request in 1921 for Grant to examine a skull found in basement construction in The Pas, Manitoba, is the earliest such request for assistance from an anatomist with anthropological interests (Albanese 2006a).

Grant was asked to examine a skeleton in 1956, alleged to be that of Tom Thomson, one of Canada's most famous northern wilderness painters, who had died under suspicious circumstances in 1917. Local friends of the artist rejected the explanation that he simply fell out of his canoe and drowned; they also averred that his body was not removed from the temporary grave on Canoe Lake in southern Ontario and that the family got the wrong body or none at all. In 1956, deliberate exhumation at Canoe Lake of a skeleton complete with an alleged bullet hole excited considerable interest. The thoughtful consideration then given to site formation processes is impressive:

> Old hazel nuts and rotted vegetation were found with the bones. Had the grave been shallower one might assume rodents had found their way to the coffin and the remains. (Sharpe 1970: 36)

The care taken in 1956 by Dr. Noble Sharpe, Medical Director of the Ontario Attorney-General's Laboratory, in showing that the skeleton was not that of Tom Thomson is impressive still today. He personally assisted with the exhumation, noting surface topography, plant cover, burial depth, artifact type, and preservation. He sifted the sand, maintained a chain of custody, and performed both a radiological examination with an expert and a differential diagnosis with a neuropathologist of the alleged bullet hole compared to surgical trephination. He also obtained opinions from Grant as to age, sex, race, height, and probable time of death and/or burial, conducted photographic superimposition, evaluated the dentition, and finally assessed burial site transformation processes.

A 1953 case in British Columbia elicited a similarly high quality of investigation involving anthropological expertise. Known as the "Babes in the Wood Case," two children's skeletons were discovered in Stanley Park (Vancouver) along with a lather's hatchet, which had been used to kill them. A sample of vegetation taken from above the bodies yielded 5 ½ years of alternating layers of deciduous leaves and pine needles, placing the deaths somewhere around 1947. These skeletons have never been identified, despite years of examination. In 1961, Mrs. Ena von Engel-Baiersdorf sculpted likenesses of the children based on the skulls in a very early example of forensic facial reproduction. She was "an artist trained in physical anthropology at the Vienna Natural History Museum" (Stainsby 1961: 59).

The Rise of Forensic Anthropology as an Academic Discipline in Canada

While specific histories of physical anthropology in Canada simply note that forensics was being done by the 1990s (Meiklejohn 1997) or do not mention it at all (Melbye and Meiklejohn 1992), the foundations for forensic casework and research were being created in Canada by the first generation of physical anthropologists. It was shortly after the Second World War that anatomy and physical anthropology were recognized to be separate and diverging disciplines with an enduring bond sustained by forensic osteology. J. C. Boileau Grant, who has been described as a physical anthropologist in all but name (Jerkic 2001), contributed significantly to the future of forensic anthropology in Canada by nurturing the osteological interests of James E. Anderson (1926–1995). Anderson became the intellectual bridge between the two disciplines. Although medically trained, receiving his degree from Toronto in 1953, Anderson became a lecturer in Anatomy in 1956 but then, significantly, was appointed in 1958 as an assistant professor of physical anthropology, Canada's first, and trained many of the prominent osteologists who currently conduct forensic work in Canada (Jerkic 2001; Melbye 1995). Anderson's *The Human Skeleton: A Manual for Archaeologists* (1969) provides particularly useful descriptions of dental morphology. Its impact on Canadian osteology can be compared to that of Don Brothwell's *Digging Up Bones* (1963), which influenced a whole generation of skeletal biologists in Britain.

In Western Canada, a second intellectual lineage of forensic anthropologists was created by the arrival of Thomas W. McKern at Simon Fraser University, British Columbia in 1971. McKern (1920–1974) received his Ph.D. from Berkeley in 1954 under the tutelage of Theodore McCown (Steele 1975) and was greatly influenced by T. Dale Stewart, with whom he wrote the classic study of skeletal age changes of identified U.S. soldiers killed in the Pacific (McKern and Stewart 1957). McKern taught Gentry Steele, a young osteologist who studied at the University of Alberta (1971–1978), where he undertook the occasional forensic case for the Medical Examiner's Office. In the late 1970s, Steele gave a workshop on forensic anthropology to the Royal Canadian Mounted Police (RCMP) in Fort Wainwright (Alaska); Steele's influence may well have prepared the ground for Owen Beattie (see below), his successor in physical anthropology at the University of Alberta.

According to Professor Steele, who took classes from McKern before he came to Canada, McKern had contacted the RCMP in British Columbia offering to undertake forensic casework, but there is no indication he had done so before his untimely death in 1974. Nevertheless, when Mark Skinner arrived in January 1976 as McKern's successor at Simon Fraser University, the local police simply expected him to provide what McKern had offered; which he did despite being completely inexperienced in the area. Significantly, a new graduate student at Simon Fraser University, Owen Beattie, soon stepped in to teach all of McKern's graduate and undergraduate classes (including osteology). Beattie harvested anatomical specimens from the University of British Columbia. These were curated by Carlos Germann and became the Germann Pubic Symphysis Collection at Simon Fraser University (subsequently studied by Nancy Lovell in 1989).[2] Professor Beattie went on to the University of Alberta to conduct enormously publicized exhumations of members of the Franklin Expedition and is routinely involved in Canadian and international forensic cases.

Forensic Anthropology: Current Practices

The modern period of forensic anthropology, according to some, begins with the creation of the Physical Anthropology Section of the American Academy of Forensic Sciences in 1972. Involved were Ellis Kerley (1924–1998) and Clyde Snow (1928–present), each of whom played key roles in making forensic anthropology international. In 1977, the American Board of Forensic Anthropology (ABFA) was created to certify Diplomates with particular expertise. Skinner was the first Canadian to become a board-certified Diplomate in 1982, followed by Jerry Melbye in 1997.

We prefer to define maturation of the discipline by the ability of the legal fraternity in Canada to call on professional expertise in forensic anthropology to support either side in an adversarial court system; that is, both the Crown and the Defense can evaluate the forensic evidence with confidence. Canadian anthropologists played a modest role in the investigation of the murder in 1984 of Christine Jessop. Guy Paul Morin was wrongfully convicted in 1992 for this crime and was exonerated only in 1995, almost ten years after he was first arrested (King 1998). In 1990, as part of the legal run-up to the trial in 1991, Kathryne Gruspier, then a doctoral candidate, appeared for the Crown; Jerry Melbye, Ph.D.,

testified for the Defense at the Preliminary Hearing while Gruspier appeared at the Trial itself on behalf of the Defense. On June 7, 2006, two doctorally qualified forensic anthropologists (Lazenby and Skinner) appeared in the Supreme Court in British Columbia to testify as expert witnesses for the Crown and for the Defense, respectively, in a high-profile serial homicide case (Robert William Pickton). As far as we are aware, these are the only two cases in Canadian legal history in which both Prosecution and Defense counsel availed themselves of expertise in forensic anthropology. In 2002, Melbye gave a paper entitled "The Rise of a New Academic Discipline in Forensic Science," which marks a disciplinary self-awareness of the vigorous growth of our activities in the preceding decade. This is discussed in the next section.

Geography and Casework

Canada is divided into ten provinces and three territories, the majority of which have a Coroner's system (see Ranson this volume). Only Alberta, Manitoba, Nova Scotia, and Newfoundland have a Medical Examiner's system. In the latter system, practitioners must be medically qualified, whereas in the former, practitioners have varied backgrounds that typically involve police work. There seems to be no logic to the varied relationships between these jurisdictional systems and forensic anthropologists. Theoretically, of course, crime scenes are the responsibility of the police (city, provincial, and national police services exist), while bodies are handled by the Coroner or Medical Examiner. In that both human remains and their surrounds usually contain evidence of circumstances of death and individuals must also be identified, there is no national consensus as to how best to involve the broad skills of the archaeologist and the anthropologist. Sad to say, in our opinion, neither the many RCMP crime labs across Canada nor the major provincial crime labs in Ontario (Centre of Forensic Science) and Quebec (Laboratoire de Sciences Judiciaires et Médecine Légale du Québec) have full-time forensic anthropologists on staff. Presumably it is even now more cost effective to involve anthropologists on an as-needed basis. With that said, the Toronto Forensic Pathology Unit of the Office of the Chief Coroner routinely provides office space and a lot of casework to a local anthropologist.

In the following section we have deliberately chosen to name Canadian forensic anthropologists and archaeologists. In so doing, we acknowledge the choice of the lone scholar to volunteer to the community his or her forensic expertise, despite little or no remuneration and with little in the way of career advancement.

For the purpose of death investigation, Alberta is divided into northern and southern territories, each of which has identified a Consultant Forensic Anthropologist to undertake cases (in Edmonton: Beattie, assisted by Pamel Mayne Correia; in Calgary: Annie Katzenberg). Even more encouraging is the situation in Nova Scotia, which, perhaps significantly, like Alberta has a Medical Examiner's system, where Tanya Peckmann has been appointed officially as the Provincial Forensic Anthropologist—Canada's first to our knowledge. Her mandated examination of all bones found in the province is conducted in the Medical Examiner's facilities. In Saskatchewan, Ernest Walker was appointed in 2000 as a supernumerary Special Constable with the RCMP and conducts all their forensic anthropological casework. In British Columbia, allocation of casework appears to be in a state of flux. Corporal Diane Cockle with the RCMP, trained as both an archaeologist and anthropologist, performed virtually all fieldwork and examination of skeletal remains in the southern part of this province from 2004 to 2006, while Richard Lazenby at University of Northern British Columbia remains extremely busy with casework in the north of British Columbia. Skinner is involved with casework internationally, while he and his graduate students receive forensic cases regularly from the Office of the Chief Coroner. Lynne Bell, now in the School of Criminology at Simon Fraser University, is part of the team helping to create a new Centre for Forensic Research (see below).

In Manitoba, Chris Meikeljohn (the University of Winnipeg) has been a Consulting Forensic Osteologist since 1980. In central Ontario, Kathy Gruspier assists the Toronto Forensic Pathology Unit, which is housed in the same complex as the Center of Forensic Science for Ontario. With the appointment of John Albanese to the University of Windsor in 2003, additional casework to that already done by Michael Spence at the University of Western Ontario is being conducted. Spence has undertaken casework since 1979, working for at least nine municipal police departments. In Northern Ontario, where a Department of Forensic Science was created in 2004, Scott Fairgrieve and Tracy Oost conduct casework. In Eastern Ontario, Jerry Cybulski and Janet Young (The Canadian Museum of Civilization, Ottawa) have conducted casework since 1974. Shelley Saunders (McMaster University) provides similar expertise in southern Ontario. Tracy Rogers, recently appointed at the University of Toronto, Mississauga, is Canada's first tenure-track professor in forensic anthropology. Clearly, Ontario has a wealth of expertise compared to the rest of Canada. A few cases have been conducted in Newfoundland by Sunny Jerkic (Memorial University). Prince Edward Island, New Brunswick, the Yukon, Northwest Territories, and Nunavut do not apparently have resident forensic anthropological expertise.

Quebec appears to be a special case. All forensic anthropological consulting is conducted by Kathy Reichs[3] (University of Northern Carolina at Charlotte). Consultation is undertaken during her periodic visits to Montreal, where she examines remains at Laboratoire de Sciences Judiciaires et de Médecine Légale du Québec.

Database of Individuals Involved in Forensic Anthropology

Potential participants in this history were asked for their curriculum vitae as well as their views on the history of forensic anthropology in Canada. They were also asked to provide names of other Canadian practitioners unknown to the authors. The total number of respondents included in this chapter is 48, including 24 in academic posts, 13 students, 4 in museum posts, and 7 in other posts (for example, working for police or intergovernmental organization). The gender ratio of this sample is 29 females:19 males.

Reported Case Loads

Only a few forensic anthropologists routinely report the size and nature of their casework as part of their professional practice[4] in papers, publications, or on their CVs. Some practitioners (for example, Skinner) report every consultation, including nonhuman animal bones and heritage cases and, as well, differentiate recent human cases by manner of death, while others consider that only recent human cases need be counted. Consequently, one suspects that the case loads reported in Table 8.1 are not truly comparable. Note that Table 8.1 does not include mass grave work yet does include forensic entomology.

As unreliable as these numbers may be, it is clear that there are two centers of activity in Canada: Ontario and the West. Ontario has its own provincial police force and contains the Center of Forensic Science. Two factors may explain the large amount of casework in B.C. and Alberta: the legacy of Tom McKern, who directly or indirectly influenced Beattie and Skinner; also, major policing in the Western provinces is done by our national police force (RCMP). The Canadian respondents to our enquiry report working on some 1,872 cases, of which about one-third relate to recent bodies. How significant are these numbers? In 1996, Beattie reported that less than 2% of Medical Examiner cases in Alberta involved the assistance of a forensic anthropologist. In 2000, Gruspier observed that, for the period 1974 to 1998, anthropological cases at the Toronto Forensic Pathology Unit represented between 1.3% and 3% of autopsies (Gruspier and Chiasson 2000: 2). These authors remark that "the actual number of anthropological cases being done by an anthropologist in the office is approximately one-third of the 20 to 40 cases which come in per year" (ibid.); in other words, pathologists and odontologists are contributing their expertise to cases that could also include an anthropologist. Interestingly, there is no trend at the Toronto Forensic Pathology Unit for an increase in the number of anthropological cases for the period

Table 8.1 Domestic casework (as of June 1, 2006).

Name	Job	Total/Comments
Albanese	academic	occasional
Beattie	academic	236 + 13 court appearances
Cockle	police/student	89 (60 nonhuman, 15 heritage, 4 acc/suic, 10 homi)
Curtin*	academic (USA)	sporadic over 22 years, 9 in last 3 years
Cybulski	museum	105 + 2 court appearances
Dupras*	academic (USA)	25
Fairgrieve	academic	76 + 4 court appearances
Gruspier	professional consultant	>477 (+ 10 court appearances)
Heathcote*	academic (USA)	4
Hillier	student	2 homicide excavations
Jerkic	academic	23
Katzenberg	academic	43
Komar	academic (USA)	12 + 3 court appearances (242 + 9 in U.S.A.)
Lazenby	academic	>50 (31 human, 8 homicides) + 1 court appearance
Meiklejohn	academic	144
Melbye	academic (Can/USA)	69 (Katzmarzyk 2001)
Oost	academic	10 (many entomological)
Peckman	academic	>20
Pietrusewsky*	academic (USA)	30
Rogers	academic	68 + 4 court appearances
Saunders	academic	"3–4 per year since the late 1980s"
Skinner	academic	358 (144 forensic, 56 homicides) + 13 court appearances
Spence	academic	65 (24 recent, 20 in field) + 3 court appearances
Stratton	academic	21
Wilson	academic	4

*Canada-trained but not resident

1974 to 1998; this is unlike the general tendency, Canada-wide, for anthropological casework to have increased dramatically over the past decades (see below). This subject needs better evaluation.

In addition, many Canadian forensic anthropologists work internationally, typically on mass graves or mass disasters. It is difficult to assess the exact number of cases undertaken by single practitioners,

because bodies are typically processed by teams. Nevertheless, Table 8.2 gives some indication of the scale of Canadian involvement in other countries.

Clearly, most of the Canadian contribution to fieldwork in mass disasters and mass graves internationally is being done by such students and young professionals as Congram, Gruspier, Katzmarzyk, and Mundorff rather than tenured faculty staff.

Table 8.2 International casework.

Name	Job	Operational Theatre(s)	Notes
Bassendale	ICMP[1]	Bosnia	student at Lukavac
Beattie	mostly PHR[2]	Cyprus, Somalia, Rwanda, Abkhazia/Georgia	
Cockle	RCMP	Thailand Tsunami	
Congram	ICTY, RCLO	Bosnia, Croatia, Iraq, Kosovo, Costa Rica	professional and student
Fernandez	ICTY,[3] ICMP, UNV[4]	Bosnia, East Timor	court appearance
Gruspier	ICTY, UNTAET[5]	Kosovo, East Timor, Cambodia	anthropologist
Katzmarzyk	ICTY, OMPF,[6] ICMP	Bosnia	Manager Lukavac
Komar	ICTY, ICMP, PHR, RCLO[7]	Bosnia, Kosovo, Iraq	
Kosalka	ICMP, Kenyon[8]	Thailand, WTC, Bosnia	student
Lazenby	consultant	Guatemala	initiating field school
Melbye	UN Review Panel		ICTY investigations
Mundorff	OCME-NYC[9]	WTC, Thailand	professional and student
Prevost	ICMP	Bosnia	student at Lukavac
Scott	Kenyon	WTC, New Orleans	student
Skinner	PHR, ICMP	Afghanistan, Bosnia, East Timor, Serbia	seconded to UNHCHR, UNTAET
Skinner, Matt	UNV	East Timor	student
Stratton	PHR	Cyprus	student then

1. International Commission on Missing Persons (Lukavac Re-association Center)
2. Physicians for Human Rights
3. International Criminal Tribunal for the former Yugoslavia
4. United Nations Volunteer
5. United Nations Transitional Administration in East Timor
6. Office of Missing Persons and Forensics, United Nations Mission in Kosovo
7. Regional Crimes Liaison Office, Iraq
8. Office of the Chief Medical Examiner, New York City
9. Kenyon International Emergency Services—disaster response

Temporal Trends in Academic Communication

Our first task was to define Canadian content. Besides students and faculty who work in Canada, we include those Canadians working abroad on a permanent or part-time basis and foreign academics trained or training in Canada. The period under consideration includes 30 years, commencing in 1978 with the first publications on forensic science by a Canadian anthropologist (Michael Wilson) and includes items in press as of June 1, 2006. Publications include peer- and non-peer-reviewed items as well as reports to such major agencies as ICTY, PHR, and ICMP but exclude book reviews. A copy of *Bibliography of Canadian Content Publications in Forensic Anthropology* containing some 160 citations is located at www.sfu.ca/archaeology/dept/fac_bio/skinner/index.htm. We also consider "presentations," which include all communications ranging from formal symposium lectures to talks to lay audiences. In both publications and presentations, we sought temporal trends in the proportion of forensic communications relative to nonforensic.

The number of publications (as defined above) per year is shown in Figure 8.1. Excluding those "in press," in the first 20 years up to 1997, 54 publications appeared—a rate of 2.7 per year. In the following nine years up to 2006, 93 publications appeared—a rate of 10.3 per year. Thus, in the latter third of the review period, the rate of forensic publications in Canada increased by 280%. This sounds encouraging for the discipline. However, comparing the number of respondents who supplied CVs (48) with the total number of publications judged to be forensic in content (ca. 147), the average number of publications in forensic anthropology (*sensu lato*) per individual career is only three. Interestingly, during the same two time periods, the average number of different authors/publication in any one year barely changed from 1.56 to 1.62, suggesting no dramatic increase in team efforts. However, note that, in 2006, the ratio of multiauthored publications peaked, indicating the recent replacement of lone efforts with teams of death investigators including anthropologists. Another factor must be the occurrence of large-scale investigations of mass graves confronted by such organizations as Physicians for Human Rights under the direction of William Haglund, who purposefully involved internationals including Canadians, and the effects of the World Trade Center disaster, which, perforce, involved large numbers of various investigators.

Clearly, however, relatively few practitioners listed in Table 8.1 publish their extensive experience, to the detriment of the discipline both in casework and theoretical developments. One must recognize, however, that those whose work has been conducted under the aegis of international criminal courts may be prevented by confidentiality

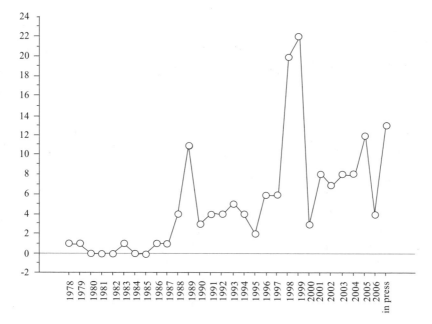

Figure 8.1 Publications with forensic content per year.

agreements from publishing detailed accounts of their findings.

We also examined the ratio of specifically forensic presentations and publications to an author's general productivity. In both cases, about 40% relate to forensic anthropology. It can be concluded that, as we saw above in the low average number of career publications in forensic anthropology, for most Canadian biological anthropologists who report any forensic involvement, forensic anthropology remains, if not a sideline, their subordinate calling. Those scholars whose publications are in forensics more often than not include John Albanese, Scott Fairgrieve, Debra Komar, Amy Mundorff, and Tracy Rogers, individuals who have chosen early in their careers to specialize in forensic anthropology.

Characterizing the Recent History of Forensic Anthropology in Canada

History will decide what efforts and which publications by Canadians were most significant for the discipline in the long run. It was teasingly remarked that when, in the 1980s, it became politically difficult in Canada to excavate First Nations' skeletal remains, Jerry Melbye cannily shifted to forensic anthropology (Knight 2006). But, as noted below, Melbye was already teaching forensics at the beginning of the decade. The major historical change in reported casework was the deployment of Canadians into foreign locales, mostly in the late 1990s.

Forensic Archaeology

Major publications in forensic archaeology include those by Skinner and Lazenby (1983) and Skinner (1987). Although field practices internationally may have been positively affected by these efforts (Luis Fondebrider and Jon Sterenberg, personal communication 2006), there is disappointingly little published evidence that forensic archaeology has increased in Canada apart from sporadic cases undertaken by Skinner and Michael Spence (University of Western Ontario). The latter archaeologist has conducted 13 field recoveries of bodies and recent skeletons with surviving soft tissue (Michael Spence, personal communication 2007), indicating local acceptance of his expertise. More encouraging is the recent appearance of the first Canadian article on remote sensing of mass graves by means of spectral analysis (Kalascka and Bell 2006) and the first book specifically on forensic archaeology (Dupras et al. 2006), which, given its American debut, may have a higher visibility and

influence. "Archaeology" is said to have been performed on the Pickton "pig farm" crime scene in British Columbia in 2002–2004 (Girard 2002), but a full account has yet to be published. The much-publicized use of conveyor belts at this scene was introduced much earlier at the dreadful Hinton Train Collision in 1986 (Stratton and Beattie 1999). Indeed, conveyor belts were also utilized at Ground Zero in New York City 2001. Another indication that, at least in foreign locales, forensic archaeology is becoming more commonplace than it is in Canada, is shown by Skinner's coauthored publications on guidelines for bioarchaeological monitors of mass grave investigations (2003), on how to allocate different kinds of forensic scientists at mass graves (Skinner and Sterenberg 2005), and a proposed typology of mass graves (Jessee and Skinner 2005).

Forensic Anthropology

A valiant but rather strained effort by Skinner (1988) to apply joint probability theory to skeletal identification has been completely obviated, one notes thankfully, by DNA-based identifications. Our inability to estimate elapsed time since death with any precision prompted us to promote forensic entomology at sites involving skeletons (Skinner et al. 1988); this is now routine in Canada thanks to the exemplary efforts of Gail Anderson and her students (reviewed in Anderson 2001). A review of research published from 1989 to 1996 reveals a number of routine articles on skeletal biology applied in a forensic context relieved only by the first articles on diagenetic changes at the histological level (Bell et al. 1993; Bell, Skinner, and Jones 1996). This period in Canadian forensic anthropology clearly fits within Kuhn's descriptions of scientists' efforts in the midst of a prevailing paradigm:

> Mopping up operations are what engage most scientists throughout their careers. They constitute what I am calling here "normal science." (Kuhn 1977: 24)

In 1997, things began to change. The impending revolution in identification methodology based on replication of biomolecules from bones was introduced to Canadian forensic anthropology by Yang and associates' (1997) important article on the removal of polymerase chain reaction (PCR) inhibitors. The very influential book on forensic taphonomy by Haglund and Sorg appeared in the same year; as we already noted, Haglund was instrumental in assisting several Canadian forensic anthropologists into international work at that time. Not coincidentally, a series of articles by Debra Komar and Owen Beattie appeared around this time describing their field simulations of taphonomic processes at the Ellerslie Research Facility, University of Alberta Farms, Edmonton, Alberta (Komar 1999; Komar and Beattie 1998a, 1998b). A similarly important work by Kathy Reichs, who had started to work on Quebec cases, appeared in 1998. Scott Fairgrieve, drawing on his commitment to forensic casework and teaching at Laurentian University, brought out a book of case studies in 1999, authored largely by Canadians, which showed for the first time the breadth of high-quality work being conducted in Canada.

A new means of tracking individual migration life history from detailed histological bone chemistry analysis was introduced in 2001 by Bell and coworkers. A new work on forensic taphonomy appeared in 2002, edited by Haglund and Sorg, that contained two articles by Canadians. So pervasive was the influence of this volume that, in Serbia at least, the phrase "forensic taphonomy" was substituted by interpreters for "forensic archaeology"—a compliment to the editors that seemed disrespectful to correct.

At this time, bodies of Kosovar Albanians buried in Serbia, including the suburbs of Belgrade,

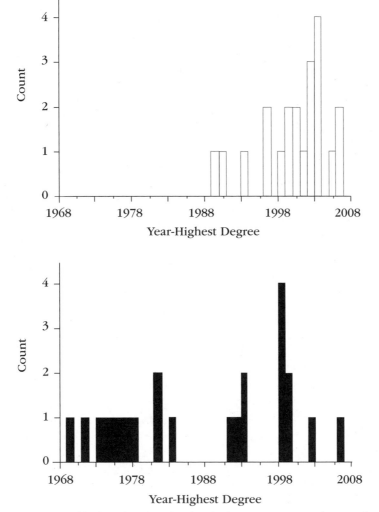

Figure 8.2 Thesis topic of highest degree undertaken by forensic practitioner by year: forensic above, nonforensic below (see text for further details).

began to be exhumed, as described in several ICMP monitor's reports written by Skinner (e.g., 2001). The ensuing years saw the publication of many articles and reports written about mass graves and mass disasters, including the World Trade Center and the 2004 Boxing Day Tsunami (Cockle, Andrews, and Thompson 2005). Fieldwork, concentrating on innovative archaeological techniques, was described in Skinner, Alempijevic, and Djuric-Srejic (2003) and in a series of articles in 2003 by Mundorff and Steadmen and in 2004 by Cockle, Andrews, and Thompson (2005). Noteworthy at this time is Debra Komar's critical review (2003) of success in reconstructions of age at death, sex, and stature of victims from Srebrenica, Bosnia, and Herzegovina conducted by anthropologists and pathologists drawn from a variety of countries. The results were properly sobering. Several articles by Tracy Rogers (2004) and Rogers and Allard (2004) signaled her appointment to the University of Toronto in 2001. Marking the shift from classical to DNA-based identifications, including cold cases, are recent articles by Torwalt and associates (2005) and Katzenberg and colleagues (2005).

Standards and Professionalism

Apart from noting the dramatic increase in peer-reviewed and other publications in recent years in forensic anthropology, another way to examine the increasing professionalism of forensic anthropological practitioners is to examine thesis topics of the highest degree (usually Ph.D.) over time to see whether the practitioner specialized in forensics as a student. The results are shown in Figure 8.2 (p. 97).

In 1989, Sabine Stratton produced the first thesis (Masters level) in Canada with a specific forensic content. The first Canadian doctorate in forensic anthropology was awarded to Debra Komar in 1999; notably, both of these were at the University of Alberta. Most forensic theses among our respondents are at Masters level, and the majority of these have been awarded outside Canada.

As current Chair of the Anthropology-Medical-Odontology Section (AMO) (created in 1995) of the Canadian Society of Forensic Science, Jerry Cybulski reports that currently there are 95 AMO members, including 16 anthropologists. Four others belong to the Medical Section for unclear reasons (Jerry Cybulski, personal communication 2007).

Training Opportunities in Canada

Jerry Melbye introduced the first course in forensic anthropology in 1981 at the University of Toronto, followed in 1983 by Mark Skinner, who introduced a course at Simon Fraser University. This course coincided with the publication of the field text for police officers, *Found! Human Remains* (Skinner and Lazenby 1983), which has been used in many course offerings across Canada.

There are dozens of undergraduate students and a handful of graduate students currently enrolled in programs across Canada. Individual courses and/or Minors in forensic anthropology are offered at times in a number of Canadian institutions (Table 8.3). Larger programs that emphasize

Table 8.3 Some of the Canadian institutions offering individual courses and/or minors in forensic anthropology.

Province	University/Other
Newfoundland	Memorial
New Brunswick	St. Thomas—offers a Minor
Ontario	Lakehead—several courses McMaster Trent Ontario: Institute of Technology
Manitoba	Manitoba
Saskatchewan	Saskatchewan (plus a 5-day noncredit course)
British Columbia	Simon Fraser Victoria

Table 8.4 Larger programs in forensic anthropology offered in Canada.

Province	Comment about Courses in Forensic Anthropology
Nova Scotia	In about 1996, Paul Erickson (Saint Mary's University) introduced basic courses in forensic anthropology. This resulted in 2000 in a formal agreement with the RCMP to offer a stand-alone Forensic Sciences Diploma Program. In 2001, 25 students enrolled (University Affairs January 2001: 7).
Ontario	The University of Toronto has led the way in teaching forensic anthropology. In 1997 Jerry Melbye created a B.Sc. Program in Forensic Science at Mississauga. Tracy Rogers succeeded him in 2001. Under her direction, University of Toronto Mississauga (UTM) has one of the most complete undergraduate forensic anthropology streams in Canada, with an introductory course, a field school emphasizing forensic archaeology, and a full-year case-based class that culminates in a mock trial under the cross-examination of an Ontario Crown Attorney. They also offer a course in the use of demonstrative aids for the presentation of expert testimony in collaboration with Biomedical Communications. Dr. Rogers has been involved in the development of a graduate forensic science program at UTM, which will give students the option of completing a Masters in either Anthropology or Forensic Science, depending on their inclination and long-term goals. She is one of the few people in Canada who teaches forensic anthropology at the graduate level, supervising graduate research in this field (Tracy Rogers personal communication).
	University of Windsor offers field and lab courses in forensic anthropology and forensic science.
	Laurentian University has an entire Department of Forensic Science, directed by a forensic anthropologist Scott Fairgrieve. Scott writes: "Yesterday (01/06/06) we just graduated our first class of the new Hons. B.Sc. in Forensic Science at Laurentian University. There were 12 students graduating with this degree in areas including Forensic Anthropology, Forensic Analytical Chemistry and Instrumentation, Forensic Psychology, and, as a single specialization, Forensic Science" (Scott Fairgrieve personal communication)
British Columbia	Simon Fraser University Centre for Forensic Research—Simon Fraser University has been a leader in the field of forensic science since the 1970s and was one of the first universities in North America to offer forensic entomology, biological anthropology, and forensic archaeology as a service to the police community. Graduate training at the Master's and Doctorate level is offered. Since this time, Simon Fraser University has been at the forefront of research in these areas and is now developing a Centre for Forensic Research (CFR). The current level of investment in the Centre itself is about $3.5 million and includes imaging suites, several secure laboratories to process entomological and biological materials safely, and the recent hiring of two new faculty. Opened in the fall of 2007, the Centre bridges the Departments of Archaeology and School of Criminology and will act as a nucleus for the expansion of research in Forensics between these two departments and others within Simon Fraser University, including botany and molecular biology. The Centre routinely accepts casework but is designed to enhance research capability in these forensic sciences.

forensic anthropology, often within a forensic science focus, are also available (Table 8.4).

Conclusion

Despite Jerry Melbye's lament at the beginning of this work, there do appear to be many people doing a great deal of forensic anthropology in Canada. It is not all homicides, and it is not all in Canada. Large-scale operations in foreign locales are now dominating expansion of the field in terms of training and publications. Some of our graduates are finding employment in Firearms and Tool Mark Examiners sections of Canada's provincial and federal crime labs. An emerging career strategy is for completed Masters degree students to work professionally for several years before returning to academe.

The core role of forensic anthropology as an applied science is to identify individuals from detailed knowledge of skeletal anatomy, which can yield reliable indications of age, sex, ancestry, and stature. Such knowledge provides a guide to more reliable means of identification based on such antemortem data as dental and medical records. All such methods have now been surpassed by the enormously more accurate means of DNA-based identifications. Recourse to this method has been routine for about a decade, and one might expect the practice of forensic anthropology to have visibly withered during this time; but, as we have seen, quite the contrary situation is occurring. How can this be? Apart from the increasing numbers of articles, practitioners, and new Ph.D. graduates trained specifically in forensic anthropology, the discipline of forensic anthropology is broadening considerably. How does a science grow? As Kuhn (1977) has shown, one way is to introduce a whole new manner of doing or seeing things. A three-pronged paradigm shift has resulted from (1) the justly famous PCR amplification of remnant degraded DNA (see Baker this volume); (2) society's realization that locked in the organic content of our bones and teeth is a unique biochemical record of a person; and (3) even in the absence of objects bearing one's DNA (for example, toothbrushes, cervical smears), there is potentially a complete copy of our DNA shared among close biological relatives. This revolution in identification methodology is implemented on an impressive scale by the International Commission on Missing Persons, which has employed a surprising number of Canadian students both in the excavation and antemortem-postmortem review phases.

Besides noting paradigm shifts, this chapter makes clear that forensic anthropologists are redefining their roles and their discipline to keep it vibrant and relevant. One way has been by broadening scales of inquiry. This is evidenced, on the one hand, by Bell and associates' analyses of stable isotopes of bone packages within osteons (2001) and Skinner's study of variation in location of the neonatal line in dental enamel as a function of gestation length (1993) and, on the other hand, by GIS-based and spectral analyses of remotely sensed images to detect mass graves (Kalascka and Bell 2006). Typically, in the variety of cases worked on by forensic anthropologists, much time

elapses between death and discovery. The intervening time creates numerous opportunities for natural postmortem processes such as scavenging, transport, burial, decay, and discovery to affect skeletal integrity, requiring a differential diagnosis to distinguish with confidence relevant and irrelevant aspects of altered bone. Taphonomic studies as undertaken by Komar and Beattie (1998a, b, c) and Komar (1999) are important enrichments of the discipline.

One obvious way to enhance the discipline is to add international casework to domestic. Functionally, most established academic practitioners stay home and students go abroad. At least one professional forensic archaeologist (Congram) has worked internationally for several years before returning to graduate studies. Another way is to broaden our anthropological purview to include human rights issues—for example, Blau and Skinner's deliberate advocacy (2005) to investigate a neglected mass grave in East Timor. Few anthropologists consult for the Defense.[5]

The question posed at the beginning of this review asked "does the historical trajectory of the discipline demand deliberate intervention for the good of the subject?" One answer is "yes!" Despite the enthusiasm and inventiveness of its practitioners, forensic anthropology in Canada has some problems. Forensic anthropologists are still not integrated into crime labs, and their involvement is piecemeal and ad hoc. Some provinces have no local expertise, whereas others bestow titles, such as Consulting Forensic Osteologist, but provide little casework. There are almost no published accounts of the application of forensic archaeology to actual cases in Canada. With the recent exception of a report by John Albanese (2006b) to the Department of National Defence, there is virtually no link between the Canadian military and academic forensic anthropology. This situation stifles the scope for research and practice on large-scale problems such as international investigations of war crimes. Skeletal and artifactual collections of forensic materials are tiny or lacking completely in most teaching institutions. Defense counsels seem largely unaware of our expertise. Our contributions to scholarly research are too focused on casework. Moreover, the failure of many of us to publish, whether because of workload, confidentiality clauses, or sloth, is surely one cause.

Our successes center on excellence in casework and court testimony, our international involvement, and the successful deployment of our students into academic and applied posts in Canada and abroad. Fundamentally, we still face the task of changing the perception by the public and by death investigators of our role. We should be much more involved as senior managers in crime scenes and field investigation including mass disasters. We should be much more involved in cases involving fresh bodies and soft tissue. We should be seen as first responders.

Notes

1. Our chapter is based on curricula vitae received by June 2006 and should be viewed as a work in progress.

2. Skinner recalls that only Owen, who had been taught how to use the McKern-Stewart symphyseal phase casts by McKern himself, felt competent in their usage; Skinner certainly did not.

3. Kathy Reichs is also an accomplished novelist specializing in forensic mysteries.

4. The two Canadians (Skinner at Simon Fraser University and Melbye, now at the University of Texas) are Diplomates of the American Board of Forensic Anthropology and thus required to submit annual tallies of casework.

5. To date, only Gruspier and Skinner are known to have done so.

References

Albanese, J. 2006a. The Grant Human Skeletal Collection and Other Contributions of J. C. B Grant to Anthropology. www.uwindsor.ca/users/a/albanese/Main.nsf/inToc/10FF8B04FF3A317885256D88005720F6.

———. 2006b. Options for Forensic Identification of Military Personnel and Civilian Employees of the Department of National Defence, Canada. Prepared for the Department of National Defence, Canada.

Anderson, G. 2001. Forensic entomology in British Columbia: A brief history. *Journal Entomological Society of British Columbia* 98: 127–135.

Anderson, J. 1969. *The Human Skeleton: A Manual for Archaeologists*. Ottawa: National Museum of Man.

Bedford, M. E, Russel, K. F, Lovejoy, C. O, Meindl, R. S., Simpson, S. W., and Stuart-Macadam, P. L. 1993. Test of the multifactorial aging method using skeletons with known ages at death from the Grant Collection. *American Journal of Physical Anthropology* 91: 287–297.

Belford, T. 2003. Forensic science gains cachet. *The Globe and Mail*. July 14: B11.

Bell, L. S., Cox, G., and Sealy, J. C. 2001. Determining life history trajectories using bone density fractionation and stable light isotope analysis:

A new approach. *American Journal of Physical Anthropology* 116: 66–79.

Bell, L. S., Skinner, M. F., and Jones, S. J. 1996. The speed of postmortem change to the human skeleton and its taphonomic significance. *Forensic Science International* 82: 129–140.

Bell, L. S., Wong, F. S., Elliot, J. C., Boyde, A., and Jones, S. J. 1993. Postmortem changes in buried human bone. *Journal of Anatomy* 183: 196.

Blau, S., and Skinner, M. F. 2005. The use of forensic archaeology in the investigation of human rights abuse: Unearthing the past in East Timor. *The International Journal of Human Rights* 9(4): 449–463.

Boaz, N., and Spencer, F. 1981. Introduction. *American Journal of Physical Anthropology* 56: 327–334.

Brothwell, D. R. 1963. *Digging Up Bones: The Excavation, Treatment and Study of Human Skeletal Remains*. London: British Museum.

Campbell, M. F. 1970. *A Century of Crime: The Development of Crime Detection Methods in Canada*. Toronto: McLelland and Stewart.

Cockle, D., Andrews, B., and Thompson, D. 2005. Tsunami Thailand Disaster Victim Identification, RCMP mission January 2005. *Identification Canada* 28(3): 4–15.

Dudar, J. C., Waye, J. S., and Saunders, S. R. 2003. Determination of a kinship system using ancient DNA, mortuary practice, and historic records in an Upper Canadian pioneer cemetery. *International Journal of Osteoarchaeology* 13: 232–246.

Dupras, T. L., Schultz, J. J., Wheeler, S. M., and Williams, L. J. 2006. *Forensic Recovery of Human Remains: Archaeological Approaches*. Boca Raton, FL: CRC Press.

Fairgrieve, S. I. (ed.) 1999. *Forensic Osteological Analysis: A Book of Case Studies*. Springfield, IL: Charles C. Thomas.

Girard, D. 2002. Vancouver Eastside missing women—Digging for evidence at B.C.'s notorious pig farm: Archaeologists sift through the debris of an alleged serial killer. *thestar.com*. www.missingpeople.net/digging_for_evidence_at_b.htm (accessed 7/24/2008).

Gruspier, K. L., and Chiasson, D. A. 2000. 25 Years of forensic anthropology in the Forensic Pathology Unit, Office of the Chief Coroner for Ontario, Toronto. Presented at the 52nd *Annual Meeting of the American Academy of Forensic Sciences*, Reno, Nevada.

Haglund, W. D., and Sorg, M. H. (eds.). 1997. *Forensic Taphonomy: The Postmortem Fate of Human Remains*, Boca Raton, FL: CRC Press.

——— (eds.). 2002. *Advances in Forensic Taphonomy: Method, Theory, and Archaeological Perspectives*. Boca Raton, FL: CRC Press.

Jerkic, S. M. 2001. The influence of James E. Anderson on Canadian physical anthropology, in L. Sawchuck and S. Pfeiffer (eds.), *Out of the Past: The History of Human Osteology at the University of Toronto*, pp. 1–8. Toronto: University of Toronto.

Jesse, E., and Skinner, M. F. 2005. A typology of mass graves and mass-grave related sites. *Forensic Science International* 152(1): 55–59.

Kalascka, M., and Bell, L. S. 2006. Remote sensing as a tool for the detection of clandestine mass graves. *Canadian Society of Forensic Science Journal* 39: 1–13.

Katzenberg, M. A., Oetelaar, G., Oetelaar, J., FitzGerald, C., Yang, D., and Saunders, S. R. 2005. Identification of historical human skeletal remains: A case study using skeletal and dental age, history and DNA. *International Journal of Osteoarchaeology* 15(1): 61–72.

Katzmarzyk, C. 2001. The academic career of Dr. Jerry Melbye, in L. Sawchuk and S. Pfeiffer (eds.), *Out of the Past: The History of Human Osteology at the University of Toronto*: CITD Press (http://citdpress.utsc.utoronto.ca/osteology/Katzmarzyk.html).

King, J. 1998. The ordeal of Guy Paul Morin: Canada copes with systemic injustice. *Champion Magazine*. National Association of Criminal DefenseLawyers.www.nacdl.org/public.nsf/championarticles/19980808?opendocument (accessed 7/24/2008).

Knight, D. 2006. A tribute to Dr. Jerry Melbye. http://uweb.txstate.edu/~fm14/tributes/Dean_Knight.htm?00339d58 (accessed 7/24/2008).

Komar, D. 1999a. Forensic Taphonomy of a Cold Climate Region: A Field Study in Central Alberta and a Potential New Method of Determining Time Since Death. Doctoral thesis, University of Alberta.

———. 1999b. The use of cadaver air scent detection dogs in locating scattered, scavenged human remains: Preliminary field test results. *Journal of Forensic Sciences* 44(2): 405–408.

———. 2003. Lessons from Srebrenica: The contributions and limitations of physical anthropology in identifying victims of war crimes. *Journal of Forensic Sciences* 48(4): 713–716.

Komar, D., and Beattie, O. 1998a. Postmortem insect activity may mimic perimortem sexual assault clothing patterns. *Journal of Forensic Sciences* 43(4): 792–796.

———. 1998b. Identifying bird scavenging in fleshed and dry remains. *Canadian Society of Forensic Science Journal* 31(3): 177–188.

———. 1998c. Effects of carcass size on decomposition rates of sun and shade exposed carrion. *Canadian Society of Forensic Science Journal* 31(1): 35–43.

Kuhn, T. S. 1977. *The Essential Tension: Selected Studies in Scientific Tradition and Change*. Chicago: University of Chicago Press.

Kurki, H. 2005. Use of the first rib for adult age estimation: A test of one method. *International Journal of Osteoarchaeology* 15: 342–350.

Leyton, E. 2003. *Hunting Humans: The Rise of the Modern Multiple Murderer* (2nd ed.). New York: Carroll and Graf.

Lovell, N. C. 1989. Test of Phenice's technique for determining sex from the os pubis. *American Journal of Physical Anthropology* 79(1): 117–120.

Lucas, D. 1996. *Lab Guide for the Investigator*. The Center of Forensic Sciences. Northern Ontario, Canada.

McKern, T., and Stewart, T. D. 1957. *Skeletal Age Changes in Young American Males, Analyzed from the Standpoint of Age Identification*. Technical Report EP-45, Environmental Protection Research Division, Quartermaster Research and Development Center, U.S. Army, Natick, Massachusetts.

Meiklejohn, C. 1997. Canada, in F. Spencer (ed.), *History of Physical Anthropology: An Encyclopedia*, pp. 245–250. New York: Garland.

Melbye, J. 1995. Dr. James E. Anderson (obituary). *The Connective Tissue* 11: 11.

Melbye, J., and Meiklejohn, C. 1992. A history of physical anthropology and the development of evolutionary thought in Canada. *Human Evolution* 4(3): 49–55.

Mundorff, A. Z. 2004. Identification issues: The World Trade Center experience, in Capstone Document: *Mass Fatality Management of Incidents Involving Weapons of Mass Destruction. Prepared by U.S. Army Soldier and Biological Chemical Command, Military Improved Response Program and the Department of Justice, Office of Justice Programs, Office for Domestic Preparedness*: 35 (U.S. government document).

Mundorff, A. Z., and Steadman, D. W. 2003. Anthropological perspectives on the forensic response at the World Trade Center disaster. *General Anthropology* 10(1): 2–5.

Nafte, M. 2000. *Flesh and Bone: An Introduction to Forensic Anthropology*. Durham, NC: Carolina Academic Press.

Ousley, S. D., and Jantz, R. L. 1998. The forensic data bank: Documenting skeletal trends in the United States, in K. J. Reichs (ed.), *Forensic Osteology* (2nd ed.), pp. 441–458 Springfield, IL: Charles C. Thomas.

Peckmann, T. 1998. *Burials from an Historic Hudson Bay Cemetery at Fort Frances, Ontario: A Case Study in Applied Forensic Osteology*, Ontario Ministry of Citizenship, Culture and Recreation Conservation Archaeology Report, Northwestern Region Report, #17.

Reichs, K. J. (ed.). 1998. *Forensic Osteology: Advances in the Identification of Human Remains* (2nd ed.). Springfield, IL: Charles C. Thomas.

Rogers, T. L. 2004a. Recognizing inter-personal violence: A forensic perspective, in M. Roksandic (ed.), *Violent Interactions in the Mesolithic: Evidence and Meaning*, pp. 9–21, British Archaeological Reports.

———. 2004b. Crime scene ethics: Souvenirs, teaching material, and artifacts. *Journal of Forensic Sciences* 49(2): 307–311.

Rogers, T. L, and. Allard, T. T. 2004. Expert testimony and positive identification of human remains through cranial suture patterns. *Journal of Forensic Sciences* 49(2): 203–207.

Sharpe, N. 1970. The Canoe Lake mystery. *Canadian Society of Forensic Science Journal* 3(2): 34–40.

Skinner, M. F. 1987. Planning the archaeological recovery of evidence from recent mass graves. *Forensic Science International* 34: 267–287.

———. 1988. Method and theory in deciding identity of skeletonized human remains. *Canadian Society of Forensic Science Journal* 21: 114–134.

———. 2001. *Petrovo Selo Exhumations, Federal Republic of Yugoslavia*. ICMP Observers Report. International Commission on Missing Persons Forensic Program.

Skinner, M. F., Alempijevic, D., and Djuric-Srejic, M. 2003. Guidelines for international forensic bioarchaeology monitors of mass grave exhumations. *Forensic Science International* 134: 81–92.

Skinner, M. F., and Dupras, T. 1993. Variation in birth timing and location of the neonatal line in human enamel. *Journal of Forensic Sciences* 38: 1379–1386.

Skinner, M. F., and Lazenby, R. A. 1983. *Found! Human Remains: A Field Manual for the Recovery of the Recent Human Skeleton*. Burnaby, B.C.: SFU Archaeology Press.

Skinner, M. F., and Sterenberg, J. 2005. Turf wars: Authority and responsibility for the investigation of mass graves. *Forensic Science International* 151: 221–232.

Skinner, M. F., Syed, A., Farrel, J., and Borden, J. H. 1988. Non-human animal and insect factors in decomposition of a homicide victim. *Canadian Society of Forensic Science Journal* 21: 71–81.

Stainsby, D. 1961. Mystery of the "Babes in the Wood" murder. *Weekend Magazine* 11(40): 4.

Steele, D. G. 1975. Thomas W. McKern (Obituary). *American Journal of Physical Anthropology* 43: 160–164.

Stratton, S. U. 1989. Forensic Implications of Acetabular Morphological Variation. Masters thesis. University of Alberta.

Stratton, S. U., and Beattie, O. B. 1999. Mass disasters: Comments and discussion regarding the Hinton Train Collision of 1986, in S. I. Fairgrieve (ed.), *Forensic Osteological Analysis: Case Studies in Forensic Anthropology*, pp. 267–286. Springfield, IL: Charles C. Thomas.

Titley, K. C., Pynn, B. R., Chernecky, R., Mayhall, J. T., Kulkarni, G. V., and Ruffman, A. 2004. The Titanic disaster: Dentistry's role in the identification of an "unknown child." *Journal of the Canadian Dental Association* 70(1): 24–28.

Torwalt, C., Murga, K., Epp, J., Balachandra, A. T., Daoudi, Y., Lee, D. A., and Smith, B. C. 2005. Cervical smears as an alternative source of DNA in the identification of human skeletal remains. *Canadian Society of Forensic Science Journal* 38(3): 165–169.

Yang, D. Y., Eng, B., Dudar, J. C., Saunders, S. R., and Waye, J. S. 1997. Removal of PCR inhibitors using silica-based spin columns: Application to ancient bone. *Canadian Society for Forensic Sciences Journal* 30: 1–5.

Young, D. A. 1968. *The Mounties*. Toronto: Hodder and Stoughton.

9

THE DEVELOPMENT AND CURRENT STATE OF FORENSIC ANTHROPOLOGY: AN AUSTRALIAN PERSPECTIVE

Denise Donlon

The history of forensic anthropology in Australia is very closely linked to the history of physical anthropology and anatomy. In this chapter, I concentrate on the early practitioners who made a major contribution to the field. This perspective investigates possible reasons why the discipline of forensic anthropology was so slow to develop in Australia. As with any discipline that deals with human remains, ethical issues are important in the history and the current practice of the discipline. These issues are discussed particularly in light of the use of collections of Aboriginal skeletal remains.

The last 15 years have seen significant advances in the field. Thus new developments in the discipline, such as advances in education and training, are briefly discussed, and the roles of various forensic societies and associations in the development of forensic anthropology are also examined. Employment of forensic anthropologists are outlined, along with examples of court cases in which forensic anthropologists acted as expert witnesses.

Forensic anthropology is sometimes confused with or overlaps with closely related disciplines such as archaeology and osteology. Forensic archaeology is concerned mainly with the search for and the recovery of remains. This chapter concentrates on forensic anthropology rather than archaeology, because the latter discipline is young

and was recently covered by Blau (2004). *Forensic osteology* is used here to mean the same thing as *forensic anthropology*.

Early Practitioners: The Anatomists

Practitioners of forensic anthropology in the six Australian states or territories were initially found in university departments of anatomy. In the state of New South Wales, for example, the coroner and police always called on the services of the Professor of Anatomy at The University of Sydney to give advice on the identification of skeletonised remains. A famous example was the "Pyjama girl" case. Found in 1934, a girl's body had been partially buried, charred, and dressed in yellow silk pyjamas and remained unidentified for ten years (Coleman 1978). During that time, her remains were examined in detail by Professor Arthur Burkitt, Challis Professor of Anatomy from 1925 to 1954. This examination included the description of some bones, X rays and also detailed anthropometric investigation of her facial features, which were compared with those of suspected victims (Figure 9.1).[1] The Pyjama Girl was preserved in formalin and placed on display in The University of Sydney's Department of Anatomy museum in an attempt to identify her. In 1944, the Pyjama Girl was formally identified

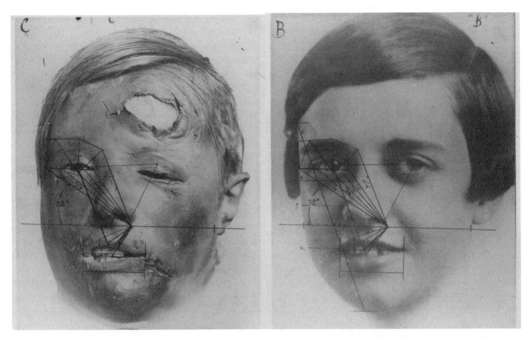

Figure 9.1 Early facial comparison by Professor A. Burkitt; the "Pyjama girl" (*left*) and Philomena Morgan (*right*) (photographs used with permission of the Shellshear Museum).

as Linda Agostini, and her husband was found guilty of manslaughter.

Probably the most outstanding pioneer in forensic anthropology in Australia was Neil Macintosh, Challis Professor of Anatomy at The University of Sydney from 1955 until 1973 (Figure 9.2). Macintosh had broad interests, which included general anatomy and the anthropology of the Australian Aborigines (Larnach and Macintosh 1966, 1967: Macintosh 1949, 1952, 1965). He was on good terms with Police Commissioners and heads of the Criminal Investigation Bureau (CIB) (of which he was an honorary consultant) in NSW from the 1950s through to the 1970s (Elkin 1978), providing them with advice on identification of skeletal remains as well as on methods of recovering remains from burials (Macintosh 1972). The police brought skeletal remains directly to the University, and pathologists from the Sydney City Morgue would ask for his advice on cases that were skeletonised or decomposed. Working alongside Macintosh during the 1960s and 1970s were Dr. Len Freedman (Senior Lecturer) and Mr. Stan Larnach (Curator of the Shellshear Museum). Their work involved the anatomy and anthropology of Aboriginal remains from the east coast of New South Wales (Freedman 1964; Larnach 1974; Larnarch and Freedman 1964, Larnach and Macintosh 1966, 1967, 1970, 1971; Macintosh and

Larnach 1973). Forensic anthropology consultation and research continues today at The University of Sydney by physical anthropologist Dr. Denise Donlon and students in the Shellshear Museum (Chiu and Donlon 2000; Croker and Donlon 2006; Robinson et al. 2006).

Practitioners such as Macintosh were in constant communication with international scholars working in the area of forensic anthropology. For example, Macintosh was particularly friendly with American anthropologists T. D. (Dale) Stewart and W. W. (Bill) Howells. In 1972, T. D. Stewart was invited to Australia to participate in the Grafton Elliot Smith Centenary Celebration (Stewart 1974). At this conference a paper on forensic anthropology was given by Godfrey Oettle (a NSW forensic pathologist) and Stan Larnach (1974). This may have been the first conference paper given in Australia that refers directly to forensic anthropology. Stewart then traveled around Australia with the help of Macintosh, visiting the police in Canberra and in Adelaide (Macintosh 1972).

The 1960s and 1970s saw international visitors to Australia whose aim was to examine the Aboriginal collections and whose publications are now used in forensic anthropological work. The visiting anthropologists included Ales Hrdlička, Eugene Giles (Giles and Elliot 1962), William Howells (1973), and Michael Pietrusewsky (1990).

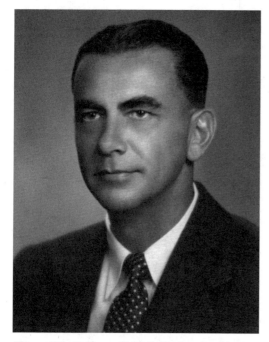

Figure 9.2 Professor N. W. G. Macintosh, a pioneer in Australian forensic anthropology (photograph taken in 1955 and used with permission of Mrs. N. W. G. Macintosh).

However their interests were not so much in forensic anthropology as in biological anthropology, human evolution, and dispersal. Macintosh, Larnach, and Freedman were motivated by Giles and Elliot's paper and Howells's work on racial identification to apply similar methods to the collection of Aboriginal remains, specifically those from the east coast of New South Wales (N.S.W.) (Macintosh and Larnach 1973).

In these early days, personnel in other Australian anatomy departments also gave opinions on cases involving skeletonised remains. There were those who took a particular interest in forensic anthropology (although it may not have been called that at the time). At The University of Queensland, Dr. Walter Wood (Senior Lecturer in Anatomy), acted as a consultant for the Queensland Government Forensic Pathology Unit assisting with the identification of unknown skeletonized human remains from 1972 until 2001. Wood analyzed Aboriginal skeletal remains from the Broadbeach burial ground (Smith, Brown, and Wood 1981; Wood 1968, 1998) and was also involved with the identification of WWII Australian servicemen in Papua New Guinea while working there as a medical practitioner. In addition, he wrote a chapter on forensic osteology in a legal book concerned with

the role of the expert witness (Wood 1993, Wood, Briggs, and Donlon 2002).

In Victoria, medical practitioners involved in forensic anthropology include Dr. W. H. Mollison, who was the Coroner's Surgeon and Lecturer in Forensic Medicine and Anatomy at The University of Melbourne from 1893 until 1943. In the 1930s, Frederick Wood Jones, Professor of Anatomy at The University of Melbourne, had a particular interest in skeletal remains. In 1945, Dr. Les Ray joined the Department of Anatomy at The University of Melbourne and also provided forensic advice to the police and Coroner (Ray 1959). From the mid-1970s until the early 1990s, advice on forensic cases was provided very much on an ad hoc basis by such people as Dr. Geoff Kenny (Senior Lecturer in Anatomy and curator of the Anatomy Museum at The University of Melbourne), as well as Associate Professor Chris Briggs (Lecturer in Anatomy, The University of Melbourne). From 1995 until 2005, Briggs provided a 24 hour, on-call consultancy service until Dr. Soren Blau began in 2005 in a full-time position at the Victorian Institute of Forensic Medicine, where her role is concerned with both domestic cases and disaster victim identification (Blau 2006). In the 2000s, Dr. Catherine Bennett, a physical anthropologist in the Department of Epidemiology, also provided advice on the identification of Aboriginal and non-Aboriginal remains (Bennett 1995).

In South Australia, much of the early skeletal identification was undertaken by Frederick Wood-Jones (1931) and A. A. Abbie (1976), Professors of Anatomy at The University of Adelaide and also physical anthropologists. More recently Maciej Henneberg (Wood-Jones Professor of Anatomy and Physical Anthropology at The University of Adelaide) provided forensic anthropology services. Henneberg was involved in a number of criminal cases, including the high-profile Falconio murder case (*R. v Murdoch* [2005] NTSC 78 (15/12/05) and Snowtown murders (Stephan and Henneberg 2006). Similarly, Dr. Carl Stephan (Lecturer in Anatomy at The University of Queensland) was involved in cases of CCTV comparisons for the FBI, South Australian and N.S.W. police. Stephan and Henneberg, along with others, have published extensively on facial approximation (Henneberg, Stephan, and Simpson 2003; Stephan and Henneberg 2001, 2004; Stephan, Henneberg, and Simpson 2003; Stephan et al. 2005).

Before the 1980s, the majority of work in Western Australia (W.A.) was performed by David Allbrook, Professor of Anatomy at The University of Western Australia (Allbrook 1961). Allbrook was followed by Dr. Len Freedman, who provided a free service to the Coroner, W.A. Police, and pathologists in the 1980s. In the early 1990s, Freedman passed the responsibility for forensic and coronial work to his student, Dr. Alanah Buck, now the full-time forensic anthropologist at the Department of Health's PathWest Centre (Buck et al. 2000).

In the Australian Commonwealth Territory (ACT) there was no medical school until very recently and relatively little demand for an anthropologist owing to the small population (approximately 300,000). Consultation on cases was done by Dr. Alan Thorne and Dr. Marc Oxenham, both of the Australian National University. In the smallest state, Tasmania, there has never been an in-house forensic anthropologist, probably because of the small population. Many of the cases in the Northern Territory involve the separation of ancient Aboriginal remains from recent Aboriginal and non-Aboriginal remains. In the 1970s, Thorne identified Aboriginal remains from under the old casino in Darwin (Cantwell 2000). More recently, identification of Aboriginal remains was undertaken by Dr. Ken Mulvaney, an archaeologist with the Aboriginal Areas Protection Authority (Ken Mulvaney, personal communication 2006).

Reasons for the Slow Development

The slow development of forensic anthropology in Australia is probably the result of a number of factors: the small population and homicide rate in Australia, the nonrepatriation of the war dead, and a lack of relevant skeletal collections, as well as difficult ethical issues involved in dealing with human remains.

Small Caseloads

As a result of the small population in Australia only a relatively small number of cases require a forensic anthropologist. The homicide rate in Australia is low compared with other countries, especially the United States (U.S.). There are around 350 homicides per year in Australia with only 1 in 50 buried (Blau 2004). This means that for each state/territory (of which there are six) there are about 50 homicides per year and roughly one buried body per state per year. In N.S.W., which has the greatest population, approximately 10 skeletonised human cases are examined by a forensic anthropologist each year (Donlon 2003).

The War Dead

Another factor in the slow development may relate to the Australian protocols for identification and burial of the war dead, which, until recently, meant that the identification and burial of any skeletonised remains was always made off-shore. Until the Vietnam War, all Australian servicemen and women were buried in the theatre of war in which they died. Thus approximately 102,239 Australians from World Wars I and II and the Korean War are buried, mainly in war graves, in Belgium, Crete, Egypt, France, Indonesia, Korea, Malaysia, Papua New Guinea, Thailand, Singapore, Solomon Islands, Turkey, and the United Kingdom (www.awm.gov.au/research/infosheets/war_casualties.asp). This situation is quite different from that of the U.S., where the mission was, and continues to be, to repatriate all of the war dead to the U.S. (www.jpac.pacom.mil/). In the United States, unlike in Australia, the skeletonised remains are examined by physical anthropologists for the purpose of identification, but, in addition, much research has been carried out on those remains since they are of known age, ancestry, sex and stature, thus providing an excellent source of data for forensic research (e.g., McKern and Stewart 1957; Trotter and Gleser 1958). Although the protocols for identification and burial of the war dead have changed in Australia, there have not been (and will probably never be) the numbers of skeletal remains examined to allow for the generation of large databases.

The Importance of Skeletal Collections and Ethical Issues

As pointed out by Walker (2000), dealing with human remains often involes a conflict among beliefs, usually religious, over the proper treatment of the dead and the value that scientists place on the data that might be collected from human remains. Such conflicts have arisen in Australia with the collection and use of Aboriginal skeletal remains for research, as well as, more recently, with coroner's cases.

In Australia there is an almost total lack of collections of Australians of European and Asian origin—the two major population groups in Australia. Thus practitioners must rely on research done in the United States or Europe, which is not always relevant to the population mix here. Although there are still large collections of Aboriginal skeletal remains in Australia, accessing them for research is problematic (Donlon 1994). Australian anthropologists have utilized research undertaken on collections in Australia and Europe. Focus, however, has been on collections from the U.S., because they include large collections of Caucasoids (for example, Terry collection in Washington, D.C.

and Hamann-Todd collection at the Cleveland Museum of Natural History) (İşcan 1988).

Of significant importance to forensic anthropology has been the research done on Australian Aboriginal collections. These collections resulted mainly from the discovery of remains by members of the public but also by archaeological excavation. Those reported to the police initially became forensic cases, then later were sent to state museums with smaller collections being housed in universities. Such collections were investigated by various anthropologists and anatomists for their Ph.D.s[2] and specific research papers (for example, early researchers/anatomists mentioned above and some relevant to forensic anthropology).[3]

At the same time as interest was growing in forensic anthropology in the 1980s and 1990s, Aboriginal skeletal remains, which had typically been the source of much research, were becoming increasingly unavailable. This was as a result of efforts by Aboriginal communities to have remains repatriated to the appropriate communities (Donlon 1994). State museums and universities around Australia drew up policies for the management of Aboriginal remains held in these institutions. All these policies restricted access to remains for research. More recently, research in physical anthropology that is useful for forensic work has moved toward using published data (Pardoe 1999; Wright 1996). Particularly useful publications around this time were manuals written for the identification of Aboriginal versus non-Aboriginal remains (Hope and Littleton 1995; Thorne and Ross 1986).

Professional associations such as the Australian Archaeological Association (AAA) and the Australian and New Zealand Forensic Science Society (ANZFSS) have codes of ethics for use by researchers. AAA's code of ethics deals specifically with Aboriginal remains. It states: "Members acknowledge the special importance to Indigenous peoples of ancestral remains and objects and sites associated with such remains. Members will treat such remains with respect" (www.australianarchaeologicalassociation.com.au/codeofethics.php). In addition, those wishing to do research using Aboriginal skeletal remains today must request permission from the appropriate local Aboriginal community. The code of ethics for the ANZFSS is concerned with the provision of evidence by expert witnesses (www.anzfss.org.au/code_of_ethics.htm). The Heritage Office of N.S.W. also has ethical and legal guidelines on the management of human remains (Bickford, Donlon, and Lavelle 1998). In Australia, all those wishing to do research into human remains must submit

their proposals to the ethics committees of their institutions.

The preceding examples illustrate that the use of skeletal collections, both Aboriginal and non-Aboriginal, is highly regulated and somewhat difficult to access for the purposes of research in forensic anthropology.

Today: Education, Professional Organizations, Employment, Disaster Victim Identification, and Court Work

The 1990s saw acceleration in the growth of forensic anthropology in Australia. This was probably due to four factors:

1. the growth of courses/training in forensic science, more than likely related to the enormous interest generated by the media;

2. an increase in the number of forensic anthropologists participating in conferences;

3. employment of anthropologists in forensic institutions;

4. an increase in terrorist activities, especially in the Asia-Pacific region (for example, the Bali bombings (see Briggs and Buck this volume);

5. the use of anthropologists and archaeologists as expert witnesses in court (see Henneberg this volume).

Education in Forensic Anthropology and Archaeology

There was a proliferation of forensic science courses in Australia in the 1990s and 2000s. The first university undergraduate science anatomy program for students majoring in forensic osteology was offered at The University of Queensland from 1990–2001. Today courses in forensic anthropology and osteology are offered at The University of Sydney, The University of New England, The University of Adelaide, and the Australian National University.

Professional Organizations and Conferences

Since the late 1990s the representation of forensic anthropologists presenting at conferences of forensic associations has increased, possibly because of the increase in the number of those becoming qualified in the discipline.

The Australian Academy of Forensic Science (AAFS). This association had its foundational meeting in Sydney in 1967. The academy initially included lawyers, medical practitioners, scientists, sociologists, police officers, and government officials. Foundation members included N.W.G. Macintosh (Professor of Anatomy, University of Sydney), who was a member of the AAFS Council and the Executive and Editorial Committees from 1967 until 1973. The academy publishes a journal entitled *Australian Forensic Science.*

The Australian and New Zealand Forensic Science Society (ANZFSS). The ANZFSS was formed in 1971 with the aim of bringing together scientists, police, criminalists, pathologists, and members of the legal profession actively involved with the forensic sciences. The Society's objectives are to enhance the quality of Forensic Science, providing both formal and informal lectures, discussions, and demonstrations encompassing the various disciplines within the science (www.anzfss.org.au/history.htm). The introduction of the Registered Forensic Practitioner Scheme was approved at the ANZFSS Annual General Meeting in 1998 but was put on hold owing to the lack of applications. Every two years the association holds an international symposium. The first symposium to include a session on forensic anthropology held in Sydney in 1996 with American anthropologists William Bass and Diane France invited as keynote speakers. All symposia since (except for 2002 in Canberra) have held an anthropology session. The most recent symposium in Fremantle, in April 2006, had the largest session yet, with standing room only for some presentations (ANZFSS 2006).

The Australasian Society for Human Biology (ASHB). The ASHB was formed in 1996 owing to the efforts of Charles Oxnard, then head of the School of Human Biology at The University of Western Australia. The majority of Australian biological anthropologists belong to this society. Nevertheless, it is a very small society of a few hundred members, and it is only in the last three or four years that forensic sessions were included in their conferences, with sessions in Auckland in 2003 (ASHB 2003) and Canberra in 2004 (ASHB 2004).

The National Institute of Forensic Science (NIFS). In 1973, a Committee of Enquiry was established by the Attorney General Senator the Honorable Lionel Murphy to investigate the need for a national forensic institution (Davey 2002). This committee laid the foundations for the NIFS, which had its first formal meeting in 1991. The

NIFS has provided a small amount of funding for individuals and training in forensic anthropology and archaeology.

Forensic anthropology was a latecomer to participating in conferences of the associations mentioned above. With no specific forensic anthropology (or even physical anthropology) association, forensic anthropologists tend to spread themselves rather thinly among these associations.

Employment of Forensic Anthropologists

This section examines the recent inclusion of anthropologists and/or archaeologists in forensic institutions for the first time. It also updates and extends developments in forensic archaeology since Blau's 1994 article.

Today forensic anthropologists are employed in forensic institutions/mortuaries in most states' capital cities. In New South Wales, Dr. Denise Donlon has been employed as consultant in forensic anthropology to the N.S.W. Department of Forensic Medicine in Sydney since 1995. Her work includes casework involving identification, recovery and excavation, court work, and training (Donlon 2003, In press). In Victoria, Dr. Soren Blau is employed as the first full-time forensic anthropologist at the Victorian Institute of Forensic Medicine in the Human Identification Services. Her work includes domestic casework, evidence presentation in court, and overseas training programs in Disaster Victim Identification (DVI). Since 2002, Dr. Ellie Simpson has been employed at Forensic Science South Australia, where her position involves casework as well as limited radiography and also case managements for autopsies (Simpson 2005; Simpson and Henneberg 2002). In Western Australia, Dr. Alanah Buck works in the forensic pathology department at PathWest. This was initially a part-time appointment (1995) but later converted to a full-time position (2002). Her work includes casework, evidence presentation in the Supreme Court, and an increasing role in the training of law enforcement officers. This increase in duties illustrates how the role of the anthropologist has expanded in W.A. In Queensland today, most of the search, recovery, and analysis of remains is done by Dr. Donna McGregor, a police officer with a background in archaeology and anthropology (McGregor, Wood, and Brenknell 1996) and Ms. Debra Whelan at the John Tonge Centre in Brisbane.

All the above-mentioned employed forensic anthropologists are women. What could be the reason for this dominance of women in this field?

Possibilities include a female bias toward studies in biological sciences and areas of social justice. It may also be that men are looking elsewhere in forensic science, perhaps to better paid and more full-time jobs. It is possible that forensic anthropology, as with some areas of archaeology, is seen as lab-based rather than field-based work and therefore "women's work" (Phillips 1998). A more positive view is that it reflects a lack of discrimination toward women working in science generally, particularly outside universities.

In 2000, the Australian Defence Forces recruited a forensic anthropologist into the Royal Australian Air Force Specialist Reserves. The role of the anthropologist is to assist with the recovery and examination of remains of servicemen and women killed in previous wars, especially WWII in Papua New Guinea (Donlon, Duflou, and Griffiths 2000), as well as more recent incidents, such as the recovery of the unknown sailor from HMAS *Sydney* on Christmas Island (Donlon 2006a) and the crash of the Sea King helicopter on Nias Island, Indonesia, in 2005 (Donlon 2006b).

In forensic archaeology, it appears that the police and other authorities are increasingly using archaeologists for excavation but not necessarily for searching for graves. Police first used archaeologists in the excavation of graves in 1988 (McDonald and Ross 1990). Since then they have occasionally used archaeologists in the search for clandestine graves such as that of Samantha Knight (Macdonald 1999).[4] The N.S.W. Coroner has also requested the assistance of archaeologists in the exhumations of Sally-Ann Huckstepp and various Aboriginal deaths in custody.

Australian anthropologist Carl Stephan and archaeologist Tim Anson assisted in the excavation and identification of remains in Iraq (Tim Anson, personal communication 2006). The Australian Federal Police employ Katie Oakley, a forensic officer with a background in archaeology/anthropology, who has assisted in the exhumation of graves in the Solomon Islands as part of Regional Assistance Mission to the Solomon Islands (Oakley 2005; see Archer and Dodd this volume). In 1990–1991, Richard Wright worked for the Attorney General's Special Investigations Unit, in charge of the discovery and excavation of three graves in the Ukraine dating from 1942 and relating to the Holocaust (Wright 1996). From 1997 to 2000 he was contracted by International Criminal Tribunal for the Former Yugoslavia (ICTY) as Chief Archaeologist. His team exhumed some 1,600 bodies from some 80 graves at 15 sites and also located another 21 mass graves. The mass graves were exhumed for humanitarian rather than evidentiary purposes (Wright, Hanson, and Sterenberg 2005). The preceding cases illustrate that interest in the recovery of remains is increasing (Briggs and Wood 1998).

Disaster Victim Identification

Recently, a number of terrorist acts and disasters occurred in the Australasian region. The associated Australian deaths resulted in the production of the Australasian Disaster Victim Identification (DVI) Procedures (Australasian DVI Standards Manual 2004) by a combination of Australian Government agencies. The resulting manual includes protocols for anthropologists (Buck 2004) participating in a specialist team in the field.

The Forensic Anthropologist and Archaeologist as Expert Witnesses

In most cases of simple identification of ancestry, age, sex, and stature, the evidence of forensic anthropologists is accepted and rarely goes to court. Exceptions may occur when the remains are not complete, as in the case of *The Queen v. Keir* (*R. v. Keir* [2002] NSWCCA 30, 28/2/2002) and *The Queen v. Carter* 2000 (*R. v. Carter* [2000] VICCCA, 15/2/00).

Recent cases involving forensic anthropologists have comprised various methods of facial recognition identification. Such cases involved identification of refugees (*SHJB v. Minister for Immigration and Multicultural and Indigenous Affairs* 2003 FCA [2003] 22/5/03) and alleged robbers (*R v. Tang* [2004] NSWCCA, 24/5/06). These areas of identification are, however, very controversial and focus on the question of whether facial recognition, facial mapping, and body mapping constitute a field of "specialised knowledge" (*R v. Tang* [2004] NSWCCA, 24/5/06; *Murdoch v. The Queen* [2007] NTCCA, 10/1/07; Stephan this volume).

The Future

Forensic anthropology in Australia has been retarded by the small amount of casework and the lack of skeletal collections representing the major population groups in the country. Some of these problems may be overcome by using data from new technologies such as imaging of the living and of cadavers (e.g., Blau 2006). However, differences in legislation between the different states may limit the utility of such research. Other research will involve the collection of data, such as stature, from the living. Standardizing the data collected from casework will allow for setting up a database of metric and nonmetric observations on Australian skeletal remains that will further assist with identification.

There will probably be an increase in funding for research into facial and body recognition to assist in the identification of possible terrorists. Notwithstanding these new developments, there will always be a need for experts in the identification of ancient Aboriginal remains in order that they may be eliminated from police enquiries. As for employment, it is likely that a small number of anthropologists and archaeologists will be taken into forensic institutions, the police forces, and possibly also into the Australian Defence Forces.

Australia does not have a professional society equivalent to the American Academy of Forensic Science, which accredits forensic scientists. The ANZFSS has an accreditation scheme, but it is on hold, because of the lack of applications during the last four years. No doubt accreditation will eventually happen, but it may be slow in coming. In 2006, the executive of the Senior Managers of Australian and New Zealand Forensic Laboratories (SMANZFL) supported the formation of a Scientific Advisory Group (SAG) made up of forensic anthropologists, mortuary managers, forensic odontologists, and forensic entomologists. The formation of such an advisory group has the potential to significantly augment the professionalism of forensic anthropology in Australia.

What of our future forensic anthropologists? There is a danger that, given the lack of skeletal collections in Australia and the tendency of students to take the "easy" path of a generalized forensic science degree, they will not have the depth of knowledge and experience needed, especially to act as experts. In spite of this, the current employment status of forensic anthropologists in institutions in all states bodes well. Forensic pathologists, coroners, and police will no doubt recognize the contributions that the forensic anthropologist can make to the identification of skeletal remains and increasingly to the identification of the living.

Acknowledgments

Given the lack of published material, I wish to acknowledge many people for discussion and information: Catherine Bennett, Soren Blau, Chris Briggs, Alanah Buck, Maciej Henneberg, Julia Horne, Katie Oakley, Colin Pardoe, Ellie Simpson, Alan Thorne, Darryl Tuck, Wally Wood, Richard Wright, and particularly Ann Macintosh and Sarah Magnell, who helped me greatly with my literature search.

Notes

1. The photograph of Macintosh was taken by his wife, and she has given me permission to include it. The photographs of the "Pyjama Girl" have appeared in the press, and her body was on display to the public. Photographs of her are also currently on display in the Justice and Police Museum in Sydney.

2. Bennett 1995; Brown 1982; Collier 1990; Donlon 1990; Pardoe 1984; Rao 1966; Webb 1984.

3. These include Berry and Berry 1967; Davivongs 1963a, 1963b; Kellock and Parsons 1970; Pietrusewsky 1990; Ray 1959; van Dongen 1963; Wood 1920.

4. In August 1986, 9-year-old Samantha Knight disappeared from a Sydney suburb. It was not until August 2001 that Michael Guider (already in prison for pedophile offenses) was charged with Samantha's murder. In July 2003, Guider finally told police where he had buried Knight's body. Her remains, were, however, never located, believed to have been disturbed during earlier building works.

References

Abbie, A. A. 1976. Morphological variation in the adult Australian Aboriginal, in R. L. Kirk and A. G. Thorne (eds.), *The Origin of the Australians*, pp. 211–214. Canberra: AIAS.

Allbrook, D. 1961. The estimation of stature in British and East African males. *Journal of Forensic Medicine* 8(1): 15–28.

ANZFSS Conference Proceedings of the 18th International Symposium of the Forensic Sciences. 2006 (April). Fremantle.

ASHB. 2003. Proceedings of the Australasian Society for Human Biology, Auckland. 2004. *Homo-Journal of Comparative Human Biology* 54(1): 71–88.

———. 2004. Proceedings of the Australasian Society for Human Biology, Canberra. 2005. *Homo-Journal of Comparative Human Biology* 56(2): 263–302.

Australasian DVI Standards Manual. 2004. Draft. Adelaide Research and Innovation Pty Ltd, Australasian Disaster Victim Identification Committee, Emergency Management Australia and the Commonwealth of Australia.

Bennett, C. M. 1995. Morphology of the Major Limb Bones of South Australian Aborigines. Ph.D. thesis, La Trobe University.

Berry, A. C., and Berry, R. J. 1967. Epigenetic variation in the human cranium. *Journal of Anatomy* (London) 101: 361–379.

Bickford, A., Donlon, D., and Lavelle, S. 1998. *Guidelines for the Management of Human Skeletal Remains under the Heritage Act 1977*, Heritage Office of N.S.W.

———. 1999. *Skeletal Remains: Guidelines for the Management of Human Skeletal Remains under the Heritage Act 1977*. N.S.W. Heritage Office.

Blau, S. 2004. Forensic archaeology in Australia: Current situations, future possibilities. *Australian Archaeology* 58: 11–14.

———. 2006. Ridges and furrows: Re-examining the pubic symphyses as an anthropological ageing technique. Conference Proceedings of the 18th International Symposium of the Forensic Sciences April 2006, Fremantle.

Briggs, C. A., and Wood, W. B. 1998. Recovery of Remains, in J. G. Clement and D. L. Ranson (eds.), *Craniofacial Identification in Forensic Medicine: Appendix I*, pp. 267–271. Sydney: Arnold Publishers.

Brown, P. 1982. Coobool Creek: A Prehistoric Australian Hominid Population. Unpublished Ph.D. thesis, Australian National University, Canberra.

Buck, A. 2004. DVI Forensic Anthropology Procedures. Appendix K. *Australasian DVI Standards Manual*: 127–130.

Buck, A. M., Cooke, C., de la Motte, P., and Knott, S. 2000. Homicide or suicide? A jigsaw of incinerated human remains *Medical Journal of Australia* 173: 606–607.

Cantwell, A. 2000. Who knows the power of his bones: Reburial Redux. *Annals of the New York Academy of Sciences* 925: 79–119.

Chiu A., and Donlon, D. 2000. The value of dental metrics in the assessment of race and sex in Caucasoids and Mongoloids. *Dental Anthropology* 14(2): 20–39.

Coleman, R. 1978. *The Pyjama Girl*. Melbourne: Hawthorn Press.

Collier, S. 1990. Sexual Dimorphism and Economy in Modern Human Populations. Unpublished Ph.D. thesis, University of New England, Armidale.

Croker, S., and Donlon, D. 2006. Human or non-human: Possible methods for the identification of bone fragments. Poster. Conference Proceedings of the 18th International Symposium of the Forensic Sciences April 2006, Fremantle.

Davey, A. 2002. Reflections on the gestation of NIFS. *The Forensic Bulletin*: 7–8.

Davivongs, V. 1963a. The pelvic girdle of the Australian Aborigine: Sex differences and sex determination. *American Journal of Physical Anthropology* 21: 443–456.

———. 1963b. The femur of the Australian Aborigines. *American Journal of Physical Anthropology* 21: 457–467.

Donlon, D. 1990. The Value of Postcranial Nonmetric Variation in Studies of Global Populations in Modern Homo sapiens. Unpublished Ph.D. thesis, University of New England, Armidale.

———. 1994. Aboriginal skeletal collections and research in physical anthropology: An historical perspective. *Australian Archaeology* 39: 1–10.

———. 2000. The value of infracranial nonmetric variation in studies of modern *Homo sapiens*: An Australian focus. *American Journal of Physical Anthropology* 113: 349–368.

———. 2001. Excavation of the old European cemetery, Christmas Island: A possible site for the grave of the unknown sailor of the *HMAS Sydney*. Report prepared for Royal Australian Navy.

———. 2003. Diversity revealed: 10 years of anthropological casework based in New South Wales, Australia. Proceedings of the *Australasian Society for Human Biology*, Auckland. Abstract. *Homo-Journal of Comparative Human Biology*: 151–152.

———. 2006a. 1945 Beaufighter and 2005 Sea King crashes: Archaeological and anthropological methods of recovery and analysis Presentation at the *ANZFSS Symposium* Fremantle.

———. 2006b. Identification of the unknown sailor from HMAS *Sydney*. Presentation at the Australian Society for Human Biology conference, Melbourne, December.

———. In press. Forensic anthropology in Australia: A brief history and review of casework, in M. Oxenham (ed.), *Forensic Approaches to Death, Disaster and Abuse*. Sydney: Australian Academic Press.

Donlon, D., Duflou, J., and Griffiths, G. 2000. Recovering the Australian war dead from PNG and forensic anthropology standards. Presentation at the Australian Archaeology Conference, Beechworth, Victoria.

Elkin, A. P. 1978. N.W.G. Macintosh and his work. *Archaeology & Physical Anthropology in Oceania* 13(2 & 3): 85–142.

Freedman, L. 1964. Metrical features of Aboriginal crania from coastal New South Wales Australia. *Records of the Australian Museum* 26(12): 309–325.

Giles, E., and Elliot, O. 1962. Race identification from cranial measurements. *Journal of Forensic Science* 7: 147–156.

Henneberg, M., Stephan, C. N., and Simpson, E. 2003. Human face in biological anthropology: craniometry, evolution and forensic identification, in M. Katsikitis (ed.), *The Human Face: Measurement and Meaning*, pp. 29–48. Dodrecht, Netherlands: Kluwer Academic Publishers.

Hope, J., and Littleton, J. 1995. *Finding Out about Aboriginal Burials*, Hurlstone Park, N.S.W.: Mungo Publications for the Darling Basin Commission.

Howells, W. W. 1973. *Cranial Variation in Man: A Study by Multivariate Analysis of Patterns of Difference among Human Populations*, Vol. 67. Cambridge, MA: Papers of the Peabody Museum, Harvard University.

İşcan, M. Y. 1988. Rise of forensic anthropology. *Yearbook of Physical Anthropology* 31: 203–230.

Joint POW/MIA Accounting Command (JPAC). 2006. www.jpac.pacom.mil

Kellock, W. L., and Parsons, P. A. 1970. Variation of minor non-metrical cranial variants in Australian Aborigines. *American Journal of Physical Anthropology* 32: 408–431.

Larnach, S. L. 1974. An examination of the use of discontinuous cranial traits. *Archaeology & Physical Anthropology in Oceania* 9(3): 217–225.

Larnach, S., and Freedman, S. L. 1964. Sex determination of Aboriginal crania from coastal New South Wales. *Records of the Australian Museum* 26: 295–308.

Larnach, S., and Macintosh, N. W. G. 1966. The craniology of the Aborigines of coastal New South Wales. *The Oceania Monographs* 13: 5-94.

———. 1967. The use in forensic medicine of an anthropological method for the determination of sex and race in skeletons. *Archaeology and Physical Anthropology in Oceania* 2(2): 155–161.

———. 1970. The craniology of the Aborigines of Queensland. *Oceania Monographs* No. 15.

———. 1971. The mandible in eastern Australian Aborigines. *The Oceania Monographs* 17: 3–34.

Mcdonald, J. J. 1999. Excavation at Berry Island, N.S.W. Unpublished report for the N.S.W. Police.

Mcdonald, J. J., and Ross, A. C. 1990. Helping the police with their enquiries: Archaeology and politics at Angophora reserve rock shelter. N. S. W. *Archaeology in Oceania* 25(2): 114–121.

McGregor, D., Wood, W. B., and Brecknell, D. J. 1996. Soil accumulation of by-products of decomposition. *Australian Journal of Forensic Science* 28: 67–71.

Macintosh, A. 1972. Correspondence to N. W. G. Macintosh on 1 December 1972. Held in the archives of the Shellshear Museum, Department of Anatomy and Histology, University of Sydney.

Macintosh, N. W. G. 1949. Survey of possible sea routes available to the Tasmanian Aborigines. *Rec. Queen Victoria Museum, Launceston* 2(3): 123–144.

———. 1952. Stature in some Aboriginal tribes in southwest Arnhem Land. *Oceania* 22(3): 208–215.

———. 1962. Correspondence to Howells 21 June 1962. Held in the archives of the Shellshear Museum, Department of Anatomy and Histology, University of Sydney.

———. 1965. The physical aspects of man in Australia, in R. and C. Berndt (eds.), *Aboriginal Man in Australia*, pp. 29–70. Sydney: Angus & Robertson.

———. 1972. The recovery and treatment of bone, in D. J. Mulvaney (ed.), *Australian Archaeology:* *A Guide to Field and Laboratory Techniques*, pp. 77–85. Canberra: AIAS.

Macintosh, N. W. G., and Larnach, S. L. 1973. A cranial study of the Aborigines of Queensland with a contrast between Australian and New Guinea crania, in R. L. Kirk (ed.), *The Human Biology of Aborigines of Cape York*, pp. 1–12. Canberra: AIAS.

McKean, D. 2006. Crime shows lead charge on forensics, Higher Education Supplement. *The Australian* July 5: 36.

McKern, T. W., and Stewart, T. D. 1957. Skeletal age changes in young American males, analyzed from the standpoint of identification. *Headqu QM Res and Dev Command*, Tech Rep EP-45 Natick, Massachusetts.

Oakley, K. 2005. Forensic Archaeology and anthropology: An Australian perspective. *Forensic Science, Medicine, and Pathology* 1(3): 169–172(4).

Oettle, T. H. G., and Larnach, S. L. 1974. The identification of Aboriginal traits in forensic medicine, in A. P. Elkin and N. W. G. Macintosh (eds.), *Grafton Elliot Smith: The Man and His Work*, pp. 103–108. Sydney: Sydney University Press.

Pardoe, C. 1984. Prehistoric Human Morphological Variation in Australia. Unpublished Ph.D. thesis, Australian National University, Canberra.

———. 1999. *The Skeletal Provenancing Project: Results and Evaluation*. Australian Archaeological Association Conference, Mandurah, W.A. December 9–12.

Phillips, C. 1998. Answering the old boys' club: Developing support systems for women archaeologists, in M. Casey, D. Donlon, J. Hope, and S. Welfare (eds.), *Redefining Archaeology: Feminist Perspectives*, pp. 63–67. Canberra: ANH Publications, RSPAS, Australian National University.

Pietrusewsky, M. 1990. Cranial variation in Australian and pacific populations. *American Journal of Physical Anthropology* 82: 319–340.

Rao, P. D. 1966. The Anatomy of the Distal Limb Segments of the Aboriginal Skeleton. Unpublished Ph.D. thesis, University of Adelaide, Adelaide.

Ray, L. J. 1959. Metrical and non-metrical features of the clavicle of the Australian Aboriginal. *American Journal of Physical Anthropology* 17: 217–226.

Robinson, M., Donlon, D. Houang, M., Harrison, H. Wolf, G. H., and Stammberger, H. 2006. Observed variations of the paranasal sinuses by computed tomography in Melanesian skulls: A forensic perspective. Poster. Conference Proceedings of the 18th International Symposium of the Forensic Sciences, April, Fremantle.

Simpson, E. 2005. Morphological age estimation, in J. Payne-James, R. Byard, T. Cory and C. Henderson (eds.), *Encyclopedia of Forensic and Legal Medicine*, pp. 119–123. Oxford: Elsevier.

Simpson, E., and Henneberg, M. 2002. Variation in soft tissue thickness on the human face and their relationship to craniometric dimensions. *American Journal of Physical Anthropology* 118: 121–133.

Smith, P., Brown, T., and Wood, W. B. 1981. Tooth Size and Morphology in a Recent Aboriginal Population from Broadbeach, South East Queensland. *American Journal of Physical Anthropology* 55(4): 423–432.

Stephan, C. N., and Henneberg, M. 2001. Building faces from dry skulls: Are they recognised above chance rates? *Journal of Forensic Science* 46(3): 432–440.

———. 2004. Predicting mouth width from inter-canine width. A 75% rule. *Journal of Forensic Sciences* 48(4): 725–727.

———. 2006. Recognition by forensic facial approximation: Case specific examples and empirical tests. *Journal of Forensic Science* 156 (2–3): 182–191.

Stephan, C. N., Henneberg, M., and Simpson, E. 2003. A prediction of nose projection and pronasale position in facial approximation: A test of published methods and a new guideline. *American Journal of Physical Anthropology* 122: 240–250.

Stephan, C. N., Penton-Voak, I. S., Clement, J. G., and Henneberg, M. 2005. Ceiling recognition limits of two-dimensional facial approximations constructed using averages, in M. Marks and J. Clement (eds.), *Computer Graphic Facial Reconstruction*, pp. 199–219. Burlington, MA: Elsevier Academic Press.

Stephan, C. N., Penton-Voak, I. S., Perrett, D. I., Tiddeman, B. P., Clement J. G., and Henneberg, M. 2005. Two-dimensional computer generated average human face morphology and facial approximation, in M. Marks and J. Clement (eds.), *Computer Graphic Facial Reconstruction*, pp. 105–127. Burlington, MA: Elsevier Academic Press.

Stewart, T. D. 1974. Perspectives on some problems of early man common to America and Australia, in A. P. Elkin and N. W. G. Macintosh (eds.), *Grafton Elliot Smith: The Man and His Work*, pp. 14–135. Sydney: Sydney University Press.

Thorne, A. G., and Ross, A. 1986. *The Skeleton Manual*. Sydney: NPWS and Police Aborigine Liaison Unit.

Trotter, M., and Gleser, G. C. 1958. A re-evaluation of estimation based on measurements of stature taken during life and of long bones after death. *American Journal of Physical Anthropology* 16: 79–123.

van Dongen, R. 1963. The shoulder girdle and humerus of the Australian Aborigine. *American Journal of Physical Anthropology* 21: 469–488.

Walker, P. L. 2000. Bioarchaeological ethics: A historical perspective on the value of human remains, in M. A. Katzenberg and S. R. Saunders (eds.), *Biological Anthropology of the Human Skeleton*, pp. 3–40. New York: Wiley Liss.

Webb, S. 1984. Prehistoric Stress in Australian Aborigines. Unpublished Ph.D. thesis, Australian National University, Canberra.

Wood, W., Briggs, C., and Donlon, D. 2002. Forensic osteology, in I. Freckelton and H. Selby (eds.), *Expert Evidence* 3/601–3/802. North Ryde: Thomson Lawbook Co.

Wood, W. B. 1968. An Aboriginal burial ground at Broadbeach Queensland: Skeletal material. *Mankind* 6(12): 681–686.

———. 1993. Forensic osteology, in I. Freckelton and H. Selby (eds.), *Expert Evidence* 3-601–3-797. North Ryde: The Law Book Company Ltd.

———. 1998. Radiographic study of the Broadbeach Aboriginal dentition. *American Journal of Physical Anthropology* 107(2): 211–219.

Wood, W. Q. 1920. The tibia of the Australian Aboriginal. *Journal of Anatomy* 54: 232–257.

Wood-Jones, F. 1931. The non-metrical character of the skull as criteria for racial diagnosis. *Journal of Anatomy* (London) 68: 323–330.

Wright, R. 1996. Uncovering genocide. War crimes: The archaeological evidence. *International Network on Holocaust and Genocide* 11(3): 8–11.

Wright, R., Hanson, I., and Sterenberg, J. 2005. The archaeology of mass graves, in J. Hunter and M. Cox (eds.), *Forensic Archaeology: Advances in Theory and Practice*, pp. 137–158. London: Routledge.

Wright, R. V. S. 1992. Correlation between cranial form and geography in *Homo sapiens*: CRANID— A computer program for forensic and other applications. *Archaeology in Oceania* 27(3): 128–135.

HISTORICAL PERSPECTIVES ON FORENSIC ANTHROPOLOGY IN INDONESIA

Etty Indriati

This chapter first presents the current status of forensic anthropology in Indonesia, including education, and then discusses research and case applications that have contributed to the historical development of this field in that region. These studies reveal low levels of sexual dimorphism in many traits and suggest that traditional methods used for sexing in biological anthropology may not apply to Indonesian remains. Training opportunities in forensic anthropology are outlined, and various forensic anthropological cases in Indonesia are described in order to contribute to the body of knowledge of casework from different parts of the world. The role of forensic anthropology in disaster victim identification (DVI) is discussed in light of the numerous disasters that have affected Indonesia over the last ten years. Indonesian laws affecting human identification and the necessary cooperation between forensic anthropology and forensic pathology, police, forensic odontology, and molecular biology are described. Finally, the future direction of forensic anthropology in Indonesia is considered.

Forensic Anthropology in Indonesia: Current Status

Forensic anthropology covers a wide range of interdisciplinary studies and involves various institutions to implement its theories. Although knowledge in forensic anthropology covers skeletal and dental anatomy and biological sciences in general, the application of forensic anthropology to casework requires the collaboration of law enforcement agencies, dentists, and the local authorities where remains are discovered or exhumed. In Indonesia, this complex relationship is often not supported by sufficient infrastructure, thus limiting the contributions forensic anthropology makes to investigation involving human remains. In 1984, Rathburn and Buikstra (1984: 5) stated that probably very few have heard of forensic physical anthropology. Although this might have been the case 23 years ago in the United States, today forensic anthropology is more widely recognized there. However, this is not the case in Indonesia. A lack of structural organization and funding resources to facilitate having a forensic anthropologist work in the event of disaster, exhumation, or identification of unknown human remains causes underutilization of forensic anthropology. As a result, cases of skeletal remains in Indonesia may not be referred to a forensic anthropologist. However, forensic pathologists and police personnel often consult forensic anthropologists in certain provinces in Indonesia where personal relationships have been built through working on various cases. Thus, in

Indonesia, forensic anthropology is utilized when the contributions that forensic anthropology can make to cases are understood by forensic pathologists, forensic dentists, and police.

Education

Several Indonesian universities offer introductory courses in forensic anthropology to students enrolled in medicine, biology, anthropology, and archaeology courses. In medical faculties, forensic anthropology is taught in conjunction with forensic medicine. Courses in archaeology may include forensic anthropology within the context of excavation techniques of human skeletal remains. In biology and anthropology, forensic anthropology is taught in conjunction with human variation and human evolution. With a small number of forensic anthropologists working in several universities in Indonesia, the development of this field is not optimal, though training and workshops on human identification among interested students are occasionally delivered, especially in conjunction with training in dealing with mass disasters. Thus, forensic anthropology in Indonesia has generally been viewed as assisting with the identification of human skeletal remains, a specific application that requires the teamwork of forensic pathologists, police, forensic odontologists, and molecular biologists. Forensic anthropologists working in universities in Indonesia occasionally examine trophy skulls from remote islands or naturally mummified remains that have emerged from a sandy beach and that turn out to be archaeological remains.

Although viewed as "bone experts," consultations with forensic anthropologists based at universities in Indonesia are not limited to skeletal identification. The forensic anthropologist may also provide opinions on a range of problems associated with identification (see Forensic Anthropology Cases in Indonesia, below). Thus, forensic anthropology in Indonesia would probably be better defined broadly as human individuation utilizing biological anthropological traits in a medico-legal context.

Studies on Human Variation in Indonesia

Individuation can be conducted only when population traits are studied. Western literature has offered a large amount of data and methods of individuation (that is, sexing and aging) using human groups far removed from Indonesia as subjects. As a result, Indonesian human skeletal remains do not always fit the standard criteria for sexing and aging offered in the Western literature. Based on research undertaken by the author, sexing os coxae, for instance, indicates that male and female Indonesians show a low degree of dimorphism (Indriati 2007). Indonesian female and male pelvises overlap in the width of the greater sciatic notch. This is inconsistent with standard Western literature, where males have been described as having wide and females as having narrow greater sciatic notch. The same is true for the subpubic angle; Indonesian male and female subpubic angles both tend to be wide, inconsistent with the narrow subpubic male and wide subpubic female in standard physical anthropological literature. In the skull, Indonesians also tend to have less dimorphism in the morphology of the supra orbital ridge in that males do not always have a pronounced supraorbital ridge. Unlike the low degree of sexual dimorphism in the cranium and the pelvis, there is a higher degree of variation in Indonesian statures. Some villages in Central Java in the remote mountainous regions, for example, have populations with an average stature of 140 cm, whereas city dwellers have an average stature of 165 cm. The diverse array of volcanic and vertical geography might have contributed to the vast human variation.

For example, a study of stature of Indonesian students in Yogyakarta in the 1990s showed that females were 7% shorter than males. This contrasts to studies of other human groups worldwide in which female stature is 3–12% shorter than that of a male (Indriati 2002; Nguyên 1981). The average stature of an Indonesian male student living in Yogyakarta was found to be 165.4 cm and that of a female 153.7 cm (n = 253). Sacral index (sacral width/length) in Indonesians is quite high, reaching 105.6 cm (males) and 108.7 cm (females) (Dewi, Indriati, and Suryadi 2003) and indicates quite low sexual dimorphism of 2.8%. This is in contrast to the sacral indices in other human groups worldwide that are quite dimorphic sexually (Table 10.1). In addition, the superior inlet exhibits inconsistency of shape and does not always fit the Western literature, which portrays the male superior pelvic inlet as more heart-shaped, whereas the female superior pelvic inlet is more rounded. Regardless of sex, the transverse diameter is almost always a bit larger than the anteroposterior diameter, which is in the category of the gynekoid pelvic girdle, typical of the female pelvis (Caldwell and Moloy 1933; Caldwell, Moloy, and D'Esopo 1934). Although

Table 10.1 Sacral indices for males and females from different populations (after Wilder 1920 in Bass 1987).

Population	Male	Female	Sexual Dimorphism
Black	91.4	103.6	11.7%
Egyptian	94.3	99.1	4.8%
Andamanese	94.8	103.4	8.3%
Australians	100.2	110.0	8.9%
Japanese	101.5	107.1	5.2%
Europeans	102.9	112.4	8.4%

the values sometimes overlap between male and female, the greater sciatic notch is a common skeletal trait for identifying sex using the pelvis, and its value is higher in the female, as reported by many workers.[1] The greater sciatic notch averages 525 in males (however, many male greater sciatic notches are close to 606) and 787 in females in Indonesian remains, with a range of 35–673 in males and 70–937 in females (Indriati 2007). Thus, based on Indriati's 2007 study on Indonesian pelvic bones, one can conclude that a greater sciatic notch of 707 or larger indicates a female, and below 707 a male, in an Indonesian population. This greater sciatic notch value is higher than the values documented by Buikstra and Mielke (1985) of approximately 303 and 606 in male and female, respectively.

Indonesians' facial and body shapes and sizes have been studied (Indriati 2004), and the results exhibit no consistent correlations between facial shapes and body types among Javanese (later referred to as simply Indonesian) people. The facial shape is unique and varied, and about 50% is pentagonal both in males and females, followed by elliptic, oval, rhomboid, and round in decreased order of frequency (following the facial shape categories of İşcan 1993). However, some relationships occur between facial and body size. For instance, there is a positive correlation between facial height (crinion to menton) and stature, significant at 95% confidence statistically. This strong correlation can be used to construct formulae for facial height in facial reconstruction, using regression analysis (facial height = 0.068 [stature] + 7.687 ± 3.801 cm).

Indriati's study (2004b) on Indonesian faces, by applying regression analysis, resulted in the development of various formulae to reconstruct facial soft tissue metrically (see also Stephan this volume):

A. To reconstruct eyes,
1. biocular diameter = 7.23 + 0.83 (nose breadth) + 0.86 cm
2. interocular diameter = 1.43 + 0.57 (nose breadth) + 0.68 cm

B. To reconstruct ears,
1. length of ear = 0.018 (stature) + 3.100 ± 1.167 cm
2. ear breadth = 1.88 + 0.26 (lip length) ± 0.43 cm

C. To reconstruct lips,
1. lip length = 2.26 + 0.23 (biocular diameter) + 0.92 cm
2. lip to lip distance = - 0.12 + 0.33 (menton subnasale length) + 0.66 cm
3. philtrum Length = 12.73 – 1.61 (menton to subnasale length) + 1.72 cm

D. To reconstruct nose,
1. nose breadth = 1.50 + 0.22 (biocular diameter) + 0.94 cm
2. nasal root breadth = 0.44 + 0.23 (lip length) + 0.45 cm

Based on George's assessment (1993), although it is impossible to predict the details of the eye, nose, ear, and lips from the skull, one can accurately position these features within and around their bony substrate. This positioning alone may be enough to create the approximation needed for recognition (George 1993). Further results of Indriati's study (2004b) of Indonesian faces noted that, seen laterally, most noses are elevated (in contrast to horizontal or prolapsed), with the tip of the nose higher than the base of alae nasi. This suggests that the shape and the direction of the nasal spine are elevated in the skull. The nasolabial groove tends to be concave among Javanese Indonesians. Most Indonesians have free lobule ears, their ear protrusion is strong, and the horizontal profile of the face is weak. When radiographs and photographs are superimposed, the useful anatomical landmarks are nasal aperture, orbital outlines, right and left gonion, as well as gnathion. The Indonesian facial types are mostly pentagonal (reaching 50%), whereas Caucasian facial outlines are mostly oval, or longer superoinferiorly.

The right and left ectocanthion and labrale inferior form a facial triangle useful to start sketching facial reconstruction. The proportion of orbitonasal shows that the distance between endocanthion is about equal to the distance between alare (alae nasi). The vertical imaginary line cutting the medial iris is the same line of chelion (lateral lip), when pupils look directly forward. Most Indonesians are brachycephalic (short-headed). The distance of the eyes is equal to the width of the eye. In other words, the distance from right to left endocanthion equals that of the ectocanthion-endocanthion. The important superimposition landmarks for facial photograph and radiograph superimposition are right and left gonion and gnathion to reconstruct the lower face; nasal aperture

to reconstruct nasal breadth; gnathion to reconstruct the chin area; orbital bone outline to reconstruct endocanthion and exocanthion of the eyes; zygomatic arch to reconstruct the cheeks; and frontal sinus to reconstruct glabella and thus root of nasal; the second premolars are used to define the length of the lips.

Indriati's study (2004b) of Indonesian faces shows that roentgenographs can be superimposed with photographs in order to evaluate skull and facial structures, when their ratios are 1:1 and both images are taken using Frankfurt Horizontal Plane position. This suggests that ideally, frontal cephalograms should be taken for identification purposes for each individual when applying for a driver's license, passport, or any government related identification card. Because the majority of Indonesians lack medical and dental records, such cephalograms should be nationally archived in order to preserve these data. Shape and volume of frontal sinuses are unique in each individual; thus, having a frontal cephalogram would be useful for future needs of identification (Figure 10.1).

Forensic Anthropological Cases in Indonesia

Indonesian law requires a police request in order for human skeletal remains to be examined. However, in the wake of a disaster, human identification can be done by health workers without a police request. This follows the World Health Organization's doctrine of right to health care (1949) and the declaration of health for all (2000), which were adapted into Indonesian law as the Health Law Number 23 (1992, point 53) (Poernomo 2006). There is also a law regarding human identification in cases involving unnatural death including homicide, suicide, accidents, and disasters, in which autopsies are conducted by a physician as required by law in the *Kitab Undang-Undang Hukum Pidana dan Kitab Undang-Undang Hukum Acara Pidana* (Book of Criminal Law), No. 2, 2002 (Poernomo 2006).

In Indonesia, a forensic anthropologist is usually consulted by a department of forensic medicine or directly by the police department. Human skeletal remains sporadically come into the hands of forensic anthropologists working in universities, which may be from archaeological contexts (e.g., Indriati 2001a) or homicides.

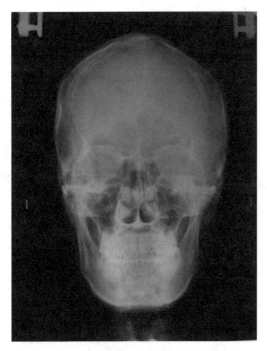

Figure 10.1 Frontal cephalograph of a 22-year-old Indonesian male shows deviation of nasal septi and different size and shape of right and left frontal sinuses useful for individuation.

Although, traditionally, forensic anthropology involves examining human skeletal remains in cases involving questions about identification, the application of forensic anthropology in Indonesia does not limit itself in this type of work.

Seroanthropology using ABO blood groups and dermatoglyphy to determine paternity are also done within the domain of forensic anthropology. Forensic anthropologists may also be involved in the assessment of body parts. For instance, in a suicide bombing, it was shown that body fragmentation patterns were different between the suicide bomber (who usually bodily carries the bomb) and the victims. The blast of the explosion disintegrates the torso and widely scatters the head and extremities of the bomber. In contrast, the fragmentation in victims is more random. Forensic facial identification using superimposition techniques is also undertaken by forensic anthropologists in Indonesia in order to match antemortem photographs and the (sometimes) disfigured head and face resulting from a suicide bombing.

The forensic anthropologist may also be consulted on cases of robbery in which images of the offender captured on a closed-circuit television (CCTV) are compared with the body outline of a possible suspect (Maciej Henneberg, personal communication 2006). The overall body outline comparison is used instead of facial identification, because robbers almost always wear masks. The forensic anthropologist may also be consulted on the use of facial disguises such as fake mustaches, beards, and wigs. In cases such as these, frontal and lateral photographs in Frankfurt horizontal plane must be taken, and attention should be drawn to morphological comparisons of eye slanting, nasal root flatness/protrusion, location of epicanthic fold (if any, whether it is medial, lateral), ear shape, and shape of the superior border of the lips. In addition, the distance between the eyes and overall shape of the head may aid identification in the presence of other facial disguises.

Other examples of skeletal remains that may be analyzed by forensic anthropologists in Indonesia, similar to other parts of the world, include decapitations, aborted fetuses, and archaeological or naturally mummified remains.

Indriati (2003) solved a case of decapitation through individuation in which a body was discovered in a city and a head was discovered in another city a month later. Measurements of particular vertebrae (the seventh cervical—C7—and the first thoracic—T1) resulted in congruency of the head and the body, through less than 1 mm difference in measurements of C7–T1 in 5 variables (Indriati 2000). Despite vertebral congruency, supporting evidence that the remains of the head and the body belonged to the same individual included the age at death (approximately 11–13 years) based on unfused epiphyses on the vertebrae and humerus. The dentition also supported this result. In addition, the estimated stature of this forensic case was 143.22 cm +/- 4.25 cm, applying the formula of (2.68.humeral length x 22.4 cm.) + 88.19. This stature is within the range of 12–13.5 years old in human growth (Boyd 1980).

Fetal remains, typically those associated with abortions during late pregnancy, are not uncommon cases. In the analysis of fetal skeletal remains Fazekas and Kosa (1978) summarize several questions that need to be answered (Table 10.2). Indriati (1999) applied four formulae to identify fetal ages in forensic cases and showed that the best-fit formula for Indonesian fetal remains is the method proposed by Ohtsuki (1977), based on Japanese fetal remains. In the case from Kedu (below), the Ohtsuki method (1977) was the closest fit for the age determination (Indriati 1999), and other Indonesian cases involving the analysis of fetal remains have been consistently resolved using Ohtsuki's method.

The Kedu Case. The author received decomposed remains in a bottle containing 200 cc of 10% formaldehyde from the Police Department of Kedu, Central Java. Examination yielded 72 pieces

Table 10.2 Questions to be considered when analyzing fetal skeletal remains (after Fazekas and Kosa 1978).

1. Are the bones human or animal?
2. If the bones proved to be of fetal origin, what is their lunar age? Do the maturity, body length, and age of the fetus correspond to the gestational age of the suspected human?
3. Could the fetus have been viable at birth, or was it born prematurely, in a nonviable state?
4. Could the fetus have originated from the suspected woman whose pregnancy was terminated in the incriminated way and time?
5. Did the investigation furnish data indicating the circumstances or the possible cause of death?
6. How much time may have elapsed between the interment of the fetus and its discovery?

of bone from one individual. The apparent proportion of the cranial bones to the extremities and the unfused secondary ossification center were used to identify that the bones were human. Four different methods were used to determine the age of the fetal remains. Mehta and Singh's 1972 method resulted in a fetal age of 6–6.5 months; the Ohtsuki method (1977) yielded an age of 6.5–7 months, and Fazekas and Kosa's 1978 method resulted in an age of 6–8 months. The Olivier and Pineau (1957) method yielded an age of 6.5–9.25 months. The postmortem interval might have been short, because soft tissue (including ligamentous attachments) and hair were present. After the written report was submitted, the police reported that the fetus had been removed from the abdomen of a decomposed pregnant woman in the autopsy room. The suspect's boyfriend confessed that the woman had been seven months pregnant and that they had gone to an unskilled abortionist, which led to the death of the girlfriend.

In addition to age determination using bone measurements in fetal remains, forensic anthropologists may also apply dental eruption schedules for age determination in children and adolescents. The decapitation case mentioned earlier had a dental eruption of almost all permanent teeth, except for the third molars, and his permanent canines were partially erupted. A study of permanent tooth eruption in Javanese children aged 12–13 years (n = 175) showed eruption of all permanent teeth except for the third molar. However, 25% of the children had partially erupted upper and lower canines (Indriati 2001b). An age range of 12–13 years was determined for the individual in the decapitated case based on an assessment of the fusion stages of the vertebral corpus and humeral head epiphyses. This result was in accordance with the dental eruption schedule of Javanese children aged 12–13 years.

Disaster Victim Identification in Indonesia and the Roles of Forensic Anthropology

Only a handful of forensic anthropologists practice in Indonesia, and they work mostly in universities. This is unfortunate, since natural and human-made disasters requiring human identification frequently occur in Indonesia (Table 10.3). Earthquakes are common in Indonesia because of its geographic location at the juncture of four active tectonic plates and its position in the Eurasian Circumpacific ring of fire, where hundreds of active volcanoes provide a constant threat of possible eruption. The large and dense nature of Indonesia's population increases the probability of large numbers of deaths in the wake of any earthquake, flood, volcanic eruption, or tsunami. Examples of recent disasters that have severely affected Indonesia include the earthquake in Yogyakarta and Klaten, which rated nearly 6.2 on the Richter scale and resulted in about 6,000 deaths on May 27th, 2006. Also in 2006, an eruption of hot mud in Sidoarjo, eastern Java, associated with fuel-mining activities by the P. T. Lapindo Brantas company, resulted in more than 5,000 people becoming homeless, because houses and agricultural fields were completely covered by hot mud. Toward the end of 2006, two significant accidents occurred. An Adam's airplane crashed near Kalimantan, killing nearly 100 people, and a boat sank off near Banjarnegara, killing more than 400 people. In February 2007, more than five days of floods in Jakarta caused the evacuation of over 156,000 families from their homes, and communal diseases such as diarrhea and itchy skin spread quickly. Again in the month of February, a twister hit Lempuyangan, Yogyakarta, and caused damage to houses and facilities within a heavily populated area. In addition to natural disasters, human-made disasters such as bombings and riots have occurred in recent years (Table 10.3).

The role of forensic anthropology in identifying victims of disaster is not always well understood in Indonesia. In some cases, forensic anthropologists may not be consulted at all, because most disaster victims are not skeletonized, and many people continue to assume that forensic anthropologists deal only with human skeletal remains. However, a recent disaster involving a plane crash that resulted in burnt soft tissue with exposure of the bones highlighted the important role of forensic anthropology for assistance in individuation. On March 7th 2007, a Boeing 737-400 approached Yogyakarta airport for landing too fast and ignited, causing the death of 21 individuals, 16 of whom were Indonesians and 5 who were Australian.

A forensic anthropologist separated the 5 Caucasian from the 16 Mongoloid remains through assessment of skull and dental characteristics and further narrowed down the remains into two female and three male Caucasian and six female and ten male Mongoloid. The assessment of ancestry and sex narrowed down the comparison between postmortem and antemortem data in the reconciliation. Positive identifications were undertaken using dental and medical records. All Mongoloid (Indonesian) remains had been identified and released to the families the day after the disaster. The remains of the five Caucasian (two females and three males) were positively identified

Table 10.3 Disasters in Indonesia 1980–2007 (adapted and modified from Umar 2006).

Disaster	Year
1. Mount Galunggung	1980
2. Food poisoning, west Jakarta	1981
3. Harbor fire, Tanjung Priok, north Jakarta	1981
4. Gas leak, Tanjung Priok, Jakarta	1982
5. Earthquake, west Java	1983
6. Hotel fire, Jakarta	1985
7. Plane crash, Krawang, west Java	1985
8. Toll road crash	1985
9. Flood, Atmajaya hospital, Jakarta	1986
10. Explosion, Fatmawati hospital, Jakarta	1987
11. Train crash, Bintaro, Jakarta	1987
12. Tanjung Priok riots, isolation in Koja hospital, Jakarta	1987
13. Food poisoning, Jakarta's factory	1988
14. Earthquake, Flores	1991
15. Riots, Jakarta	1992
16. Flood, Jakarta	1991–1992
17. Tsunami, Lombok	1993
18. Earthquake, Liwa	1993
19. Mount Merapi eruption, Yogyakarta	1995
20. Earthquake, Kerinci	1995
21. Riots, PDIP political party, Jakarta	1996
22. Earthquake and Tsunami, Biak	1997
23. Earthquake, south Sulawesi	1997
24. Ethnic riots, Pontianak	1997
25. Earthquake, Bengkulu	1997
26. Ethnic riots, Sampit	2001
27. Displaced persons in Madura, Poso, west and east Nusa Tenggara, Papua, west Java, central Java, Maluku, north Sulawesi	2001
28. Drought, Sampang, Borneo	2001
29. Mount Papandayan eruption	2002

Table 10.3   *Continued*

Disaster	Year
30. Train crash, Brebes, central Java	2002
31. Land slide, east Java	2002
32. Flood, north Sumatra	2002
33. Flood, Pekalonogan and Semarang	2002
34. Religious conflicts and riots, Ambon	1999–2002
35. Religious conflicts and riots, Palu, southeast Sulawesi	1999–2002
36. Riots, Papua	1999–2002
37. Terrorist bombing, 32 times, Jakarta	1998–2002
38. Political riots, Jakarta	1998–2002
39. Two weeks flood, Jakarta	2002
40. Displaced migrant workers, Nunukan	2002
41. Terrorist bomb, Bali	2002
42. Terrorist bomb, Marriot Hotel, Jakarta	2003
43. Explosion in Chemical Factory, Gresik, east Java	2004
44. Terrorist bomb, Australian embassy in Jakarta	2004
45. Earthquake, Karang Asem, Bali	2004
46. Earthquake, Nabire, 2 times	2004
47. Earthquake and tsunami, Aceh	2004
48. Earthquake, Palu, southeast of Sulawesi	2004
49. Drought, east Nusa Tenggara	2005
50. Earthquake, west Java	2005
51. Landslide in trash dump, Bandung	2005
52. Earthquake, Nias and Simulue	2005
53. Train crash, Tg Barat, Jakarta	2005
54. Mandala air crash, Medan	2005
55. Bomb, Bali	2005
56. Budi Asih hospital, Jakarta	2005
57. Earthquake of 6.2 richter scale, Yogyakarta and Klaten (600 deaths)	2006
58. Hot muds covering hundreds of kilometers area in Sidoarjo	2006
59. Air crash, Adam's Air, near Kalimantan (100 deaths)	2006
60. Boat sank, Senopati, Banjarnegara (400 deaths)	2006
61. A week of big floods, affecting most of central Jakarta	2007
62. Twister, Lempuyangan Yogyakarta	2007
63. Air crash, Garuda Indonesian Airlines, Yogyakarta	2007

on the third day postdisaster following the delivery of antemortem data brought by the Australian authorities.

Indonesia, with 18,000 islands and more than 250 languages spoken by 215 million inhabitants, continues to increase in population. Because Indonesia is made up of provinces, government-coordinated relief efforts and organized handling of dead bodies are difficult. With vast islands and unevenly distributed habitations around the country and merely 62 years of independence, Indonesia has struggled not only in its infrastructure, economic, and sociopolitical development but also in managing its resources, particularly with the recent decentralization of provinces from Jakarta. In various governmental institutions, a disaster unit is present, but each is incomplete in terms of its human and capital resources. An organization appointed by the central government *Bakornas (Badan Koordinasi Nasional-National Coordination Body)* was formed in 2000 as an institution responsible for coordinating relief efforts in the wake of disasters. In addition, the Department of Health and the national Police signed a memorandum of understanding to work together and formed the National Team of Disaster Victim Identification, divided into four teams covering 27 provinces. However, the lack of funding and interdepartmental and interprovincial human resources does not always enable forensic anthropologists to work together as a team on site where human remains are recovered.

As discussed above, taking a frontal cephalograph is suggested as a possible tool to assist identification in the future. The cephalographs would ideally be stored centrally rather than locally. The victims of the December 2004 tsunami who were killed while taking a vacation in Thailand could have their medical and dental records retrieved from their home countries for identification purposes, but this was not possible for the tsunami victims in Aceh (see Black this volume). In addition to few people having medical or dental records in Aceh, 75% of the region was damaged, and the majority (140,000, or 75%) of the population died as a result of the event. This vast area of damage highlights the effects of not having medical records preserved locally. Clearly, there is more work to be done in enhancing the roles of forensic anthropologists both in disaster victim identification and other areas where identification is required, as well as in addressing concerns regarding appropriate infrastructure and funding. Emergency financial support during the acute phase may be drawn from regional governments at the province level, central government, national police

and health department, and later on from various other resources.

Forensic Anthropology in Indonesia: Future Directions

Though merely a handful of forensic anthropologists are available in Indonesia, a wide range of identification cases not limited to skeletal remains have been conducted. Sporadic interest from students to pursue forensic anthropology as a career and the unavailability of positions after graduation make the development of forensic anthropology in Indonesia a difficult task. Team work and close collaboration among academics, physicians, and police and health personnel are necessary to carry out human identification following death resulting from crimes and/or disasters. Although efforts toward that direction have begun to emerge through various DVI workshops and seminars, no formal supporting infrastructure and organizational networking with administrative and funding support from the government have been developed. The formation of the national DVI team needs to be followed up with adequate recruitment of forensic anthropologists, forensic odontologists, molecular biologists, and forensic pathologists in each region. Adequate funding from an established source should be available for operational costs ideally supported by local and central governments for handling work in human identification.

Though Reichs (1986) defines forensic anthropology as the identification of human skeletal remains within a legal context, forensic anthropology should not limit its identification scope merely to skeletal remains, since various identification modes emerge through cases such as paternity, facial matches of old and new photographs, facial disguise, CCTV whole-body outline, and body fragmentation in suicide bombings. For this reason, the definition of forensic anthropology should be placed in a broader context, such as human identification and individuation in medico-legal situations utilizing biological traits that are not restricted to human remains or human skeletal remains. Because identification cases are sporadic and do not follow a continuous predictable event, there appears to be no need for the forensic anthropology practitioner in Indonesia to be certified as yet. Many cases are consulted informally and confidentially, and some cases turn out to be archaeological remains. Ideally, forensic anthropologists, forensic pathologists, and forensic odontologists as well as molecular biologists, law enforcement agencies, and local governments should work hand in hand. Such collaboration would allow authorities to see improved results in human identification in both domestic and disaster situations.

Acknowledgments

I thank Dr. Soren Blau and Dr. Douglas Ubelaker for the invitation to write this chapter and the anonymous reviewers for their comments, which helped to improve this paper. Thanks also to my forensic pathological colleagues, Dr. Hastri, Dr. Purnomo, Dr. Agung, Dr. Oktavinda, Dr. Eddy, Dr. Musadeq, Dr. Peter, Dr. Alphons, Dr. Surjit, Dr. Lipur, Dr. Mukhlis, and Dr. Yoni, of various institutions in the Mabes Polri, Polda Metro Jaya, Polda Jateng, Polda Jatim, UGM, Unpad, Unair, UI, and the Indonesian DVI team for their discussions during our sporadic reunions. My thanks also go to my medical students in the international program at UGM, who have been working with me on various research projects related to human identification.

Note

1. Bass 1987; Buikstra and Mielke 1985; Buikstra and Ubelaker 1994; Indriati 2004a; Krogman 1962; Krogman and İşcan 1986; Olivier 1969; Phenice 1969; Ubelaker 1991.

References

Bass, W. M. 1987. *Human Osteology: A Laboratory and Field Manual* (3rd ed.). Columbus, MO: Missouri Archaeological Society.

Boyd, E. 1980. *Origins of the Study of Human Growth*. Portland: University of Oregon Health Sciences Center Foundation.

Buikstra, J. E., and Mielke, J. H. 1985. Demography, diet and health, in R. I. Gilbert and J. H. Mielke (eds.), *The Analysis of Prehistoric Diets*, pp. 359–422. New York: Academic Press.

Buikstra, J. E., and Ubelaker, D. H. 1994. *Standards for Data Collection from Human Skeletal Remains*. Fayetville: Arkansas Archaeological Survey Research.

Caldwell, W. E., and Moloy, H. C. 1933. Anatomical variations in the female pelvis and their effect in labor with a suggested classification. *American Journal of Obstetrics and Gynecology* 26: 479–505.

Caldwell, W. E., Moloy, H. C., and D'Esopo, D. A. 1934. Further studies on the pelvic architecture. *American Journal of Obstetric Gynecology* 28: 482–492.

Dewi, A., Indriati, E., and Suryadi, E. 2003. *Dimorfisme seksual sacrum pada rangka di Laboratorium Anatomi Fakultas Kedokteran Universitas Gadjah Mada. Indeks sacra dan sudut midlateral sacral.* Sexual dimorphism of the sacrum on skeletal remains housed at the Laboratory of Anatomy, Embryology, and Anthropology. B. I. Ked. 35(1): 23–29.

Fazekas, I. Gy., and Kosa, F. 1978. *Forensic Fetal Osteology*. Budapest: Akademiai Kiado.

George, R. M. 1993. Anatomical and artistic guidelines for forensic facial reconstruction, in M. Y. İşcan and R. P. Helmer (eds.), *Forensic Analysis of the Skull: Craniofacial Analysis, Reconstruction, and Identification*, pp. 229–246. New York: Wiley-Liss.

Indriati, E. 1999. The roles of forensic anthropology in fetal death investigation. *Berkala Ilmu Kedokteran* 31(3): 181–187.

———. 2000. Individuation in decapitation through vertebral congruence (*Penentuan individu pada penggal kepala dengan kongruensi vertebra*). *Berkala Ilmu Kedokteran* 32(3): 147–154.

———. 2001a. Human skeletal remains from a bronze kettledrum: Prehistoric Indonesia. Paper presented at the Australasian Society for Human Biology, Sydney, December 10–14.

———. 2001b. Permanent tooth eruption in Javanese Children. *Berkala Ilmu Kedokteran* 33(4): 237–248.

———. 2002. Stature in Yogyakarta's student and prehistoric Balinese circa 1,000 A.C. *Berkala Ilmu Kedokteran* 34(1): 1–7.

———. 2003. (*Individuasi pada penggal kepala dengan skaning vertebra C7-T1*). Individuation in decapitation by C7-T1 vertebral scanning. *Berkala Ilmu Kedokteran* 35(3): 143–149.

———. 2004a. *Antropologi Forensik. Identifikasi Rangka Manusia dalam Konteks Hukum.* Yogyakarta: Gadjah Mada University Press.

———. 2004b. Human faces: Facial profile and metric for individuation in forensic anthropology. Unpublished research report funded by Gadjah Mada University Society, Faculty of Medicine, Yogyakarta.

———. 2007. Sexual dimorphism of the pelvic girdle: Pelvimetry and pelvic types in Javanese skeletal remains. *Berkala Ilmu Kedokteran* 39(1): 14–22.

İşcan, M. Y. 1993. Introduction of techniques for photographic comparison: Potential and problems, in M. Y. İşcan and R. P. Helmer (eds.), *Forensic Analysis of the Skull: Craniofacial Analysis, Reconstruction, and Identification*, pp. 57–70. New York: Wiley-Liss.

Krogman, W. M. 1962. *The Human Skeleton in Forensic Medicine.* Springfield, IL: Charles C. Thomas.

Krogman, W. M., and İşcan, M. Y. 1986. *The Human Skeleton in Forensic Medicine* (2nd ed.). Springfield, IL: Charles C. Thomas.

Mehta, L., and Singh, H. M. 1972. Determination of crown-rump length from fetal long bones: Humerus and femur. *American Journal of Physical Anthropology* 36: 165–168.

Nguyên-Thi-Ánh-Tuyé't. 1981. Body height and weight in two rural groups of Indonesians on Java. *Berkala Bioanthropologi Indonesia* II(2): 47–92.

Ohtsuki, F. 1977. Developmental changes of the cranial bone thickness in the human fetal period. *American Journal of Physical Anthropology* 46: 141–154.

Olivier, G. 1969. *Practical Anthropology.* Springfield, IL: Charles C. Thomas.

Olivier, G., and Pinneau, H. 1957. Comparison entre les mensurations sur le squellete et sur le vivant. *Revue Anthropologique* 3: 1–16.

Phenice, T. W. 1969. A newly developed visual method of sexing the os pubis. *American Journal of Physical Anthropology* 30: 297–302.

Poernomo, S. 2006. Pengalaman dalam pelaksanaan DVI pada bencana massal di Indonesia. Paper presented at the DVI workshop, Monash University, Padjajaran University and Indonesian National Police. November 27th, Bandung.

Rathburn, T. A., and Buikstra, J. E. 1984. The role of the forensic anthropologist, in T. A. Rathburn and J. E. Buikstra (eds.), *Human Identification*, pp. 5–14. Springfield, IL: Charles C. Thomas.

Reichs, K. J. 1986. Introduction, in K. J. Reichs (ed.), *Forensic Osteology: Advances in the Identification of Human Remains*, pp. xv–xxxi. Springfield, IL: Charles C. Thomas.

Ubelaker, D. H. 1991. *Human Skeletal Remains* (2nd ed.). Washington, D.C.: Taraxacum.

Umar, R. D. 2006. *Kebijakan Depkes dalam sistem penanggulangan bencana gawat darurat terpadu.* DVI workshop, Monash University, Padjajaran University and Indonesian National Police. November 27th, Bandung.

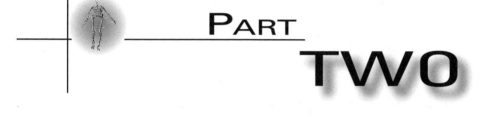

PART
TWO

FORENSIC ARCHAEOLOGY

11

THE SEARCH FOR AND DETECTION OF HUMAN REMAINS

Thomas D. Holland and Samuel V. Connell

Forensic human skeletal analysis frequently begins in the dirt. The systematic recovery, to include the complete documentation of "archaeological" contexts, is every bit as critical to the successful identification of the remains as are the remains themselves. This fact tends to be overlooked by physical anthropologists operating in academic environments concerned with humans at the population level, as well as researchers trained on museum collections and other curated resources for which the source and recovery context of the material being analyzed is either unimportant or may not be fully (or accurately) documented. It goes without saying, therefore, that any training regimen in forensic anthropology and forensic archaeology should begin with a thorough understanding of methods for locating buried human remains.

When Alfred Kroeber (1916: 20) said that "the proof is in the spade," he was simply articulating the fundamental weakness of archaeology as a science—namely, the difficulty in reconciling academic models with a prehistoric past to any degree of certainty. Only through careful and systematic excavations, Kroeber argued, was there hope of establishing a verifiable nexus between the past and the present.

Humans have in fact been recovering the remnants of the past for centuries. What sets archaeology apart from the casual collection of cultural detritus, however, is the systematic manner in which it is pursued, at least when it is done well. Indeed, British archaeologist Sir Mortimer Wheeler said, "the excavator without an intelligent policy may be described as an archaeological food-gatherer, master of skill, perhaps, but not creative in the wider terms of constructive science" (1956: 152).

The value of archaeologists in the realm of forensics can be categorized colloquially into two broad contributions: (1) archaeologists are good at systematically finding things that are buried; and (2) they are good at systematically recovering what they find. The latter contribution will be discussed in detail in Chapter 12 (Cheetham and Hanson this volume) and will be discussed here only to the extent that it overlaps with the topic of human remains location.

Traditional Methods

Buried human remains (such as those commonly of interest to forensic anthropologists and forensic archaeologists) typically are found either through accident (for example, construction activities, erosion, and so on) or through the recognition of surface indicators during an intentional search. The basic techniques of intentional searches have remained the same for the last several hundred years, and, more recently, new techniques involving remote sensing have been developed. In the United States, archaeological work often is characterized by three phases: survey, testing, and recovery. The phase system is well suited to traditional archaeological projects where multiple sources of funding and multiyear recovery schedules are often in place. In contrast, however, the phase system often applies poorly to forensic recoveries where time, budget constraints, and legal urgency may not allow for the individual phases to be kept discrete and may require that the process be compressed into a single recovery effort. Nevertheless, it is conceptually useful to consider the search for buried human remains within the traditional phase concept.

Traditional Survey Methods

Traditional survey involves the systematic inspection of a large surface area, often hundreds of square meters or even square kilometers, for the presence of surface indicators of subsurface features. Historically, surveys have relied on one or more of the five senses, principally sight, touch, and smell, employed unaided. For buried remains, the survey is most commonly made on foot, although wheeled vehicles or even aircraft

might be employed under certain circumstances. For example, during our search for missing service members in Southeast Asia, helicopters have been utilized to interpret altered topography. As an extension, aerial photography might also be used, especially in situations involving vast areas or hostile or relatively inaccessible terrain, but, in any case, the underlying principle remains the same: the detection and recognition of surface indicators that past experience has demonstrated are correlated to some degree with the subsurface presence of human remains.

A typical pedestrian survey involves the searchers walking a circumscribed area in a systematic fashion, such as a "skirmish" line or linear transects spaced at regular intervals (Figure 11.1). Various search patterns can be employed—for example, S-shapes, zigzags, and/or spirals. The "pattern" of the search is not as important as is the completeness. The distance between two transects is site- and context-specific and may be dictated by physical constraints such as topography and vegetation. A 2–3-meter interval works well in most cases; however, in flat terrain and/or low vegetation, wider intervals might be employed, provided that they allow the searchers to readily identify common surface indicators of buried remains. When indicators are encountered, such as disturbances in the soil,

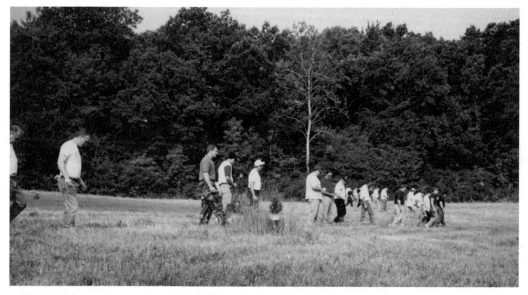

Figure 11.1 Typical pedestrian surface surveys involve searchers systematically walking the suspected burial area while noting indicators of possible buried remains. Parallel transects, spaced at 2–3-meter intervals, work well under most conditions. Common surface indicators of a burial include mounded earth; depressions; areas of increased or unusual plant, animal, or insect activity; differential moisture retention; and inexplicable changes in the floral community.

clothing, or remains appearing to be human in nature, the searchers should mark the area with survey flags, survey tape, or some other means, and continue the search. At the completion of the survey, marked areas of interest can be revisited, and the indicators that were marked can be reevaluated within the context of all the marked areas within the search area.

Surface indicators of buried remains typically reflect physical and chemical changes to the surface as the result of a burial pit being dug. For example, human burials often can be detected by the presence of either a mound, usually associated with more recent inhumations, or a depression, resulting from settling and compaction of the burial pit over time (Morse, Duncan, and Stoutamire 1983; also Killam 1990). With interments involving humans, a secondary slump near the center of the pit depression may result from the collapse of the thoracic cavity over time. In addition, physical alteration of the surface may lead to drying cracks around the perimeter of the burial pit as the result of differential moisture retention between the fill and the surrounding soil matrix. The vegetation may also show differences as weed pioneers colonize the newly disturbed soil. These pioneers often are replaced with a succession of plant species that may differ markedly from the established

floral regime in the general area. Chemically, the soil in the burial pit is enriched by the decomposition of the body and the aeration of the soil during the inhumation process and typically manifests in a darkened or stained soil that may be visible on, or near, the ground surface. This chemical change, combined with the physical change, has the effect of creating a small, self-sustaining system whereby the richer, looser pit fill traps and holds more moisture that encourages animal, insect, and plant activity, which further aerates and enriches the soil. The results of this self-sustaining system often remain visible as soil stains hundreds or thousands of years later (Figure 11.2).

In situations involving incidental inhumations, such as burials in mudslides or resulting from floods and other natural events, some physical changes may not be readily recognizable. Similarly, in cases where remains are deposited on the surface and become covered by sediment built up over time, there will be no evidence of a burial pit or unnatural disturbance to the soil.

Another survey approach for forensic cases is the use of a cadaver dog. Cadaver dogs are trained to detect the odor of decomposing human remains, ignoring other animal remains, and alert their handlers to their location (Rebmann, Koenig, and David 2000). They can locate remains scattered on

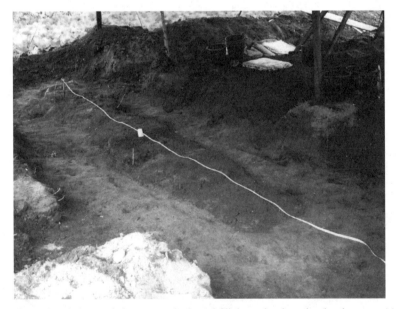

Figure 11.2   Physical and chemical changes to the burial fill, brought about by the decomposition of human remains and the aeration of the soil during inhumation, often are manifested as burial "stains." Burial stains, such as the one demarcating a mass grave in North Korea dating to circa 1950, may persist for hundreds or thousands of years.

the surface or buried shallowly below it and are particularly useful when a search area is loosely defined but too large for a pedestrian search.

The purpose of traditional survey methods is to narrow down a large search area to a manageable number of smaller areas of interest that can then be subjected to a more thorough examination. Consequently, a good survey should be reductive without excluding any reasonable feature of forensic interest.

Testing

Testing seeks to take the reduced set of interest points and reduce them further, with the goal of identifying a specific location for full-scale excavation and recovery. Like the survey, testing typically involves the use of one or more of the human senses, but unlike the survey, the purpose of testing is to extend the range of those senses below the ground surface. Subsurface indicators of a burial mirror many of those found on the surface. They also include features such as buried organic material, which is surface vegetation that is incorporated into a subsurface context as the result of digging and back-filling a pit, and inverse stratigraphy, which is the disruption and disarrangement of normal soil layers as the result of back-filling activities.

Testing actually constitutes the initial examination, commonly called "ground-truthing," of the areas of interest identified through the survey. Unlike the relatively large areas encompassed by the survey, testing is limited to smaller, well-circumscribed areas. A wide variety of procedures fall under the definition of testing. Many of these— for example, pH analysis of the soil, organic-content analysis of the soil, and gas detection—are not discussed here, because they are less frequently used, harder to interpret, and tend to be more time consuming. Instead, the focus is on the more traditional methods of subsurface testing: probing, coring, and limited excavation.

Probing. Probing is the least technical of the traditional subsurface testing procedures, but it is fast and inexpensive to accomplish. It involves the use of a metal probe, commonly 1–2 m in length, which is inserted into the ground for the purpose of assessing soil compaction (Figure 11.3). As with all the survey and testing procedures, probing is best accomplished in a systematic fashion, with probe insertions being made at regular intervals (for example, 20 cm) along a transect that initiates and terminates on either side of the suspected burial location. By beginning and ending outside the suspected pit location, one can readily detect the relative compaction of the natural soil matrix as opposed to (generally looser) burial fill. Since the insertion of a probe can be damaging to any human remains or other fragile evidence encountered, it is the detection of the burial fill—not the detection of buried remains themselves—that is the goal. The

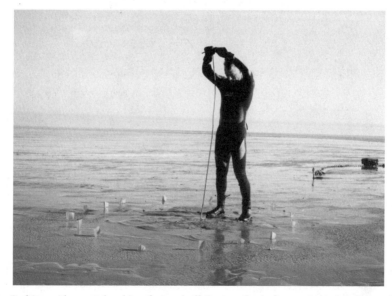

Figure 11.3 Probing with a metal rod is a fast and efficient method of assessing subsurface soil compaction. By probing in a systematic fashion, one can readily detect differences between loose burial fill and the more compact surrounding soil matrix.

depth of insertion should be sufficient to detect differences in soil compaction but should not be so deep as to run the risk of damaging any buried evidence. Often several parallel or perpendicular transects may be required to adequately assess the area under consideration.

Coring. Coring is similar to probing in that it involves the insertion of a metal coring tube into the soil, but unlike a solid probe, the soil corer has a metal tube attached to the end. (Augur coring devices, which effectively "drill" a hole into the ground, are not recommended in forensic cases due to the high potential for significant damage to any buried remains encountered). When the coring tube is inserted into the soil and then removed, it brings with it a cylindrical plug, or core, of soil (Figure 11.4). By removing and examining cores of subsurface soil along a transect that initiates and terminates on either side of the suspected burial location, one can infer the actual stratigraphy. In addition, the soil cores may be examined for other burial related features and materials such as buried organics or even possible fragments of human remains or clothing.

Soils tend to be arranged in distinct, orderly layers called *horizon*s. Intrusive pits such as burials effectively mix or invert the stratigraphic components when they refill. In addition, surface organic material (for example, leaves, grass, twigs) may incidentally become buried in the process.

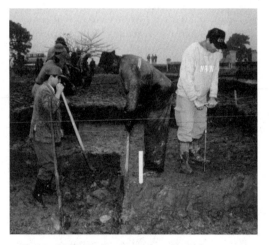

Figure 11.4 Coring is similar to probing except that it allows the actual examination of small plugs of subsurface soil. The archaeologist shown surveying a Vietnam War era aircraft crash in northern Vietnam was able to determine the subsurface distribution of the 30-year-old wreckage field by noting the presence or absence of residual jet fuel trapped in the clay soil.

The detection of these mixed or inverted stratigraphic elements and buried organics in a soil plug removed during coring is an indication only that a subsurface disturbance is present and that additional work is required to determine the nature of the disturbance.

Limited Excavation. Limited excavation is the most intuitive means of subsurface testing in that it involves actually digging holes. Indeed, the dividing line between testing and recovery often is difficult to discern, and in many forensic cases the former evolves seamlessly into the latter with no clear procedural demarcation. Testing, however, is really a continuation of the systematic procedure that began with the identification of possible surface indicators. The function of testing is to further narrow down the area of interest so that recovery resources can be applied more efficiently. Limited excavation can be categorized into three broad techniques: shovel testing, trenching, and limited block excavation.

- *Shovel testing*: Shovel testing is the quickest, least expensive, and least rigorous of the limited excavation techniques. It involves the excavation of small holes, often the width and depth of a shovel blade, for purpose of examining a larger area of subsurface soil than can be achieved with a soil corer. As with probing or coring, shovel testing is best accomplished in a systematic fashion, with the tests applied along transects that begin and end outside the suspected burial area in order to establish a basis of comparison between the native soil context and the possible burial fill.

- *Trenching*: Trenching, both manually and with heavy equipment (such as a backhoe), is also a quick and efficient means to examine the subsurface for possible indicators of a burial; however, considerably more care must be exercised to avoid destroying the context and material evidence associated with any burial encountered. As with the other methods, the key to successful trenching is to accomplish it in a systematic fashion. Instead of probe holes or shovel tests placed at discrete points along one or more transects, trenching is effectively the removal of the uppermost soil layers along the entire transect. To achieve maximum coverage of the suspected burial area, parallel trenches should be spaced no farther apart than the minimum suspected width of the burial pit. Depending on

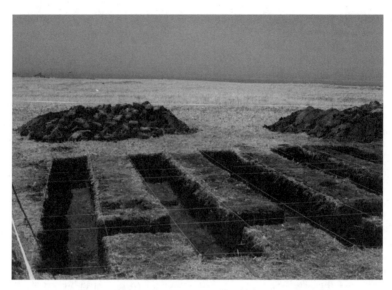

Figure 11.5 Systematically excavated trenches, and parallel cross-trenches, are an effective means to examine large areas of subsurface soil. The burial location of a U.S. Air Force RB-29 crewman, shot down over Yuri Island, Russia, in 1959, was readily identified using well-placed trenches that exposed the outline of the burial pit intruding into the undisturbed subsurface soil matrix.

the nature of the underlying soil strata, cross-trenches running perpendicular to the initial set of parallel trenches may be required (Figure 11.5).

- *Limited Block Excavation*: Limited block excavation is effective when the suspected burial area is relatively small and circumscribed and can be undertaken either by hand or with the aid of a mechanical excavator. As with the typical block excavation of traditional archaeological excavation, limited block excavation can be an effective means of systematically exposing subsurface indicators of intrusive activities. Just as with the spacing of cross-trenches, the size and the placement of excavation blocks should be suited to the size and the configuration of the suspected burial area. Often, block excavation follows directly from trenching when the latter reveals subsurface anomalies that require further investigation (Figure 11.6).

Regardless of the testing method employed, the goal remains the same: to expose the underlying soil strata for the purpose of detecting disturbances related to intrusive activities such as the digging of a burial pit. Once such areas are detected, they can be evaluated, and recovery resources can be applied effectively.

Remote Sensing

In addition to the more traditional testing measures, numerous geophysical studies (Bevan 1998; Cheetham 2005; Clark 1996; Conyers 2004; Wiseman and El-Baz 2007) have documented the ability of geophysical instrumentation to detect and map near-surface features without the removal of the uppermost soil strata, and thus expand the archaeologist's ability to detect burial contexts beyond that limited by the traditional use of the five human senses. A clear benefit to remote sensing is that, as its name implies, it is remote and therefore non-, or at least minimally, intrusive. This can be important when searches must be conducted in areas of cultural, ethnic, or political sensitivities.

Remote sensing technologies should not be misinterpreted as "bone-finders." All remote sensing techniques function by detecting differences between two or more media, usually different soil strata. In practical terms, this means that if there is uniform underground soil composition, or if the soil composition exhibits a patterned distribution (for example, discernable strata), then remote sensing techniques can document any intrusive features as *anomalies*. In these cases, the analyst is relying on the remote sensing equipment to isolate stratigraphic differences that do not exhibit the same pattern as the subsurface surroundings do. Historically these disturbances were detected

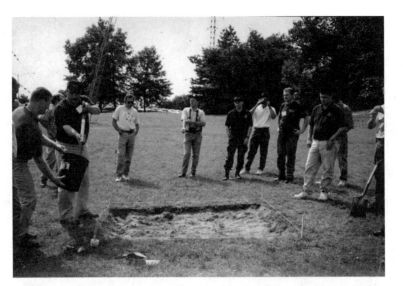

Figure 11.6 Limited block excavation as a testing procedure has the advantage of easily leading directly into full-scale recovery. The key is to systematically remove only the uppermost soil layers in order to expose evidence of intrusive pits.

only through the traditional survey and testing techniques outlined above (or through accidental exposure), but under the right geomorphological conditions, geophysical instruments may be able to detect and resolve differences in subsurface composition and pattern without recourse to soil removal (Clark 1996; Conyers 2006). How these differences are made manifest, however, varies depending on the material in question, the surrounding environment, and the equipment being used.

Many detailed treatments of geophysical instrumentation can be found (Bevan 1998; Cheetham 2005; Clark 1996; Conyers 2004), including those dealing specifically with forensic archaeological work (Buck 2003; Dupras et al. 2006). The main points to understand are that the geophysical principles used by each piece of equipment are different in their application and that context-specific background knowledge about the recovery locations is a critical presurvey step. Because of the complexity of this equipment, geophysical experts are increasingly, although perhaps not yet commonly, being called on to consult in finding the location of interments in historical cemeteries (Conyers 2006). Three different but widely used remote sensing technologies are outlined below: the soil resistivity meter, the cesium magnetometer, and the ground-penetrating radar (GPR).

Soil Resistivity. The remote sensing technique of soil resistivity is based on the demonstrated tendency of soil to differentially resist (or conduct) electrical currents. The resistivity of a given soil matrix depends on a number of factors, including the structure and the morphology of the soil and its water and ion content. The presence of impermeable constituents in the soil, such as volcanic rock, or more permeable soil structures, such as features excavated into the sterile horizon, will also alter the flow of electricity through the ground (Clark 1996: 27–63). By passing a known current through a circumscribed section of a suspected burial site, variations in current, which are read using a resistivity meter, can be used to infer the presence of natural and cultural subsurface anomalies. Disturbances in the soil that result from soil compaction (for example, floors, paths) or loosening (for instance, burials) can be detected during resistivity surveys, although burial pits often constitute relatively "small" anomalies within the range of potential subsurface disturbances. Complications can also arise when the soil in the survey area has been disbursed by modern building and agriculture (Bevan 1996: 72–73), or where other sources of electrical current, such as underground cables, are present.

The resistivity meter is commonly employed using steel or copper-clad electrodes (Figure 11.7). As a general rule, the distance between the electrode poles is roughly the depth below the ground surface that the equipment will measure. As with the traditional survey techniques of probing, coring,

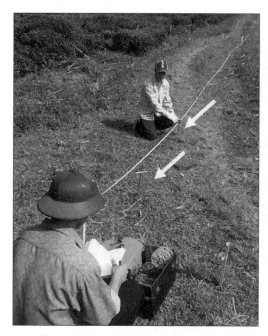

Figure 11.7 Soil resistivity testing can be accomplished with minimal equipment. A resistivity survey of a site in Vietnam illustrates readings being taken along transects with the electrodes (arrows) spaced at 2-m intervals.

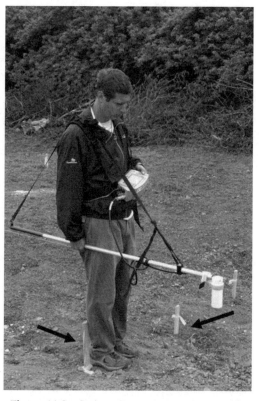

Figure 11.8 Cesium magnetometers are portable and readily usable by single investigators. Note that the readings are being taken at 1-m intervals marked by wooden stakes.

and trenching, resistivity readings should be taken along transects that begin and end outside the suspected burial area for the purpose of establishing baseline values. Readings may be imported into a database and plotted using commercially available graphing software, or by hand onto a contour density map.

Magnetometry. Burials often can be detected by analyzing changes in the magnetic field in a given area. Magnetometers are devices which measure field variations in the earth's magnetosphere. The metal detector is the most common means of conducting magnetic surveys and detects local spikes in an induced electric field. Owing to their ubiquity and intuitive nature of their use, metal detectors will not be discussed here. There are several types of magnetometers, FLUXGATE and CESIUM GRADIOMETERS being among the most common in archaeology. In recent years, cesium-vapor magnetometers (a type of alkali-vapor magnetometer) have come to be the dominate type used by forensic anthropologists owing to their sensitivity and speed of use. Cesium-vapor magnetometers use a photon emitter and a cesium-vapor chamber to detect energy quanta, specifically energy quanta related to anomalies in the earth's magnetic field at any given point on the ground surface.

Subsurface magnetic anomalies can result from subsurface inclusions (especially metal objects) or from changes in the magnetic polarity of individual soil particles that result when soil is disturbed or mixed. One-person hand-carried cesium-vapor magnetometers are available (Figure 11.8), and the actual survey consists of systematically walking over the suspected burial site and surrounding area to detect local variations in the magnetic field. As with all of the survey procedures, magnetic data should be collected in a systematic fashion, such as along transects or a discrete grid nodes. Data can be collected in continuous mode and downloaded to commercially available postprocessing software for analysis. Most magnetic-field gradient surveys can also be performed in the same grid established for the soil resistivity assays and researchers may find it cost effective to simultaneously conduct two or more types of remote sensing surveys on a site, although level grassy environments are ideal for magnetic data collection (Clark 1996: 114). As with soil resistivity data, magnetometer data may be rendered as contour density maps.

Unlike soil resistivity meters, magnetometers are largely unaffected by differentials in the retention of moisture in soil (Bevan 1983: 50; Clark 1996: 64–98). However, there are a number of potential obstacles to conducting a magnetic survey in an alleged burial area. For example, in more populated areas, purported burial sites may be contaminated with sources of modern magnetic surface interference such as electrical wires, underground pipes, and non-incident-related metal surface objects. One way to mitigate this problem is to conduct a metal-detector survey prior to the magnetometer survey to detect and, when possible, to remove all metal objects found at or near the ground surface. In addition, the underlying magnetization of bedrock material, called *thermoremnant magnetization*, may make magnetic surveying of an area impossible (Scollar 1965), particularly when the underlying magnetization of bedrock material in the study area overwhelms subtle gradients triggered by cultural anomalies (Dorbin and Savit 1988: 651). In these difficult cases, carefully measuring the magnetic susceptibility of the near-surface soil deposits may be more productive (Clark 1996: 116). There is also the factor of solar diurnal variation in the earth's magnetic field which alters readings over the course of a day, a problem that is mitigated by continually standardizing the readings using a control point outside the area being surveyed or, in smaller areas, by simply completing the survey quickly.

Ground-Penetrating Radar (GPR). Ground-penetrating radar (sometimes known as subsurface interface radar, or SIR) operates by directing a short, controlled, electromagnetic pulse into the ground and then measuring the time required for the pulse to be reflected back to a radio receiver. Since the signal's propagation time is a constant, any variation in the time required for the signal to leave the radio transducer and be reflected back to the receiver is a function of the depth and the density of objects that the pulse encounters as it passes through the ground (Conyers 2004; Conyers and Goodman 1997; Vaughan 1986). It follows that GPR surveys work best when the underlying soil strata are relatively uniform and the subsurface anomalies occur abruptly, meaning that intrusive features such as burials are readily apparent (Conyers 2006) (Figure 11.9).

Earlier GPR systems involved numerous pieces of heavy equipment and employed ground-contact transducer sleds that often required extensive site preparation to ensure a relatively smooth ground surface on which to drag the sled. The amount and the nature of the equipment limited the usability of GPR in many search locations and conditions. Also, failure to properly prepare the ground surface prior to conducting the survey often resulted in numerous data-acquisition errors. Modern systems can now be mounted on a wheeled cart capable of transiting uneven terrain without introducing significant data-acquisition errors. In addition, the cart can be equipped with a survey wheel that measures distance traveled over the survey area (Figure 11.10), thus facilitating accurate and systematic coverage of

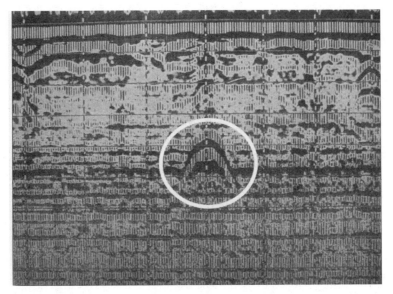

Figure 11.9 Ground-penetrating radar data showing the relatively uniform horizontal bands representing undisturbed soil strata and the characteristic hyperbolic "echo" (white circle) of a burial.

the survey area. Most of the modern GPR systems allow collected data to be viewed in real time as each line scan is produced as well as allowing the data to be uploaded to post-processing software. Different radar transducers, or antennae, capable of generating different frequency signals (for example, 400 MHz and 900 MHz) are available. The choice of antenna is dictated by the geomorphology at the site and the nature and depth of the target to be detected. Lower frequency antennae, for example, send relatively longer waves into the ground that generally provide deeper penetration, but with lower resolution. Conversely, higher frequency antennae typically sacrifice sensing depth for greater resolution. The 400-MHz antenna generally provides good resolution to a depth of 3.0 to 4.0 m, whereas the 900-MHz antenna is useful to approximately 1.0 m. It should be emphasized, however, that local conditions, such as moisture content, often dictate actual penetration depths.

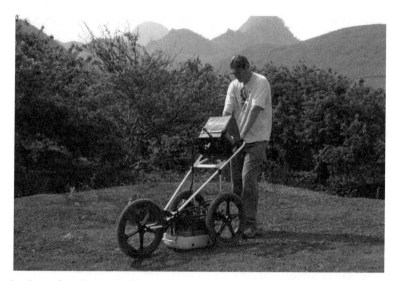

Figure 11.10   Ground-penetrating radar equipment is increasingly becoming more portable. Many of the devices now are cart-mounted and can be used with minimal ground-surface preparation.

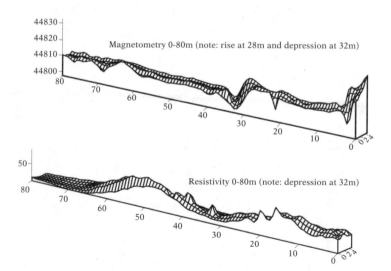

Figure 11.11   The combination of two or more remote-sensing techniques, such as magnetometry and soil resistivity, allows for subsurface anomalies to be recognized that might go unnoticed or be misinterpreted based on a single line of evidence.

Postprocessing

Any survey, but especially those involving remote sensing techniques, is only as good as the analyst's ability to postprocess the data. Although analysis can be a long-term endeavor, a number of simple techniques exist for viewing the data that allow it to be interpreted efficiently and quickly after the survey takes place or even directly in the field, facilitating on-the-spot adjustments to survey or excavation strategies. These techniques are obviously essential in the forensic world, where no one can afford to wait for the consulting expert to analyze and interpret data.

Both soil resistivity and magnetometry data can be converted to three-dimensional x, y, z coordinates and imported into an off-the-shelf computer mapping program for easy viewing (Figures 11.11

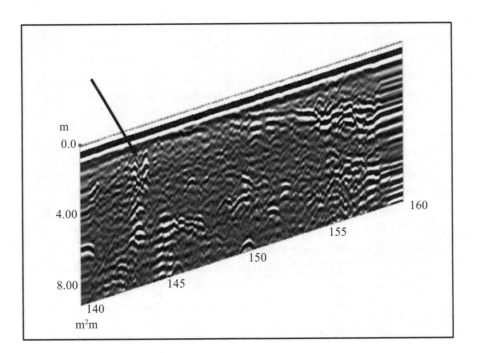

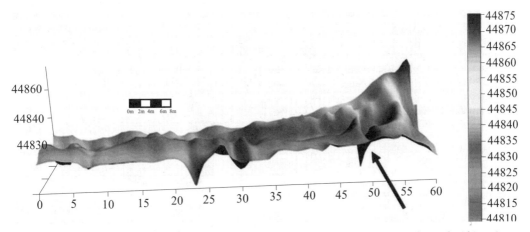

Figure 11.12 Anomalies identified by ground-penetrating radar and magnetometer located within a 2-m radius. Note the radar hyperbola and the dipolar gradient readings where the intrusive feature is located.

and 11.12). If a grid survey was employed during the survey, then one can simply overlay the data maps generated by the two techniques for quick analysis. There are a number of other techniques, such as filtering out the extreme high and low readings, that can be used to isolate the gradients that are important for the analysis.

As with the traditional survey techniques, remote sensing surveys should seek to reduce the area that will require ground-truthing, in the form of test trenches or limited block excavations, but they should not be so exclusive as to erroneously eliminate actual buried remains. Data filters should thus be set at a level to achieve this end, but since remote sensing analysis operates by detecting differences in the subsurface matrix (which may represent the presence of an intrusive cultural anomaly or feature), most surveys result in the detection of numerous anomalies. Consequently, the placement of test excavations may best be determined by assumptive hypothesis; that is, whenever two or more of the three pieces of instrumentation register an anomaly at one location, there is a stronger likelihood that a subsurface feature exists and is not a figment of data acquisition.

Conclusion

The application of archaeological methods and procedures to the detection of buried human remains has been slow to mature. Although forensic anthropology has emerged over the last 40 years as a viable subdiscipline of anthropology, the recognition of forensic archaeology as a distinct specialty has lagged behind. This is changing.

Buried human remains are best located by the application of methodical, systematic procedures. Many of these procedures (probing, coring, searching for surface indicators) have changed very little over the last hundred years or so. Other procedures, such as magnetometry, ground-penetrating radar, and soil resistivity, represent more recent developments and offer great promise. These remote procedures carry the added benefit of being less intrusive and therefore more appropriate in areas where political, cultural, or ethical concerns may otherwise be constraints.

References

Bevan, B. W. 1983. Electromagnetics for mapping earth features. *Journal of Field Archaeology* 10(1): 47–54.

———. 1996. Geophysical exploration in the US National Parks. *Northeast Historical Archaeology* 25: 69–84.

———. 1998. *Geophysical Exploration for Archaeology: An Introduction to Geophysical Exploration*. Midwest Archaeological Center, Special Report No. 1. Lincoln, Nebraska.

Buck, S. C. 2003. Searching for graves using geophysical technology: Field tests with ground penetrating radar, magnetometry, and electrical resistivity. *Journal of Forensic Sciences* 48(1): 5–11.

Cheetham, P. 2005. Forensic geophysical survey, in J. Hunter and M. Cox, M. (eds.), *Forensic Archaeology: Advances in Theory and Practice*, pp. 62–95. London: Routledge.

Clark, A. 1996. *Seeing Beneath the Soil: Prospecting Methods in Archaeology* (rev. ed.). London: Routledge.

Conyers, L. B. 2004. *Ground-Radar for Archaeology*. Walnut Creek, CA: AltaMira Press.

———. 2006. Ground-penetrating radar techniques to discover and map historic graves. *Historical Archaeology* 40(3): 64–73.

Conyers, L. B., and Goodman, D. 1997. *Ground-Penetrating Radar: An Introduction for Archaeologists*. Walnut Creek, CA: AltaMira Press.

Dorbin, M. B., and Savit, C. H. 1988. *Introduction to Geophysical Prospecting*. New York: McGraw-Hill.

Dupras, T. L., Schultz, J. J., Wheeler, S. W., and Williams, L. J. 2006. *Forensic Recovery of Human Remains: Archaeological Approaches*. Boca Raton, FL: CRC Press.

Killam, E. W. 1990. *The Detection of Human Remains*. Springfield, IL: Charles C. Thomas.

Kroeber, A. L. 1916. Zuni potsherds. *American Museum of Natural History, Anthropological Papers* 18(1): 20.

Morse, D., Duncan, J., and Stoutamire, J. 1983. *Handbook of Forensic Archaeology and Anthropology*. Tallahassee, FL: Rose Printing.

Scollar, I. 1965. A contribution to magnetic prospecting in archaeology. *Archaeo-Physika* 1: 21–92.

Rebmann, A., Koenig, M., and David, E. 2000. *Cadaver Dog Handbook*. Boca Raton, FL: CRC Press Inc.

Vaughan, C. J. 1986. Ground-penetrating radar surveys used in archaeological investigations. *Geophysics* 51(3): 595–604.

Wheeler, M. 1956. *Archaeology from the Earth*. Oxford: Clarendon Press.

Wiseman, J. R., and El-Baz, F. (eds.). 2007. *Remote Sensing in Archaeology*. New York: Springer.

12

EXCAVATION AND RECOVERY IN FORENSIC ARCHAEOLOGICAL INVESTIGATIONS

Paul N. Cheetham and Ian Hanson

The chess board is the world, the pieces are the phenomena of the universe, the rules of the game are what we call the laws of Nature. (Huxley 1909)

Why involve archaeologists in forensics? This chapter discusses practical reasons. Archaeologists have expertise in untangling the seemingly chaotic structure[1] of scattered and buried features, artefacts, and deposits. They have specifically developed strategies for managing and organising the spatial and temporal control and analysis of complex sites—investigating buried landscapes whose rules are the laws of nature, as Huxley describes above. Few agencies historically in charge of crime-scene and forensic cases have recognized both the complexities of these buried environments and the need for an archaeologist's specialist skills in uncovering "hidden" evidence. Pathologist Sir Sydney Smith in 1924 saw "something of the worries of an archaeologist" when excavating a mass grave during a murder investigation in Cairo (Smith 1959: 71), and pathologist Keith Mant realised the spatial control required in exhumations and the effects of taphonomy on remains and evidence while recovering the bodies of missing servicemen in postwar Germany (Mant 1987). It was Stuart Kind (1987) of the Forensic Science Service who noted the similarities between crime investigation and archaeology—that both constructed hypotheses from fragmentary evidence, determined events along time lines, and required a basic understanding of principles of evidential identification, deterioration, and change.

The realisation of what archaeology brings to forensic studies is still limited globally but has spread as professional archaeologists and anthropologists have applied themselves to mainstream forensic questions in cases ranging from North, Central, and South America, the United Kingdom, Australia, and international war crimes investigations (for example, Bass 1978; Davis 1992; Hunter, Roberts, and Martin 1996; İşcan 1988; Morse, Crusoe, and Smith 1976; Skinner 1987; Spennemann and Franke 1995). What is clear is that *any* archaeologist or anthropologist engaging in forensic work must adapt to a medico-legal framework, which may involve time constraints and evidential and information controls that are outside his or her usual realm of experience.

Concepts

There are several issues to consider in approaching archaeological excavation and recovery of forensic investigations. One is that archaeology and archaeologists are conceptualized and defined very differently, depending on where and how they exist.

Archaeologists who excavate salvage/rescue sites for commercial companies, who excavate "classical sites" focussing on structures, who undertake excavation in Europe, Central America, or Southeast Asia all have different approaches and understanding of how techniques and archaeological methodology should apply to fieldwork. Archaeologists may come from various anthropological, historical, geographical, or hard-science backgrounds. In forensic archaeological work, investigators should apply a "histiographical" approach to understanding how the requirements of an investigation will be affected by a particular methodological or theoretical approach. The fact that there is no standard approach to archaeological fieldwork globally has implications for fieldwork that takes place in a legal framework—a framework (that many do not commonly encounter in their everyday work) with serious ramifications for archaeologists in terms of the interpretation, definition, and presentation of archaeological evidence. Conversely, forensic archaeologists need to be aware of the cultural, social, political, legal, and historical agendas in their work—things that many archaeologists are well aware of from their understanding of a subjective past. Archaeologists operating in a forensic context are experienced and competent field archaeologists, in the same way that a forensic pathologist is a specialist pathologist.

What constitutes experience and competence when it comes to forensic archaeology? Even the differences between a forensic archaeologist and a forensic anthropologist are not clear (for example, see Skinner, Alempijevic, and Djuric-Srejic 2003). Few attempts to define these things at a practical level have been undertaken, even though defining competence and experience is important for the expert witness process. In the U.K., the Council for the Registration of Forensic Practitioners has begun to develop some definitions for these concepts for forensic archaeology (CRFP 2006).

In legal terms, archaeologists may undertake recovery of burials in the context of domestic homicide and other police support work (such as recovering buried stolen goods, weapons, or ransom money and civil cases such as boundary disputes [Hunter 1996: 99]), international humanitarian identification, international criminal investigation for war crimes tribunals, and recovery after disasters. The requirements for recovery in each situation will be different, depending on the legal system within which the archaeologists find themselves. In domestic murder cases, archaeologists may find themselves defined as scientists fulfilling one task in a formal legal system, assisting a pathologist at scene or providing a statement and expert witness testimony in court.

In a humanitarian exhumation where the missing are recovered from a mass grave, the archaeologist may be the only scientist undertaking many combined aspects of a field exercise—including search, location, recovery, and analysis, recovering bodies to return to families—with no legal obligation to provide testimony or reports. Often the archaeologist does not direct the process, as is the case in normal excavations, but is managed as a scientific element within a judicial, medico-legal, and investigative hierarchy and strategy (see Wright and Hanson this volume; Skinner and Sterenberg 2005; Wright, Hanson, and Sterenberg 2005).

Crime-scene protocols governing the responsibilities and therefore the activities of the forensic archaeologist often vary from scene to scene, even within national boundaries and common legal systems; for example, the 43 police forces in England and Wales will likely use scientific support differently. An archaeologist may be brought in to advise and implement a recovery strategy at the start of a case or to assist a pathologist in a recovery after the fact, with, frustratingly little influence over some aspects of the recovery process. In some international contexts, the archaeologist may direct the scientific element of a mass-grave excavation or aircraft crash site, coordinating a range of experts that are drawn into the archaeologist's domain of the buried environment.

What remains important in any investigation involving excavation and recovery is that the archaeologist at the outset of involvement clearly defines his or her responsibilities, as well as whom to report to and how to report.

The Search Never Ends

The process of planning, explaining, and organising the process of fieldwork should be broken into manageable modules along a timeline. The practice of using standard operating procedures is common in many professions, such as in fire brigades and the armed forces, and now also for the forensic archaeological process (Cox et al. 2007). Such procedures are necessary for basic training, implementation, and understanding of the inexperienced; for the experienced professional, they become merely prompts and reminders. Thus for the competent forensic archaeologist, there should be no processual distinction among search, location, and recovery. After one pinpoints a site and deals with the search, identification, and recovery of surface material, the process of excavation is one of continuing the search to locate and define bodies and artefacts (evidence) and features or deposits (which also have strong evidential value) in ever more focused spatial units defined by the surviving anthropogenic and environmental stratigraphy. The definition of spatial and temporal evidential perimeters from a wide regional to a (potentially) microscopic resolution is a key element of archaeological assistance in forensics, as is the appropriate recording of this process (see below). An important element of developing this concept of continuity over time and space is the significance placed on it by the criminal justice system in terms of evidence control and also of data exchange and management of the investigative process.

Requirements of Forensic Archaeology in Excavation and Recovery

The investigational aims and benefits of archaeological involvement in forensic work at the scene (as discussed by Hanson 2007; Haglund 2001; Haglund, Connor, and Scott 2001; Hunter et al. 1994; Juhl 2004) include:

- Sequencing and dating of events
- Providing evidence for identification of the dead
- Identifying ethnic, religious, and/or cultural groups
- Assisting in the determination of manner and cause of death
- Determining where the dead are from
- Determining whether the dead have been moved after death
- Reconstructing the crime scene
- Linking crime scenes
- Determining perpetrators' actions
- Determining evidence of perpetrator identity

The (often) short time from deposition to excavation means there is usually good archaeological evidential survival, along with the possibility to reconstruct events in time very accurately. The "Pompeii premise" holds that events sealed by burial within a very short time frame and found in the archaeological record are verifiable by other evidential means such as witnesses, aerial imagery, and video (Cox et al. 2007; Hanson 2004). Indeed, the ability to understand burial

preservation and the expertise to deal with human remains are primary reasons for involving archaeologists in forensic excavation. The requirements of forensic investigations have guided the demands now placed on archaeology in these situations. Thus the involvement of archaeologists and forensic scientists in cases such as the Srebrenica massacre in Bosnia informed criminal investigators of what could be recovered from buried crime scenes— for instance, by recording vehicle tracks and marks, detecting and analyzing foreign soils in secondary burials, and recognizing multiple stratigraphic deposits in graves demonstrating grave reuse (Brown 2006; Cox et al. 2007; Hanson 2004). Such skills and procedures provide support to investigators in areas outside their expertise, for example in:

- Recognizing disturbed soil
- Removing soil and dealing with safety issues of soil stability
- Advising on the usefulness and correct application of heavy earth-moving machinery
- Recording the location of objects in 2D and 3D and representing them in plans, computer-based images, and photography
- Showing understanding and competence in excavating human remains
- Recognizing when to use other experts, such as soil scientists, botanists, and those with dating expertise
- Managing large teams of scientists (after Wright, Hanson, and Sterenberg 2005)
- Defining the excavation and recovery process within a crime-scene context
- Reporting on forensic archaeological matters

These procedures are based on foundational archaeological processes and principles, as discussed (mainly in the form of case studies) in Cox and associates (2007), Hunter and Cox (2005), Wright, Hanson, and Sterenberg (2005), Hanson (2004), and Connor and Scott (2001). A key element is that the field archaeologist is able to simultaneously excavate and interpret and to quickly establish the stratigraphic sequence and its relevance and distribution for each site. Little has been published on the practical techniques for achieving these goals; some are discussed below.

The flexibility that is naturally required of an archaeologist in investigating every unique site becomes, importantly, in forensic cases, an ability to adapt to the procedures of different agencies managing the crime scene. Such adaptability is critical to developing the experience that will allow archaeologists to demonstrate and to provide scientific support in forensics that expands the ability of investigations to optimise data capture during excavation and recovery. The onus is often on the forensic archaeologist to prove to investigators that he or she has constructive input or has revealed something of interest—often this is something that investigators will not recognize or appreciate on their own.

The key considerations that archaeologists need to make investigators aware of within the investigative excavation and recovery framework are these:

- Spatial extent of the scene (often best achieved through open-area excavation)
- Site-formation processes affecting the time frame of interest
- Stratigraphy reflecting events at scene relevant to the specific investigation (including any bodies that can be viewed as a deposit)
- Identification of physical evidence within deposits, such as hairs, fibres, and/or shell cases and demonstration of their relevance to the case
- Identification of physical evidence on surfaces, such as hairs, fibres, toolmarks, and/or prints and demonstration of their relevance to the case
- Identification of taphonomic influences to evidence and bodies
- Determination of strategies for optimum recording and recovery of such evidence
- Determination of strategies for sampling deposits to collect such evidence
- Appreciation of the accumulation of evidence in a reverse examination of a sequence of archaeological features and deposits that reflects moving back through time
- Identification of the needs for conservation of recovered evidence
- Ensuring that planning and recording formats and measures are suitable to produce competent archaeological reports for courts

Archaeologists therefore need appropriate methods to demonstrate not only to a prosecutor and a court but also to investigators while still at scene that their evidence is relevant and sound. Much depends on an archaeologist's awareness of the particular medico-legal investigative structure and the scientific potential of the evidence. Often this comes down to enlightening a single senior investigator in charge of scenes or cases and the ability of the archaeologist to persuade this person of the veracity of his or her findings.

Similarities and Differences between Archaeologist and CSI

Archaeological approaches can inform the investigative process (and vice versa) in ways that are both practical and strategic. For example, the cordons and grids used to delineate the crime scene impose artificial boundaries on the landscape to control access and to allow systematic search and recording. However, such visual two-dimensional boundaries can limit the ability of both investigators and archaeologists to "see" the landscape. The pleasing symmetry of a grid or an inner and outer crime-scene boundary can inhibit defining the relevant area of criminal events or the relevant archaeological record. Although gridding a site is an excellent way to delineate a landscape for systematic searches, it is of limited assistance for domestic murder scenes of small scale, given time and space restrictions, when a pair of datum points will suffice. On a disaster recovery scene such as a plane crash, an outer cordon set to control access to the scene and define evidential distribution can become obsolete overnight, when strong winds blow documents, clothing, and personal effects 300 metres past the cordon, and dogs carry remains away.

There are differences between archaeologists' and investigators' approaches to photography. Archaeologists have a formalised approach in terms of the symmetry of how shots are framed, while taking shots that provide the clearest overall images and allow additional interpretation by others. A panoramic overview is often presented. Crime-scene photographers, in contrast, record from formal views and angles to demonstrate a common, repeated approach. Their images illustrate a limited concept of the vertical, without the wide angle that an archaeological image will present. The scales used in crime-scene photographs would not be adequate for many archaeological site photographs. For many investigators, the main evidential record for a scene is the photograph, with the crime-scene sketch as a supplement; for archaeologists, the plan is the primary record, and photographs supplement the interpretive build-up of single-, multiple-context, and phase plans. The use of archaeological plans has now extended into police work and is often done by accident investigation teams, but this development is not systematic, and so the archaeologist may have to do all or part of the surveying and plan drawing.

There are lessons in the detail of archaeological recording that can be learned by investigators; but these lessons are often overlooked, especially since many criminal cases are solved quickly and do not need the long-term interpretations or review that many archaeologists ask of their data.

How archaeologists and investigators justify their actions is another important part of any investigation. Both seek objective analyses in what is also a subjective process. Police teams, for example, have standard procedures, forms, and logs. Within this structure, they have an incident and policy-change logbook in which to record when and why there were changes to the standard procedures; thus they have a written record to justify their actions in court. The entire reporting process is controlled by the crime-scene manager to minimise reporting conflicts among officers. Archaeologists, however, often operate in a more egalitarian way, with all team members filling out forms—but they would benefit greatly from formalising the recording of methodology and policy in an incident and policy-change logbook. Control of recording by one archaeologist on a large forensic excavation team is often appropriate as a way to limit interpretive conflicts and errors (see Cox et al. 2007). A checklist of evidential considerations for forensic archaeologists (as is issued to crime-scene investigators, or CSIs) would be very beneficial, but such a checklist does not exist at present.

The complexity of many forensic excavations (especially mass-grave work) makes continual record-taking essential. Photographic working shots are an essential way to record archaeological excavation method; they allow excavation processes to be reviewed and errors to be checked. Increasingly, using photographs and video to record process and methodology (not just evidential shots) is encouraged on crime scenes; for any complex archaeological excavation, it is vital. Whenever one records 10,000 survey points and collects 2,000 pieces of evidence on a mass-grave excavation, there will be errors in records, labelling, and documentation. Process-recording photography can allow such inconsistencies to be resolved. Thus it is important is that an error-checking quality assurance process exists and is implemented.

The repetition of forms may seem onerous to archaeologists and investigators, but it allows errors to be spotted and rectified or noted. Archaeologists have something to learn from the exhibits officer who controls the error-reduction process for the crime-scene manager. At the same time, defensive tactics of searching for procedural errors to attack evidence has led to a basic lack of flexibility in recording crime scenes. The best way to counteract this problem may be to state the error rate discovered when checking records and describe this as normal (based on the scale of the scene and the volume of documentation generated).

Variations in Methodology

The great variations in the requirements of different investigations provide concern for archaeologists. Policies and regimes change, and work that was originally undertaken only for humanitarian reasons may be reviewed or required by the courts at a later date. Data from excavations undertaken to return victims to families may be subsequently required as evidence in tribunals, where they will be critically analysed under a new set of criteria. For this reason, it is necessary to define standards of fieldwork in terms of appropriate and inappropriate techniques in a sense not normally deemed necessary in nonforensic archaeological excavations. Archaeologists excavating in a forensic setting must presume that any work done may be scrutinised and used by a court of law and thus should be of a standard acceptable to those courts,[2] whatever the original motivation for commissioning the work. When the archaeological record is used as forensic evidence, all work must be undertaken according to methods that are in general practice, that are peer reviewed, that minimise evidential loss and destruction, and that are defensible as processual methods in court. All results must be able to be independently checked and verified.

In the end, it may be the courts rather than archaeologists who decide what archaeological standards and techniques are suitable for forensic work. Huxley's "laws of nature" establish a firm basis for determining appropriate archaeological methods in that context, and the principles of geological and archaeological stratigraphy provide some universal rules for interpreting the archaeological record in forensic cases. Stratigraphic understanding is the key to demonstrating scientific rigour in forensic archaeological excavation. The stratigraphic identification and excavation of individual archaeological contexts, along with the systematic recording of these using plans and matrices, can fulfil the requirements for scientific evidence required by the courts. Methods that arbitrarily remove stratigraphic boundaries, or that do not record systematically, destroy evidence and are liable to be exposed as doing so.

Two excavation methods in common usage are pedastalling—the digging of a grave by removing the surrounding material so as to leave the body on a sort of artificially created mortuary table—which allows access but destroys the grave structure, and excavating in spits—removing arbitrary thicknesses of material across the whole of an area in horizontal slices—which will mix soils (and the evidence contained in them) from different stratigraphic units, thereby limiting stratigraphic understanding, the ability to record in plans and sections, and the recovery of human-made features. These methods are fine to use in some circumstances, but too often they are used simply because they are the "conventional" approach and convenient and straightforward to undertake. But when stratigraphic units are not identified or individually excavated, evidence is lost. So why are these methods conventional? A sort of "chicken and egg" theory may be operating here: many archaeologists are simply not used to identifying or excavating stratigraphy. The methods they use during excavation do not allow for stratigraphic exposure, and therefore stratigraphic understanding is limited. Without that understanding, methods for maximising stratigraphic exposure will never be instituted. In forensic contexts, there is *always* stratigraphy in the form of cut features, surfaces, and deposits that intrude into previously established deposits and strata.

Stratigraphic excavation is the cornerstone of the recovery of evidential data in archaeological and forensic archaeological excavation. It is the source of the evidence used to establish, sequence, and demonstrate past events and to independently date these events with a precision that (at present) surpasses all other methods. And so the crux of the whole recovery process—given that archaeological excavation is inherently destructive—is this: a missed stratigraphic unit not only destroys evidence, its stratigraphic relevance cannot be established and, potentially, its existence cannot even be realised by the excavator or anybody else, which ultimately could result in perpetrators not being convicted. In such cases, lack of stratigraphic recording and understanding becomes a gift for defence lawyers, allowing them to raise questions of reasonable doubt, whereas the evidence already destroyed could have provided "proof" of innocence for the accused.

Debate at the institutional level about the efficacy of particular methods has not occurred thus far—nor have the methodologies of excavation and recovery used by archaeologists in forensic cases as yet been thoroughly examined or challenged in any national or international courts. Why? Many criminal investigators, lawyers, and judiciaries are not aware of the role that archaeological methods play in the criminal and forensic field in the same way that they know about the applicability of other methods, such as the rules of chain of custody or fingerprinting. No doubt, in the future, archaeological methods and data will need to prove themselves in court to be valid for forensic purposes.

What methods, then, are appropriate? A flexible strategy is needed. When asked how they know what are the best methodological approaches for a site, archaeologists will respond "you do it from experience" or "you use standard excavation methods." But these responses offer scant help to graduates and archaeologists seeking to develop their skills in forensic studies, and, without additional explanation, they are difficult arguments to sustain under cross-examination. One should aim to have a "tool box" of techniques and methods that can be applied in the right circumstance.

Competent forensic archaeologists, however, do not spend a great deal of time calculating moves; their experience leads them to rapidly understand a site and the methods required. There are a number of standard methods—such as stratigraphic excavation, levelling, spitting, single-context planning, and half-sectioning (see Barker 1987; Harris 1979; Roskams 2001),which are frequently used. Experience comes into play when standard methods are perceived as too limiting for maximising data recovery or crime-scene reconstruction, because the site presents archaeological or environmental extremes that are out of the ordinary. In forensic cases, these challenges may be logistical in nature, such as when deep mass graves in Bosnia penetrate the water table and require remedial engineering works; they may be due to the recent nature of the archaeology with, for instance, grave features extending into the vegetative layers and O horizon of the relevant stratigraphy; or they may involve adjusting methodology to take account of active bio-turbation in the soil horizons that displaces evidential material downward. Any method used must be justifiable to the management of the investigative process and also to any court or critical review.

Demonstrating and knowing, however, what methods are appropriate to a forensic investigation (which often involves burials) are difficult tasks for practitioners, because relatively little of any detail has been published on the practical processes of archaeological excavation or the pros and cons of these techniques (for examples see Cox et al. 2007; Hanson 2004; Joukowsky 1980; United Nations 1991). Although critical discussion has occasionally taken place in field archaeology (Droop 1915; Harris, Brown, and Brown 1993; Wheeler 1954), many writers and organisations describe methods that should be used as "standard," "appropriate," or "demonstrably fit for purpose" (for example, see IFA 2001) without explaining what these phrases mean, and they use methods out of convention rather than suitability. This approach may not stand up under critical review in court, because it leaves archaeologists without definitive standards. Indeed, one could claim that the definition of standards has been avoided in archaeology generally to limit criticism over differing views on excavation methods historically undertaken and the now unacceptable level of data recovery they reflect, but such avoidance of the issue is not possible for forensic work in an inquisitive judicial domain.

Archaeologists as Facilitators for Multidisciplinary Investigation

The developing field of forensic archaeology is one of an increasing number of scientific specialties identified as useful for certain investigations. Archaeologists who view their knowledge of the natural sciences as giving them a "jack of all trades" status within their profession need to carefully reconsider this position in the forensic arena. Archaeologists are usually very good at identifying anomalies, the unusual, a wide range of evidence types, and the potential relevance of data at a scene. But pressures from investigators to rationalise costs and personnel at the crime scene often lead to demands that one specialist (such as the archaeologist, geologist, or palynologist) undertake sampling and recovery of evidence that falls outside his or her level of expertise. This should be resisted, since few archaeologists have the qualifications or experience to undertake the role of anthropologist or another specialty and defend themselves in court as experts in such an area. Although the archaeologist typically may use many experts in scene analysis, his or her role in forensic terms should primarily be limited to advising investigators on what other experts may be

needed to maximise evidential identification and recovery.

Internationally, archaeologists have often led the scientific management and recovery of mass graves, because they have been the most experienced and suitable professionals to make sense of these large-scale scenes. The skills required in these situations can often be learned from working on the type of complex, stratified urban excavations found on construction sites, where archaeologists must also deal with financial and time constraints, health, safety, staff welfare issues, logistics, and machinery and engineering problems. In domestic cases, the crime-scene manager and scientific support deal with many of these issues. Any murder, mass murder, or disaster scene is such a complex investigative environment that a multidisciplinary approach, especially in terms of the finding and recovering of evidence by scientific specialists, is vital; it is no surprise, then, that archaeologists have become key personnel in the identification of potential evidence and are often the specialists best equipped to deal with it.

Conclusion

The use of archaeology and archaeologists in criminal, humanitarian, and disaster excavation and recovery is slowly being incorporated into the standard operating procedures, management strategies, and tactics of practical scene investigations. Thus it is becoming increasingly important to synthesise forensic archaeological practice and understanding nationally and internationally into the processes of crime-scene management, auditing, error reduction, evidential control, and custody management. At the same time, the benefits of wide-spectrum processual and analytical approaches to the methodologies and the interpretations that archaeologists bring to burial scenes, scatters, and disasters provide vital new approaches for investigators that maximise evidential identification and recovery and contribute to crime-scene and event reconstruction. Archaeologists are becoming important facilitators within the practice of multidisciplinary forensic science, but they need to standardise their forensic methodologies and approaches to ensure that the work they undertake can be justified; and they should assume that all cases of excavation and recovery in the forensic arena may end up in court. Archaeologists, moreover, have a responsibility to inform the forensic community of strategies that will maximise evidential recovery and archaeological potential on the chessboard of forensic excavations.

Notes

1. The stratified nature of buried geological, environmental, and archaeological layers, features, and deposits, and their direct relation to dating events and sequencing activity, is still not grasped by many involved in criminal and human rights investigation; often the ground is seen as the surface of a sea of mud that has no more definable structure and subtlety than the perceived nature of the oceans.

2. Of course, these standards can be debated; standards of evidential control enforced on U.K. domestic murder scenes are different, for example, from those of an international tribunal. Perhaps a key argument is that precedents in both national and international law are developing so that citizens of any country might be indicted and seized for trial in an international or national court for crimes committed abroad—for instance, see the Zardad case (BBC 2005). Optimum evidential recovery seems a logical approach as global cases begin to outline some common approaches to crime-scene recovery.

References

Barker, P. 1987. *Techniques of archaeological excavation*. Batsford: London.

Bass, W. 1978. Exhumation: The method could make the difference. *FBI Law Enforcement Bulletin* 47(7): 6–11.

BBC. 2005. *Afghan warlord guilty of torture*. http://news.bbc.co.uk/1/hi/uk/4693239.stm (accessed 29/12/06).

Brown, A. 2006. The use of forensic botany and geology in war crimes investigations in NE Bosnia. *Forensic Science International* 16(3:) 204–210.

Connor, M., and Scott, D. D. 2001. Paradigms and perpetrators, *Journal of Historical Archaeology* 35(1): 1–6.

Council for the Registration of Forensic Practitioners. 2006. *Annual review 2005/6*. London: CRFP.

Cox, M., Flavel, A., Hanson I., Laver, J., and Wessling, R. (eds.). 2007. *The Scientific Investigation of Mass Graves*. Cambridge: Cambridge University Press.

Davis, J. 1992. Forensic Archaeology. *Archaeological Reviews from Cambridge* 11(1): 152–156.

Droop, J. P. 1915. *Archaeological Excavation*. Cambridge: Cambridge University Press.

Haglund, W. D. 2001. Recent mass graves, an introduction, in W. D. Haglund and M. H. Sorg (eds.), *Advances in Forensic Taphonomy*, pp. 243–261. Boca Raton, FL: CRC.

Haglund, W. D., Connor, M., and Scott, D. D. 2001. The archaeology of contemporary mass graves, *Journal of Historical Archaeology* 35(1): 57–69.

Hanson, I. 2004. The importance of stratigraphy in forensic investigation, in K. Pye and D. J. Croft (eds.), *Forensic Geoscience: Principles, Techniques and Applications*, pp. 39–47. London: Geological Society, Special Publications.

———. 2007. Forensic archaeology: Approaches to international investigations, in M. Oxenham (ed.), *Forensic Approaches to Death, Disaster and Abuse*. Perth: University of Western Australia Press.

Harris, E. C. 1979. *Principles of Archaeological Stratigraphy*. London: Academic Press.

Harris, E. C., Brown, M. R., and Brown, G. J. 1993. *Practices of archaeological stratigraphy*. London: Academic Press.

Hunter J. R., 1996. Locating buried remains, in J. R. Hunter, C. A. Roberts, and A. Martin (eds.). *Studies in Crime: An Introduction to Forensic Archaeology*, pp. 87–100. London: Routledge.

Hunter, J. R. and Cox, M. 2005. *Forensic Archaeology: Advances in Theory and Practice*. London: Routledge.

Hunter, J. R, Heron, C, Janaway, R. C, Martin, A. L, Pollard, A. M., and Roberts, C. A. 1994. Forensic archaeology in Britain. *Antiquity* 68: 758–769.

Hunter, J. R., Roberts, C. A., and Martin, A. (eds.). 1996. *Studies in Crime: An Introduction to Forensic Archaeology*. Routledge: London.

Huxley, T. H. 1909. A liberal education, in A. L. F. Snell (ed.), *Autobiography and Selected Essays by Thomas Henry Huxley*. Chicago: Riverside College Classics.

Institute of Field Archaeologists (IFA). 2001. *Standard and Guidance for Archaeological Excavation*. Reading: IFA.

İşcan, M.Y. 1988. Rise of forensic anthropology. *American Journal of Physical Anthropology* 31(9): 203–229.

Joukowsky, M. 1980. *A Complete Manual of Field Archaeology*. Upper Saddle River, NJ: Prentice Hall.

Juhl, K. 2004. The contribution by (forensic) archaeologists to human rights investigations of mass graves. *AmS-Nett* 5. Stavenger: Museum of Archaeology.

Kind, S. S. 1987. *The Scientific Investigation of Crime*. Harrogate: Forensic Science Services.

Mant, A. K. 1987. Knowledge acquired from postwar exhumations, in A. Boddington, A. N. Garland, and R. C. Janaway (eds.), *Death, Decay and Reconstruction: Approaches to Archaeology and Forensic Science*, pp. 65–78. Manchester: Manchester University Press.

Morse, D., Crusoe, D., and Smith, H. G. 1976. Forensic Archaeology. *Journal of Forensic Science* 21(2): 323–332.

Roskams, S. 2001. *Excavation*. Cambridge: Cambridge University Press.

Skinner, M. 1987. Planning the archaeological recovery of evidence from recent mass graves. *Forensic Science International* 34: 267–287.

Skinner, M., Alempijevic, D., and Djuric-Srejic, M. 2003. Guidelines for international forensic bio-archaeology monitors of mass grave exhumations. *Forensic Science International* 134(3): 81–92.

Skinner, M., and Sterenberg, J. 2005. Turf wars: Authority and responsibility for the investigation of mass graves. *Forensic Science International* 151(2-3): 221–232.

Smith, Sir S. 1959. *Mostly Murder: An Autobiography*, pp. 71–73. London: Harrap Ltd.

Spennemann, D. H., and Franke, B. 1995. Archaeological techniques for exhumations: A unique data source for crime scene investigations. *Forensic Science International* 74: 5–15.

United Nations (UN). 1991. Model protocol for disinterment and analysis of skeletal remains, in *Manual on the Effective Prevention and Investigation of Extra-Legal, Arbitrary and Summary Executions*, pp. 30–41. New York: United Nations.

Wheeler, Sir M. 1954. *Archaeology from the Earth*. Oxford: Oxford University Press.

Wright, R., Hanson, I., and Sterenberg, J., 2005. The archaeology of mass graves, in J. R. Hunter and M. Cox (eds.), *Forensic Archaeology: Advances in Theory and Practice*, pp. 137–158. London: Routledge.

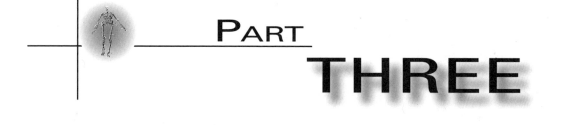

PART
THREE

FORENSIC ANTHROPOLOGY

13

DIFFERENTIATING HUMAN FROM NONHUMAN SKELETAL REMAINS

Dawn M. Mulhern

One of the first questions faced by a forensic anthropologist is whether the remains are human or nonhuman. When complete or partial bones are present, gross analysis of morphological features can often be used to confirm or rule out human remains. Extreme fragmentation makes morphological analysis more difficult if not impossible and may require microscopic, biochemical, or DNA analysis. This chapter explores the morphological features that can be used to distinguish human from nonhuman bone and identifies the most common examples of misidentification. Next, it investigates microscopic techniques for distinguishing human from nonhuman bone. Finally, it discusses biochemical analyses.

Gross Analysis

Macroscopically and microscopically, human bone is most similar to the bone of other mammals, and therefore the most likely source of confusion is between human and nonhuman mammalian species. In a forensic context, one must take into account the local context and consider what species are most likely to be present in that area. The unique combination of a very large brain case, orthognathic face (that is, with a nonprojecting jaw), and adaptations to bipedal locomotion in humans provides many morphological differences

between humans and nonhuman mammals that are useful for distinguishing individual skeletal elements. In addition to morphological differences, subadult human bones can be distinguished from adult mammalian bones that are similar in size by the presence of unfused or partially fused epiphyses. A number of sources for archaeologists provide illustrated atlases comparing and describing the differences between human and nonhuman bone (Cornwall 1956; Gilbert 1973; Olsen 1973; Schmid 1972); some of the most important differences are summarized below.

Skull

Compared to that of other mammals, the human cranial vault is very large relative to body size; also, the human cranium has a more domed shape and thinner cortex compared to that of other mammals. The frontal, temporal, and occipital bones fuse in early childhood in humans but remain as separate elements in many mammals (Cornwall 1956). In addition, the human vault exhibits gracile muscle attachment sites and lacks sagittal and nuchal crests. A notable exception is the large mastoid process, which serves as an attachment site for the sternocleidomastoid muscle that functions in swiveling and tilting the head in humans to accommodate a vertical posture. The foramen magnum is also centrally located in the cranial base; this differs from quadrupeds, in which the foramen magnum is more posteriorly situated.

The mandible is short anterior-posteriorly in humans, resulting in a lack of prognathism. The coronoid process is only slightly higher than the mandibular condyle. In some mammals, the coronoid process is much more superiorly located compared to the condyle (horse, cow, deer, sheep, rabbit, bear, beaver) and is also located much more anteriorly in humans compared to other mammals (Schmid 1972).

Dentition

Human teeth are easily differentiated from the teeth of most other mammals owing to size and morphology. Humans exhibit small canines with apical wear, lack a diastema, and have nonsectorial premolars. Human premolars and molars have low, rounded cusps adapted to an omnivorous diet; these are easily distinguished from the teeth of herbivores and carnivores. Other mammals with similar molar form include bears and pigs; however, bears have much larger teeth than humans, and pigs have four premolars and three molars, whereas humans have two premolars and three molars. The first three premolars are sectorial (and therefore have a sharp cutting edge) in pigs and the three molars are larger than human teeth. The only possible point of confusion is between the fourth premolar in a pig and a human molar (Byers 2005).

Vertebral Column

The human spine is characterized by an S-shaped curve that accommodates a vertical posture. In addition, the vertebral bodies gradually increase in size from the superior to the inferior aspect of the vertebral column, owing to the need to support increasingly more weight. This pattern is not as dramatic in quadrupeds, since compression forces from gravity are similar throughout the spine. The number of vertebrae differs among mammals—for example, members of Order Carnivora have 1–3 more thoracic vertebrae and 1–2 more lumbar vertebrae than humans do (Cornwall 1956).

Compared to that of other mammals, the human atlas exhibits shallower occipital condyles and a much smaller distance between the facets for the occipital and axis. The human axis has a short, stout odontoid process. The spinous processes of the cervical vertebrae are often bifid in humans. In addition, spinous processes are short in humans compared with those of other mammals, because they do not support the massive musculature needed by quadrupeds in the neck and back. In humans, all the spinous processes are oriented inferiorly. Quadrupeds have an anticlinal thoracic vertebra with a vertical spinous process; all other spinous processes are inclined toward it, caudally for the cervical and upper thoracic spine and cranially for the spinous processes of the lower thoracic and lumbar spine (Cornwall 1956). Human vertebral bodies are shorter and broader compared to those of other mammals of comparable size.

Ribs

The human rib cage is broad and shallow, like that seen in apes. In general, mammals have a horizontal posture that is characterized by a narrow, deep thorax. The curvature of the ribs is therefore different in humans and most mammals, with human ribs exhibiting a more pronounced curve. Furthermore, ungulates have bony rib elements that connect the anterior end of the vertebral ribs with the sternum (Stewart 1979).

Pelvis

The morphology of the human pelvis is unique, owing to bipedal locomotion. The ilium is broad and ventrally wrapped in humans, in contrast to the elongated, dorsally located ilium in quadrupedal mammals. The pubic symphysis is rarely fused in humans. The sacrum is broad and wedge-shaped in humans; it is generally narrower in other mammals. The coccyx in humans takes the place of the tail vertebrae found in other mammals.

Shoulder Girdle

The human clavicle is long and robust, because the upper limbs are located on the sides of the body. The retention of a clavicle is a primitive trait in mammals. In addition to primates, other mammalian orders that exhibit functional clavicles include insectivores, rodents, and bats. Although ape clavicles are similar in size and morphology to human clavicles, mammals that are most likely to be found in a forensic context and that would potentially be confused with humans based on size either have reduced clavicles or lack clavicles completely.

The human scapula is triangular in shape, with a large infraspinous fossa. Nonhuman scapulae exhibit a much smaller postspinous fossa relative to the size of the bone. Also, the human scapula is longest perpendicular to the spine, whereas other mammals exhibit scapulae that are longest along the axis of the spine (Figure 13.1).

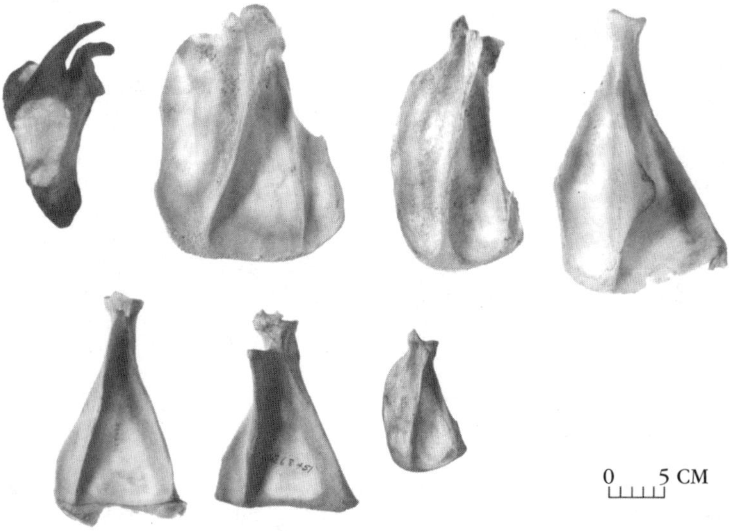

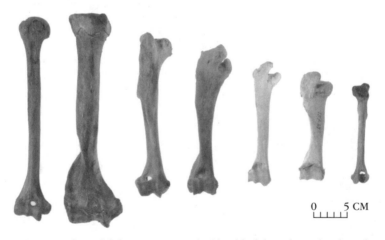

Figure 13.1 Scapula of an adult human compared with a black bear, large dog, hog, deer, domestic sheep, and small dog (*left to right*) (photos previously published in Ubelaker 1989 as Fig. 63; courtesy D. H. Ubelaker and Taraxacum Press).

Figure 13.2 Humerus of an adult human compared with a black bear, large dog, hog, deer, domestic sheep, and small dog (*left to right*) (photos previously published in Ubelaker 1989 as Fig. 63; courtesy D. H. Ubelaker and Taraxacum Press).

Long Bones

In general, long bones in humans are more slender and are not as rugose (that is, exhibit less pronounced muscle markings) than long bones in other mammals. The articular surfaces of human long bones are also flatter with less of a sculpted appearance than other mammalian bones (Figures 13.2 and 13.3). The head of the humerus in humans is hemispherical, allowing a wide range of motion in the shoulder. This feature is found in suspensory primates, but other mammals have flatter humeral heads. The greater tubercle of the humerus is small in humans but is very prominent, whereas in other mammals, such as cows, deer, sheep, and pigs, the tubercle extends superiorly to the humeral head. The capitulum is prominent in the human humerus, to accommodate the enhanced mobility of the radial head. In most quadrupeds, the radius also articulates with the trochlea. The coronoid process is more prominent and the olecranon fossa is less prominent

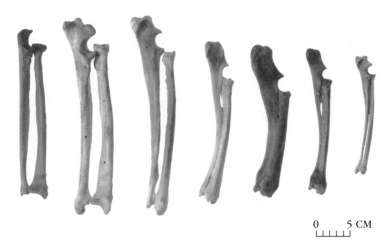

0   5 CM

Figure 13.3 Radius and ulna of an adult human compared with a black bear, large dog, hog, deer, domestic sheep, and small dog (*left to right*) (photos previously published in Ubelaker 1989 as Fig. 63; courtesy D. H. Ubelaker and Taraxacum Press).

in humans than in quadrupeds. A supratrochlear foramen is found in pigs, wolves, foxes, bears, and rabbits. An entepicondylar foramen is present in some mammals, such as raccoons, weasels, otters, pumas, and bobcats (Cornwall 1956; Olsen 1973). The human ulna has a very short olecranon process, again allowing a wider range of motion in the elbow than typical of most

mammals. In quadrupeds, the olecranon process is extended, providing more leverage for the triceps. The radius and ulna are fused together in some mammals, such as the goat, horse, and pig (Olsen 1973).

The femur is long and the shaft is medially angled in humans. Compared to that of other mammals, the human femoral shaft has a smaller

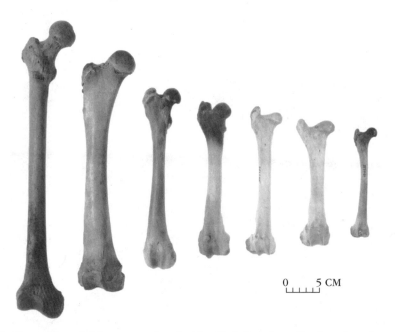

0   5 CM

Figure 13.4 Femur of an adult human compared with a black bear, large dog, hog, deer, domestic sheep, and small dog (*left to right*) (photos previously published in Ubelaker 1989 as Fig. 63; courtesy D. H. Ubelaker and Taraxacum Press).

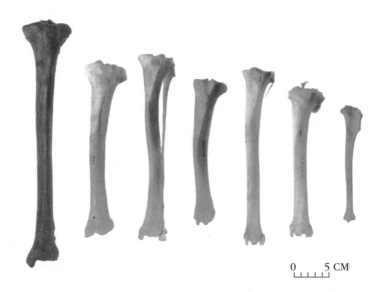

Figure 13.5 Tibia of an adult human compared with a black bear, large dog, hog, deer, domestic sheep, and small dog (*left to right*) (photos previously published in Ubelaker 1989 as Fig. 63; courtesy D. H. Ubelaker and Taraxacum Press).

circumference for its length. The human femur exhibits a robust head and a long neck. The angle between the neck and the shaft is greater in humans compared to most quadrupedal mammals (Figures 13.4 and 13.5). The attachment site for the leg extensors, *linea aspera*, is well developed in humans (Cornwall 1956). A lateral lip is present on the anterior aspect of the distal femur; this feature of the distal articular surface helps hold the patella in position during the force of a striding gait. The proximal and distal articular surfaces of the tibia are flat and platform-like, to accommodate the weight of a biped. The tibia and fibula are fused together in some mammals but not in those that would generally be confused with human.

Hands and Feet

Unlike most mammals, humans retain the primitive trait of five digits. The heads of the metacarpals and the metatarsals are rounded, allowing extensive mobility of the digits. The articular surfaces

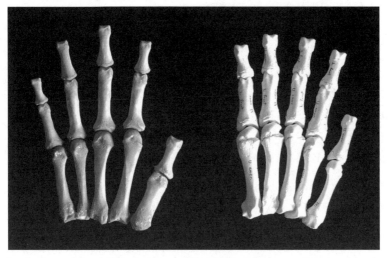

Figure 13.6 Comparison of an adult human hand (*left*) with the front paw of a young bear (*right*), including metacarpals, proximal and middle phalanges.

of the hand and foot phalanges in humans are flatter than in other mammals and lack a median ridge. The first digit of the human hand is opposable. The first metatarsal is more robust than the other metatarsals in humans. The tarsal bones in humans are robust owing to bipedal locomotion. In particular, the talus has a very flat, platform-like superior articular surface.

Bear paws and human hands and feet exhibit similarities that may lead to confusion, particularly in cases where a bear paw is partially fleshed and lacks the claws (Stewart 1959). Bears exhibit larger carpals than humans, with a fused navicular and lunate. In the hand, the second or third metacarpal is longest in the human, whereas the fourth metacarpal is longest in the bear (Stewart 1979). The differences between the metacarpals and the phalanges of a human and bear are shown in Figure 13.6, on the previous page.

In the foot, the first human metatarsal is more robust than the others, whereas in the bear all five metatarsals are comparable in robusticity. The second metatarsal is longest in humans, and the fourth metatarsal is longest in the bear (Gilbert 1973). The distal ends of the phalanges exhibit deeper grooves in the bear. Bears also exhibit sesamoid bones on the heads of all of the metacarpals and metatarsals, whereas humans typically have sesamoid bones only on the head of the first metatarsal (Hoffman 1984).

Radiographic Analysis

Chilvarquer and colleagues (1987) conducted a comparative radiographic analysis of long-bone patterns in human and nonhuman bones. They found that the trabeculae of the spongy bone in human long-bone midshafts define spaces with a circular or oblong pattern and sometimes show homogeneous but sparse distribution, whereas the trabecular pattern in nonhuman bone is more homogeneous and dense. In addition, human bone often lacks a clear border between the cortical and the trabecular bone, whereas a well-defined border is often present in nonhuman bone. Finally, nonhuman bones are characterized by small, spicule-like invaginations from the cortex into the trabecular bone and the penetration of nutrient canals into the midshaft. A test of this method on 20 samples resulted in the correct classification in 86.8% cases by archaeologists and 81.9% by dentists (ibid.).

Microscopic Analysis

Extreme fragmentation of skeletal remains poses a significant problem in a forensic context, even in terms of determining whether the bones are human. Microscopic analysis may provide useful information in differentiating human from nonhuman bone when gross differences are not observable. Differences in bone microstructure among species have been recognized in numerous studies dating back to the mid-19th to the early 20th century, ranging from a study of vertebrates by Quekett (1849) that included several histological drawings to a comparative histological atlas by Foote (1916), which included low magnification drawings of hundreds of specimens. Enlow and Brown (1956, 1957, 1958) published a large comparative study identifying the histological patterns observed in major vertebrate groups, including both fossil and recent taxa. This large study, although the most comprehensive of its kind, is descriptive. For the past several decades, quantitative assessments of histological variables in mammalian bone[1] and human bone[2] have also contributed to the comparative literature.

The overall pattern of bone microstructure may be useful in a forensic context, particularly in ruling out human bone. Mammalian bone includes both lamellar and fibrolamellar (also called plexiform, or laminar) bone. Lamellar bone may be observed as concentric layers of bone around the outside and the inside of the bone circumference, or as discrete units of concentric layers surrounding a Haversian canal (also known as a Haversian system, or secondary osteon). Fibrolamellar bone is characterized by a network of woven bone that is laid down quickly and filled in more slowly by lamellar bone, often resulting in a regular, rectangular pattern (Figure 13.7).

Large mammals including many artiodactyls (for example, cows, sheep, pigs, and deer) have bone diameters that grow quickly and exhibit mostly fibrolamellar bone, with Haversian bone primarily near muscle attachments. Sometimes the blood vessels in fibrolamellar bone anastomose and are surrounded by layers of lamellar bone, resulting in the creation of primary osteons (Currey 2002). Primary osteons are distinguished from secondary osteons by the lack of a reversal line. As illustrated in Figure 13.8, the arrangement of these primary osteons is often linear, with multiple rows, or bands, of these structures. The primary osteons may also eventually be replaced by some secondary osteons. This pattern is common in mammalian bone but uncommon in human bone (Mulhern and Ubelaker 2001).

Ubelaker (1989) used the presence of osteon banding to identify a large bone fragment as nonhuman. The fragment was initially identified by authorities as human, because it had a

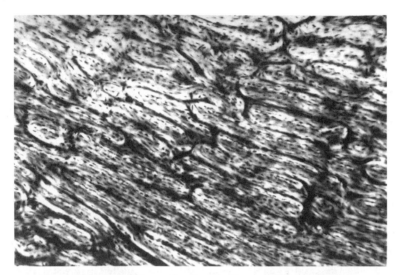

Figure 13.7   Sheep femur showing plexiform, or fibrolamellar bone.

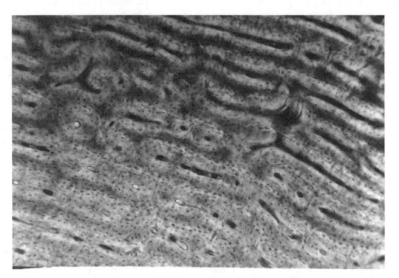

Figure 13.8   Fibrolamellar bone, including osteon banding in the femur of a miniature swine.

pseudoarthrosis held together with a surgical plate. Microscopic analysis of the fragment revealed a pattern of alternating osteon bands, including both primary and secondary osteons, and lamellar bone. The fragment was most likely from a large dog, with the surgical work performed by a veterinarian.

Foote (1916) reports the distribution of bone types as important bone structures in nonhuman mammalian bone ($n = 133$), adult human bone ($n = 139$), and human fetal bone ($n = 7$). Lamellar bone is an important structure in 48% of the nonhuman sample, 92% of the adult human sample,

and 100% of the fetal human sample. Plexiform bone is an important structure in 50% of the nonhuman bone, 8% of the adult human bone, and 100% of the fetal human bone. Haversian systems are important in 82% of the nonhuman sample, 100% of the adult human sample, and 0% of the fetal human sample. Plexiform bone is more common in nonhuman mammals; however, one should note that it is commonly found in fetal human bone. Although Foote provides drawings of plexiform bone in the adult sample, the occurrence of this pattern in adult humans is very rare and is not reported elsewhere in the literature.

In general, large mammalian bones that could be confused with human bones based on size can be ruled out as human if the overall pattern is plexiform, including a more laminar structure or the presence of multiple osteon rows, or bands.

As indicated in Foote's research, Haversian systems are common in both human and nonhuman bone. In primates and carnivores, for example, Haversian bone generally replaces primary bone (Currey 2002). Haversian systems can be isolated, scattered or densely packed, depending on various factors, including chronological age and mechanical demands. If such a pattern is encountered and plexiform bone is absent, human bone cannot be ruled out. Haversian bone is shown in Figure 13.9.

An obvious question is whether microstructural variables, such as osteon number or size, could be used to distinguish different species. Osteon density is partially age dependent and therefore a poor candidate for distinguishing interspecies differences. Differences in microstructural measurements including osteon size and Haversian canal size need to be explored further. The current literature includes a number of quantitative studies on nonhuman bone including taxa that could be important in a forensic context (Albu, Georgia, and Georoceneau 1990; Georgia et al. 1982; Jowsey 1966; Martiniaková, Vondráková, and Fabiš 2003; Mori et al. 2005), but most have very small sample sizes. In addition, many of these studies report different dimensions requiring conversion to a common variable for comparison. A comparative study by Jowsey (1966) of rats, cats,

dogs, rhesus monkeys, and cows suggests that osteon size increases with body size, but sample sizes range from 2 to 6, bringing into question the results of the study. In addition, there is little overlap in the literature in the nonhuman species studied, and where overlap does exist, results are not always consistent. For example, Jowsey (1966) reported a mean Haversian canal perimeter of 85 m in the femora of 4 dogs. Georgia and colleagues (1982) found a mean Haversian canal diameter of 48.5 m in a sample of 25 dog femora. When converted to area, these values are 0.0006 mm^2 and 0.0018 mm^2, respectively. The smallest reported mean Haversian canal size in a sample of human femora ($n = 33$) is 0.0015 mm^2 (Singh and Gunberg 1970). This means that the value reported by Georgia and colleagues (1982) is within the lower end of the human range, but the value reported by Jowsey (1966) falls outside the human range. Additional studies are needed for all nonhuman taxa, particularly those like the dog with such extensive variability in body size. Caution should be exercised when citing such studies in a forensic case.

Owsley, Mires, and Keith (1985) used bone microstructure to help determine the origin of several unknown bone fragments that potentially belonged to a homicide victim. The suspect in the case claimed that the bone fragments found in his truck belonged to a deer that he had shot. The bone fragments from the truck were compared with bone from the victim's humerus as well as a deer humerus. Osteon density and Haversian canal diameter were consistent with the human bone and

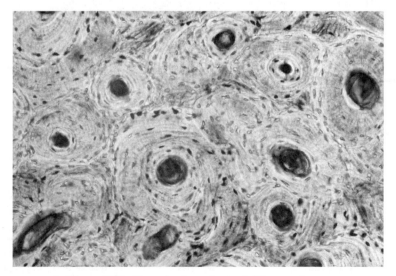

Figure 13.9 Haversian bone in an adult human femur.

inconsistent with deer bone. In this case, the comparison with the victim was important, because the values for osteon density and Haversian canal diameter observed in the deer do not fall outside the human range, but they were not comparable to this particular individual.

In a case involving numerous, small unknown bone fragments, Stout and Ross (1991) used cortical thickness and a lack of plexiform bone to rule out bone from larger mammals and used osteon size to rule out dog bone. Further, the cortical thickness and the orientation of the osteons suggested that the fragments were from the skull. This information, in conjunction with evidence from DNA and chemical analysis, was used to convict the murder suspect, even though the body of the victim was never recovered.

Catteneo and colleagues (1999) found that quantitative microscopy was more accurate than standard microscopy and more reliable than immunological and DNA techniques for distinguishing human and nonhuman bone subject to burning. Discriminant function equations were developed for microstructural variables, including osteon and Haversian canal dimensions, based on the humeri and femora of 15 human bones and 20 nonhuman bones, including 5 cows, 6 sheep, 6 pigs, 1 horse, 1 dog, and 1 cat. The test sample of 11 human bones and 10 nonhuman bones (4 cows, 2 horses, 2 pigs, and 2 sheep) resulted in correct classification of all samples. The best discriminating factor was Haversian canal size. Standard morphological analysis resulted in the incorrect classification of 1 human bone as nonhuman and 1 nonhuman bone as human. The presence of human albumin was detectible in 5 out of 11 burned human bones, although it was detectible in all 11 unburned control samples. Mitochondrial DNA was not detectible in any of the burned bones, although it was present in all of the unburned control samples.

Biomolecular Methods

Biomolecular methods are also potentially important for distinguishing human and nonhuman bone and are useful for identifying species. Ubelaker, Lowenstein, and Hood (2004) applied a technique developed by Lowenstein (1980) for identifying human albumin to a sample of 3 human and 3 nonhuman bones. The technique involves extracting protein from the bone and then conducting a solid-phase double-antibody radioimmunoassay. Rabbit antisera were exposed to albumins or sera from different known species. The resulting species-specific antibodies were then allowed to bind to antigens in the bone protein samples. Radioactive antibodies were used to identify the strongest reactions, which indicated species-specific relationships. All 6 samples were correctly identified as human or nonhuman, although some protein depletion was noted in the 1 human sample of archaeological bone. In addition, a deer sample was tested for species-level identification and was successfully distinguished from other nonhuman species, including cow, deer, dog, goat, and pig. One benefit of this method is that only a small bone sample (200 mg or less) is required.

Techniques involving repetitive mitochondrial DNA markers have been used successfully in wildlife forensics for identifying the species of an unknown sample, including a variety of game and commercial species such as pig, cow, sheep, deer, moose, elk, bear, and turkey (Guglich, Wilson, and White 1994; Murray, Clymont, and Strobeck 1995). Techniques that apply the use of restriction enzymes are potentially preferable to DNA sequencing methods, because they are faster and more cost-efficient.

Conclusion

Depending on the extent and the preservation of the remains present, a variety of methods are available for distinguishing human and nonhuman bone. As the least invasive and most cost-effective choice, gross analysis should be attempted first. In many cases, the morphology of human bone can be detected, even in fragmentary remains. Specifically, an experienced osteologist can identify the evidence for a large cranium and physical features related to bipedal locomotion in human remains. If differences are not observable using gross analysis, then radiographic, microscopic, or biomolecular techniques may be required. The trabecular pattern of bone, pattern of histological structures, and size and number of histological structures have the potential to provide additional information about the origin of a bone. At present, histological methods provide a stronger basis for rejecting a particular bone as human than for identifying an unknown fragment as definitely human. Finally, biomolecular methods offer the possibility of species-specific identification. As these methods improve, they will likely prove invaluable for cases of highly fragmented remains. A thorough understanding of the benefits and limitations of each of these methods is essential for achieving the level of certainty needed in a forensic context.

Notes

1. Albu, Georgia, and Georoceneau 1990; Burr 1992; Georgia and Albu 1988; Georgia et al. 1982; Havill 2004; Jowsey 1966, 1968; Martiniaková, Vondráková, and Fabiš 2003; Mori et al. 2005; Mulhern and Ubelaker 2003, 2006; Schaffler and Burr 1984; Singh, Tonna, and Gandel 1974.

2. Cho et al. 2002; Currey 1964; Eriksen 1991; Evans 1976; Kerley 1965; Pirok et al. 1966; Singh and Gunberg 1970; Stout and Paine 1992; Thompson 1980.

References

Albu, I., Georgia, R., and Georoceneau, M. 1990. The canal system in the diaphysial compacta of the femur in some mammals. *Anatomischer Anzeiger* 170(3-4): 181–187.

Burr, D. 1992. Estimated intracortical bone turnover in the femur of growing macaques: Implications for their use as models in skeletal pathology. *The Anatomical Record* 232: 180–189.

Byers, S. N. 2005. *Introduction to Forensic Anthropology*. Boston: Pearson.

Catteneo, C., DiMartino, S., Scali, S., Craig, O. E., Grandi, M., and Sokol, R. J. 1999. Determining the human origin of fragments of burnt bone: A comparative study of histological, immunological and DNA techniques. *Forensic Science International* 102: 181–191.

Chilvarquer, I., Katz J. O., Glassman, D. M., Prhihoda, T. J., and Cottone, J. A. 1987. Comparative radiographic study of human and animal long bone patterns. *Journal of Forensic Sciences* 32(6): 1645–1654.

Cho, H., Stout S. D., Madsen, R. W., and Streeter, M. A. 2002. Population-specific histological age-estimating method: A model for known African-American and European-American skeletal remains. *Journal of Forensic Sciences* 47(1): 13–18.

Cornwall, I. W. 1956. *Bones for the Archaeologist*. London: Phoenix House.

Currey, J. 1964. Some effects of ageing in human Haversian systems. *Journal of Anatomy* 98(1): 69–75.

———. 2002. *Bones: Structure and Mechanics*. Princeton, NJ: Princeton University Press.

Enlow, D. H., and Brown, S. O. 1956. A comparative histological study of fossil and recent bone tissues, Part I. *The Texas Journal of Science* VII(4): 405–443.

———. 1957. A comparative histological study of fossil and recent bone tissues, Part II. *The Texas Journal of Science* IX(2): 186–214.

———. 1958. A comparative histological study of fossil and recent bone tissues, Part III. *The Texas Journal of Science* X(2): 187–230.

Eriksen, M. F. 1991. Histological estimation of age at death using the anterior cortex of the femur. *American Journal of Physical Anthropology* 84: 171–179.

Evans, F. G. 1976. Mechanical properties and histology of cortical bone from younger and older men. *Anatomical Record* 185: 1–12.

Foote, J. S. 1916. *A Contribution to the Comparative Histology of the Femur*. Washington, D.C.: Smithsonian Contributions to Knowledge 35(3).

Georgia, R., and Albu, I. 1988. The Haversian canal network in the femoral compact bone in some vertebrates. *Morphologie et Embryologie (Bucur)* 34(3): 155–159.

Georgia, R., Albu, I., Sicoe, M., and Georoceneau, M. 1982. Comparative aspects of the density and diameter of Haversian canals of diaphyseal compact bone of man and dog. *Morphologie et Embryologie (Bucur)* 28(1): 11–14.

Gilbert, B. M. 1973. *Mammalian Osteo-archaeology: North America*. Springfield, MO: Missouri Archaeological Society.

Guglich, E. A., Wilson, P. J., and White, B. N. 1994. Forensic application of repetitive DNA markers to the species identification of animal tissues. *Journal of Forensic Sciences* 39(2): 353–361.

Havill, L. M. 2004. Osteon remodeling dynamics in Macaca mulatta: Normal variation with regard to age, sex and skeletal maturity. *Calcified Tissue International* 74: 95–102.

Hoffman, J. M. 1984. Identification of nonskeletonized bear paws and human feet, in T. A. Rathbun and J. E. Buikstra (eds.), *Human Identification: Case Studies in Forensic Anthropology*, pp. 96–106. Springfield, IL: Charles C. Thomas.

Jowsey, J. 1966. Studies of Haversian systems in man and some animals. *Journal of Anatomy* 100(4): 857–864.

———. 1968. Age and species differences in bones. *Cornell Veterinarian* 58: 74–94.

Kerley, E. R. 1965. The microscoic determination of age in human bone. *American Journal of Physical Anthropology* 35: 171–184.

Lowenstein, J. M. 1980. Species-specific proteins in fossils. *Naturwissenschaften* 67: 343–346.

Martiniaková, M., Vondráková, M., and Fabiš, M. 2003. Investigation of the microscopic structure of rabbit compact bone tissue. *Scripta Medica* 76(4): 215–220.

Mori, R., Tetsuo, K., Soeta, S., Sato, J., Kakino, J., Hamato, S., Takaki, H., and Naito, Y. 2005. Preliminary study of histological comparison on the growth patterns of long-bone cortex in young calf, pig and sheep. *The Journal of Veterinary Medical Science* 67(12): 1223–1229.

Mulhern, D. M., and Ubelaker, D. H. 2001. Differences in osteon banding between human and nonhuman bone. *Journal of Forensic Sciences* 46(2): 220–222.

———. 2003. Histologic examination of bone development in juvenile chimpanzees. *American Journal of Physical Anthropology* 122(2): 127–133.

———. 2006. Bone microstructure in juvenile chimpanzees. Abstract. *American Journal of Physical Anthropology* Supp. 42: 135.

Murray, B. W., Clymont, R. A., and Strobeck, C. 1995. *The Journal of Forensic Sciences* 40(6): 943–951.

Olsen, S. J. 1973. *Mammal Remains from Archaeological Sites. Part 1: Southeastern and Southwestern United States.* Cambridge, MA: Peabody Museum.

Owsley, D. W., Mires, A. M., and Keith, M. S. 1985. Case involving differentiation of deer and human bone fragments. *Journal of Forensic Sciences* 30(2): 572–578.

Pirok, D. J., Ramser, J. R., Takahashi, H., Villanueva, A. R., and Frost, H. M. 1966. Normal histological, tetracycline and dynamic parameters in human, mineralized bone sections. *Henry Ford Hospital Medical Bulletin* 14: 195–218.

Quekett, J. 1849. On the intimate structure of bone as composing the skeleton in the four great classes of animals, viz. mammals, birds, reptiles and fishes. *Transactions of the Microscopical Society of London* 2: 40–42.

Schaffler, M. B., and Burr, D. B. 1984. Primate cortical bone microstructure: relationship to locomotion. *American Journal of Physical Anthropology* 65: 191–197.

Schmid, E. 1972. *Atlas of Animal Bones: For Prehistorians, Archaeologists and Quaternary Geologists.* Amsterdam: Elsevier Publishing Company.

Singh, I. J., and Gunberg, D. L. 1970. Estimation of age at death in human males from quantitative histology of bone fragments. *American Journal of Physical Anthropology* 33: 373–382.

Singh, I. J., Tonna, E. A., and Gandel, C. P. 1974. A comparative histological study of mammalian bone. *Journal of Morphology* 144: 421–438.

Stewart, T. D. 1959. Bear paw remains closely resemble human remains. *FBI Law Enforcement Bulletin* 28(11): 18–21.

———. 1979. *Essentials of Forensic Anthropology.* Springfield, IL: Charles C. Thomas.

Stout, S. D., and Paine, R. R. 1992. Histological age estimation using rib and clavicle. *American Journal of Physical Anthropology* 87: 111–115.

Stout, S. D., and Ross, L. M. 1991. Bone fragments a body can make. *Journal of Forensic Sciences* 36(3): 953–957.

Thompson, D. D. 1980. Age changes in bone mineralization, cortical thickness and Haversian canal area. *Calcified Tissue International* 31: 5–11.

Ubelaker, D. H. 1989. *Human Skeletal Remains: Excavation, Analysis, Interpretation* (2nd ed.). Washington, D. C.: Taraxacum.

Ubelaker, D. H., Lowenstein, J. M., and Hood, D. G. 2004. Use of solid-phase double-antibody radioimmunoassay to identify species from small skeletal fragments. *Journal of Forensic Sciences* 49(5): 924–929.

14

Dating of Anthropological Skeletal Remains of Forensic Interest

Shari Forbes and Kimberly Nugent

Traditional areas of research in forensic anthropology have dealt with variation in sex and population affinity and with estimation of age and stature for purposes of identification (Işcan 1998; Roberts 1996). Although the importance of these subjects has in no way diminished, additional topics have become increasingly visible over the last decade. Emerging areas of forensic anthropology focus on factors relating to the context of crime scenes, such as taphonomy (Aturaliya and Lukasewycz 1999), animal scavenging (Morton and Lord 2006), bone trauma (Symes et al. 2002), and time since death determinations (İşcan 1998). Of these newly developing areas, the determination of time since death (postmortem interval) has proven to be among the most challenging.

The initial determination of postmortem interval can assist in distinguishing between modern and ancient bones (Nafte 2000). Establishing whether skeletal remains are of forensic significance is of prime importance in determining whether a criminal investigation will be launched (Jarvis 1997; Knight and Lauder 1969). In a forensic context, establishing the postmortem interval of skeletal remains is important in providing investigators with a time frame in which the person may have disappeared, thus increasing the likelihood of a positive identification (Forbes 2004). It also plays a key role in determining the final movements of a victim and identifying potential suspects within the investigation (Pollard 1996).

Owing to its importance in forensic investigations, determination of postmortem interval of skeletal remains has been researched extensively by anthropologists and other disciplines in the forensic community. Early studies focused on morphological characteristics, such as bone consistency, weight, and specific gravity, as a means for differentiating modern and ancient bones (Berg 1963; Berg and Specht 1958). However, such techniques achieved limited success, and the focus soon shifted to studying chemical and immunological characteristics of bone, which proved more successful in distinguishing the two groups.

Of the numerous chemical and immunological studies conducted over the last 50 years, most have focused on the organic components of bone, bone extracts, and bone diagenesis (Collins et al. 2002; Cook and Heizer 1952; Hare 1976; Knight and Lauder 1969; Yoshino et al. 1991). Many of these studies, while initially unsuccessful, provided the basis for future research and further development of the techniques (Knight 1968, 1969; Knight and Lauder 1969). The major limitation encountered in these pioneering studies was an inability to account for the effect of environmental variables on bone degradation.

Radioisotope studies provided a means for overcoming such barriers and have recently become the most extensively researched methods for dating skeletal remains (Taylor et al. 1989; Tuniz, Zoppi, and Hotchkis 2004; Wild et al. 2000; Zoppi et al. 2004). Radioisotope measurements have the advantage of being more readily quantifiable than other techniques and are less affected by environmental variations. Although radiocarbon dating has been around for more than half a century, the technique has recently found new success in forensic investigations (Ubelaker 2001). Although a large range of alternative dating techniques have been investigated over the years, radioisotope methods appear to be the most reliable and are the current focus in forensic anthropology.

This chapter provides an overview of the morphological, chemical, immunological, and radioisotope dating techniques investigated within the last 60 years and their potential application to the field of forensic science.

Morphological Studies

Several early studies in the field of forensic pathology attempted robust dating estimates based on the morphological and physical characteristics of soft-tissue remains (Berg 1963; Knight 1968; Knight and Lauder 1967, 1969). The pathologist would commonly estimate postmortem interval using characteristics such as the cooling of the body temperature (algor mortis), fixation of hypostasis (livor mortis), and stiffening of the muscles (rigor mortis). Once the early postmortem period had passed, autolytic and putrefactive changes were used but provided a less than accurate estimation of postmortem interval (Knight 1968). Typically, within the first five years postmortem, fragments of ligaments, tendons, skin, hair, and cartilage are still observed on the decomposed remains. Yet soft tissues are prone to environmental modifications and do not generally survive the decomposition process, rendering the use of morphological characteristics in dating human remains problematic over time. As an alternative, scientists turned to skeletal material, which is generally more resistant to the postmortem decomposition process. Some changes in bone appearance and morphology provide indicators of time since death. After several decades, for example, the bone may exhibit a spotty discoloration and an overall soapy texture in addition to the presence of small pieces of collagenous tissue. Over a century after death, bone may appear light and crumbling in nature.

Chemical Studies

In addition to morphological studies, chemical studies were employed in an attempt to apply more scientific principles and objectivity to time since death estimations (Knight 1968, 1969; Knight and Lauder 1969). Initial studies investigated both organic and inorganic constituents of bone (Cook and Heizer 1952). A study by Berg and Specht conducted in 1958 was considered to be the first comprehensive attempt at using chemical methods to date skeletal remains (Berg and Specht 1958). A range of tests was investigated with varying results. The test for carbonate by reaction with hydrochloric acid produced a lively reaction when testing petrified bone but gave only a weak reaction for younger samples (Berg 1963). Conversely, analysis of younger samples under a mercury vapor lamp produced an intense blue-violet fluorescence that weakened as the age of the sample increased. A decline in fluorescence was also correlated with a gradual loss in affinity for the chemicals indophenol and a higher susceptibility to Nile Blue. All these techniques were, however, subjective and not sufficiently reliable. Tests involving determination of specific gravity and superconductivity gave similar results and were not considered useful as a stand-alone method for dating recent bone material (Berg 1963; Berg and Specht 1958; Facchini and Pettener 1977).

Although Berg and Specht's research identified many parameters for investigation, some of the techniques (including Nile Blue staining, dichloroindophenol staining, and reaction with acid) were considered to be too sophisticated for most users and not practical for crime-scene investigation (Knight and Lauder 1969). An attempt was therefore made to develop methods that were neither time-consuming nor expensive. A range of chemical techniques was investigated by Knight and Lauder (Knight 1968, 1969; Knight and Lauder 1967, 1969) in order to differentiate between "modern" (<70–100 years) and "ancient" (>70–100 years) bone (Knight and Lauder 1969). Although these definitions are not constant across different jurisdictions, these dating periods were used in the United Kingdom at the time of the research to determine whether further investigations were required by the Home Office. Some of the original methods were found to be useful in distinguishing between "modern" and "ancient" remains and were further developed and used by other researchers in the field both nationally and internationally (Facchini and Pettener 1977; Jarvis 1997).

A chemical analysis, known as the semimicro Kjeldahl technique, was used to analyze nitrogen content in bone and demonstrated a progressive decrease in nitrogen levels with postmortem age. Samples less than 50 years old (and therefore considered to be of forensic interest) contained a nitrogen content of more than 3.5 gm%. The results were consistent with an earlier study by Berg (1963) that showed nitrogen levels of more than 3.6 gm% for bone samples up to 40 years old (Knight and Lauder 1967, 1969). However, a lack of samples in both the time interval of interest (0–50 years) and the interval immediately preceding it (50–100 years) rendered the results insignificant.

A more recent study, which aimed to enhance this technique, investigated nitrogen levels in long bones interred for a period of 26–90 years (Jarvis 1997). The study was later improved on by incorporating bones that had deposition times that fell within the period of forensic interest. The methodology focused only on long bones and used a macro Kjeldahl technique that eliminated the errors associated with sample handling. The results further confirmed both the Berg (1963) and Knight and Lauder (1967, 1969) studies, which demonstrated a general decrease in total nitrogen content with time since deposition.

The fluorescence of bone has limited value as a confirmatory test but may provide useful information in combination with other indicators (Knight and Lauder 1969). Fluorescence under ultraviolet light is a measure of the organic constituents remaining in the bone material, and as these constituents are lost, fluorescence weakens considerably. Samples of forensic interest will generally contain a sufficient organic component so as to provide intense bluish-white fluorescence across the entire cross-section of the surface, even when recovered from a range of deposition environments (Facchini and Pettener 1977). The use of spectrofluorimetry (a type of electromagnetic spectroscopy that analyzes fluorescence from a sample) improves the subjectivity associated with this method, because it reduces spectral interference in the region where emission occurs, by employing a reflection grating rather than a filter. In addition, it allows both qualitative and quantitative determinations of fluorescence.

In addition to testing and further developing Berg and Specht's methodologies, Knight and Lauder also pioneered their own methods for dating remains (Knight and Lauder 1967, 1969). Studies involving the quantification of amino acids demonstrated a decline with postmortem age. As proteins in buried bones hydrolyze over time, they are released as amino acids that are ultimately lost to the environment as the postmortem age increases (Knight 1968, 1969). The presence of numerous amino acids (generally seven or more) demonstrates a high probability that the bone is less than 100 years old, and if proline and hydroxyproline are present then the bone may be closer to 50 years old. A bone in excess of 100 years old is not likely to contain more than three or four amino acids.

Benzidine testing of bone surface was also investigated and demonstrated that a strong positive reaction will occur in recent bone samples (Knight and Lauder 1969; Facchini and Pettener 1977). The intensity of the reaction will decrease with time, and a negative result indicates a bone sample in excess of 150 years old. Since the test relies on the presence of blood, the results are susceptible to alterations in different environmental conditions and the rapid loss of blood remnants. However, once these factors are taken into account, the benzidine reaction can supply a useful indicator for dating skeletal remains of forensic interest.

An alternative analysis dependent on the presence of blood is luminol testing. Luminol is a solution that produces a bluish-white light following a reaction with hydrogen peroxide in the presence of blood. The light can be visualized and photographed in the dark and is routinely used in forensic investigations to expose traces of blood (Jackson and Jackson 2004). In bone samples that have a recent time of death, the chemiluminescence produced will be intensive. As with the benzidine test, the intensity will decrease as the age of the bone increases, owing to the loss of hemoglobin proteins (Introna, Di Vella, and Campobasso 1999). A negative result is indicative of older bone samples. Luminol testing is perhaps the most recent development in chemical techniques used to date skeletal remains. The method provides a good correlation between the levels of intensity of the chemiluminescence with the difference in time since death of the bones. Objectivity of the method is achieved through the use of image analysis procedures that provide quantitative determination of the intensity and the distribution of the chemiluminescence reaction (Introna, Di Vella, and Campobasso 1999). In the present study, gray-level classification of the image was utilized to provide a more objective analysis of luminol; this is a common procedure available in the menu option of all image-enhancement software.

A range of analytical techniques have recently been investigated including X-ray diffraction, which can determine the crystalline structure of bone (Bartsiokas and Middleton 1992), and Raman spectroscopy (a technique used in condensed matter physics and chemistry to study vibrational, rotational, and other low-frequency modes in a system), which can identify the organic and inorganic components (Bertoluzza et al. 1997). Unfortunately, all studies have suffered from a lack of bone samples in the time interval of interest. Although further research with appropriate samples may yield more successful results, the accuracy achieved by these methods is generally not sufficient for practical use in forensic investigations.

Immunological Studies

The following section details the types of immunological studies undertaken to investigate postmortem interval, including gel diffusion testing, fat estimations, histological examinations, and colorimetry and ion-exchange chromatography.

Gel Diffusion Test

Immunological techniques have focused on the detection of residual serological activity of bone protein as an indicator of postmortem bone age (Berg 1963; Camps and Purchase 1956; Castellano, Villanueva, and von Frenckel 1984; Knight 1969; Knight and Lauder 1967, 1969). Immunological reactions between bone powder and antihuman rabbit serum were evaluated using precipitation times, and a gel diffusion test was performed (modified from Ouchterlony's method 1948 and 1958). Based on positive reactions, Camps and Purchase (1956) reported date estimates within the first 10 years postmortem, whereas Knight and Lauder (1969) and Knight (1969) reported an age of origin of less than 5 years using this technique. Berg (1963) quoted a bone age of up to 50 years if the protein precipitation was delayed and weak, but a rapid reaction most likely indicated an age of less than 20 years. Inconsistent results between studies were attributed to the quality of the antiserum and strength of the bone extracts (Knight 1969; Knight and Lauder 1969). Expanding on this earlier research, Castellano, Villaneuva, and von Frenckel (1984) demonstrated an important correlation between loss of both protein and lipids with postmortem aging of skeletal remains. Protein content, in particular zinc, which was hypothesized by the authors to be linked to protein in some way, displayed strong regression values and standard errors between 3–9 years, depending on the confidence intervals used.

Note that even though these methods offer potential for further investigations, the quality of the intact protein is questionable, since protein decomposition commences immediately after death (Collins et al. 2002; Hare 1976; Knight and Lauder 1969; Wiechmann, Brandt, and Grupe 1999). Recently, the reliability of immunological techniques to postmortem bone dating has been discussed (Brandt, Wiechmann, and Grupe 2002; Lendaro et al. 1991), and inconsistent findings are thought to have resulted from nonspecific reactions of serum against bone, soil contamination, and the presence of false-positives arising from unknown contaminating antigens.

Fat Estimations

Expanding on the work of Gangl (1936), various studies have attempted to correlate the fat content of bone with postmortem age (Berg 1963; Castellano, Villanueva, and von Frenckel 1984; Cook and Heizer 1952; Knight and Lauder 1969). Work by Buerger and Maestre in 1962 (Castellano, Villanueva, and Frenckel 1984) showed a decrease in bone lipid within 8–10 years postmortem. Berg (1963) also provided evidence that fat content decreases with bone age; however, Knight and Lauder failed to confirm this correlation in their 1969 study. More recently, Castellano, Villanueva, and von Frenckel (1984) validated the findings of both Buerger and Maestre (Castellano, Villanueva, and von Frenckel 1984) and Berg (1963), documenting a sharp decrease in bone triglycerides over time. Moreover, they successfully detected lipids in bones a century old.

Histological Examinations

Studies have well described the histological features of skeletal decomposition (Ascenzi 1955; Kerley 1965; Piepenbrink 1986; Yoshino et al. 1991); however, there has been less success in attributing postmortem age using histological bone sections. Knight and Lauder failed to obtain significant results in their 1969 study, ascertaining that it was technically impossible to analyze bone extracts unless undecalcified samples were available. The most promising results stemmed from Berg's research (1963), wherein he was able to assign robust age estimates based on fat remnants found within compact bone. Through the course of the postmortem decay process, marrow may be converted into adipocere, which then diffuses into the Haversian canals of femoral bones. For several decades thereafter, cross-sections provide a visible indicator of bone age. A bone cavity filled with adipocere indicates a bone age of less than 30 years postburial, whereas scanty adipocere material suggests a maximum bone age of 50 years. The use of this technique is limited, however, since both age and contents of the burial environment influence results.

Colorimetry and Ion-Exchange Chromatography

Knight and Lauder (1969) modified a technique first described by Moores, Spackman, and Stein in 1958 and Ho in 1965 in which bone powder was resuspended in dilute acid. The optical density of the resulting supernatant was analyzed and subjected to ion-exchange chromatography. Results demonstrated a promising correlation between bone color and age, but the technique did not prove reliable for routine use. Furthermore, no relationship between free amino acids and postmortem bone age was apparent, since results failed to identify more than a few free amino acids among the ten samples analyzed.

Environmental Conditions

The previously discussed investigations have attempted to establish methods for dating bone that would be less dependent on environment than on time. Unfortunately, burial surroundings, climate, and taphonomic conditions all influence postmortem decomposition processes. These variations, in turn, affect the reliability of dating techniques. Ambient temperature, humidity, moisture, soil pH, and geological events (erosion, flooding) are some of the more obvious abiotic environmental pressures encountered (Berg 1963; Hare 1976; Knight and Lauder 1969; Piepenbrink 1986). The effect of these factors on decomposition and skeletonization has been discussed extensively in the literature (Haglund and Sorg 1997; Micozzi 1991; Rodriguez and Bass 1985) and are not considered here. Biotic agents that have been found to play a significant role in dating skeletal remains include microorganisms and plants.

Biotic Factors

Arguably, the most common mechanism of postmortem bone deterioration is the product of microorganisms, in particular fungi and bacteria (Bell, Skinner, and Jones 1996; Child 1995; Collins et al. 2002; Marchiafava, Bonucci, and Ascenzi 1974; Piepenbrink 1986; Yoshino et al. 1991). Microbial activity affects morphological structure and chemical composition of bone and has been shown to occur very soon after death and in any burial condition (Bell et al. 1996; Collins et al. 2002).

Characteristic features of bone deterioration by microorganisms include bone staining, tunneling, demineralization, and fluorochroming and vary with the type of invading microorganism (Bell et al. 1996; Marchiafava et al. 1974; Piepenbrink 1986; Yoshino et al. 1991). These combined effects may lead to misinterpretations of postmortem history and thus compromise the accuracy of skeletal dating techniques available at this time.

Plants may be found growing in and among skeletal remains, particularly in clandestine burial environments. Although the discipline is still in its preliminary stages, to date the use of plant roots/indicators in establishing postmortem bone dates has found some success (Quatrehomme et al. 1997; Willey and Heilman 1987). Root cross-sections, branch growth, and root damage have been outlined as possible indicators of postmortem interval (PMI). Roots that are contacting or penetrating bones may be cross-sectioned and their annual rings counted in order to establish a minimum postmortem time frame. If the surrounding burial environment has been disturbed, the damaged roots may produce a permanent scar or point of reference, from which the annual growth rings may be counted. Finally, a relationship between annual growth (longitudinal and radial) and branch length (originating from the point of contact with remains) can be estimated and a time frame for growth established.

Radioisotope Studies

The use of radioactive isotopes to date archaeological bone material is not a new technique. Since its introduction in 1949, radiocarbon dating has been used extensively to estimate the approximate age of ancient remains (Ubelaker 2001). Although the technique predominantly uses the collagen fraction of bone, other fractions, including osteocalcin, have been investigated (Ajie and Kaplan 1990). Uranium-series dating has also found some success (Grun et al. 2005; Pike, Hedges, and van Calsteren 2002), although both methods are hampered by the relatively large errors associated with determining an accurate time since death (van Calsteren and Thomas 2006). Although predominantly used for archaeological investigations, modern-era activities have allowed the use of radioisotopes for dating bone samples of forensic interest.

Between 1950 and 1963, extensive nuclear weapons tests caused a high level of radiocarbon (^{14}C) to be released into the atmosphere, particularly in the Northern Hemisphere (Hua 2004; Tuniz, Zoppi, and Hotchkis 2004). During this time, the atmospheric radiocarbon level almost doubled compared to the reference level recorded in 1890 (Libby et al. 1964; Reimer, Brown, and Reimer 2004). Following the implementation of the Nuclear Test Ban Treaty in 1963, the atmospheric ^{14}C level has decreased exponentially to a concentration approximately 10% higher than the level recorded prior to nuclear testing (Hua 2004; Tuniz, Zoppi, and Hotchkis 2004). This higher concentration, known as the "bomb pulse," was initially used to assess the potential hazard of ^{14}C in medical use (Libby et al. 1964) and is now recognized as being a useful parameter in distinguishing pre-bomb from postbomb organic remains (Ubelaker 2001; Ubelaker and Houck 2002). As part of the biological cycle, both plants and animals (including humans) have incorporated the bomb ^{14}C via the food chain (Geyh 2001; Ubelaker and Buchholz 2006). Therefore, this temporal change may be used to date skeletal remains that are less than 50 years postmortem and therefore of forensic significance (Tuniz et al. 2004; Ubelaker, Buchholz, and Stewart 2006; Zoppi et al. 2004).

The earliest study to utilize bomb pulse dating in a forensic context was that conducted by Taylor and associates (1989). The study identified three different time periods based on ^{14}C data that could be used for estimating time since death of skeletal remains. Specifically, these intervals were classed as (1) pre-1650 period, (2) 1650–1950 period, and (3) post-1950 period, which was the period of interest in the study. Owing to the broad categories devised, the study was successful in differentiating modern from nonmodern bones. However, limitations of the technique included the length of time required to analyze samples, the amount of bone required, and the inability to provide a post-mortem interval estimation referring to a specific year.

Further attempts to date the collagen fraction of recent bone samples by means of bomb radiocarbon demonstrated more precise ranges (from approximately 3 years to several decades) compared to the earlier study (Geyh 2001). Additional corrections were made to account for the cessation of ^{14}C uptake in adult humans at the age of 19. However, even with these corrections, the ranges were not considered sufficiently precise to be used in forensic cases. This can be attributed to the relatively long carbon turnover rates of bone collagen compared to other bone fractions (Ubelaker, Buchholz, and Stewart 2006; Wild et al. 1998).

Lipids from bone and bone marrow have been shown to provide a more reliable estimate of the time of death for recent bone samples using ^{14}C measurement (Wild et al. 1998, 2000). In instances where the bone lipid has completely degraded, or is not recoverable, hair or dental tissue can also provide a reliable estimate (Geyh 2001; Ubelaker, Buchholz, and Stewart 2006; Wild et al. 1998). With the selection of appropriate material (that is, material with a rapid carbon turnover rate), the radiocarbon bomb-pulse method appears to be the most accurate method currently available for dating skeletal remains that are considered to be of forensic significance. The technique has successfully been employed in forensic casework to clearly distinguish between ancient remains and more recent remains that warrant a forensic investigation (Ubelaker, Buchholz, and Stewart 2006; Ubelaker and Houck 2002). It is not possible to comment on whether the method was accepted in court testimony, because neither case went to court.

The fallout from nuclear weapons testing led to the contamination of the environment with additional radioisotopes such as strontium-90 (^{90}Sr) (Papworth and Vennart 1984). Investigations of ^{90}Sr activity in bones have demonstrated significant differences in concentration between prebomb and postbomb skeletal remains (Maclaughlin-Black et al. 1992). The method is simple to use compared to radiocarbon techniques and is reliable in determining whether an individual died pre- or post-1950 (Neis et al. 1999). However, samples tend to suffer from groundwater contamination following burial in soil. The technique requires further investigation in order to correlate the ^{90}Sr burden with the postmortem interval of skeletal tissue.

A more recent method has been proposed for dating human skeletal material and involves the measurement of lead-210 (^{210}Pb) and polonium-210 (^{210}Po) concentrations in bone (Swift 1998). The relatively short half-life of ^{210}Pb makes it an ideal radioisotope for forensic analyses. Further, it is an abundant isotope in the environment, and its ratio with ^{210}Po can be quantitatively measured with accuracy. Preliminary studies suggest that there is a correlation between certain radionuclide content and time since death and an intercorrelation between trace elements and time since death of recent skeletal material (Swift 1998; Swift et al. 2001). Specifically, trace lead levels from a historical period were shown to be higher than the concentrations observed for both recent bone samples and ancient bone samples. Higher levels of incidental lead ingestion from sources such as lead plumbing and paints common until the 1930s provide the most likely explanation.

Further studies have confirmed these findings and have also identified significant differences between patterns of radionuclide concentrations and trace element concentrations in different types of bones (Howard et al. 2006). Ongoing studies have shown that the combination of activity concentration values for ^{210}Po, ^{238}U (uranium-238), and ^{226}Ra (radium-226) can potentially separate bones derived from individuals who have died in archaeological (>150 years ago), historical (75–149 years ago), and recent (<75 years ago) periods. Furthermore, radionuclide activity concentrations, and calcium content in bones, from the archaeological era are generally higher than those from more recent eras (Howard, Meyer, and Forbes 2006). The results of these current studies have shown great potential for the use of radioisotopes other than radiocarbon and will likely shape the future for skeletal dating techniques.

Conclusion

In many investigations, the time since death estimation provided by the anthropologist will more likely be based on experience in particular regional/environmental contexts than any of the above-mentioned techniques. However, such estimations may vary considerably among anthropologists owing to the subjectivity involved in analyzing the remains. The need for objective and accurate methods for dating skeletal remains continues to be acute, and considerable research has been focused in this area. Determining whether human skeletal remains are of possible or of definite forensic interest should be done prior to any death investigation; this will ultimately shape the course of that investigation.

Original attempts at dating skeletal remains using morphological and physical characteristics were not successful and led to the investigation of chemical characteristics instead. Although many chemical techniques were employed and some success was achieved, the majority of studies yielded contradictory results. Immunological studies proved equally inaccurate, and all techniques suffered from the unknown effects of environmental parameters. Recent radioisotope studies have shown the most promise, and further studies in this area will potentially provide an accurate method for dating skeletal remains of forensic significance.

The need for accurate dating methods has become more apparent in recent years as forensic anthropologists are called on to investigate deaths resulting from genocide, war crimes, and crimes against humanity (Schmitt 2002). Commonly, mass graves are identified many years after the event, and the exact postmortem interval of the exhumed human remains may be unknown. A precise method for estimating time since death of such skeletal remains would provide invaluable assistance to war crime tribunals and ultimately assist in the prosecution of war criminals.

In all criminal investigations, regardless of their nature, the estimation of time since death is one of the most important variables present. Although methods exist for estimating this time frame in the early postmortem period, accurate techniques applied to the subsequent (skeletal) postmortem period are lacking. For this reason, research in the field of forensic anthropology should continue to focus on the important task of estimating postmortem interval of forensically significant skeletal remains.

References

Ajie, H. O., and Kaplan, I. R. 1990. AMS radiocarbon dating of bone osteocalcin. *Nuclear Instruments and Methods of Physics Research B* 52: 433–437.

Ascenzi, A. 1955. Some histological properties of the organic substance in Neandertalian bone. *American Journal of Physical Anthropology* 13: 557–566.

Aturaliya, S., and Lukasewycz, A. 1999. Experimental forensic and bioanthropological aspects of soft tissue taphonomy: 1. Factors influencing postmortem tissue desiccation rate. *Journal of Forensic Sciences* 44: 893–896.

Bartsiokas, A., and Middleton, A. P. 1992. Characterization and dating of recent and fossil bone by X-ray diffraction. *Journal of Archaeological Science* 19: 63–72.

Bell, L. S., Skinner, M. F., and Jones, S. J. 1996. The speed of postmortem change to the human skeleton and its taphonomic significance. *Forensic Science International* 82: 129–140.

Berg, S. 1963. The determination of bone age, in F. Lundquist (ed.), *Methods of Forensic Science*, pp. 231–252. New York: Wiley and Sons.

Berg, S., and Specht, W. 1958. Untersuchungen zur Bestimmung der Liegezeit von Skeletteilen. *Verhandlungen der Deutschen Gesellschaft für Innere Medizin* 47: 209–241.

Bertoluzza, A., Brasili, P., Castri, L., Facchini, F., Fagnana, C., and Tinti, A. 1997. Preliminary results in dating human skeletal remains by raman spectroscopy. *Journal of Raman Spectroscopy* 28: 185–188.

Brandt, E., Wiechmann, I., and Grupe, G. 2002. How reliable are immunological tools for the detection of ancient proteins in fossil bones? *International Journal of Osteoarchaeology* 12: 307–316.

Camps, F. E., and Purchase, W. B. 1956. *Practical Forensic Medicine*. London: Hutchinson.

Castellano, M. A., Villanueva, E. C., and von Frenckel, R. 1984. Estimating the date of bone remains: A multivariate study. *Journal of Forensic Sciences* 29(2): 527–534.

Child, A. M. 1995. Towards an understanding of the decomposition of bone in the archaeological environment. *Journal of Archaeological Science* 22: 165–174.

Collins, M. J., Nielsen-Marsh, C. M., Hiller, J., Smith C. I., and Roberts, J. P. 2002. The survival of organic matter in bone: A review. *Archaeometry* 44(3): 383–394.

Cook, S., Heizer, R. 1952. The fossilization of bone: Organic components and water. *Reports of the University of California Archaeological Survey* 17: 1–24.

Facchini, F., and Pettener, D. 1977. Chemical and physical methods in dating human skeletal remains. *American Journal of Physical Anthropology* 47: 65–70.

Forbes, S. L. 2004. Time since death: A novel approach to dating skeletal remains. *The Australian Journal of Forensic Sciences* 36: 67–72.

Gangl, I. 1936. Alterbestimmung fossiler Knochenfunde auf chemische Wege. *Österreichische chemische Zeitung* 39: 79–82.

Geyh, M. A. 2001. Bomb radiocarbon dating of animal tissues and hair. *Radiocarbon* 43: 723–730.

Grun, R., Stringer, C., McDermott, F., Nathan, R., Porat, N., Robertson, S., Taylor, T., Mortimer, G., Eggins, S., and McCulloch, M. 2005. U-series and ESR analyses of bones and teeth relating to the human burials from Skhul. *Journal of Human Evolution* 49: 316–334.

Haglund, W. D., and Sorg, M. H. 1997. Method and theory of forensic taphonomy research, in W. D. Haglund and M. H. Sorg (eds.), *Forensic Taphonomy: The Postmortem Fate of Human Remains*, pp. 13–26. Boca Raton, FL: CRC Press.

Hare, P. E. 1976. Organic geochemistry of bone and its relation to the survival of bone in the natural environment, in A. Behrensmeyer and A. P. Hill (eds.), *Fossils in the Making: Vertebrate Taphonomy and Paleoecology*, pp. 208–219. Chicago: The University of Chicago Press.

Ho, T-Y. 1965. Amino acid composition of bone and tooth proteins in Late Pleistocene Mammals. *Proceedings of the National Academy of Sciences* 54: 26–31.

Howard, S. J., Meyer, J., and Forbes, S. L. 2006. Estimating time since death from human skeletal remains by radioisotope and trace element analysis. *Proceedings of the 18th International Symposium on the Forensic Sciences,* Perth, Australia.

Hua, Q. 2004. Review of tropospheric bomb 14C data for carbon cycle modeling and age calibration purposes. *Radiocarbon* 46: 1273–1298.

Introna, F., Jr., Di Vella, G., and Campobasso, C. P. 1999. Determination of postmortem interval from old skeletal remains by image analysis of luminol test results. *Journal of Forensic Sciences* 44: 535–538.

İşcan, M. Y. 1998. Progress in forensic anthropology: The 20th century. *Forensic Science International* 98: 1–8.

———. 2001. Global forensic anthropology in the 21st century. *Forensic Science International* 117: 1–6.

İşcan, M. Y., and Loth, S. R. 1997. The scope of forensic anthropology, in W. G. Eckert (ed.), *Introduction to Forensic Sciences*, pp. 343–369. Boca Raton, FL: CRC Press Inc.

Jackson, A. R. W., and Jackson, J. M. 2004. *Forensic Science*. Harlow, England: Pearson Prentice Hall.

Jarvis, D. R. 1997. Nitrogen levels in long bones from coffin burials interred for periods of 26–90 years. *Forensic Science International* 85: 199–208.

Kerley, E. 1965. The microscopic determination of age in human bone. *American Journal of Physical Anthropology* 23(2): 149–164.

Knight, B. 1969. Methods of dating skeletal remains. *Medicine, Science and the Law* 9: 247–252.

———. 1968. Estimation of the time since death: A survey of practical methods. *Journal of Forensic Science* 8(2): 91–96.

Knight, B., and Lauder, I. 1967. Practical methods of dating skeletal remains: A preliminary study. *Medicine, Science and the Law* 7(4): 205–208.

———. 1969. Methods of dating skeletal remains. *Human Biology* 41(3): 322–341.

Lendaro, E., Ippoliti, R., Bellelli, A., Brunori, M., Zito, R., Citro, G., and Ascenzi, A. 1991. Brief communication: On the problem of immunological detection of antigens in skeletal remains. *American Journal of Physical Anthropology* 86: 429–432.

Libby, W. F., Berger, R., Mead, J. F., Alexander, G. V., and Ross, J. F. 1964. Replacement rates for human tissue from atmospheric radiocarbon. *Science* 146: 1170–1172.

Maclaughlin-Black, S. M., Herd, R. J. M., Wilson, K., Myers, M., and West, I. E. 1992. Strontium-90 as an indicator of time since death: A pilot investigation. *Forensic Science International* 57: 51–66.

Marchiafava V. Y., Bonucci, E. Y., and Ascenzi, A. Y. 1974. Fungal osteoclasia: A model of dead bone resorption. *Calcified Tissue International* 14(1): 195–210.

Micozzi, M. S. 1991. *Postmortem Change in Human and Animal Remains: A Systematic Approach.* Boca Raton, FL: CRC Press.

Moores, S., Spackman, D. H., and Stein, W .H. 1958. Chromatography of amino acids on sulfonated polysterene resins. *Analytical Chemistry* 30: 1185–1190.

Morton, R. J., and Lord, W. D. 2006. Taphonomy of child-sized remains: A study of scattering and scavenging in Virginia, USA. *Journal of Forensic Sciences* 51: 475–479.

Nafte, M. 2000. *Flesh and Bone: An Introduction to Forensic Anthropology.* Durham, NC: Carolina Academic Press.

Neis, P., Hille, R., Paschke, M., Pilwat, G., Schnabel, A., Niess, C., and Bratzke, H. 1999. Strontium 90 for determination of time since death. *Forensic Science International* 99: 47–51.

Ouchterlony, O. 1948. *In vitro* method for testing toxin producing capacity of diphtheria bacteria. *Acta pathologica et microbiologica Scandinavica* 25: 186–191.

———. 1958. Progress in allergy. *Basel* 5: 1.

Papworth, D. G., and Vennart, J. 1984. The uptake and turnover of ^{90}Sr in the human skeleton. *Physics in Medicine and Biology* 29: 1045–1061.

Piepenbrink, H. 1986. Two examples of biogenous dead bone decomposition and their consequences for taphonomic interpretation. *Journal of Archaeological Science* 13: 417–430.

Pike, A. W. G., Hedges, R. E. M., and van Calsteren, P. 2002. U-series dating of bone using the diffusion-adsorption model. *Geochimica et Cosmochimica Acta* 66: 4273–4286.

Pollard, A. M. 1996. Dating the time of death, in J. Hunter, C. Roberts, and A. Martin (eds.), *Studies in Crime: An Introduction to Forensic Archaeology*, pp. 139–155. London: Routledge.

Quatrehomme, G., Lacoste, A., Bailet, P., Grevin, G., and Ollier, A. 1997. Contribution of microscopic plant anatomy to postmortem bone dating. *Journal of Forensic Sciences* 42: 140–143.

Reimer, P. J., Brown, T. A., and Reimer, R. W. 2004. Discussion: Reporting and calibration of post-bomb ^{14}C data. *Radiocarbon* 46: 1299–1304.

Roberts, C. A. 1996. Forensic anthropology 1: The contribution of biological anthropology to forensic contexts, in J. Hunter, C. Roberts, and A. Martin (eds.), *Studies in Crime: An Introduction to Forensic Archaeology*, pp. 101–121. London: Batsford.

Rodriguez, W. C., and Bass, W. M. 1985. Decomposition of buried bodies and methods that may aid in their location. *Journal of Forensic Sciences* 30: 836–852.

Schmitt, S. 2002. Mass graves and the collection of forensic evidence: genocide, war crimes, and crimes against humanity, in W. D. Haglund and M. H. Sorg (eds.), *Advances in Forensic Taphonomy: Method, Theory, and Archaeological Perspectives*, pp. 277–292. Boca Raton, FL: CRC Press.

Swift, B. 1998. Dating human skeletal remains: Investigating the viability of measuring the equilibrium between 210Po and 210Pb as a means of estimating post-mortem interval. *Forensic Science International* 98: 119–126.

Swift, B., Lauder, I., Black, S., and Norris, J. 2001. An estimation of the post-mortem interval in human skeletal remains: A radionuclide and trace element approach. *Forensic Science International* 117: 73–87.

Symes, S. A., Williams, J. A., Murray, E. A., Hoffman, J. M., Holland, T. D., Saul, J. M., Saul, F. P., and Pope, E. J. 2002. Taphonomic context of sharp-force trauma in suspected cases of human mutilation and dismemberment, in W. D. Haglund and M. H. Sorg (eds.), *Advances in Forensic Taphonomy: Method, Theory, and Archaeological Perspectives*, pp. 403–434. Boca Raton, FL: CRC Press.

Taylor, R. E., Suchey, J. M., Payen, L. A., and Slota, Jr., P. J. 1989. The use of radiocarbon (14C) to identify human skeletal materials of forensic Science Interest. *Journal of Forensic Sciences* 34: 1196–1205.

Tuniz, C., Zoppi, U., and Hotchkis, M.A.C. 2004. Sherlock Holmes counts the atoms. *Nuclear Instruments and Methods in Physics Research B* 213: 469-475.

Ubelaker, D. H. 2001. Artificial radiocarbon as an indicator of recent origin of organic remains in forensic cases. *Journal of Forensic Sciences* 46: 1285–1287.

Ubelaker, D. H., and Buchholz, B. A. 2006. Complexities in the use of bomb-curve radiocarbon to determine time since death of human skeletal remains. *Forensic Science Communications* 8: 1.

Ubelaker, D. H., Buchholz, B. A., and Stewart, J. E. B. 2006. Analysis of artificial radiocarbon in different skeletal and dental tissue types to evaluate date of death. *Journal of Forensic Sciences* 51: 484–488.

Ubelaker, D. H., and Houck, M. M. 2002. Using radiocarbon dating and paleontological extraction techniques in the analysis of a human skull in an unusual context. *Forensic Science Communications* 4: 4.

van Calsteren, P., and Thomas, L. 2006. Uranium-series dating applications in natural environmental science. *Earth-Science Reviews* 75: 155–175.

Wiechmann, I., Brandt, E., and Grupe, G. 1999. State of preservation of polymorphic plasma proteins recovered from ancient human bones. *International Journal of Osteoarchaeology* 9: 383–394.

Wild, E., Golser, R., Hille, P., Kutschera, W., Priller, A., Puchegger, S., Rom, W., and Steier, P. 1998. First 14C results from archaeological and forensic studies at the Vienna Environmental Research Accelerator. *Radiocarbon* 40: 273–281.

Wild, E. M., Arlamovsky, K. A., Golser, R., Kutschera, W., Priller, A., Puchegger, S., Rom, W., Steier, P., and Vycudilik, W. 2000. 14C dating with the bomb peak: An application to forensic medicine. *Nuclear*

Instruments and Methods in Physics Research B 172: 944–950.

Willey, P., and Heilman, A. 1987. Estimating time since death using plant roots and stems. *Journal of Forensic Sciences* 32(5): 1264–1270.

Yoshino, M., Kimijima, T., Miyasaka, S., Sato, H., and Seta, S. 1991. Microscopical study on estimation of time since death in skeletal remains. *Forensic Science International* 49: 143–159.

Zoppi, U., Skopec, Z., Skopec, J., Jones, G., Fink, D., Hua, Q., Jacobsen, G., Tuniz, C., and Williams, A. 2004. Forensic application of 14C bomb-pulse dating. *Nuclear Instruments and Methods in Physics Research B* 223-224: 770–775.

ANALYSIS OF COMMINGLED HUMAN REMAINS

John Byrd and Bradley J. Adams

Commingling is a problematic aspect of many anthropological analyses. Regardless of whether the context is archaeological, such as a Native American ossuary, or forensic, such as an aircraft crash, commingling of human remains will complicate every facet of the process from recovery to final disposition. With the exception of an early article by Charles Snow (1948) that outlines protocols used in the anthropological analysis of American war dead from World War II, the subject of commingling has only relatively recently been discussed in detail, for example, by Ubelaker (2002), Byrd and Adams (2003), Adams and Konigsberg (2004), and Adams and Byrd (2006, 2008), all of which provide comprehensive lists of references on the topic.

When dealing with commingled assemblages, only properly trained individuals should participate in all phases of the project. In the field, the recovery should be directed by archaeologists or archaeologically trained forensic anthropologists familiar with the excavation and documentation of human remains and associated evidence. In the laboratory, two primary objectives will be to sort the bones into specific individuals and quantify the number of dead. When feasible (such as with modern mass casualties), a major component of the effort will also be the positive identification of victims. Only experienced osteologists should be

used for these undertakings, or the results may be incomplete or incorrect.

Scale of the Incident

The complexity of a commingled assemblage is clearly dependent on the overall number of dead involved in the incident and the preservation of the remains. It is possible to broadly categorize commingling into two types: small-scale and large-scale.

Small-scale commingling is much easier to deal with and exists when (1) there are not many disassociated portions and/or (2) the number of individuals is small. Even in cases where the overall number of individuals is large (such as a mass grave), the degree of commingling may still be considered to be small-scale, especially if the skeletal elements are mostly articulated on their recovery. In this context, careful excavation must be exercised in order to preclude intermixing of individuals during the recovery effort. In other small-scale situations, there may be extensive mixing of skeletal elements or body parts, but there are only a few individuals represented. This creates a situation in which it may be feasible to re-associate the parts to specific individuals with great confidence. Adams and Byrd (2006), for example, present a case example of small-scale commingling resulting from the crash of a helicopter with two individuals aboard. In this case, it was possible to use gross techniques to confidently re-associate almost all the extensively commingled and fragmentary skeletal elements.

Large-scale commingling involves large numbers of individuals whose bodies are mixed in what can be taken as a random manner (although formal analysis may reveal patterning). It may also be the case that the number of individuals alone is not daunting, but extreme fragmentation greatly complicates the process and magnifies the scale of the analytical undertaking. With extensive fragmentation it can be the case that the majority of the body parts cannot be associated by traditional (that is, gross) means and therefore cannot be attributed to any individual. The remains recovered from the World Trade Center attacks in New York City in 2001 represent an example of large numbers of individuals and extreme body fragmentation. In this case, 2,749 individuals were killed, and more than 20,000 human remains of varying sizes and preservation states were recovered (Mundorff 2008; Mundorff et al. 2008). Large-scale commingling often necessitates a greater reliance on DNA analysis and presents numerous logistical challenges.

Field Recovery

In any scenario resulting in the discovery of commingled human remains, there must be a thoroughly documented and controlled retrieval process in order to preserve contextual evidence from the field (Cheetham and Hanson this volume; Dirkmaat and Adovasio 1997; Haglund 2002; Hochrein 2002; Reineke and Hochrein 2008; Schmitt 2002; Skinner 1987; Skinner, Alempijevic, and Djuric-Srejic 2003; Skinner, York, and Connor 2002). If one does not account for spatial data, many important associations may be lost. Successful accomplishment of this step will greatly assist in the laboratory analysis and ensure that secondary commingling is not caused as a result of careless recovery techniques. The same care is necessary in the laboratory to make sure that the important recovery scene information is preserved. For example, the maintenance of field provenience through specimen labeling is recommended in order to preserve field context data. It is most frequently in the laboratory that the number of individuals represented will be estimated, portions will be re-associated to specific individuals, and, within the forensic context, remains will be identified and returned to the next of kin. Without proper field recovery protocols, all facets of the laboratory process will be greatly complicated.

Laboratory Sorting

Depending on circumstances of death and deposition, the condition of the commingled remains may range from fleshed to skeletonized, and from intact to fragmentary. Thermal alteration, such as cremation or burn trauma, may add yet another facet to the complexity of the analysis (Bass and Jantz 2004; Kennedy 1996; Warren 2008; Warren and Maples 1997; Warren and Schultz 2002). When working with mutilated, fleshed human remains, one may only with difficulty be able to grossly recognize the full extent of commingling. In some traumatic events it is possible for body parts from one individual to become attached to and/or embedded into the body of another individual. Although radiography has traditionally been used for identification purposes, it can also be a useful tool in the recognition of commingling, depending on the type of incident and preservation of the bodies (Blau, Robertson, and Johnston 2008; Goodman and Edelson 2002; Viner 2008). A preliminary radiographic evaluation of fleshed body parts (perhaps at an initial triage station) may be warranted to detect commingling through the identification of excessive number of body parts, for example, and to assist in the sorting process. This is especially true in regard to contemporary situations when rapid scene response is possible, such as an aircraft crash or terrorist bombing. In these situations, every fragment of bone and soft tissue should be initially considered as a separate specimen unless it can be shown to be attached by soft tissue or to conjoin to another piece. *The simple fact that portions are recovered together from the field and are bagged as a unit is not conclusive evidence that they originated from the same person.*

Sorting Commingled Remains

For the sorting process, it is commonly the job of the physical/forensic anthropologist to "rebuild" the individuals to the greatest extent possible. An early discussion of sorting that is still germane can be found in the article by Charles Snow (1948). Snow advocated a systematic approach to sorting that utilized gross methods such as pair matching, articulation, and process of elimination in a series of steps. Today, the analysis of DNA profile data provides another powerful stage in the sorting process (Budimlija et al. 2003; Mundorff et al. 2008) that was not available to Snow. As DNA technology becomes more rapid and cost effective, it is proving to be more commonplace in the resolution of commingling. Without a doubt, one can imagine many examples of "unidentifiable" or "un-associable" human remains from past events that would today be resolvable thanks to the advent of DNA analysis.

The sorting guidelines exemplified in this chapter provide an objective and sound basis for gross, metric, and molecular analysis. It is important that systematic procedures are utilized and appropriately documented. Many scenarios, especially those involving dry bone, will be amenable to several gross techniques (biological profile, visual pair matching, checking articulations, process of elimination, robusticity, and taphonomy), one metric technique (osteometric comparison), and, when appropriate and feasible, DNA analysis. The majority of these sorting procedures are not stand-alone techniques. For best results, they should be used in conjunction with one another. For example, a combination of articulation, process of elimination, and taphonomy may provide strong evidence of association, but any of these alone may be insufficient. In addition, osteometric comparison (Byrd 2008; Byrd and Adams 2003) may provide an objective manner of segregating two elements hypothesized to originate from different individuals. It is worth reiterating that extensive fragmentation will hinder most gross techniques and necessitate a greater reliance on the use of DNA analysis, regardless of the scale of the incident.

The gross and metric sorting procedures can be accurately and objectively applied to most instances of small-scale commingling. They are also very useful for large-scale commingling situations, but discriminating power is likely to be reduced in many circumstances as the number of skeletal elements grows (for example, differences in size and shape may not be as apparent when the number of individuals increases). Large-scale commingling also introduces many logistical problems regarding analysis, such as laboratory space and data management issues (Byrd et al. 2003). Most of the procedures recommended in this chapter require considerable laboratory bench space. These procedures also require the assignment of specimen numbers that need to be physically associated with each body part. The data generated during the analytical process must be compiled, stored, and then retrieved as needed in support of analyses. Data management and analysis is best done on computers, but there is still a need to develop software to automate the process.

Conjoining Fragmentary Remains

The first step of the sorting process involves determining element representation. As part of this step, fragmentary remains should be conjoined (for example, glued together) to the greatest extent possible, since this will assist in the overall segregation process. Bones should then be sorted by element type, side, and size (for instance, all right femora should be organized from smallest to largest). Grouping elements by age criteria (for example, lack of epiphyseal fusion) may also be helpful at this stage of the sorting process. All provenience information collected during the recovery effort should be maintained, because it may become critical during the analytical process. Furthermore, it is not unusual for articulated body portions to be recovered together (for instance, right arm and hand, and these associations should be maintained as a unit throughout the analysis as long as there is confidence in their association. Once these initial steps are completed, the formal sorting techniques can be systematically applied.

Biological Profile (Age, Sex, and Stature)

The human aging process is characterized by roughly 25 years of skeletal and dental development followed by decades of degradation, popularly referred to as "aging." This aging process is reflected in numerous places in the skeleton (see Rogers this volume) and can be a critical clue in the sorting process (Schaefer 2008). Teeth erupt according to a relatively uniform schedule over the first 18 years of life (see Clement this volume). Epiphyses are open during the early periods of rapid growth but eventually close in a gradual manner. The closing of epiphyses, usually complete by the mid-20s, can be scored on an ordinal scale, as in the classic study by McKern and Stewart (1957). Other areas of the skeleton, including the pubic symphyses, the auricular surfaces, and the sternal ends of the 4th ribs, exhibit gradual degradation throughout life. This degradation has been studied and presented as series of stages by anthropologists (Brooks and Suchey 1990; İşcan, Loth, and Wright 1984, 1985; Lovejoy et al. 1985). Advanced age is often reflected by the presence of arthritic lipping and resorption of bone in areas such as the joints.

Age estimates derived from various specimens can be used in the sorting process to separate bones of demonstrably different ages. For example, an innominate aged at 40 to 50 years can be confidently sorted apart from a humerus with a proximal epiphysis unfused. A cranium with the second molars fully formed and the third molars unerupted with incomplete root formation could be sorted apart from the innominate but not from the humerus.

In addition to the informative role that skeletal age markers may play in the sorting process, there may also be sorting clues based on the individual's sex or stature that can be of assistance. For example, a pelvis that is clearly female can often be segregated from all crania that are conclusively male. Similarly, it may be possible to objectively segregate long bones that have widely divergent stature estimates. Regarding stature, osteometric comparison (see below) will provide a more robust method of sorting based on metric data.

Visual Pair Matching

Visual pair matching refers to the association of homologous (that is, left-right) elements based on similarities in morphology. In many instances, the right and left sides will be mirror images of each other. This concordance can be exploited in the process of sorting commingled remains through the recognition of paired bones from the same individual. Visual pair matching is arguably among the most reliable and accurate methods available to the anthropologist sorting commingled remains, especially when the population size is manageable. The level of reliability is, however, contingent on the experience of the analyst. Regular training and proficiency testing are recommended.

Note that pair matching refers to the same element type (for example, right and left humeri). Visual matching of different skeletal elements (for instance, a humerus and a femur) based on morphology is not recommended owing to the subjective nature of the procedure. Visual matching of different element types using information such as robusticity and taphonomy may be possible in cases of small-scale commingling, as discussed below.

The basic procedure for visual pair matching is to hold the two specimens in question side by side and to evaluate their concordance. The specimens should be observed from different angles. It is advised to look at the comparison critically, attempting to note discrepancies that make their association untenable. This can be done by formally comparing the size (that is, length and width), followed by the overall shape, then the shape of any processes, then the shape of articular facets, and so forth. Figure 15.1 provides illustrations of the method at work. The more corresponding features there are, the greater the confidence that can be placed in the association. However, one distinct difference can lead to the segregation of two specimens. Note the differences in overall length, the development of the deltoid tuberosity, and the shape of the distal condyles in Figure 15.1c, which should lead to the conclusion that these are not a pair-match.

Preliminary research (Adams 1996; Adams and Konigsberg 2004) tested the reliability of visual pair matching with an archaeological skeletal collection housed at the University of Tennessee, Knoxville. Two commingled scenarios were simulated, one from a sample of 15 individuals and one from a sample of 30 individuals (note that only a 60% recovery was simulated in order to ensure that not every element would have a true pair represented). Only tibiae, femora, and humeri were

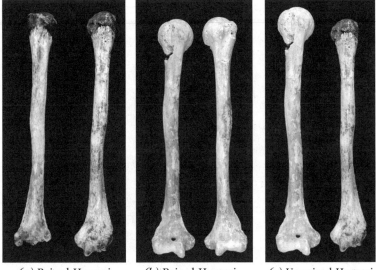

(a) Paired Humeri   *(b)* Paired Humeri   *(c)* Unpaired Humeri

Figure 15.1   Two pairs of humeri depicted in *a* and *b*, with a comparison between nonassociated bones in *c*.

tested, and the samples consisted of both complete and fragmentary elements from both adults and subadults. Results of the 15 individual groups showed that all femora were matched correctly, all tibiae were matched correctly, and one pair of humeri was incorrectly identified. Results of the 30 individual tests revealed that the following were not accurately recorded: one pair of humeri and one pair of tibiae. All femora were correctly pair-matched. Although the limited results of this test are encouraging, one suspects that this high matching frequency may change if the sample size is substantially increased, since variation among individuals may not be as obvious. Furthermore, even minimal fragmentation can obliterate key areas used for identifying a match and be cause for errors.

Articulation

Skeletal specimens that are adjoining elements can be associated or sorted by assessing their articulation, or formation of a congruent joint or juncture with another element. The basis for this form of analysis is the fact that articulating skeletal elements grow together as moving parts. Unless the

individual suffers a pathological condition, the articulations will show a good fit in terms of size and shape. Some skeletal articulations require tighter concordance than others. Although articulation is one of the best methods for gross sorting, the confidence in an agreeable articulation as evidence of true association will vary according to how much concordance is actually required for the two bones to fit together. Table 15.1 provides a ranking of major skeletal articulations in terms of the confidence placed in a positive result (note that this table is based on the experience of the authors). Although an agreeable articulation does not guarantee a true association, a poor articulation is taken as proof of nonassociation.

Through articulation it may be possible to systematically sort much of a commingled assemblage, especially in small-scale incidents. As with most techniques, large-scale commingling will greatly complicate the process. When feasible, the best area to initiate the "rebuilding" process is often with the pelvis or vertebrae. From here the various elements can be added. Problems with articulation arise from the lack of a close fit between some elements, such as between the arm and the torso. The articulation between the humeral head and

Table 15.1 Table of articulations, with indication of degree of confidence in a fit. Articulations classed as "low" cannot serve as evidence of a good match but do have some potential for excluding very poor fits (from Adams and Byrd 2006).

High	Moderate	Low
Cranium, mandible	Cranium, atlas	Ribs, thoracic vertebrae
Vertebrae	Tibia, fibula	Manubrium, clavicle
5th lumbar vertebra, sacrum	Femur, tibia	Humerus, scapula
Humerus, ulna	Innominate, femur	
Innominate, sacrum	Patella, femur	
Tibia, talus	Navicular (scaphoid), radius	
Ulna, radius	Carpals[†]	
Metatarsals*	Carpals, metacarpals	
Metacarpals*		
Tarsals		
Tarsals, metatarsals		

*The 1st metacarpal and 1st metatarsal do not articulate closely with the others and are to be regarded as "low" confidence so far as their articulation with the others is concerned.
†The articular surface of the pisiform is too small to articulate with confidence.

the glenoid fossa of the scapula is not very diagnostic, nor is there an obvious way to articulate the scapula to the rest of the body. Linking arms, scapulae, and clavicles to torsos can be difficult or impossible based solely on articulation. Other elements, such as ribs, may also be challenging to associate based on articulation. As with all the procedures described in this chapter, greater confidence is granted to results that lead to exclusions. The power of exclusion is based on the fact that in some circumstances one can definitively show that two specimens cannot have originated from the same individual, whereas consistency between specimens demonstrates only the *possibility* that they originated from the same individual.

Size and Shape/Osteometric Comparison

There are strong correlations among the sizes of the bones of the skeleton. Thus, a large humerus is associated with a large femur and a large metatarsal. This allometric reality can be exploited in the sorting process by formally comparing the sizes of two bones. Osteometric comparison is a technique that uses statistical models to objectively compare size and shape relationships between elements through measurement data (Buikstra, Gordon, and St. Hoyme 1984; Byrd 2008; Byrd and Adams 1999, 2003). This technique, unlike the others described in this chapter, may be relatively unfamiliar to many anthropologists who deal with commingled human remains.

Osteometric comparison removes subjective judgment calls and provides a solid statistical basis for segregation. The strength of this technique is that it can be used to sort remains that could not be segregated through other means, such as pair matching and articulation. It is also amenable to situations in which the remains are fragmentary. One must realize that the real strength of osteometric comparison is to recognize *inconsistent* relationships that lead to exclusionary sorting (that is, consistency between elements alone is often not sufficient evidence for association). Naturally, some elements exhibit greater correlations in size with one another than with others. In most instances, it is not possible to osteometrically segregate individuals with similar body proportions, which could prove problematic for large-scale incidents. Thus, the power of the method is determined by the inherent allometric relationships among the skeletal elements as well as the size diversity of the commingled individuals (Byrd 2008; Byrd and Adams 2003).

Osteometric sorting utilizes a reference dataset composed of measurements collected from known individuals. The reference data used for osteometric sorting comprise primarily postcranial measurements. These include the standard measurements found in the Forensic Databank at the University of Tennessee, Knoxville (Moore-Jansen, Ousley, and Jantz 1994), as well as new measurements designed specifically for fragmented bones. Details regarding the reference data and new measurements are presented in Byrd and Adams (2003). The dataset is composed of pooled individuals representing both sexes and several ancestral groups. The reference dataset is continually growing as additional metric data are collected.

To apply the technique, regression models are derived that provide the comparative means for assessing the relationship between two elements (Byrd 2008; Byrd and Adams 2003). It has been found that the best regression models were created when the measurement values were converted to natural logarithms. The available measurements on a bone are simply summed, and the natural logarithm of this sum is the value used in simple bivariate regression statistical models.. Since length measurements typically show the highest correlations with one another, models including length measurements perform best. The addition of breadths and girth measurements into the indices offers a slight but measured improvement in the statistical models. A surprising finding is that models utilizing several breadth and girth measurements, with no length measurements, often perform nearly as well as those including lengths (Byrd and Adams 2003). This fact has great significance when working with fragmented assemblages. Error rates for the method as a whole, using the 90% prediction interval, have been found to be approximately 5%. A more thorough discussion of the technique is presented by Byrd (2008) and Byrd and Adams (2003), along with several regression models.

Currently, osteometric comparison is limited in its utility based on limited access to the reference data and the tedious process of customizing regression models. However, this method is superbly suited to computer automation. One hopes that software will be developed whereby all available measurement values for the case specimens are entered in advance, and all relevant comparison results can be produced as the analysis proceeds, without having to generate the statistical models for each comparison as separate steps for the anthropologist. As specimens are sorted apart by the various methods described in this chapter, they can be eliminated from consideration in the software application.

Robusticity or "Build"

Snow (1948) mentioned body "build" as one of the characteristics used to individualize commingled skeletal remains. Indeed, every experienced osteologist recognizes that short, stocky bodies can be distinguished from tall, slender ones by observation of the skeleton. Further, persons with heavy musculature, often described as robust, exhibit characteristics not shared with more gracile individuals. Bones showing the signs of hypertrophy (for example, larger girth, more pronounced muscle attachment sites) can be successfully sorted from their atrophied counterparts. Where a small number of individuals with widely divergent builds are commingled, this method alone has the potential to resolve the problem.

The problem with this approach resides partly with the nature of human variation and partly with the lack of any systematic procedure to follow during its execution. Humans vary along a continuum from stout to thin, from tall to short, and from robust to gracile. Thus, where commingled assemblages include remains of numerous individuals, the likelihood of encountering ambiguous results during comparisons is great. Comparisons involving elements of the upper body with those of the lower body (that is, the humerus compared to the tibia) will be most difficult to resolve. The method is further confounded by the lack of control over its application to an assemblage. Snow (1948) never elaborated on its use but rather left it up to the reader to decide how it should be used. Because the method is entirely subjective (in its current state), lacking explicit criteria for consideration, it does not lend itself to the determination of general error rates.

The authors advocate the use of this method under tightly controlled circumstances. Body-build characteristics should be brought into consideration when the other primary methods have been exhausted, leaving multiple specimens yet to be resolved. This approach does not negate the subjectivity of the method, but it does limit the odds of drawing erroneous or inexplicable conclusions. Many of the features associated with robusticity will be picked up in the other procedures, such as pair matching and osteometric comparison.

Taphonomy

Skeletal remains are often commingled long after their initial deposition. One example is the relatively recent discovery by Vietnamese farmers of the wreckage of an aircraft that crashed during the Vietnam War. With the best of intentions, the farmers gathered the bones they found in and around the wreckage, placed them in bags, and then turned them over to local government authorities (Adams and Byrd 2006). Bones of United States servicemen killed during the Korean conflict were exhumed by the North Korean government, warehoused for an unspecified period of time, and then commingled (whether intentionally or not) at a later time (Pokines et al. 2002). Remains of Bosnians placed in mass graves by their Serb neighbors were exhumed at a later date with power excavators, loaded on dump trucks, and moved to new locations where they were redeposited with no attempt to keep individual sets of remains discrete (Skinner, York, and Connor 2002). In all these instances, one expects that taphonomic processes could have left distinctive patterns on individual sets of remains during the period immediately following initial deposition. Where this has occurred, the patterns can be exploited during the sorting process.

Exposure of the skeleton to these variables at the level of the microenvironment creates the taphonomic patterns that can be used in the sorting process. Skeletons resting in different locations within a grave can be exposed to sediments with different micromorphological properties. Dark, fine-grained sediment tends to darken bones, whereas coarse-grained sands tend to produce lighter colors. Wet conditions leave bones with greater mass (owing to the lack of leaching, as well as the addition of moisture) than do dry conditions. Bones left on the surface are subject to weathering in a manner not observed in buried bones. Common symptoms of surface exposure are cortical exfoliation, loss of color (bleached appearance), cracking, and loss of bone mass. Proximity to artifacts or other nonbone materials can mark the skeleton. Deposition next to burning materials, for example, can cause color change owing to thermal alteration and/or exposure to charcoal and smoke (see Thompson this volume). The long-term deposition of metal artifacts next to bone can produce distinctive patterns. Copper artifacts tend to create a green stain and also tend to promote preservation of the bone. Steel artifacts tend to leave oxidation stains on bone. Although stains that are found on single-bone specimens are not helpful in the sorting process, stains are often produced across multiple articulating bones; thus alignment of such stains can be powerful evidence of an association of two or more bones.

However, drastic taphonomic differences may also be observed on the remains of the same individual owing to traumatic disarticulation (such as may occur from dismemberment or an aircraft crash) and a variable burial context. In these situations, portions of a single individual may be dispersed into very different contexts. The most significant point to be made concerning taphonomic patterns is that they are the result of idiosyncratic circumstances. The processes that produce these patterns can affect whole skeletons or only portions of a skeleton. Taphonomic patterns must be used with considerable caution in the sorting process, since the circumstances that create observable patterns can just as easily affect portions of adjacent skeletons as the elements of a single skeleton (all other things being equal).

Process of Elimination

Process of elimination suggests that bones may be assigned to a specific individual, because that element is exclusively represented by an individual, or can be conclusively excluded from all other potential individuals. This technique may be very useful in small-scale commingling, but as the number of individuals increases it usually becomes problematic to narrow the list of potential candidates to a single individual. In most cases, it is essential to complete all other methods of sorting prior to utilizing process of elimination. After these methods have been exhausted, duplicated elements may remain that can be associated with a specific individual through exclusion from all other possible options. An accurate accounting of the number of individuals involved in the incident, when possible, will also greatly facilitate the use of process of elimination as a sorting technique.

DNA Profile Data

Over the past decade, the ability to obtain DNA from skeletal remains has become a powerful tool for anthropologists sorting commingled remains (see Baker this volume). DNA is typically derived from one of two primary sources, nuclear DNA (nucDNA) or mitochondrial DNA (mtDNA). Obtaining useful data from these sources involves the application of widely varying laboratory methods, and interpretation of the results requires awareness of the special considerations attached to each method. The reader is encouraged to utilize published resources such as *Forensic DNA Typing* by John Butler (2005) and to regularly consult with experts in the field of forensic DNA analysis.

For purposes of sorting commingled remains, nucDNA and mtDNA each have strengths and weaknesses. nucDNA is most commonly utilized by analysis of Short Tandem Repeat (STR) markers (Butler 2005). The development of commercial

kits for STR analysis has made this form of DNA analysis relatively fast, inexpensive, and reliable. The analysis of STRs also has the advantage of individualization—random match probabilities are typically low enough to merit only minimal concern. The STR profile from a set of remains can be compared to a sample from a missing individual, and a match is grounds for a positive identification. This is one approach currently utilized by the United States Department of Defense, which collects blood samples from all active duty service members and stores them at the Armed Forces DNA Repository for future use (Department of Defense Directive No. 5154.24). When family reference samples must be utilized for comparison to the DNA profile from the remains, interpretation of results is more complex. This arises from the fact that individuals inherit half of their nucDNA from each parent and thus will not exhibit an exact match to any family member (excluding identical twins). If STR DNA typing is used, profiles obtained from direct reference samples (such as toothbrushes or medical specimens from the missing person) can be directly compared to profiles obtained from the remains. Kinship analysis can aid in comparing DNA profiles obtained from two or more family reference samples to those obtained from the remains. Perhaps the greatest weakness of nucDNA testing is the difficulty involved in obtaining a usable DNA profile when remains are poorly preserved, resulting in a partial or no DNA profile. In these cases, analysts will often resort to mtDNA testing.

The advantage of mtDNA over nucDNA is its preponderance in remains. Mitochondria are organelles found outside the nucleus of a cell. There may be up to 1,000 mitochondria per cell and several thousand copies of mtDNA in each mitochondrion (Bogenhagen and Clayton 1974). The higher copy number leads to a greater probability of obtaining a usable mtDNA sequence from poorly preserved remains. mtDNA testing has become routine for testing degraded or low DNA content samples such as hair, ancient bones, and teeth. The greatest weakness of mtDNA is that it is not individualizing and thus cannot be used as a unique identifier. Repeated types are commonly observed in large populations. Studies have shown that there are relatively common mtDNA types found within Hypervariable Regions I and II and that matches between unrelated people are not uncommon (Holland and Parsons 1999; Melton et al. 2001). In cases where mtDNA testing is used, finding fewer discrete sequences than the number of individuals estimated by anthropological techniques in the laboratory analysis (see section below on Quantification) can possibly indicate the existence of one or more random matches.

Measures that can be taken to mitigate the risk of a false association during mtDNA testing include: an accurate assessment of the number of individuals involved in the incident; prompt and comprehensive collection of family reference samples; and the utilization of multiple confirmatory lines of evidence when making initial sorting decisions. Regardless of which DNA testing method is used, sample selection is best assessed by the forensic anthropologist responsible for the case in conjunction with an expert in the field of forensic DNA analysis. One of the risks inherent in the use of either nucDNA or mtDNA is the chance of spurious matches resulting from sample contamination, so strict protocols must be followed to prevent such occurrences. Samples should be carefully chosen so that they will: (1) provide information relevant to the sorting process and subsequent identification; (2) not destroy evidence critical to the overall analysis (for example, gunshot wound or significant landmark needed for analysis); and (3) yield useful DNA data, given that some sample locations have better success than others. Needless sampling or samples of excessive size are to be discouraged, because they often destroy evidence and waste the resources of the DNA laboratory.

Quantification

It is often the job of the physical/forensic anthropologist to determine the number of individuals represented in cases involving commingled human remains. This process usually occurs after the conjoining and sorting process is complete. The most common technique utilized for this assessment is the Minimum Number of Individuals (MNI) determined from skeletal elements. Regardless of the context (forensic or archaeological), anthropologists frequently use the MNI value in their reports as the estimate of individuals represented. Although the MNI may provide an accurate representation of the actual number of individuals, it is also subject to bias and misleading results. When the recovery of skeletal elements falls below 100%, the MNI may not be an accurate indicator of the true death population. When appropriate, a more accurate technique may be the Most Likely Number of Individuals (MLNI) for the quantification of commingled human remains (Adams and Konigsberg 2004, 2008). The MLNI is a simple modification of the Lincoln Index (LI), a technique that has been effectively described in the zooarchaeological literature (Allen and Guy 1984; Fieller and Turner 1982; Ringrose 1993; Turner 1980,

1983). The main difference between the MNI and the MLNI is that the MNI provides only an estimate of the recovered assemblage and does not account for taphonomic loss. If the recovery of major body portions is less than 100%, the resulting number estimates associated with the MNI will reflect this bias and produce an underestimate of the actual number of individuals. The MLNI, in contrast, accounts for taphonomic data loss and provides an estimate of the true population size that may be more accurate. Because of their importance, specific details are provided for the MNI and the MLNI below.

Minimum Number of Individuals (MNI)

The MNI is the most popular method of quantification in any type of commingled osteological analysis. For interpreting population size from a skeletal assemblage, the MNI (as the name suggests) presents the minimum number of individuals that contributed to the sample. To deal with fragmentary body parts, specific segments of an element (for example, proximal humerus) can be used for the calculation of the MNI. Every fragment must share a specific landmark to ensure that fragments of the same element are not counted as two distinct individuals. For example, an adult proximal humerus fragment and an adult distal humerus fragment cannot be counted as two different people unless they duplicate a landmark, such as the deltoid tuberosity, since they could otherwise be parts from the same person. An exception to this is possible if there are obvious age discrepancies between the two portions. The basic principle of an MNI estimate is to avoid counting the same individual twice.

Although there are variations involved with the calculation of the MNI, the most popular method employed by anthropologists is simply a report of the most frequently observed element. This is obtained by simply sorting elements into lefts and rights and then taking greatest number as the estimate. It is equivalent to assuming that all of the less frequently observed bones are paired with the more frequently observed bones. For example, if there were 23 left humeri, 19 right humeri, 36 left femora, and 29 right femora, the MNI would be 36. This indicates that a minimum of 36 individuals would have to be present in the commingled assemblage to account for this number of bones (based on the count of left femora).

In some instances, the MNI will not provide an accurate estimate of the original population. The MNI simply states how many individuals would have been necessary to provide the *recovered* skeletal elements but says nothing about the *original* number of bodies. If the recovery of major skeletal elements nears 100%, then the MNI will be an accurate representation; otherwise, it may be of limited value for the interpretation of osteological assemblages. Consider a hypothetical scenario in which 100 individuals were placed in a mass grave. At some point, the remains were disturbed (intentional or otherwise), resulting in commingling. Decades later, the site was excavated in order to identify those that were killed, although it is unknown to the excavators exactly how many individuals were originally interred. Taphonomic forces had acted on the site, and the recovery did not represent 100 complete skeletons (that is, there was commingling, unpaired elements, miscellaneous portions were missing, and so on). Based on the most frequently encountered element (for instance, the number of right femora), the MNI derived from this site was determined to be 80 individuals. Based on this MNI estimate, 20 individuals are not accounted for, which could have serious consequences in the identification process.

Most Likely Number of Individuals (MLNI)

The Lincoln Index (LI) was first developed for population studies of living animals based on capture-recapture techniques and was later adapted for application to zooarchaeological faunal assemblages. The Most Likely Number of Individuals (MLNI) is a simple modification of the LI, which provides less bias in the estimates resulting from small sample sizes. The MLNI provides a maximum likelihood estimate. For this reason, emphasis is given to the calculation of the MLNI instead of the LI. The reader is encouraged to review the articles by Adams and Konigsberg (2004, 2008) for additional information regarding both the LI and MLNI. The key feature for the use of the MLNI with skeletal remains is that accurate estimates of the original population can be derived from samples in which taphonomic biasing and data loss have occurred in a random manner. This is of particular utility with archaeological samples or in forensic situations when remains have been exposed to random taphonomic forces. In addition to providing point estimates with the MLNI, one can also calculate confidence intervals.

When working with skeletal elements, the MLNI is calculated based on pair matching (see section above on Sorting). Pair matching involves the comparison of right and left elements to determine if they are from a single individual. Since the pair matching step should be completed during the sorting process, the data should be readily available for calculation of the MLNI. In theory, any paired element in the body could be used for calculation of the MLNI. In practice, though, particular parts of the skeleton will be more useful than others. Important criteria to consider for choosing appropriate skeletal elements are their size, presence of distinct morphological traits, potential for age and sex determination, and likelihood of survival.

An estimate of the original death assemblage based on the MLNI represented by a specific skeletal element (for example, femora) is

$$\mathrm{MLNI} = \frac{(L+1)(R+1)}{(P+1)} - 1$$

where L = left bones, R = right bones, and P = pair-matches.

For example, take a scenario where there are 64 right femora, 51 left femora or vice versa femora, and 44 femur pairs. Calculation of the MLNI indicates a maximum likelihood estimate of 74 individuals. In this same example, the MNI would be only 64 individuals. Furthermore, it is possible to present confidence intervals with the MLNI. Using the example above, an approximate 95% confidence interval is 71 to 79 individuals. The specifics involved in calculation of confidence intervals around the MLNI estimate using a hypergeometric probability function (available in most spreadsheet software programs) are thoroughly discussed by Adams and Konigsberg (2004, 2008). As might be expected, the confidence bounds get tighter as the recovery rate of elements approaches 100%, but the MLNI has been shown to perform very accurately when the recovery of elements exceeds 50%.

The primary danger involved with the use of the MLNI for quantification from skeletal elements is the misidentification of pairs. Because of the multiplicative nature of this technique, it is more vulnerable than other methods are to fragmentation and misinterpretation of paired skeletal elements. In extremely fragmentary situations, pair matching may be impossible, and the MLNI should not be calculated. Currently, the best option in highly fragmentary situations would be a MNI estimate, but this should not be considered a true count of the original death population.

Identification and Ethical Considerations with Commingled Remains

In any type of mass casualty event, one of the critical analytical goals is the identification of the dead.

When bodies are relatively complete and there is access to antemortem information, identification by traditional means (for example, radiographic and fingerprint) may be relatively straightforward and rapid. When bodies are highly decomposed, fragmentary, and/or skeletal remains are commingled, this task becomes more difficult (Kontanis and Sledzik 2008). It may be possible to positively identify a fragment of a maxilla to a specific individual through dental records. It may also be possible to positively identify a fragment of a hand based on fingerprints. The identification of other very small, nondiagnostic fragments may be more challenging and may rely almost entirely on DNA analysis. Obviously, the sorting process described above and the victim identification process are closely related. The linkage of an unidentified fragment with another portion that has been positively identified will, as a result, positively identify the newly linked piece.

At the onset of any analysis involving commingled remains, one must establish baseline parameters and protocols. Decisions need to be made early on in the process to determine the scope of the effort. With contemporary events there are also ethical considerations during the analysis and identification effort and in dealing with families of the deceased. Some complicated and sensitive issues to consider include:

- Will every fragment of bone and soft tissue be analyzed, or is there a size parameter that will be used (for example, only fragments >1 cm)? Laboratory policies and procedural decisions will need to be made regarding the scope of DNA testing and to determine which remains should be considered candidates for molecular analysis. If the decision is made to attempt identification of all fragments, regardless of their size, DNA testing will likely be the only means of re-association and identification for many specimens.

- Is the goal to identify every person, to re-associate and identify every fragment, or to do both? These are complicated but related issues. For example, if some amount of remains can be positively attributed to every individual involved in a mass casualty incident, how much effort should then be expended to associate additional unidentified portions to these individuals?

- How will "unidentifiable" bones (for example, calcined bones) and degraded soft tissue (for instance, poorly preserved skin fragment) be treated? Will the decision be made to destroy certain material as medical waste or will everything be retained? In many scenarios it will not be possible to positively link every fragment to a specific individual, regardless of the time and effort expended. One option is to retain everything and have some type of a group designation. This acknowledges the fact that the remains could have originated from any number of people involved in the incident and provides an option for their inclusion in a memorial or common grave.

Such decisions are crucial to the identification effort and, as such, will dictate the effort put into the process of sorting and re-associating fragments. There are serious and long-lasting implications for not only scientific endeavors but also victims' next of kin, especially as this relates to mass fatality incidents. There are no universal answers to these questions, and decisions will be incident specific, perhaps largely based on input by and wishes of the affected families as well as budgetary and other logistical constraints. In most mass fatality incidents, it usually falls to the medical examiner or coroner's office with jurisdictional control to make the final determination regarding the identification effort.

Conclusion

The sorting of commingled skeletal remains is a necessary step in the forensic identification process. The complexity of the problem requires that it be addressed by highly skilled forensic/biological anthropologists utilizing a careful, systematic approach. Under ideal conditions, the anthropologist will engage a combination of field, morphological, and DNA profile data such that each sorting decision will be informed by multiple lines of evidence. Reliance on a single line of evidence, to include DNA profiles, is not recommended. Only through persistent application of multiple lines of evidence will the practitioner be able to maximize the accurate sorting of remains and subsequently support individual identification.

References

Adams, B. J. 1996. The Use of the Lincoln/Peterson Index for Quantification and Interpretation of Commingled Human Remains. Master's Thesis: Department of Anthropology, University of Tennessee, Knoxville.

Adams, B. J., and Byrd, J. E. 2006. Resolution of small-scale commingling: A case report from the Vietnam War. *Forensic Science International* 156(1): 63–69.

Adams, B. J., and Byrd, J. E. 2008. *Recovery, Analysis, and Identification of Commingled Human Remains.* Totowa, NJ: Humana Press.

Adams, B. J., and Konigsberg, L. W. 2004. Estimation of the most likely number of individuals from commingled human skeletal remains. *American Journal of Physical Anthropology* 125(2): 138–151.

———. 2008. How many people? Determining the number of individuals represented by commingled human remains, in B. J. Adams and J. E. Byrd (eds.), *Recovery, Analysis, and Identification of Commingled Human Remains,* pp. 241–256. Totowa, NJ: Humana Press.

Allen, J., and Guy, J. B. M. 1984. Optimal estimations of individuals in archaeological faunal assemblages: How minimal is the MNI? *Archaeology in Oceania* 19: 41–47.

Bass, W. M., and Jantz, R. L. 2004. Cremation weights in east Tennessee. *Journal of Forensic Sciences* 49(5): 901–904.

Blau, S., Robertson, S., and Johnston, M. 2008. Disaster Victim Identification: New applications for postmortem computed tomography. *Journal of Forensic Sciences* 53(4): 1–6.

Bogenhagen, D., and Clayton, D. A. 1974. The number of mitochondrial deoxyribonucleic acid genomes in mouse L and human HeLa cells. *Journal of Biological Chemistry* 249: 7991–7995.

Brooks, S., and Suchey, J. M. 1990. Skeletal age determination based on the os pubis: A comparison of the Acsádi-Nemeskéri and Suchey-Brooks methods. *Human Evolution* 5(3): 227–238.

Budimlija, Z. M., Prinz, M. K., Zelson-Mundorff, A., Wiersema, J., Bartelink, E., MacKinnon, G., Nazzaruolo, B. L., Estacio, S. M., Hennessey, M. J., and Shaler, R. C. 2003. World Trade Center human identification project: Experiences with individual body identification cases. *Croatian Medical Journal* 44(3): 259–263.

Buikstra, J. E., Gordon, C. C., and St. Hoyme, L. 1984. The case of the severed skull: Individuation in forensic anthropology, in T. A. Rathbun and J. E. Buikstra (eds.), *Human Identification: Case Studies in Forensic Anthropology,* pp. 121–135. Springfield, IL: Charles C. Thomas.

Butler, J. 2005. *Forensic DNA Typing.* Burlington, MA: Elsevier Academic Press.

Byrd, J. E. 2008. Models and methods for osteometric sorting, in B. J. Adams and J. E. Byrd (eds.), *Recovery, Analysis, and Identification of Commingled Human Remains,* pp. 199–200. Totowa, NJ: Humana Press.

Byrd, J. E., and Adams, B. J. 1999. Sorting commingled human remains. Paper presented at Advances in Personal Identification in Mass Disaster, Hickam AFB, Hawai'i.

———. 2003. Osteometric sorting of commingled human remains. *Journal of Forensic Sciences* 48(4): 717–724.

Byrd, J. E., Adams, B. J., Leppo, L. M., and Harrington, R. J. 2003. Resolution of large-scale commingling issues: Lessons from CILHI and ICMP. Paper presented at the 55th Annual Meeting of the American Academy of Forensic Sciences, Chicago, Illinois.

Dirkmaat, D. C., and Adovasio, J. M. 1997. The role of archaeology in the recovery and interpretation of human remains from an outdoor forensic setting, in W. H. Haglund and M. H. Sorg (eds.), *Forensic Taphonomy: The Postmortem Fate of Human Remains,* pp. 39–64. Boca Raton, FL: CRC Press.

Fieller, N. R. J., and Turner, A. 1982. Number estimation in vertebrate samples. *Journal of Archaeological Science* 9: 49–62.

Goodman, N. R., and Edelson, L. B. 2002. The efficiency of an X-ray screening system at a mass disaster. *Journal of Forensic Sciences* 47(1): 127–130.

Haglund, W. D. 2002. Recent mass graves, an introduction, in W. D. Haglund and M. H. Sorg (eds.), *Advances in Forensic Taphonomy: Method, Theory, and Archaeological Perspectives,* pp. 243–261. Boca Raton, FL: CRC Press.

Hochrein, M. J. 2002. An autopsy of the grave: Recognizing, collecting, and preserving forensic geotaphonomic evidence, in W. D. Haglund and M. H. Sorg (eds.), *Advances in Forensic Taphonomy: Method, Theory, and Archaeological Perspectives,* pp. 45–70. Boca Raton, FL: CRC Press.

Holland, M. M., and Parsons, T. J. 1999. Mitochondrial DNA sequence analysis: Validation and use for forensic casework. *Forensic Science Review* 11: 21–50.

İşcan, M. Y., Loth, S. R., and Wright, R. K. 1984. Metamorphosis at the sternal rib end: A new method to estimate age at death in white males. *American Journal of Physical Anthropology* 65: 147–156.

———. 1985. Age estimation from the rib by phase analysis: White females. *Journal of Forensic Sciences* 30: 853–863.

Kennedy, K. A. 1996. The wrong urn: Commingling of cremains in mortuary practices. *Journal of Forensic Sciences* 41(4): 689–692.

Kontanis, E., and Sledzik, P. 2008. Resolving commingling issues during the medicolegal investigation of mass fatality incidents, in B. J. Adams and J. E. Byrd (eds.), *Recovery, Analysis, and Identification of Commingled Human Remains,* pp. 317–336. Totowa, NJ: Humana Press.

Lovejoy, C. O., Meindl, R. S., Pryzbeck, T. R., and Mensforth, R. P. 1985. Chronological metamorphosis of the auricular surface of the ilium: A new method for the determination of adult skeletal age at death. *American Journal of Physical Anthropology* 68(1): 15–28.

McKern, T. W., and Stewart, T. D. 1957. *Skeletal Age Changes in Young American Males, Technical Report EP-45*. Natick, MA: Headquarters Quartermaster Research and Development Command.

Melton, T., Clifford, S., Kayser, M., Nasidze, I., Batzer, M., and Stoneking, M. 2001. Diversity and heterogeneity in mitochondrial DNA of North American populations. *Journal of Forensic Sciences* 46(1): 46–52.

Moore-Jansen, P. M., Ousley, S. D., and Jantz, R. L. 1994. Data Collection Procedures for Forensic Skeletal Material. Knoxville: University of Tennessee, Department of Anthropology.

Mundorff, A. Z. 2008. Anthropologist directed triage: Three distinct mass fatality events involving fragmentation of human remains, in B. J. Adams and J. E. Byrd (eds.), *Recovery, Analysis, and Identification of Commingled Human Remains*, pp. 123–144. Totowa, NJ: Humana Press.

Mundorff, A. Z, Shaler, R., Bieschke, E., and Mar-Cash, E. 2008. Marrying anthropology and DNA: Essential for solving complex commingling problems in cases of extreme fragmentation, in B. J. Adams and J. E. Byrd (eds.), *Recovery, Analysis, and Identification of Commingled Human Remains*, pp. 285–300. Totowa, NJ: Humana Press.

Pokines, J. T., Berg, G. E., Adams, B. J., Bunch, A. W., Byrd, J. E., Holland, T. D., Belcher, W. R., and Leney, M. D. 2002. How not to stage a burial: Lessons from North Korea. Paper presented at the 54th Annual Meeting of the American Academy of Forensic Sciences, Atlanta, Georgia.

Reineke, G., and Hochrein, M. 2008. Pieces of the puzzle: F.B.I. Evidence Response Team approaches to scenes with commingled evidence, in B. J. Adams and J. E. Byrd (eds.), *Recovery, Analysis, and Identification of Commingled Human Remains*, pp. 31–56. Totowa, NJ: Humana Press.

Ringrose, T. J. 1993. Bone counts and statistics: A critique. *Journal of Archaeological Science* 20: 121–157.

Schaefer, M. 2008. Patterns of epiphyseal union and their use in the detection and sorting of commingled remains, in B. J. Adams and J. E. Byrd (eds.), *Recovery, Analysis, and Identification of Commingled Human Remains*, pp. 221–240. Totowa, NJ: Humana Press.

Schmitt, S. 2002. Mass graves and the collection of forensic evidence: Genocide, war crimes, and crimes against humanity, in W. D. Haglund and M. H. Sorg (eds.), *Advances in Forensic Taphonomy: Method, Theory, and Archaeological Perspectives*, pp. 277–292. Boca Raton, FL: CRC Press.

Skinner, M. 1987. Planning the archaeological recovery of evidence from recent mass graves. *Forensic Science International* 34(4): 267–287.

Skinner, M., Alempijevic, D., and Djuric-Srejic, M. 2003. Guidelines for international forensic bio-archaeology monitors of mass grave exhumations. *Forensic Science International* 134(2-3): 81–92.

Skinner, M. F., York, H. P., and Connor, M. A. 2002. Postburial disturbance of graves in Bosnia-Herzegovina, in W. D. Haglund and M. H. Sorg (eds.) *Advances in Forensic Taphonomy: Method, Theory, and Archaeological Perspectives*, pp. 293–308. Boca Raton, FL: CRC Press.

Snow, C. E. 1948. The identification of the unknown war dead. *American Journal of Physical Anthropology* 6: 323–328.

Turner, A. 1980. Minimum number estimation offers minimal insight in faunal analysis. *OSSA* 7: 199–201.

———. 1983. The quantification of relative abundances in fossil and subfossil bone assemblages. *Annals of the Transvaal Museum* 33: 311–321.

Ubelaker, D. H. 2002. Approaches to the study of commingling in human skeletal biology, in W. D. Haglund and M. H. Sorg (eds.), *Advances in Forensic Taphonomy: Method, Theory, and Archaeological Perspectives*, pp. 331–351. Boca Raton, FL: CRC Press.

Viner, M. 2008. The use of radiology in mass fatality events, in B. J. Adams and J. E. Byrd (eds.), *Recovery, Analysis, and Identification of Commingled Human Remains*, pp. 145–184. Totowa, NJ: Humana Press.

Warren, M. W. 2008. Detection of commingling in cremated human remains, in B. J. Adams and J. E. Byrd (eds.), *Recovery, Analysis, and Identification of Commingled Human Remains*, pp. 185–198. Totowa, NJ: Humana Press.

Warren, M. W., and Maples, W. R. 1997. The anthropometry of contemporary commercial cremation. *Journal of Forensic Sciences* 42(3): 417–423.

Warren, M. W., and Schultz, J. J. 2002. Post-cremation taphonomy and artifact preservation. *Journal of Forensic Sciences* 47(3): 656–659.

16

THE ASSESSMENT OF ANCESTRY AND THE CONCEPT OF RACE

Norman J. Sauer and Jane C. Wankmiller

Physical anthropologists have long been interested in the biological relationships of past and present populations. In bioarchaeology, establishing biological affinity elucidates crucial historical processes, including migration patterns. Methods also exist for estimating population affinity of individual specimens—a process that is often useful in forensic anthropology. The assessment of ancestry, like the estimation of age, sex, and stature, is typically an expected component of a biological profile provided to law enforcement by a forensic anthropologist. Unlike sex, age and stature, however, ancestry estimation is fraught with misunderstanding, misuse, and controversy. Underlying any discussion of the assessment of ancestry and its value to forensic anthropology is the concept of race. In this chapter, we discuss the relationship between race and ancestry determination in forensic anthropology, discuss the methods developed by anthropologists to determine ancestry, and finally address some relevant philosophical and ethical issues.

The conflation of ancestry and race is typical in the anthropological literature and has a long history. In fact, physical anthropology (the parent discipline of forensic anthropology) was instrumental in establishing the concept of race and entrenching it in the American and European worldview. As Brace (1982) so aptly points out,

several personalities variously recognized as the founders of physical anthropology—John Fredrich Blumenbach, Paul Broca, Samuel Morton, Ernest A. Hooton, and Aleš Hrdlička—either defined the race classifications that have become so pervasive and accepted race as the natural condition of human variation or carried out research on human variation within the race framework. The fact that in the 1920s and 1930s the pages of the *American Journal of Physical Anthropology* were replete with articles describing the physical and behavioral characteristics of "Negroids," "Caucasoids," and "Mongoloids" is testimony to the continuation of physical anthropology's fascination with the concept of race up to World War II.

In the 1940s, it was M. F. Ashley Montagu who seriously began to question the concept of race for humans and recommended dropping the term (and associated notions) altogether (Montagu 1941, 1942, 1952). In the 1960s, Frank Livingstone (1962) applied questions raised nearly a decade earlier by Wilson and Brown (1953) about nonhuman subspecies to the human-race question. Livingstone pointed out that the discordance of physical (genetic) traits made it impossible to partition humans in any biologically meaningful way. The number and type of races anyone generated from the basis of biological variation would depend on the number and types of traits selected. A scheme founded on skin color, for example, would have no resemblance to one based on blood groups. Livingstone (and Montagu, for that matter) suggested that a better understanding of human variation would be arrived at by studying traits (or genes).

Over the past few decades, the idea of human races has fallen into disfavor among most physical anthropologists (Lieberman and Reynolds 1996; Lieberman, Kirk, and Littlefield 2003). However, physical anthropologists are not alone in their rejection of the race concept applied to humans. Recently, molecular geneticist Alan Templeton (2002) attempted to address the issue of human races using criteria that are typically applied by biologists to nonhuman animals. He set up his arguments by establishing that there are two basic models for viewing subspecies (or races): the lineage model and Sewell Wright's "F_{st} statistic." He then tested the applicability of the models using human DNA data. In the first model, according to Templeton, races are viewed as evolutionary lineages. If human races represent discrete evolutionary lineages, then there must be more interbreeding within members of each lineage than between lineages. The models test whether breeding frequency associates with major races or with proximity. The DNA data, he argues, are consistent with the proximity model (that is, humans interbreed more frequently with conspecifics, or other members of the same species, in their immediate proximity than with members of their own so-called race). The DNA evidence does not accord with the lineage model (ibid.).

Templeton has focused on the eminent geneticist Sewell Wright's statistic of diversity (F_{st}) that zoologists use to gauge whether genetic variation among groups within a species exceeds "a minimum level of differentiation" (ibid.: 35) that is sufficient to divide the taxon into smaller groups, or subspecies. An F_{st} of 0 indicates that, although individuals differ, there is no diversity among populations. An F_{st} of 1 indicates that all individuals in each local population are identical but that each population is different from all others. The traditional criterion for the existence of subspecies is an F_{st} value of 0.25–0.30. Species with an F_{st} above 0.30 are divisible into subgroups, whereas, according to Templeton, species with an index below 0.25 are not. For illustrative purposes, Templeton produces a table of sample species, some with accepted subspecies and others that cannot be subdivided. The F_{st} for humans is 0.156, which is well below the index generated for nonhuman species. Thus the human species is not divisible according to this criterion either—there are no human subspecies, or races.

If races do not exist, how then can forensic anthropologists expect to provide estimates of ancestry in their research and case reports? It is our contention that a problem exists only if ancestry is equated with race. We maintain that human variation is such that estimating a place of origin is not only reasonable but quite practical (Brace 1995). Anthropologists can often link unknown human remains to a known region of the world based on variation in skeletal morphology. The idea of race becomes relevant when this linking is associated with the assignation that is most likely in a particular cultural context. For example, one popular forensic anthropology textbook (Byers 2005: 158–159) advocates the use of "White," "Black," "Asian," "Native American," and "Hispanic" for the population of the United States.

Like attitudes toward the concept of race itself, the methods available for the assessment of ancestry have evolved. In the next section, we review a number of the methods that have been and continue to be used by forensic anthropologists to identify ancestry. Decisions about the use of terminology in this review have been difficult. Despite our belief that ancestry does not equal race, we have left the term *race* and some of the group identifiers (for example, "Caucasoid") when we feel that changing terms would change the author's meaning or intent.

History of Methods

Most of the early studies on human variation were designed to document human biological diversity. Topics ranged from the "Physical Anthropology of the American Negro" (Cobb 1942), a thorough documentation of a host of physical attributes of African Americans, to population variation among individual bones such as the scapula (Gray 1942) or vertebral column (Trotter 1929). Other early works include but are by no means limited to variation among rib lengths (Lanier 1944), sciatic notch measurements (Letterman 1941), cephalic indices (Michelson 1944), the morphology and closure of the superior orbital fissure (Ray 1955), various body dimensions (Thurstone 1947; Todd and Lindala 1928), cranial morphology (Todd and Tracy 1930), and long-bone lengths/stature (Trotter and Gleser 1952).

Many of the early publications were influenced by the 1885 introduction of anthropometry by Alphonse Bertillon, a French law enforcement officer. Anthropometry originally involved 11 measurements: the individual's height, reach, length of trunk, length and width of head, width of cheeks, length and width of right ear, length of left middle finger, length of left little finger, and length of left forearm (Bertillon 1896). Bertillon also outlined multiple other bases for comparison among people, ranging from hair texture and skin pigmentation to alveolar prognathism. Although his methods were aimed at identifying criminals who had been arrested and were likely to be repeat offenders, they set the stage for future metric analyses of the human body.

While most early physical anthropologists focused their attention on research concerning growth, development, nutrition, and other descriptive analyses of skeletal populations, a handful of pioneers began applying their knowledge of the skeleton to forensic cases (İşcan 1988). Aleš Hrdlička began assisting the FBI with cases in 1936 (Ubelaker 2000), and Wilton M. Krogman, with his 1939 publication "Guide to the Identification of Human Remains" in the *FBI Law Enforcement Bulletin*, brought the importance of anthropological skeletal analysis to the attention of the law enforcement community (Rhine 1990a). In addition to determining age at death, sex, and stature, anthropologists often provided opinions as to the possible ancestry of unidentified skeletal remains. Momentum continued to build, leading Ellis Kerley to comment in 1978: "the list of physical anthropologists who have been engaged in medico-legal activities is a long and impressive one that includes most of the major physical anthropologists of the first half of the twentieth century" (Rhine 1990a: xix).

Alice Brues (1958) highlighted some of the key skeletal features that are commonly examined by physical anthropologists in the context of a forensic investigation, including some that are used to estimate race. According to Brues, because there is no one feature on all skulls in any given racial group, the anthropologist must examine multiple features in order to accurately assess an individual's ancestry. She based her analysis on three aspects of the face: (1) soft tissue; (2) areas where soft tissue closely follows bone contours; and (3) aspects visible only on the skull itself (Brues 1958: 559). Brues was careful to point out the potential for incongruity between ancestry assessment based on skeletal remains and the "racial" category with which the individual would have identified during life (ibid.).

One of the most definitive works published during the early period of forensic anthropology involving human identification was Krogman's 1962 publication, *The Human Skeleton in Forensic Medicine*. Knowing that an anthropologist would not always be called to assist with cases, Krogman authored this book as a reference for law enforcement to become acquainted with bones and the information they can provide (Krogman 1962). Although this volume also includes information on bone growth and development, time since death, and identification techniques such as skull-image comparisons and comparative radiography, most of the book focuses on establishing the biological profile. Krogman relied on early studies that described population differences in the pelvis, scapula, long bones, and other parts of the skeleton to develop methods for race identification. He concluded that the long bones, scapula, and mandible could not be racially classified, that the pelvis had only limited applicability (70–75%), and that morphological and metric analyses of the skull tended to be useful 85–90% of the time (Krogman 1962: 206).

A number of individual studies were carried out, and several books were published on the subject of forensic anthropology during the 1970s and 1980s (e.g., Krogman and İşcan 1986; Rathbun and Buikstra 1984; Reichs 1986). However, 1990 brought about the publication of *Skeletal Attribution of Race* (Gill and Rhine 1990), the most comprehensive guide available for race identification from human skeletal remains. *Skeletal Attribution of Race* arose from a symposium at the 1984 meeting of the American Academy of Forensic Sciences that had been inspired by annual meetings of the Mountain Desert and Coastal forensic anthropologists (Rhine 1990a). Most of the methods included in the volume represent improvements on or critiques of previous research; others are presented for the first time.

We now move to a discussion of methods available to forensic anthropologists for determining ancestry from skeletal remains. The methods are grouped into metric and anthroposcopic analyses (methods that utilize visual assessment as opposed to measurements) of cranial and postcranial elements.

Cranial Morphology

The Gill and Rhine volume (1990) describes several methods that involve visual assessment of the skull. Among them is Alice Brues's technique for evaluating the shape of the nasal root. According to Brues (1990), "Negroids" tend to have nasal roots shaped like "quonoset huts" (buildings with a semicircular arched roof), "Mongoloids" have "tented" nasal roots, and the nasal roots of "Caucasoids" resemble "a church with a steeple." Though this method is appealing because it appears to be straightforward and provide immediate results, the terminology is problematic because of the potential relationship between it and racial stereotypes (Figure 16.1).

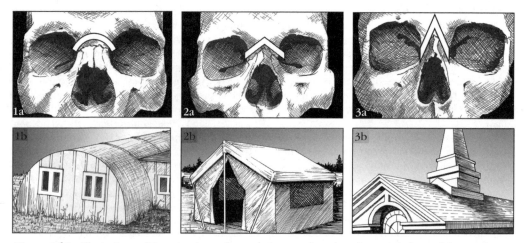

Figure 16.1 Illustrations of Brues's scheme for assessing race based on the morphology of the nasal root (Brues 1990; original illustration by J. Wankmiller). (1a) Depicts the stereotypic morphology of a Negroid over an illustration of a Quonset hut (1b); (2a) depicts the stereotypic morphology of a Mongoloid over an illustration of a tent (2b); (3a) depicts the stereotypic morphology of a Caucasoid over an illustration of a church with a steeple (3b).

Rhine (1990b) presents a "nonmetric skull racing" technique, an anthroposcopic method that incorporates a suite of cranial traits. He examined 87 complete skulls ("Anglo," "Hispanic," "Modern Amerind," Prehistoric "Amerind," "Black," and "Black casts"), all of known identity except for the prehistoric skulls, and all from the Maxwell Museum's collection (1990b: 9). Rhine's chapter includes lists of common and rare features or traits, along with illustrations, that he attributes to crania representative of each of the three groups he encounters most frequently as a forensic anthropologist working in the American Southwest ("American Caucasoid," Southwestern "Mongoloid," and American Black) (1990b). For example, a large nasal spine, parabolic dental arcade, sloping orbits, and retreating zygomatics are associated with the "American Caucasoid"; a small nasal spine, hyperbolic dental arcade, rectangular orbits, and vertical zygomatics are associated with the "American Black"; and a small nasal spine, elliptic dental arcade, rounded orbits, and projecting zygomatics are associated with the Southwestern "Mongoloid" (ibid.).

Several new methods for anthroposcopic analysis of the cranium are also presented in the Gill and Rhine volume. For example, Napoli and Birkby studied the morphology of the external auditory meatus in skulls of "Caucasoids," "Mongoloids," and individuals of mixed "Caucasoid/Mongoloid" ancestry. Their "Mongoloid" sample consisted of 35 prehistoric crania from three Western Pueblo archaeological sites in east-central Arizona, and the

"Caucasoid" and mixed "Caucasoid/Mongoloid" sample consisted of 36 modern crania from forensic cases (Napoli and Birkby 1990: 28). They concluded that the shape of the external auditory meatus differs to the extent that in "Caucasoids" and "Caucasoid/Mongoloid" admixed individuals, the oval window inside the ear canal is visible, whereas "Mongoloids" tend to have a morphology that does not allow visual inspection of the oval window (Napoli and Birkby 1990) (Figure 16.2).

Angel and Kelley (1990) studied the mandibles of 375 females and 406 males from the Terry Collection and forensic cases, evaluating them for the extent of ramus inversion and gonial flaring (Angel and Kelley 1990). Their test populations were expanded to include Blacks from a late 18th-/early-19th-century slave cemetery in Maryland, an

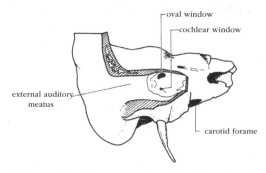

Figure 16.2 The cross-section of a right temporal bone showing the location of the oval window inside the auditory canal (from Napoli and Birkby 1990).

early-19th-century cemetery of free Blacks from Philadelphia, and several African and American (Plains) Indian mandibles. According to Angel and Kelley (1990), both ramus inversion and gonial flaring are more pronounced among Blacks than among Whites, and these differences are more pronounced among males than among females. They also note that based on morphological differences between the American Black mandibles and grouped American Indian and African mandibles, the American Black mandibles appear to exhibit some racial admixture.

Brooks and colleagues report on a nonmetric assessment of alveolar prognathism (Brooks, Brooks, and France 1990). Their sample included skulls or maxillae from a number of regions: 3 skulls from India; 17 from various Southeast Asian countries; 53 North American Indian maxillae from several sites in Nevada; 40 Arikara skulls from South Dakota; 51 American Black and 49 American White skulls (primarily from the Terry Collection); and 20 Sudanese Nubian skulls (Brooks, Brooks, and France 1990: 42). According to the authors, alveolar prognathism is marked in all their sample populations except for the American Whites. American Black and Nubian skulls are the most prognathic, but prognathism is also pronounced in North American Indians and Southeast Asians. Other methods for distinguishing among American Indians, Blacks and Whites using facial features include visual assessment of the transverse palatine suture, the zygomaticomaxillary suture, and the shapes of the mastoid process and palate (Gill 1998).

Cranial Metrics

Several anthropologists have noted variation in facial indices and head measurements among different groups of people (Cameron 1929a, 1929b, 1929c, 1930; Gill 1984; Gill et al. 1988; Iyer and Lutz 1966; Michelson 1944; Woo 1949). The discriminant function analysis introduced by Giles and Elliot (1962) provided a mechanism for cranial analysis that went beyond measurements and indices. Their work was pioneering (İşcan 1988; Kerley 1978), and it continues to inspire research.

Giles and Elliot (1962) based their work on eight cranial measurements: glabello-occipital length, maximum cranial width, basion-bregma height, maximum bi-zygomatic diameter, prosthion-nasion height, basion-nasion, basion-prosthion, and nasal breadth. From these measurements, Giles and Elliot developed four discriminant functions that would distinguish between: (1) White and American Negro males; (2) White and American Negro females; (3) White and American Indian males; and (4) White

and American Indian females. Five of these cranial measurements were also used to develop formulae for determining the sex of an individual if that is also in question (Giles and Elliot 1962: 148). The American Negro and White crania ($n = 408$) are from the Terry Collection (currently housed in the Department of Anthropology at the National Museum of Natural History of the Smithsonian Institution) and the Todd Collection (currently housed at the Cleveland Museum of Natural History). The prehistoric Indian Knoll site, for which age and sex were first assessed and published by Clyde Snow in 1948, provided the American Indian sample (Giles and Elliot 1962: 148). According to Giles and Elliot, the Indian Knoll remains were re-examined to verify the age and sex assessments in Snow's earlier work, prior to the data collection for their 1962 article. All 408 American Negro and White crania from the Terry and Todd Collections were subjected to the eight aforementioned measurements. Subsequently, the measurements of 75 males and 75 females from each of the three groups were used to create the discriminant functions. When applied to the 225 males and 225 females used in the calculations, and to 326 other individuals (not used in the initial calculations), the discriminant functions provided an accuracy rate of 82.6% for males and an 88.1% rate for females (Giles and Elliot 1962: 156). To use the method, the analyst measures an unknown skull, subjects the measurements to two algorithms, then places the resulting values along two axes on a graph (Figure 16.3). Placement on the graph indicates the most likely ancestral group. The method operates under the assumption that the skull under examination derives from one of the three populations involved in the study (Giles and Elliot 1962: 150).

In 1966, Walt Birkby tested the Giles and Elliot method against Southwestern American Indian and Labrador Eskimo populations in order to assess whether the discriminant functions could be applied to populations other than those from the original study. Birkby found that the Indian Knoll sample was not representative of all American Indians and "the determination of race by discriminant functions based only on a single American Indian sample cannot be suited with any degree of confidence on any other American Indian population" (Birkby 1966: 26). Echoing Giles and Elliot, Birkby pointed out that statistical methods may have substantially less utility when applied to populations that were not part of the sample on which the calculations or techniques were originally developed.

A further test of the Giles and Elliot discriminant functions was published by Snow and associates (1978). Where Birkby's analysis focused on

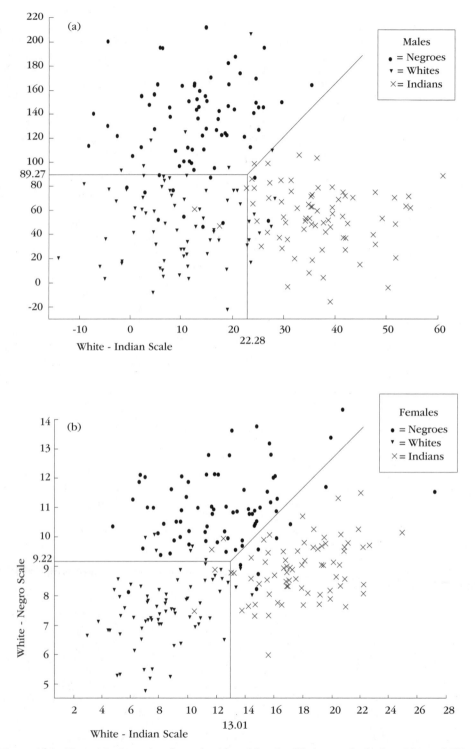

Figure 16.3 The sectioning points for males (a) and females (b) that resulted when Giles and Elliot applied their discriminant functions to the 225 males and 225 females used in the calculations (Giles and Elliot 1962: 153–154).

the four functions designed to determine ancestry, Snow and associates tested the discriminant functions that were developed to determine race and sex where both are unknown. They applied the method to a series of 52 forensic cases (individuals with known identities), and found that the functions were useful for distinguishing between White and Black skulls, but misclassified 6 out of 7 Indian crania. They concluded that the Giles and Elliot method is useful, despite its population limitations, and that the limitations may actually be minimized with further refinement of the functions (Snow et al. 1978).

The Giles and Elliot functions resurfaced in the Gill and Rhine edited volume. Fisher and Gill (1990) applied the functions to a sample of Northwestern Plains Indians. Their findings indicate that the discriminant functions are useful for determining sex, but again their utility diminishes when they are used to ascertain the ancestry of individuals from populations other than the ones in the original study. Ayers and colleagues (1990) further tested the discriminant functions by applying them to 191 modern forensic cases (representing White, Black, and Amerindian males and females). They found that their modern forensic sample was different enough from the material used to calculate the original functions to suggest a possible secular change in the United States. According to Wescott and Jantz (2005), a secular change in the cranial shape of Americans has in fact occurred over the last 150 years. They noted shifts in the locations of anatomical landmarks on the skull and concluded that the changes are likely the result of "genetic changes, improved health and nutrition, and biomechanical responses to a more processed diet" (Wescott and Jantz 2005: 240).

Other cranial metric analyses include the work of Gill and Gilbert (1990), Curran (1990), Gill and associates (1988), and Howells (1973, 1989, 1995). Drawing on earlier research (Gill 1984 and Gill et al. 1988), Gill and Gilbert (1990) present a method for measuring the midfacial skeleton of American Blacks and American Whites, with the hopes of circumventing some of the problems inherent in the Giles and Elliot functions. Incorporating a simometer (modified coordinate calipers first developed by Howells in 1973), Gill and Gilbert took six measurements of midfacial dimensions from 100 American Blacks, 125 American Whites, and 173 Amerindians. Eventually they arrived at three indices they believed were most useful for determining ancestry: maxillofrontal index, zygoorbital index, and Alpha index (Gill and Gilbert 1990). They concluded that Whites scored differently on all three indices than did Blacks and Indians, and

the last two groups produce very similar values (Gill and Gilbert 1990: 48–49).

Although Gill and Gilbert used a large American Indian sample for their study, Curran (1990) points out that their sample from the Southwest is relatively small ($n = 27$). He tested the ability of the midfacial indices to distinguish among "Caucasoids," "Negroids," and a larger sample ($n = 100$) of Southwestern American Indians. Curran reports that although the functions separate "Negroid" and "Caucasoid" crania and "Caucasoid" and Indian crania, they fail to reliably differentiate between "Negroid" and Indian crania (1990: 56).

In 1973 and 1989, W. W. Howells conducted and published two extensive studies of craniometric variation among thousands of males and females from a number of the world's populations. Subjecting the data from these studies to various statistical analyses, he concluded that subjects tend to cluster with one another by region. Howells expanded on his earlier work in 1995 by subjecting test crania to statistical analysis to see how closely they fit with selected groups from his 1973 and 1989 studies. These test crania were of known provenience and population affinity; however, he treated them as unknown in order to assess the predictive value of having large amounts of data on so many populations from around the world (Howells 1995). Howells's method and data have been major contributors to some of the most recent and progressive discriminant function analytical tools, such as *FORDISC*.

Now in its third version, *FORDISC* is an interactive computer program that allows an investigator to compare measurements of unknown remains to as many as 11 groups using 1 to 34 cranial measurements or 1 to 39 postcranial measurements (Fried and Jantz 2005). A major advantage of *FORDISC* is its capability to customize discriminant functions to a particular specimen when, for example, it is too damaged to take all of the prescribed measurements or if it is not from a population already in the database (Ousley and Jantz 1996).

Although it is based on the same principles as the Giles and Elliot discriminant functions, *FORDISC* takes into account a number of new measurements in addition to having a much larger data bank from which to draw comparisons. The data bank used to generate *FORDISC* is composed of known, contemporary samples from the Forensic Data Bank at the University of Tennessee in Knoxville, the Howells world sample, and several archaeological populations (Fried and Jantz 2005; Ousley and Jantz 2005). Ousley and Jantz (2005) contend that having data from numerous populations from various time periods may enable the program to account for secular change.

In addition to *FORDISC*, there is another computer program, *CRANID*, which calculates a linear discriminant and nearest neighbor discriminant analysis with 29 cranial measurements. The cranium is classified after comparison with 64 samples that include 3,163 crania from around the world (Wright 1992, 2007, 2008).

Dentition

In many cases, the more fragile bones of the skeleton are lost to taphonomic forces. However, teeth tend to survive the elements very well and can assist anthropologists in assessing the ancestry of unknown human remains (see Clement, this volume). Shovel-shaped incisors, for example, are among the most recognizable traits that can be associated with a particular ancestral group. Aleš Hrdlička brought shovel-shaped incisors to the attention of physical anthropologists with his 1920 publication on the trait (Hinkes 1990). He noted varying degrees of shoveling and varying frequencies of the trait among Chinese, Mongolian, Japanese, Eskimo, American Indian, American White, and American Black dentitions and concluded that American Indians tend to exhibit the trait to a greater degree than any of the other groups (Hrdlička 1920). Hinkes cites a number of other researchers who reported on observations of shovel-shaped incisors, both before and after Hrdlička's 1920 publication (see Hinkes 1990). Her 1990 chapter in the Gill and Rhine volume synthesizes all the other studies into one table, which contains a list of the samples along with the frequencies and varying degrees of shovel-shaping.

A recent publication by Lease and Sciulli (2005) discusses metric and morphological analyses of the deciduous teeth of African-American and European-American children to assess differences between these two groups. Lease and Sciulli used casts of dental arcades from children aged 2–6 years: 110 (males and females) for metric analyses and 117 (males and females) for morphological/non-metric analyses (Lease and Sciulli 2005: 57). They concluded that, on average, African-Americans' deciduous teeth are approximately 7% larger than those of European-Americans and that although European-Americans show higher frequencies and more extreme expressions of nonmetric traits on their anterior teeth, African-Americans show such variation on the posterior teeth (Lease and Sciulli 2005: 60). According to Lease and Sciulli, although children could be placed into ancestral groups as identified by their parents, those categories are not derived from the continent of origin; rather, they are social categories and are dependent on how the parents categorize themselves and their children. They also cite Dahlberg (1951), identifying other aspects of dentition that are known to be population-related, including third-molar agenesis and molar cusp pattern variation. Recent research reports population variation in the thicknesses of the enamel, dentine, and pulp of deciduous teeth (Harris, Hicks, and Barcroft 2001).

Postcranial Metrics

Historically, the femur is among the most thoroughly studied human postcranial bones. Consequently, several of the methods available for evaluating ancestry based on the postcranial skeleton involve the femur. T. Dale Stewart claimed that his 1962 publication on the anterior curvature of the femur was the first to involve the postcranium for assessing ancestry. Until that time, "squatting facets" on the anterior margins of the tibiotalar joint were the "nearest thing to such a criterion so far reported" (Stewart 1962: 49). He credits Aleš Hrdlička with the observation that "skeletons of Negroes are always to be distinguished from those of other races by the straightness of their long bones" (Stewart 1962: 49). Stewart's method involved leveling the bone using a wooden wedge beneath its proximal end and then measuring the heights above the table of: (1) the leveling points; (2) the point on the diaphysis (shaft) of the greatest anterior curvature; (3) the highest point on the cervical tubercle; and (4) the highest point on the head (Figure 16.4) (Stewart 1962: 49).

Together, these four measurements place values on both the anterior curvature of the diaphysis and the torsion of the proximal end of the bone (Stewart 1962: 49). Stewart found that Indians have the most pronounced curvature, Negroes have the least, and values for Whites fall somewhere in between. He indicated that assessing anterior femoral curvature alone is not as efficient as using it in combination with the degree of torsion for determining an individual's ancestry (Stewart 1962: 58). One must keep in mind that variation such as this may be attributable to differences in diet or activity levels and may not, in fact, reflect genetic differences.

According to Gilbert and Gill (1990), American Indians tend to have a noticeably flattened (anteroposteriorly) subtrochanteric region when compared to American Blacks and Whites. In 2005, Wescott tested the Gilbert and Gill subtrochanteric (platymeric) index, evaluating its usefulness for distinguishing among five different populations: American Indians, Polynesians, Hispanics,

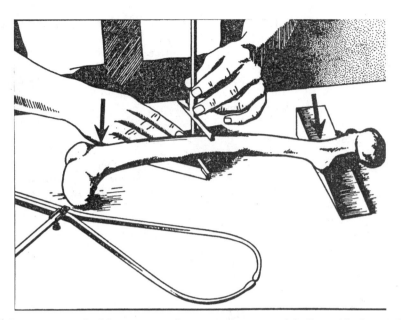

Figure 16.4   Stewart's method for measuring the anterior curvature of the femur. The bone is leveled by placing a wooden wedge beneath the proximal end (Stewart 1962: 51).

American Whites, and American Blacks (Wescott 2005: 286). He noted several limitations of the application of the platymeric index to the assessment of ancestry: (1) the shape of the proximal femur is more likely related to activity than it is to ancestry; (2) considerable intragroup variation can be attributed to sex differences rather than population differences; (3) different groups of Native Americans may exhibit very different indices; and (4) the potential for interobserver error exists in the taking of measurements (Wescott 2005: 287). After pooling the American Blacks and Whites into one sample, Wescott found that although the subtrochanteric index can be useful for differentiating Native Americans from American Blacks and Whites, its utility ends there, because the differences among Hispanics, American Blacks, and American Whites are not statistically significant, and Native Americans frequently classify as Polynesian (Wescott 2005: 289).

A third study involving metric analysis of the femur was introduced by Baker and colleagues (1990). They examined the anterior outlet of the intercondylar notch of the femur, concluding that "American Negroids" tend to have higher maximum notch heights than do "Caucasoids." Baker and associates refer to Trotter and Gleser (1952) and suggest that part of the difference in notch height may be due to the fact that "American Negroids" tend to have longer limbs than "Caucasoids" do (Baker, Gill, and Kieffer 1990: 94).

The pelvis has been found to be among the most reliable postcranial predictors of ancestry. İşcan (1983) measured three aspects (biiliac breadth, antero-posterior height, and transverse breadth) of 400 reconstructed pelves from the Terry Collection (100 of each sex-race group: American Black and White, males and females). Using the discriminant function method, İşcan found that accuracy of ancestry identification was high, 88%, in the sample used to generate the functions. This method has the same potential limitation as do the Giles and Elliot cranial metric functions in that it will not reflect secular change. The method requires whole pelves, which could be problematic if remains are incomplete. It is also age dependent, so that the age of the individual must be known or estimated to make the best use of the method.

In 1983, DiBennardo and Taylor introduced a method that combined measurements of the pelvis and femur. They took a series of 32 measurements of pelves and femora of 260 North American Whites and Blacks (65 males and females of each race) from the Terry Collection. The measurements were then subjected to multiple discriminant function analyses to test their utility in predicting the race and the sex of unknown individuals. Race and sex were taken together to provide insight as to how racial and sexual variation affect each other (DiBennardo and Taylor 1983: 306). DiBennardo and Taylor (1983: 308) report an accuracy rate of approximately 95% for predicting both sex and race. They also developed a method for assessing ancestry via discriminant function analysis of the central portion of the pelvis in isolation, with a substantially lower success rate (average of 61.2%) than when the innominate and the femur are analyzed together (ibid.).

İşcan and Cotton (1990) expanded on this methodology by adding the tibia to the analysis of the pelvis and the femur. According to İşcan and Cotton (1990: 83), until 1990, the Schulter-Ellis and Hayek (1984) method, focusing on the acetabular region and the pubis, was the only method in the literature that did not require measurements of a complete pelvis, femur, or tibia. The İşcan and Cotton method involves discriminant function analysis of 21 measurements in all: 6 from the pelvis, 7 from the femur, and 8 from the tibia (İşcan and Cotton 1990: 83). Because this technique requires fewer measurements of the same elements used in previous methods and includes the analysis of an additional element, the authors suggest it is more applicable to incomplete remains (ibid.). Whereas the pelvis and the femur are often considered the most accurate postcranial predictors of ancestry, other postcranial elements (for example, the scapula) have been analyzed for their utility in determining ancestry (Krogman and İşcan 1986).

Since the publication of *Skeletal Attribution of Race* (Gill and Rhine 1990), several authors have included ancestry determination sections in laboratory or field manuals (Bass 1995; Buikstra and Ubelaker 1994; Burns 1999; Krogman and İşcan 1986; White and Folkens 2005).

Ethics of Race/Ancestry Determination in Forensic Anthropology

Forensic Anthropology has often been called upon to substantiate typological thinking and to reinforce the type concept itself. (Williams, Belcher, and Armelagos 2005: 344)

Anthropologists have established the obvious fact that people from different parts of the world look different from one another. In fact, this systematic variation often allows anthropologists and others to be able to suggest a person's place of ancestry by looking at him or her. Physical anthropologists have expanded this understanding of human variation to the skeleton such that forensic anthropologists, by observing suites of morphological characteristics or applying measurements to various algorithms, are able to estimate place

of ancestry from skeletononized human remains, particularly the skull.

At the same time, the majority of anthropologists have rejected the concept of race applied to humans. According to Lieberman, Kirk, and Littlefield (2003: 112), 80% of cultural anthropologists and 69% of physical anthropologists disagreed with this statement: "there are biological races in the species *Homo sapiens*." Some anthropologists, most notably Goodman and Armelagos (1996), have argued that anthropologists should discredit the idea of human races and reject the notion that there are human groups that are definable by physical characteristics. They have criticized forensic anthropologists for adding credence to the idea of human races by including information about ancestry or race in their reports. To the contrary, some authors (see Cox, Giles, and Buckley 2006; Gill 1998) contend that it is essential to include the assessment of ancestry or race in a report and that it may in fact be unethical or irresponsible not to do so.

George Gill, an outspoken champion of the race concept, states that, unlike other kinds of anthropologists, forensic anthropologists do not have the luxury of ignoring the "the traditional concept of race" (Gill 1998: 295). Because they work in a context where traditional schemes of race have "clear meaning," he believes that forensic anthropologists must translate their findings into terms such as "Caucasoid" and "Black." He is strongly critical of those forensic anthropologists who deny the existence of race and who avoid using it in forensic cases.

Cox and associates (2006) present an interesting and novel justification for the identification of ancestry by forensic anthropologists. They point out that in New Zealand, the Maori believe that the remains of their ancestors "retain special importance" and that the physical remains of these ancestors need to be identified so that they can be handled in culturally prescribed ways (ibid.: 870). They state: "forensic anthropologists who refuse to identify 'race' could be seen to be placing their own beliefs over those of an indigenous group. Identification of the race and therefore ancestry of human physical remains by forensic anthropologists could be seen as an *ethical responsibility*" (emphasis added ibid.: 869). Presumably, their arguments are relevant to other Indigenous peoples.

Controversy about the existence of race in the field of anthropology and beyond presents practicing forensic anthropologists with a dilemma. Although most forensic anthropologists include some mention of ancestry (or race) as a key part of a biological profile, critics point out that this reifies an outdated and demonstrably harmful concept (see Albanese and Saunders 2006).

Williams, Belcher, and Armelagos (2005) and Goodman (1997) are among the anthropologists who believe that forensic anthropology should avoid attempts to identify either ancestry or race, because the methods used to do so are flawed and inaccurate. Williams, Belcher, and Armelagos (2005) applied discriminant function analyses using *FORDISC* 2.0 to a sample of 42 ancient Nubian crania dated from B.C.E. 350–C.E. 350. Using 12 measurements, the Forensic Data Bank series identified 12 of the 42 crania as White, 11 as Black, 3 as Japanese, 1 as Hispanic, and 1 as Native American. The remaining 14 crania "were significantly different from the population specified by *FORDISC* 2.0 (typicality p < 0.05)" (Williams et al. 2005: 342) and were considered inadequately classified. The authors conclude: "skeletal specimens or samples cannot be accurately classified by geography or by racial variation . . ." (Williams et al. 2005: 345). The authors buttress their argument with an earlier published study of Spanish crania.

In 2002, Ubelaker, Ross, and Graver reported on a study that applied *FORDISC* 2.0 to a sample of crania from 16th- and 17th-century Spain. Twenty standard measurements were taken on 95 crania, 58 of which were believed to be male and 37 female. *FORDISC* 2.0 analysis using the Forensic Data Bank option classified the crania as follows: 44% as White; 35% as Black; 9% as Hispanic; 4% as Japanese; 4% as American Indian. Williams and associates (2005) refer to this study as a second illustration of how *FORDISC* 2.0 performs poorly when asked to identify specimens from samples not already in the system.

Are forensic anthropologists faced, as Williams and associates (2005) contend, with applying methods that do not work to ascribe individuals to races that do not exist? Not necessarily. First, no forensic anthropologists we know of uses discriminant functions as the sole or primary tool for determining ancestry. In our laboratory, and from personal experience, we know that our practice is the norm: *FORDISC* 2.0 and 3.0 are used to help confirm or to raise doubts about conclusions based on morphology and context (see also Ubelaker 2002). To critique the practice of ancestry determination based on an application of discriminant function in a vacuum is naive and unwarranted. Second, as Ubelaker and colleagues (2002) and Ousley and Jantz (1996) point out, *FORDISC* does not perform well on individuals or samples that are not adequately represented in the database. Without a Nubian or Spanish sample in

the database, the system is neither expected nor designed to perform adequately.

Brace (1995), Kennedy (1995), and Sauer (1992) have all supported the no-race position yet argue that identifying place of ancestry is a legitimate and useful goal when trying to generate a biological profile and identify unknown human remains. Using estimations of region of ancestry can be a useful tool when applied to missing persons' cases. How the information is communicated to various agencies must depend on the circumstances of the individual case and its context.

Conclusion

In this chapter, we have briefly discussed the concept of race from an historical perspective to illustrate that, despite the contributions that anthropology made in the past to the establishment of traditional views of race, the prevalent view among contemporary anthropologists is that races do not exist. Having established that, we argue that current techniques are useful for assessing the region of ancestry for many individuals (Brace 1995; Sauer 1992) and that this information has potential value for identifying decomposed or otherwise unrecognizable human remains. Although it should be clear that identifying an individual's place of ancestry is not tantamount to identifying his or her race, identifying place of ancestry does allow anthropologists to predict to which race a missing person was most likely assigned (see Sauer 1992).

Ancestry evaluation is an integral part of the forensic examination. Assisting investigators with human remains identification by adding information about ancestry may facilitate and accelerate the process. Of course, caution is essential when one is offering any judgment about an individual from his or her remains, but many decades of research have shown that an understanding of systematic human variation allows the accurate (although not perfect) estimation of ancestry from the skeleton. It is our position that when reporting on ancestry investigators should avoid loaded archaic terms. However, if it is clear that an individual's ancestors are highly likely to have come from Europe, for example, then that fact should be communicated to the proper authorities.

References

Albanese, J., and Saunders, S. R. 2006. Is it possible to escape racial typology in forensic identification?, in A. Schmitt and E. Cunha (eds.), *Forensic Anthropology and Medicine: Complementary*

Sciences from Recovery to Cause of Death, pp. 281–316. Totowa, NJ: Humana Press.

Angel, J. L., and Kelley, J. O. 1990. Inversion of the posterior edge of the jaw ramus: New race trait, in G. W. Gill and S. Rhine (eds.), *Skeletal Attribution of Race,* pp. 33–39. Albuquerque, NM: Maxwell Museum of Anthropology.

Ayers, H. G., Jantz, R. L., and Moore-Jansen, P. H. 1990. Giles and Elliot race discriminant functions revisited: A test using recent forensic cases, in G. W. Gill and S. Rhine (eds.), *Skeletal Attribution of Race,* pp. 65–71. Albuquerque, NM: Maxwell Museum of Anthropology.

Baker, S. J., Gill, G. W., and Kieffer, D. A. 1990. Race and sex determination from the intercondylar notch of the distal femur, in G. W. Gill and S. Rhine (eds.), *Skeletal Attribution of Race,* pp. 91–96. Albuquerque, NM: Maxwell Museum of Anthropology.

Bass, W. M. 1995. *Human Osteology: A Laboratory and Field Manual* (4th ed.). Columbia, MO: Missouri Archaeological Society.

Bertillon, A. 1896. *Signaletic Instructions Including the Theory and Practice of Anthropometrical Identification.* Chicago: The Werner Company.

Birkby, W. H. 1966. An evaluation of race and sex identification from cranial measurements. *American Journal of Physical Anthropology* 24: 21–28.

Brace, C. L. 1982. The roots of the race concept in American physical anthropology, in F. Spencer (ed.), *A History of American Physical Anthropology: 1930–1980,* pp. 11–29. New York: Academic Press, Inc.

———. 1995. Region does not mean Race: Reality and convention in forensic anthropology. *Journal of Forensic Sciences* 40(2): 171–175.

Brooks, S., Brooks, R. H., and France, D. 1990. Alveolar prognathism contour, an aspect of racial identification, in G. W. Gill and S. Rhine (eds.), *Skeletal Attribution of Race,* pp. 41–46. Albuquerque, NM: Maxwell Museum of Anthropology.

Brues, A. M. 1958. Identification of skeletal remains. *The Journal of Criminal Law, Criminology, and Police Science* 48(5): 551–563.

———. 1990. The once and future diagnosis of race, in G. W. Gill and S. Rhine (eds.), *Skeletal Attribution of Race,* pp. 1–7. Albuquerque, NM: Maxwell Museum of Anthropology.

Buikstra, J. E., and Ubelaker, D. H. 1994. *Standards for Data Collection from Human Skeletal Remains.* Fayetteville, AR: Arkansas Archaeological Survey Research Series 44.

Burns, K. R. 1999. *Forensic Anthropology Training Manual.* Upper Saddle River, NJ: Simon & Schuster/ A Viacom Company.

Byers, S. N. 2005. *Introduction to Forensic Anthropology: A Textbook.* Boston: Pearson Education, Inc.

Cameron, J. 1929a. The facial height as a criterion of race: Craniometric studies, No. 21. *American Journal of Physical Anthropology* 13(2): 319–334.

———. 1929b. The facial width as a criterion of race: Craniometric studies, No. 22. *American Journal of Physical Anthropology* 13(2): 335–343.

———. 1929c. A study of the upper facial index in diverse racial types of mankind: Craniometric studies, No. 23. *American Journal of Physical Anthropology* 13(2): 344–352.

———. 1930. The nasal (nasion-akanthion) height as a criterion of race. *American Journal of Physical Anthropology* 14(2): 273–283.

Cobb, W. M. 1942. Physical anthropology of the American Negro. *American Journal of Physical Anthropology* 29(2): 113–223.

Cox, K., Giles, N. G., and Buckley, H. R. 2006. Forensic identification of "race": The issues in New Zealand. *Current Anthropology* 47(5): 869–874.

Curran, B. K. 1990. The application of measures of midfacial projection for racial classification, in G. W. Gill and S. Rhine (eds.), *Skeletal Attribution of Race,* pp. 55–58. Albuquerque, NM: Maxwell Museum of Anthropology.

Dahlberg, A. A. 1951. The dentition of the American Indian, in W. S. Laughlin (ed.), *Papers on the Physical Anthropology of the American Indian,* pp. 138–176. New York: Viking Fund.

DiBennardo, R., and Taylor, J. V. 1983. Multiple discriminant function analysis of sex and race in the postcranial skeleton. *American Journal of Physical Anthropology* 61: 305–314.

———. 1984. Race and sex assessment of the central portion of the innominate by discriminant function analysis (Abstract). *American Journal of Physical Anthropology* 63: 152.

Fisher, T. D., and Gill, G. W. 1990. Application of the Giles & Elliot discriminant function formulae to a cranial sample of Northwestern Plains Indians, in G. W. Gill and S. Rhine (eds.), *Skeletal Attribution of Race,* pp. 59–63. Albuquerque, NM: Maxwell Museum of Anthropology.

Freid, D., and Jantz, R. L. 2005. Classification and evaluation of unusual individuals using FORDISC. Paper presented at the annual meeting for the American Academy of Forensic Sciences, February 21–26, New Orleans, Louisiana.

Gilbert, R., and Gill, G. W. 1990. A metric technique for identifying American Indian femora, in G. W. Gill, and S. Rhine (eds.), *Skeletal Attribution of Race,* pp. 97–99. Albuquerque, NM: Maxwell Museum of Anthropology.

Giles, E., and Elliot, O. 1962. Race identification from cranial measurements. *Journal of Forensic Sciences* 7(2): 147–156.

Gill, G. W. 1984. A forensic test case for a new method of geographical race determination, in T. A. Rathbun and J. E. Buikstra (eds.), *Human Identification: Case Studies in Forensic Anthropology*, pp. 329–339. Springfield, IL: Charles C. Thomas.

Gill, G. W. 1998. Craniofacial criteria in the skeletal attribution of race, in K. J. Reichs (ed.), *Forensic Osteology: Advances in the Identification of Human Remains* (2nd ed.), pp. 293–311. Springfield, IL: Charles C. Thomas.

Gill, G. W., and Miles Gilbert, B. 1990. Race identification from the midfacial skeleton: American Blacks and Whites, in G. W. Gill and S. Rhine (eds.), *Skeletal Attribution of Race*, pp. 47–57. Albuquerque, NM: Maxwell Museum of Anthropology.

Gill, G. W., Hughes, S. S., Bennett, S. M., and Gilbert, B. M. 1988. Racial identification from the midfacial skeleton with special reference to American Indians and Whites. *Journal of Forensic Sciences* 33(1): 92–99.

Gill, G. W., and Rhine, S. (eds.). 1990. *Skeletal Attribution of Race*. Albuquerque, NM: Maxwell Museum of Anthropology.

Goodman, A. 1997. Bred in the Bone? *Sciences* March/April: 20–25.

Goodman, A. H., and Armelagos, G. J. 1996. The resurrection of race: The concept of race in physical anthropology in the 1990s, in L. T. Reynolds and L. Lieberman (eds.), *Race and Other Misadventures: Essays in Honor of Ashley Mongagu in His Ninetieth Year*, pp. 174–186. Dix Hills, NY: General Hall, Inc.

Gray, D. J. 1942. Variations in human scapulae. *American Journal of Physical Anthropology* 29(1): 57–72.

Harris, E. F., Hicks, J. D., and Barcroft, B. D. 2001. Tissue contributions to sex and race: Differences in tooth crown size of deciduous molars. *American Journal of Physical Anthropology* 115: 223–237.

Hinkes, M. J. 1990. Shovel shaped incisors in human identification, in G. W. Gill and S. Rhine (eds.), *Skeletal Attribution of Race*, pp. 21–26. Albuquerque, NM: Maxwell Museum of Anthropology.

Howells, W. W. 1973. Cranial variation in Man. Cambridge, MA: *Papers of the Peabody Museum of Archaeology and Ethnology* 67: 1–259.

———. 1989. Skull shapes and the map: Craniometric analyses in the dispersion of modern Homo. *Papers of the Peabody Museum of Archaeology and Ethnology* 79: 1–189.

———. 1995. Who's who in skulls: Ethnic identification of crania from measurements. *Papers of the Peabody Museum of Archaeology and Ethnology* 82: 1–108.

Hrdlička, A. 1920. Shovel shaped teeth. *American Journal of Physical Anthropology* 3: 429–465.

İşcan, M. Y. 1983. Assessment of race from the pelvis. *American Journal of Physical Anthropology* 62: 205–208.

———. 1988. Rise of forensic anthropology. *Yearbook of Physical Anthropology* 31: 203–230.

İşcan, M. Y., and Cotton, T. S. 1990. Osteometric assessment of racial affinity from multiple sites on the postcranial skeleton, in G. W. Gill and S. Rhine (eds.), *Skeletal Attribution of Race*, pp. 83–90. Albuquerque, NM: Maxwell Museum of Anthropology.

Iyer, V. S., and Lutz, W. 1966. Cephalometric comparison of Indian and English facial profiles. *American Journal of Physical Anthropology* 24: 117–126.

Kennedy, K. A. R. 1995. But professor, why teach race identification if races don't exist? *Journal of Forensic Sciences* 40(5): 797–800.

Kerley, E. R. 1978. Recent developments in forensic anthropology. *Yearbook of Physical Anthropology* 21: 160–173.

Krogman, W. M. 1939. A Guide to the Identification of Human Skeletal Material. *FBI Law Enforcement Bulletin* 8: 1–31.

———. 1962. *The Human Skeleton in Forensic Medicine*. Springfield, IL: Charles C. Thomas.

Krogman, W. M., and İşcan, M. Y. 1986. Assessment of racial affinity, in W. M. Krogman, and M. Y. İşcan (eds.), *The Human Skeleton in Forensic Medicine*, 2nd ed., pp. 268–301. Springfield, IL: Charles C. Thomas.

Lanier, Jr., R. R. 1944. Length of first, twelfth, and accessory ribs in American Whites and Negroes: Their relationship to certain vertebral variations. *American Journal of Physical Anthropology*, N.S. 2(2): 137–146.

Lease, L. R., and Sciulli, P. W. 2005. Brief communication: Discrimination between European-American and African-American children based on deciduous dental metrics and morphology. *American Journal of Physical Anthropology* 126: 56–60.

Letterman, G. S. 1941. Greater sciatic notch in American Whites and Negroes. *American Journal of Physical Anthropology* 28(1): 99–116.

Lieberman, L., Kirk, R. C., and Littlefield, A. 2003. Exchange across difference: The status of the race concept. Perishing paradigm: Race 1931–99. *American Anthropologist* 105(1): 110–113.

Lieberman, L., and Reynolds, L. T. 1996. Race: The deconstruction of a scientific concept, in L. T. Reynolds and L. Lieberman (eds.), *Race and Other Misadventures: Essays in Honor of Ashley Montagu in His Ninetieth Year*, pp. 142–173. Dix Hills, NY: General Hall, Inc.

Livingstone, F. B. 1962. On the non-existence of human races. *Current Anthropology* 3(3): 279–281.

Michelson, N. 1944. Studies in the physical development of Negroes III: Cephalic index. *American Journal of Physical Anthropology*, N.S. (1): 417–424.

Montagu, A. 1941. The concept of race in the human species in light of genetics. *The Journal of Heredity* 32: 243–247.

———. 1942. The genetical theory of race and anthropological method. *American Anthropologist* 44: 369–375.

———. 1952. *Man's Most Dangerous Myth: The Fallacy of Race.* New York: Harper.

Napoli, M. L., and Birkby, W. H. 1990. Racial differences in the visibility of the oval window in the middle ear, in G. W. Gill and S. Rhine (eds.), *Skeletal Attribution of Race,* pp. 27–32. Albuquerque, NM: Maxwell Museum of Anthropology.

Ousley, S. D., and Jantz, R. L. 1996. *FORDISC 2.0: Personal Computer Forensic Discriminant Functions User's Guide.* Knoxville: The University of Tennessee.

———. 2005. The next FORDISC: FORDISC 3. Abstract for a Paper presented at the annual meeting for the American Academy of Forensic Sciences, February, 21–26, New Orleans, Louisiana.

Rathbun, T. A., and Buikstra, J. E. (eds.). 1984. *Human Identification: Case Studies in Forensic Anthropology.* Springfield, IL: Charles C. Thomas.

Ray, C..D. 1955. Configuration and lateral closure of the superior orbital fissure. *American Journal of Physical Anthropology, N.S.* 13: 309–321.

Reichs, K. J. (ed.). 1986. *Forensic Osteology: Advances in the Identification of Human Remains* (2nd ed.) Springfield, IL: Charles C. Thomas.

Rhine, S. 1990a. Foreword, in G. W. Gill and S. Rhine (eds.), *Skeletal Attribution of Race,* pp. xiii–xvii. Albuquerque, NM: Maxwell Museum of Anthropology.

———. 1990b. Non-metric skull racing, in G. W. Gill and S. Rhine (eds.), *Skeletal Attribution of Race,* pp. 9–20. Albuquerque, NM: Maxwell Museum of Anthropology.

Sauer, N. J. 1992. Forensic anthropology and the concept of race: If races don't exist why are forensic anthropologists so good at identifying them? *Social Science and Medicine* 34(2): 107–111.

Snow, C. C., Hartman, S., Giles, E., and Young, F. A. 1978. Sex and race determination of crania by calipers and computer: A test of the Giles and Elliot discriminant functions in 52 forensic science cases. *Journal of Forensic Sciences* 24(2): 448–460.

Stewart, T. D. 1962. Anterior femoral curvature: Its utility for race identification. *Human Biology* 34: 49–62.

Templeton, A. R. 2002. The genetic and evolutionary significance of human race, in J. M. Fish (ed.), *Race and Intelligence: Separating Science from Myth,* pp. 31–56. Mahwah, NJ: Lawrence Erlbaum Assoc.

Thurstone, L. L. 1947. Factorial analysis of body measurements. *American Journal of Physical Anthropology, N.S.* (5): 15–28.

Todd, T. W., and Lindala, A. 1928. Dimensions of the body: Whites and American Negroes of both sexes. *American Journal of Physical Anthropology* 12(1): 35–119.

Todd, T. W., and Tracy, B. 1930. Racial features in the American Negro cranium. *American Journal of Physical Anthropology* 15(1): 53–110.

Trotter, M. 1929. The vertebral column in Whites and in American Negroes. *American Journal of Physical Anthropology* 13(1): 95–107.

Trotter, M., and Gleser, G. C. 1952. Estimation of stature from long bones of American Whites and Negroes. *American Journal of Physical Anthropology* 10: 463–514.

Ubelaker, D. H. 2000. A history of Smithsonian-FBI collaboration in forensic anthropology, especially in regard to facial imagery. *Forensic Science Communications* 2(4).

Ubelaker, D. H., Ross, A. H., and Graver, S. M. 2002. Application of forensic discriminant functions to a Spanish cranial sample. *Forensic Science Communications* 4(3): 1–6.

Wescott, D. J. 2005. Population variation in femur subtrochanteric shape. *Journal of Forensic Sciences* 50(2): 286–293.

Wescott, D. J., and Jantz, R. L. 2005. Assessing craniofacial secular change in American Blacks and Whites using geometric morphometry, in D. E. Slice (ed.), *Modern Morphometrics in Physical Anthropology,* pp. 231–245. New York: Kluwer Academic/Plenum Publishers.

White, T. D., and Folkens, P. A. 2005. *The Human Bone Manual.* Burlington, MA: Elsevier-Academic Press.

Williams, F. L., Belcher, R. L., and Armelagos, G. J. 2005. Forensic misclassification of ancient Nubian crania: Implications for assumptions about human variation. *Current Anthropology* 46(2): 340–346.

Wilson, E. O., and Brown, W.L., Jr. 1953. The subspecies concept and its taxonomic application. *Systematic Zoology* 2(3): 97–111.

Woo, J-K. 1949. Racial and sexual differences in the frontal curvature and its relation to metopism. *American Journal of Physical Anthropology, N.S.* (7): 215–226.

Wright, R. 1992. Correlation between cranial form and geography in *Homo sapiens*: CRANID. A computer program for forensic and other applications. *Perspectives in Human Biology 2/Archaeology in Oceania* 27: 128–134.

———. 2007. Guide to using the CRANID programs CR6LDA.EXE and CR6NN.EXE, *www.box.net/shared/static/n9q0zgtr1y.EXE.*

———. 2008. Detection of likely ancestry using CRANID, in M. F. Oxenham (ed.), *Forensic Approaches to Death, Disaster, and Abuse.* Queensland: Australian Academic Press.

17

ANTHROPOLOGICAL ESTIMATION OF SEX

Valeria Silva Braz

This chapter discusses the different methods involved in estimating the sex of an individual from his/her skeleton. Estimating the sex of skeletons from forensic or archaeological contexts is an essential step in the process of identifying an individual and/or developing a population biological profile. Estimation is predominantly based on the analysis of markers present on the cranium and pelvis. However, analyses of other bones can be done with varying degrees of accuracy. When estimating the sex of an individual, one must consider individual and population variation that modulates skeletal and secondary sexual characteristics development.

Sexual Dimorphism

Bone growth is hormonally and genetically controlled. The production of sexual hormones increases around the time of puberty, resulting in the development of sexually dimorphic skeletal characteristics, which appear at adulthood. Such dimorphism varies both within and among populations. After an individual has reached 18 years, sexual dimorphism is better defined, and thus sex estimation can be made with greater confidence.

Compared to other groups of primates, modern humans present far less sexual dimorphism in body and tooth (particularly canine) size. In an equal sample of 50 male and 50 female modern humans, for example, sorting accuracy is therefore reduced. Human sexual dimorphism is complex, with important behavioral, physiological, and anatomical aspects. Anatomical differences in living individuals can be extreme in some areas and more limited in others, such as the skeleton. Nevertheless, skeletal differences between males and females do exist and are therefore useful to osteologists.

In estimating sex using any skeletal element, the osteologist starts with 50% accuracy: there is a 50-50 chance the individual could be either male or female. For some elements, such as the cranium, training and experience can often allow the practitioner to correctly sort using morphological features about 80–90% of the time (Krogman and İşcan 1986). However, only *after* puberty does the skeleton become sufficiently different to be useful in sexing.

In general, the female skeleton is characterized by smaller size and gracile morphology. Thus, in a large and mixed-sex collection of bones, the largest and most robust elements with the heaviest relief are considered male and the smallest, most gracile elements, female. Normal individual variation, may, however, produce some small, gracile males and some large, robust females that compose the center of the distribution where accuracy tends to zero. For this reason, osteologists traditionally concentrate on the elements of the skull and pelvis where sex markers are the more evident.

In addition to individual variation within a population, incorrect sex identifications are sometimes made because of variation between populations. Some populations are composed of larger, heavier and more robust individuals of both sexes, and other populations are characterized by the opposite features. Because of such differences in size and robusticity, males from one population are sometimes mistaken for females in other populations, and vice versa. The osteologist must attempt to become familiar with the skeletal sexual dimorphism of the population from which unsexed material has been drawn. As in the case of aging, a careful analysis of the whole skeletal series can be a helpful approach in determining the sex of skeletal remains from a population.

Techniques Used to Estimate Sex

Techniques used to estimate the sex of an individual based on the skeleton may include visual assessment of gross morphology and/or a metric assessment of the skeletal remains.

Visual Assessment of Gross Morphology

The Pelvis. There are great differences between male and female pelvic anatomy that extend to other parts of the skeleton. The pelvis has a crucial role in locomotion and parturition. During evolution, adaptation of the human species to vertical posture, new mechanical demands, and decrease of pelvic diameter led to the sexual dimorphism observed in the modern human pelvis.

Traditional methods used to determine sex on the pelvis are based on the assumption that the sacrum and the os coxae of females are smaller and less robust than those of males (Figure 17.1). Female pelvic inlets are relatively wider than male ones. Compared with males, females have a

relatively wider greater sciatic notch and relatively longer pubic portions of the os coxae, including the superior pubic ramus. The subpubic angle, formed between the lower edges of the two inferior pubic rami, is also larger in females than in males (Figure 17.2). The pre-auricular sulcus is present more often in females than in males, and the acetabulum tends to be larger in males.

In some cases, the application of metric criteria is difficult, because the material may be too fragmentary for reliable measurements. The method proposed by Phenice (1969) is especially useful in such circumstances. In employing Phenice's method to estimate sex using pelvic bones, note that not every feature has to match the "model" of male or female. When there is some ambiguity concerning one or two of the criteria (most often in the medial aspect of the ischiopubic ramus, and least often in the ventral arc), usually one of the remaining criteria clearly attributes the specimen to a sex. After analyzing the specimen with the mentioned procedure, one must observe the more traditional features outlined previously to see if they corroborate the diagnosis—remembering that female individuals are most likely to be intermediate in displaying the Phenice parameters. Phenice's method can be applied only to fully adult material. Reported accuracy of sexing based on this method ranges from 96% to nearly 100%, but Lovell (1989) suggested that accuracy might be reduced in the case of older adult specimens.

Phenice's Protocol:

1. Orient the pubis so that its rough ventral surface faces you, and you are looking down along the plane of the pubic symphysis surface. The ventral arc is a slightly elevated ridge of bone that sweeps inferiorly and laterally across the ventral surface of the pubis, merging with the medial border of the ischiopubic ramus. The ventral arc, when present, sets off the inferior, medial corner of the pubic bone in

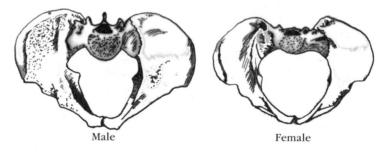

Male   Female

Figure 17.1   Sexual dimorphism in human pelvis; note the different size and shape.

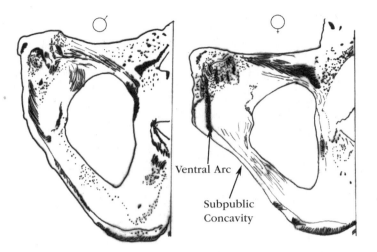

Figure 17.2   Posterior view of the pubic portion of the os coxae of both sexes.

ventral view. It is present only in females. Male os coxae may have elevated ridges in this area, but these do not take the wide, evenly arching path of the female's ventral arc or set off the lower medial quadrant of the pubis.

2. Turn the pubis over, orienting it so that its smooth, convex dorsal surface faces you and you are once again sighting along the midline. Observe the medial edge of the ischiopubic ramus in this view. Female os coxae display a subpubic concavity there; the edge of the ramus is concave in this view. Males, in contrast, do not show a

huge concavity. Male edges are straight or very slightly concave.

3. Turn the pubis 90°, orienting the symphysis surface so that you are looking directly perpendicular to it. Observe the ischiopubic ramus in the region immediately inferior to the symphysis. This medial aspect of the ischiopubic ramus displays a sharp edge in females (Figure 17.3). In males, the surface is fairly flat, broad, and blunt.

Considerations about Parturition Scars: Kelley (1979) developed a detailed analysis of the female pelvis in relation to parity status. The author

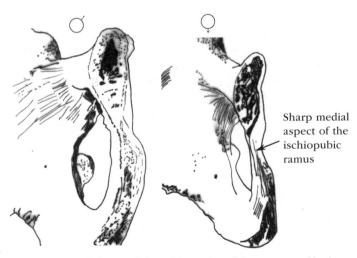

Figure 17.3   Medial view of the pubic portion of the os coxae of both sexes.

analyzed 198 complete pelves and found three significant features associated with parturition (dorsal pubic pitting, pre-auricular grooves, and interosseous grooves). Kelley's study concluded: (1) combining the aforementioned features provides the most significant indicator of parity status; (2) evidence of pregnancy and parturition can disappear over time, leaving no indication of childbirth among elderly women; (3) although the pre-auricular groove provides the best indicator of parity, researchers should be aware that pits and grooves occasionally occur in nulliparous women in the sacroiliac region (occurred in 20% of Kelly's sample); and (4) determining the number of pregnancies and children delivered is difficult through skeletal remains alone (Kelley 1979).

The study by Suchey and associates (1979) on a sample of 486 American females of known parity between the ages of 13 and 99 provides additional perspective. This research found that the correlation between dorsal pitting in the pubic bone showed only a weak correlation with evidence of full-term pregnancy. Also noteworthy was the finding that of the 148 females reported to be nulliparous (no children), 17 presented dorsal pitting of the pubis. In addition, 22 females with records of full-term pregnancy lacked the skeletal evidence of dorsal pitting. Thus, although marked dorsal pitting seems to be an excellent indicator of female sex, it is not entirely diagnostic of full-term pregnancy.

Although the pubic symphysis can produce highly accurate estimates of sex, one must consider that this part of the pelvis is highly susceptible to taphonomic alterations. Consequently, other parts of the skeleton have to be considered when estimating sex.

The Cranium. Determination of sex based on assessment of the size and the morphology of parts of the cranium follows the observation that males tend to be larger and more robust than females. Relative to female crania, male crania are characterized by greater robusticity. Male crania also display more prominent supraorbital ridges, a more prominent glabella, and heavier temporal and nuchal crest (Figure 17.4). Male frontal and parietal bones tend to be less bossed (pronounced) than female ones. Males also tend to have relatively large, broad palates, squarer orbits, larger mastoid processes, larger sinuses, and larger occipital condyles than do females. Compared to female mandibles, male mandibles are characterized by squarer chins, more gonial eversion, deeper mandibular rami, and more rugose (thick) muscle attachment points. Scaling these features has been attempted in order to reduce the subjective nature of the assessment process (Buikstra and Ubelaker 1994).

When one is using the cranium to estimate sex, one should also analyze other individuals of the same population under study. When possible, the study population should be seriated and sorted. If only one or a few individuals are being analyzed, a comparative population that is genetically and temporally close to the ones under study should be used.

Morphometric Assessments

To go beyond the traditional methods outlined above, Giles and Elliot (1963) used nine standard cranial measurements to diminish the subjectivity involved in sexing the cranium. However, a later study by Meindl and colleagues (1985) has shown that subjective assessments compared favorably to the discriminant functions of Giles and Elliot (1963). Meindl and associates (1985) found that older individuals show a more "masculine" morphology. They also suggested that one should be able to estimate overall sex ratios and age-to-sex ratios in prehistoric cemeteries from an analysis of adult burials.

Many authors studied and documented metric sexual differences in the postcranial skeleton, but these analyses are still considered less accurate than those on the pelvis and cranium.[1] The maximum diameters of the heads of femur, humerus, and radius (Table 17.1) are good indicators of sex in adults when they are far from the center of the distribution curve (overlap zone). Authors have also observed sexual dimorphism in other limb bones (Holman and Bennett 1991; İşcan, Yoshino, and Kato 1994; Purkait 2001; Wilbur 1998). According to Ubelaker (1999), these techniques predicted sex with an accuracy of 58% to nearly 100%.

The discriminant function statistic was developed by Fischer in 1940 but has since been adopted by anthropologists as a quantitative approach to estimate sex (and ancestry). Sex determination is amenable to discriminant function analysis based on the assumption that the two sexes will produce a bimodal curve. Discriminant function analysis is used to determine which continuous variables differentiate two or more naturally occurring groups.

Discriminant functions, as proposed by Giles (1970), can be used for sex inferences, but most of the equations are population specific, demanding special attention in cases of unknown ancestry. The discriminant function approach turned into a very important source for the building of a forensic database. The interactive computer program, FORDISC 3.0, developed at the University of Tennessee by Ousley and Jantz (1996), provides an interface that classifies adults by ancestry

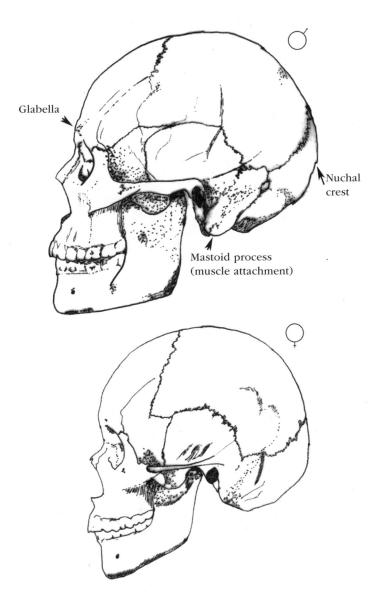

Figure 17.4 Lateral view of male and female adult skulls. The female skull represents the "female" end of female range. Observe the size and robusticity differences.

and sex using any combination of standard measurements and enables the user to customize discriminant function equations and also classify the "unknowns" (see Sauer and Wankmiller this volume). According to Ubelaker (1999), advantages for forensic purposes are (1) the flexibility that requires fewer measurements; (2) the forensic origin of the sample producing the database; and (3) the presentation of results in statistical format.

Sex Estimation of Subadults: The assessment of sex of subadult remains is a highly contested sub-

ject. Fazekas and Kosa (1978) assessed whether there was a statistically significant difference in the cranial base bones of fetal male and female specimens, and Schutkowski (1993) performed morphognostic analyses of infant mandibles. The accuracy of these studies was assessed by Ridley (2002), who concluded that there are sex differences in the mandible but not in the cranial base, based on developmental differences between males and females. The cranial base develops slower than does the mandible. The accelerated

Table 17.1 Diameter ranges of female and male femora, humeri, and radial heads from black and white North American populations (Berrizbeitia 1987; Dwight 1904–1905; Stewart 1979).

	Diameter (mm)	
	Female	*Male*
Femur	<43	>48
Humerus	<43	>47
Radius	<21	>23

growth of the mandible leads to a differentiation in the sexes, which becomes apparent at earlier stages of skeletal development.

Conclusion

The reliability of morphological skeletal characteristics to estimate the sex of an individual varies according to the remains being analyzed and the chosen parameters used to provide the estimation. Therefore, observed sexual dimorphism must be carefully used as a criterion of sexual determination applicable to all populations, especially in comparative studies. However, ongoing research has been conducted using DNA to assist with sex determination in both forensic contexts (Andréasson and Allen 2003; Kontanis and Reed 2006; Williams and Rogers 2006) and those of degraded skeletal remains (Alonso et al. 2004; Irwin et al. 2007). Combing both observable morphological features and DNA may prove to be very helpful in future studies of sex determination, especially in the examination of populations with extensive variation in the expression of sexual dimorphism.

Note

1. Black 1978; Falsetti 1995; Holman and Bennett 1991; Introna et al. 1997; Işcan and Miller-Shaivitz 1984; Lazenby 1994; Robling and Ubelaker 1997; Scheuer and Elkington 1993; Smith 1996; Steele 1976.

References

Alonso, A., Martín, P., Albarrán, C., García, P., García , O., Fernández de Simón, L., García, J., Sancho, M., Rúa, C., and Fernández-Piqueras, J. 2004. Real-time PCR designs to estimate nuclear and mitochondrial DNA copy number in forensic and ancient DNA studies. *Forensic Science International* 139(2): 141–149.

Andréasson, H., and Allen, M. 2003. Rapid quantification and sex determination of forensic evidence materials. *Journal of Forensic Sciences* 48(6): 1280–1287.

Berrizbeitia, E. L. 1987. Sex determination with the head of the radius. *Journal of Forensic Sciences* 34(5): 1206–1213.

Black, T. K. 1978. A new method for assessing the sex of fragmentary skeletal remains: Femoral shaft circumference. *American Journal of Physical Anthropology* 48: 227–232.

Buikstra, J., and Ubelaker, D. (eds.). 1994. *Standards for Data Collection from Human Skeletal Remains.* Fayetteville, AS: Archeological Survey Research Seminar Series 44.

Dwight, T. 1904–1905. The size of the articular surfaces of the long bones as characteristic of sex; an anthropological study. *American Journal of Anatomy* 4(1): 19–31.

Falsetti, A. B. 1995. Sex assessment from metacarpals of the human hand. *Journal of Forensic Sciences* 40: 774–776.

Fazekas, I. G., and Kosa, F. 1978. *Forensic Fetal Osteology.* Budapest: Akademiai Kiado.

Giles, E. 1970. Discriminant function sexing of the human skeleton, in T. D. Stewart (ed.), *Personal Identification in Mass Disasters*, pp. 99–109. Washington, D.C.: Smithsonian Institution.

Giles, E., and Elliot, O. 1963. Sex determination by discriminant function analysis of crania. *American Journal of Physical Anthropology* 21: 53–68.

Holman, D. J., and Bennett, K. A. 1991. Determination of sex from arm bone measurements. *American Journal of Physical Anthropology* 84: 421–426.

Introna, F., Di Vella, G., Campobasso, C. P., and Dragone, M. 1997. Sex determination by discriminant analysis of calcanei measurements. *Journal of Forensic Sciences* 42: 725–728.

Irwin, J. A., Leney, M. D., Loreille, O., Barritt, S. M., Christensen, A. F., Holland, T. D., Smith, B. C., and Parsons, T. J. 2007. Application of low copy number STR typing to the identification of aged, degraded skeletal remains. *Journal of Forensic Sciences* 52(6). Electronic Document: www.blackwell-synergy.com

İşcan, M. Y., and Miller-Shaivitz, P. 1984. Discriminant function sexing of the tibia. *Journal of Forensic Sciences* 29: 1087–1093.

İşcan, M. Y., Yoshino, M., and Kato, S. 1994. Sex determination from the tibia: Standards for contemporary Japan. *Journal of Forensic Sciences* 39(3): 785–792.

Kelley, M. A. 1979. Parturition and pelvic changes. *American Journal of Physical Anthropology* 51(4): 541–545.

Kontanis, E. J., and Reed, F. A. 2006. Evaluation of real-time PCR amplification efficiencies to detect PCR inhibitors. *Journal of Forensic Sciences* 51(4): 795–804.

Krogman, W. M., and İşcan, M. Y. 1986. *The Human Skeleton in Forensic Medicine* (2nd ed.) Springfield, IL: Charles C. Thomas.

Lazenby, R. A. 1994. Identification of sex from metacarpals: Effect of side asymmetry. *Journal of Forensic Sciences* 39: 1188–1194.

Lovell, N. C. 1989. Test of Phenice's technique for determining sex from the Os Pubis. *American Journal of Physical Anthropology* 79: 117–120.

Meindl, R. S., Lovejoy, C. O., Mensforth, R. P., and Don Carlos, L. 1985. Accuracy and direction of error in the sexing of the skeleton: Implications for palaeodemography. *American Journal of Physical Anthropology* 68: 79–85.

Ousley, S. D., and Jantz, R. L. 1996. Fordisc 2.0: *Personal Computer Forensic Discriminant Function.* Knoxville: The University of Tennessee.

Phenice, T. W. 1969. A newly developed visual method of sexing the Os Pubis. *American Journal of Physical Anthropology* 30: 297–302.

Purkait, R. 2001. Measurements of ulna: A new method for determination of sex. *Journal of Forensic Sciences* 46(4): 924–927.

Ridley, J. 2002. Sex Estimation of Fetal and Infant Remains Based on Metric and Morphognostic Analyses. Unpublished M.Sc. dissertation. Louisiana State University and Agricultural and Mechanical College.

Robling, A. G., and Ubelaker, D. H. 1997. Sex estimation from the metatarsals. *Journal of Forensic Sciences* 42(6): 1062–1069.

Scheuer, J. L., and Elkington, N. M. 1993. Sex determination from metacarpals and the first proximal phalanx. *Journal of Forensic Sciences* 38: 769–778.

Schutkowski, H. 1993. Sex determination of infant and juvenile skeletons: I. Morphognostic features. *American Journal of Physical Anthropology* 90: 199–205.

Smith, S. L. 1996. Attribution of hand bones to sex and population groups. *Journal of Forensic Sciences* 41: 469–477.

Steele, D. G. 1976. The estimation of sex on the basis of the talus and calcaneous. *American Journal of Physical Anthropology* 45: 581–588.

Stewart, T. D. 1979. *Essentials of Forensic Anthropology: Especially as Developed in the United States.* Springfield, IL: Charles C. Thomas.

Suchey, J. M., Wiseley, D. V., Green, R. F., and Noguchi, T. T. 1979. Analysis of dorsal pitting in the Os Pubis in an extensive sample of modern American females. *American Journal of Physical Anthropology* 51: 517–540.

Ubelaker, D. H. 1999. *Human Skeletal Remains: Excavation, Analysis, Interpretation* (3rd ed.). Washington, D.C.: Taraxacum.

Wilbur, A. K. 1998. The utility of hand and foot bones for the determination of sex and the estimation of stature in a prehistoric population from west-central Illinois. *International Journal of Osteoarchaeology* 8(3): 180–191.

Williams, B. A., and Rogers, T. L. 2006. Evaluating the accuracy and precision of cranial morphological traits for sex determination. *Journal of Forensic Sciences* 51(4): 729–735.

SKELETAL AGE ESTIMATION

Tracy L. Rogers

Age estimation is a critical component of the biological profile, as even the broadest age ranges can help focus the investigation into an unknown's identity. The narrower the age estimate, the more useful a skeletal analysis will be in reducing the number of potential missing person matches and expediting the process of positive identification. An example from the missing persons files of British Columbia, Canada, provides a useful demonstration of this principle. In October 1999, there were 1,755 reported missing people in British Columbia; 444 (25%) were female. Of those missing females, 143 were between the ages of 20 and 40 years, and, of those, 38 were nonwhite (Robin Lamb, Royal Canadian Mounted Police, personal communication 2006). In this example, an extremely broad age estimate of 20–40 years for unknown remains would be sufficient to reduce the number of prospective female matches in the missing persons files from 444 to 143.

Although restricted age ranges are desirable, they are not always feasible. The difficulty in estimating the age-at-death of a skeleton stems from the fact that our chronological age (how old we are in years) rarely corresponds exactly to our physiological age (how old our bodies appear as a result of use and wear). Skeletal aging is a variable and nonlinear process, resulting from individual health, nutrition, genetics, mechanical

wear, and exposure to environmental stressors. To encompass the scope of individual variability inherent in the aging process, skeletal age estimations are always reported in ranges, for example, 23–57 years. Depending on the technique used to approximate age-at-death, the recommended age ranges can be expected to encompass the majority of individuals in the test sample (Gilbert and McKern 1973), 95% of the range of individual variation (McKern and Stewart 1957; Suchey, Wiseley, and Katz 1986), or some other measure of inclusiveness (Lovejoy et al. 1985a).

In a forensic context it is necessary to balance a restricted age estimate, capable of eliminating some members of the missing persons list, and a broad age range that accounts for individual variation and encompasses the true age of the deceased. If the estimated age range is too large, then greater time, effort, and money will be needed to test all the potential matches for DNA identification (ID). If the age-at-death evaluation is too narrow, however, then the true age of the deceased may not be included in the estimate, causing the police to incorrectly eliminate that individual as a potential match to the remains. Either problem can have serious repercussions for a medico-legal investigation.

Excellent overviews and summaries of skeletal age indicators are available in several texts, including Buikstra and Ubelaker (1994), Bass (1995), Schwartz (1995), Cox and Mays (2000), White (2000), and Byers (2005). Juvenile remains are given detailed consideration in Fazekas and Kósa (1978) and Scheuer and Black (2000, 2004). One of the most complete treatments of skeletal age estimation is provided by İşcan's (1989) *Age Markers in the Human Skeleton.*

This chapter addresses macroscopic age-at-death estimation of unknown, human skeletal remains in a forensic context from a theoretical perspective. After outlining the primary themes and concerns associated with skeletal age indicators, I summarize major historical developments that have led to significant advances and influenced current trends. The chapter concludes with an examination of the future of skeletal age-at-death estimation.

Main Issues and Concerns

Estimating the age of skeletal remains introduces several theoretical and practical problems: (1) subadult versus adult age estimation; (2) chronological versus physiological age; (3) statistical analysis of age-related changes in the skeleton; and (4) combining information from multiple age indicators.

Subadult versus Adult Age Estimation

Because the approaches and techniques of evaluating juvenile age-at-death differ from those applied to adults, a brief evaluation of maturational stage generally precedes age estimation. Although this poses no difficulty when one is evaluating infants and children, the adolescent and young-adult periods are transitional, marked by disparate rates of skeletal development and complicated by sexual and individual variation. Adolescence is both a biologically variable period and a culturally heterogeneous experience. In a physiological sense, an adult skeleton is one in which the growth process is complete; all epiphyses are fused. Epiphyseal union is a gradual process that occurs primarily throughout the teenage years for long bones but that extends into the mid-20s and early 30s for the iliac crest (Webb and Suchey 1985) and sternal clavicle (Black and Scheuer 1996; Webb and Suchey 1985). In a cultural sense, "adult" can mean the legal determination of adulthood as established by the state, province, or country; a cultural or ethnic recognition of adulthood; or an informal acknowledgment of adult status by family or peers. One cannot assume a skeletal evaluation of "adult" will be universally or correctly interpreted by medico-legal investigators. Thus, a minimum age estimate should be provided

for all cases in which only the broadest distinction between adult and subadult is possible.

Subadult age estimation is based on development and growth, while adult skeletal age indicators are rooted in remodeling and degenerative changes (İşcan and Loth 1989). Because subadult age indicators are limited to the developmental stage in which they are active (that is, dental formation in young children, tooth eruption in middle childhood, epiphyseal fusion in later childhood and adolescence, and diaphyseal length up to the point of epiphyseal union) the progressive nature of growth and development generates more precise age ranges than is possible with adult age indicators. Maturational changes during development are largely under genetic control, although health, nutrition, and other environmental stressors do have the capacity to stunt and/or slow these processes (Johnston and Zimmer 1989; Konigsberg and Holman 1999; Lampl and Johnston 1996; Stinson 2000). Teeth are less susceptible than bone is to environmental disturbances, making teeth the preferred tissue for estimating juvenile age (Demirjian 1986). Dental formation is favored over eruption, as eruption rates vary by population and can be negatively affected by disease and poor nutrition.

Subadult age estimation is inextricably linked to the study of growth; thus research on the subject can be found in both the anthropological[1] and clinical literature.[2] The focus tends toward testing and updating age indicators. Saunders and colleagues (1992), for example, demonstrate that techniques such as those developed by Moorrees, Fanning, and Hunt (1963) and Anderson, Thompson, and Popovich (1976) can successfully be employed to estimate the age of individual juvenile skeletons, as well as to produce reliable age distributions for skeletal samples. Similarly, Crowder and Austin (2005) provide a systematic examination of epiphyseal union of the distal tibia and fibula in an effort to modernize and standardize these indicators.

Chronological versus Physiological Age and Statistical Solutions

Estimating the age of adult skeletons is based on bone remodeling and degenerative changes that result from complex interactions between mechanical stress, health, nutrition, and time. The challenge in developing a technique to estimate adult skeletal age is to identify and quantify the pattern, sequence, and rate of age-related changes, while allowing for the contributions of genetics and lifestyle that influence each person's aging process (İşcan and Loth 1989). Some researchers have argued that all skeletal age indicators are inherently unreliable owing to poor correlation between physiological and chronological age (Bocquet-Appel and Masset 1982; Jackes 2000). Jackes (2000) suggests that age may account for as little as 30% of the total amount of morphological variability observed on joint surfaces.

Traditional attempts to associate bone change with senescence use regression analysis to identify the best age-associated trend in the data, from which age-at-death ranges are produced (Aykroyd et al. 1997). This process results in techniques of skeletal age estimation that are moderately successful when applied to individuals but that demonstrate systematic bias when tested on large samples; under-aging older individuals and over-aging younger individuals, with the transition occurring at approximately 40–50 years of age (Aykroyd et al. 1997). (For examples of test results see Murray and Murray [1991], Saunders and associates [1992], and Bedford and colleagues [1993].) Similar results have been reported for some dental techniques (Solheim and Sundnes 1980). Applying these age indicators to archaeological populations in paleodemographic analyses produces age profiles that overtly mimic the reference sample (Bocquet-Appel and Masset 1982; Hoppa and Vaupel 2002; Jackes 1985, 1992, 2000), prompting several authors to recognize age estimation as "one of the most thorny problems facing human osteoarchaeology" (Mays 1998: 50).

Various solutions to these dilemmas have been sought by bioarchaeologists and forensic anthropologists. To increase accuracy, most methods have been extensively tested, and several modifications have been proposed. Methods include assessment of

- pubic symphyses,
- auricular surface,
- cranial sutures,
- rib morphology, and
- dental techniques.

To reduce the bias toward the middle caused by regression analysis, alternate approaches to data processing, such as Bayesian prediction using prior probabilities and classical correlation, are recommended (Aykroyd et al. 1997; Hoppa and Vaupel 2002; Lucy et al. 1996). Both the pubic symphysis and auricular surface have been re-evaluated using a Bayesian approach, producing results that are reliable, unbiased, and useful on individuals over 50 years of age (Hoppa and Vaupel 2002; Schmitt et al. 2002).

Combining Information from Multiple Age Indicators

Todd (1920) recommended the use of more than one indicator to assess age. His advice has been repeated over the decades as a solution to the problems of inaccuracy and bias that can result from the use of individual indicators (Brooks 1955; Lovejoy et al. 1985a). Yet McKern's (1957) analysis of the pubic symphysis, epiphyseal union, and cranial sutures reveals that random pooling of observations produces variable results, not all of them successful. Few physical anthropologists would argue the importance of evaluating all age-related criteria and combining the results in a biologically meaningful manner. Unfortunately, no common standardization, calibration, or evaluation procedures currently exist (Ritz-Timme et al. 2000), leaving the issue of combining indicators open to debate.

Gustafson's technique (1950), which scores six variables of a longitudinally sectioned tooth, was the first to combine age criteria. Several ensuing improvements were made, after testing and recalculation of Gustafson's data revealed errors in his analysis (Rösing and Kvaal 1999). Lamendin and colleagues (1992) introduced a nondestructive method using tooth translucency and periodontosis, eliminating the need for tooth sectioning. Subsequent tests on modern populations have produced results equal or superior to skeletal techniques of age estimation (Prince and Ubelaker 2002).

Acsádi and Nemeskéri (1970) proposed the "Complex Method" of combining age indicators (recommended by the Workshop of European Anthropologists 1980). Their approach utilizes four indicators: endocranial sutures, proximal humerus trabecular involution (increased marrow space at the expense of trabecular bone), proximal femur trabecular involution, and the pubic symphysis. Observers using the Complex Method must assess the pubic symphysis to determine if the individual was younger or older than 50 years. If younger, the lower limit of the age range for each indicator is selected; if approximately 50 years of age, the mean of each range is used; and if older, the upper limit of the range is selected. The resultant values are then averaged. According to Acsádi and Nemeskéri (1970), the complex method produces age assessments that are 80% to 85% accurate with a ±2.5-year margin of error.

Lovejoy and colleagues (1985a) use seriation to refine age estimates and systematically combine the results of age indicators using the multifactorial approach to produce a summary age. Their study includes the pubic symphysis (Todd's method and the authors' revisions of Todd), auricular surface, proximal femur trabecular involution, cranial sutures, and dental wear. In the multifactorial approach, all indicators are applied separately to a population, and the results are used to create an intercorrelation matrix. Principal components analysis determines the correlation of each age indicator to the first factor (assumed to represent chronological age). The correlation is the indicator's weight, with the final age of an individual determined as the weighted average of all indicators available for that specimen (Lovejoy et al. 1985a).

The authors report success with the multifactorial approach (all ages normalized inaccuracy was 7.5 and bias -5.4), as do Bedford and colleagues (1993), who used it to combine the results of four age indicators: pubic symphysis, auricular surface, proximal femur trabecular involution, and radiographic analysis of the clavicle. They conclude the multifactorial approach is superior to any single indicator. In contrast, Saunders and colleagues (1992) found that summary age essentially averaged the results they obtained from analyses of the auricular surface, sternal rib end, ectocranial sutures, and pubic symphyses. The complexity of the multifactorial approach and its failure to demonstrate an improvement over averaged results prompted Saunders and associates (1992) to conclude there was no compelling reason to use the multifactorial approach. Applying the multifactorial approach in a forensic context is problematic unless the observer uses the same indicators as Lovejoy and associates (1985a), because weightings for each indicator are derived from population data. When examining a single skeleton, a forensic anthropologist is limited to using published weightings (ibid.), which may not be appropriate given the population variability observed in several age indicators, for example, pubic symphysis (Katz and Suchey 1989). Factor analysis is most effective when weightings are calculated using the population from which the unknown remains originate (Saunders et al. 1992).

Baccino and colleagues (1999) examined the accuracy of the Suchey-Brooks pubic symphysis technique, the sternal end of the 4th rib, the Lamendin dental method, and histology of the femur, individually and in combination. They considered three means of combining data: (1) averaging the results of the four techniques; (2) a two-step procedure whereby the Suchey-Brooks age is used if the symphysis scores in one of the first three phases, and the Lamendin age is used if the pubis is in one of the later Suchey-Brooks phases; and (3) a "global" approach taking all results into

consideration and drawing on the experience of the observer. The study produced single-year age estimates to facilitate comparisons, and the results demonstrated that all three combined methods produced better age estimates than did any single method. Of the three comprehensive approaches, averaging was the least successful. Saunders and colleagues (1992) and Brooks and Suchey (1990) agree that indiscriminant averaging is not a useful approach to estimating skeletal age. According to Saunders and associates (1992), there are no shortcuts in age estimation. Combining information from several techniques involves: (1) evaluating the accuracy, range, and applicability of each method; (2) selecting the most appropriate method based on sex, population, and preservation; and (3) using the overlapping areas of the resulting age phases to identify the most likely age range, given the limitation of the techniques.

Aiello and Molleson (1993) recommend the use of general indicators (for example, epiphyseal union, joint wear, porosity, osteophytic development) or histology to determine an approximate age category, or relative age of a skeleton. Once relative age is established, the most effective techniques for that stage of senescence can be applied, such as McKern and Stewart (1957) for young adults or the pubic symphysis method of Acsádi and Nemeskéri (1970) for older adults. The latest solution is to use Bayešian statistics.[8] Clearly, there is no accepted protocol for devising a skeletal age assessment from multiple indicators; even textbook explanations vary considerably (Buikstra and Ubelaker 1994; Byers 2005; Schwartz 1995; Ubelaker 1999; White 2000).

Less controversy surrounds subadult age estimation. As White observes, "all osteologists use dental development, eruption, epiphyseal appearance, and fusion when aging immature skeletal material" (2000: 361). Nevertheless, Pfau (1991) examined the relationships among dental development, diaphyseal length, epiphyseal closure, and age-at-death, specifically examining sex and population variation, to determine the validity of combining results obtained from these variables. He concluded that dental and long-bone development are independent phenomena. The three variables are separately useful as age indicators and are complementary when combined. He has created a tripartite graph that may be used to predict chronological age from these traits (reproduced in Bass 1995). Although he recommends the use of both dental and long-bone development to assess age, he does not specify how to combine results. Based on a comprehensive examination of subadult dental age estimation, Liversidge and colleagues (1998) recommend using as many teeth as possible and calculating a mean value from the individual results.

Admissibility in Court

There is no definitive way to produce an age estimate. In a forensic context, the determining factor must always be how well the analysis will stand up in court. It must be admissible, accurate, and logical. If not, opposing counsel will attempt to have the evidence rendered inadmissible or will encourage the jury to disregard the testimony by implying that the techniques are unreliable, not generally accepted, or illogically applied. Although a forensic anthropologist may not be subpoenaed to testify strictly about the age of a skeleton, his/her report will be a matter of record and will be open to review. Poorly implemented techniques, assumptions, and contradictory or illogical summaries can be used to discredit other aspects of the analysis, some of which may be crucial to the case.

Judges use several criteria to rule on the admissibility of expert testimony, including general acceptance of the technique. In the United States, the *Daubert* factors (*United States Supreme Court in Daubert v. Merrell Dow Pharmaceuticals* 1993) provide additional guidelines for judges to consider: (1) expert testimony must be based on reliable principles and methods; (2) the theory or technique in question must have been subjected to peer review and publication; and (3) the potential or known error rates of the technique, as well as the standards controlling the operation of the technique. The research that provides the basis for the testimony must be conducted independent of the litigation and should not be undertaken expressly for the purposes of the trial (Giannelli and Imwinkelried 1999). The Canadian legal system has found these criteria useful (Rogers and Allard 2004), and similar requirements exist in other jurisdictions (Ritz-Timme et al. 2000).

Statistical means of combining age indicators provide a mathematically sound approach that is defensible, if not entirely comprehensible, to a jury. Jury comprehension of expert testimony is as important to a trial as the testimony itself. If jury members cannot understand the nature of the evidence, they will disregard it and its significance entirely (Ayd and Troeger 1999). Keeping in mind that the average jury member has a high school education, forensic anthropologists must be able to explain why and how the final age estimation was established in a manner that is clear and engaging (Ayd and Troeger 1999). Each forensic anthropologist must decide how she/he is most comfortable conveying and defending the science and conclusions of the analysis.

Major Historical Developments

İşcan and Loth (1989), İşcan (1989), Katzenberg and Saunders (2000), and Kemkes-Grottenthaler (2002), among others, provide excellent historical reviews of the development of skeletal age indicators. My concern here is with the paradigm shifts responsible for key advances in the study of age-at-death assessment of the human skeleton.

The history of skeletal age estimation mirrors theoretical developments in physical anthropology. From 1900 to 1939, the prevailing approach to research in physical anthropology was historical-descriptive and typology-driven, seeking to understand culture history and the history of human races (Armelagos and Van Gerven 2003). Although both qualitative and quantitative methods were utilized, the literature from this period consists largely of non-analytical anatomical studies (Lovejoy, Mensforth, and Armelagos 1982). Armelagos and Van Gerven (2003) define analytical analyses as those that (1) propose and test specific hypotheses; (2) address issues of process or function; or (3) attempt to place analyses into a broader theoretical context. Descriptive publications discuss sorting methods, or identification without placing results into a broader context or anatomical description (see Ubelaker this volume).

Todd (1920), who as an anatomist, laid the foundation for systematic analysis of skeletal age indicators with his groundbreaking study of the pubic symphysis (İşcan and Loth 1989), followed shortly afterward by an examination of cranial sutures (Todd and Lyon, Jr., 1924, 1925a, 1925b, 1925c). Although his analysis of the pubic symphysis is descriptive in its formulation of age phases, Todd (1920) situated his analysis within the larger context of growth and development of the pubic bone and the potential for variation in growth rates/patterns in different ancestral groups. Taking a functional approach, his goal was to understand the nature of pubic symphyseal modification to better appreciate the applicability and limits of his newly proposed technique of age estimation. The result is a 10-phase system of evaluating age-related morphological changes of the pubic symphysis, and proof that such modifications are not growth related. Unfortunately, in defining developmental phases and corresponding age ranges, Todd based his descriptions on what he considered normal variation. Divergent symphyseal faces were deemed "anomalous" and were eliminated from his sample

(Todd 1920). By artificially truncating the range of variability observed for each age, Todd introduced a bias into his technique that was not fully understood for more than 60 years (Meindl et al. 1985).

The prevailing descriptive paradigm prevented a critical examination of the nature of skeletal age indicators for almost 30 years (İşcan and Loth 1989). Physical anthropology embraced this new tool in the belief that age is correlated with skeletal changes in a predictable manner that is uniform across time and space, despite Todd's recognition of individual and population variability. In 1951 Sherwood Washburn introduced "The New Physical Anthropology," emphasizing evolutionary processes and mechanisms, and arguing for a dynamic analysis of functional anatomy, in place of static descriptions. Process, theory formulation, and hypothesis testing were all part of the equation (Armelagos and Van Gerven 2003). Shortly afterward, physical anthropology saw many of its assumptions questioned. The study of skeletal age estimation was no exception.

By the 1950s, physical anthropologists had identified a perplexing trend in their skeletally based demographic data but were at a loss to explain it. Few archaeological populations exhibited mean ages of death over 30 years of age (Brooks 1955). Finally acknowledging a potential problem with their two primary age indicators, the pubic symphysis and cranial sutures, physical anthropologists embarked on a testing and revision spree that lasted more than 40 years. Brooks, encouraged by the "dynamic approach now introduced into anthropometrical analyses" (Brooks 1955: 567), initiated the process with two questions: (1) can age estimation methods be applied to populations other than the test sample; and (2) how well do the pubic symphysis and cranial suture techniques correlate to each other? Her conclusions would not be out of place in the literature of the 1980s; the pubic symphysis has a statistically significant correlation with known age, although it has a tendency to underage older individuals, whereas cranial sutures are poorly correlated with age. McKern and Stewart (1957: 72), concerned with the "static" nature of Todd's (1920) technique, introduced a new method of evaluating the pubic symphysis based on component scoring. Emphasis was on process and a means of recognizing and incorporating variation.

During the 1960s and 1970s, a functional approach to the skeleton began to emerge, and skeletal population studies and multivariate statistical analyses were common (Armelagos and Van Gerven 2003). Physical anthropology became data driven, rather than problem directed, as

exemplified by research produced during the 1970s (Armelagos and Van Gerven 2003). The lack of predominantly theoretical papers was a glaring omission in the pages of the *American Journal of Physical Anthropology*. The creation of a Forensic Anthropology section of the Academy of Forensic Sciences in 1972 marked the beginning of modern forensic anthropology, and both the role and the scope of forensic anthropology began to change (İşcan 1988; Ubelaker this volume). The need for more exact methods of skeletal age estimation increased as forensic anthropologists became more active in casework. Although Bouquet-Appel and Masset did not bid farewell to paleodemography until 1982, physical anthropologists were accumulating sufficient evidence to recognize problems with the raw data of demographic analysis, in particular, age estimation. The belief in a single method applicable through time and across space was beginning to fade (Workshop of European Anthropologists 1980). As Stojanowski and Buikstra (2005) observe, there is value in descriptive research. The accumulation of raw data for synthesis and validation studies can lead to a complete re-evaluation of current thought and, ultimately, a paradigm shift.

In 1977 Buikstra coined the term *bioarchaeology*, introducing a holistic approach to the study of past populations. According to Armelagos and Van Gerven (2003), bioarchaeology incorporates three primary features. It (1) takes a population perspective, (2) views culture as a force both affecting and interacting with bioadaptation, and (3) provides a method for testing hypotheses involving interaction between the biological and the cultural elements of adaptation. Three themes linked to the comprehensive approach of bioarchaeology began to emerge in the literature of age estimation: (1) testing/triangulating data; (2) phase (holistic) versus component analysis of age criteria; and (3) population variation.

Triangulating data from several sources was the cornerstone of a pivotal series of articles published by Lovejoy, Meindl, Mensforth, and colleagues in 1985 (Lovejoy et al. 1985a, 1985b; Meindl and Lovejoy 1985; Mensforth and Lovejoy 1985; Walker and Lovejoy 1985). The authors advocate a systematic, objective means of combining information from several age indicators, blind testing of techniques, and a more informative method of expressing the relationship between chronological and skeletal age that states the degree and direction of bias (inaccuracy and bias, respectively). Their work, and the critiques of Bocquet-Appel and Masset (1982), ushered in the statistical revolution that marked skeletal age-estimation research of the 1990s. The continued efforts of Meindl and colleagues have been a motivating force in changing attitudes toward adult age estimation (Jackes 2000).

This team also introduced the auricular surface method of age assessment, which explicitly recognizes the superiority of some features over others and reopened the question of how best to score age indicators. Kemkes-Grottenthaler (2002) describes two systems of scoring: phase and component. The author recognizes three: phase, component, and revised phase or holistic—based on their manner of coping with atypical individuals. The earliest methods were phase analysis (Todd 1920), consisting of descriptions that corresponded to particular age ranges. The phase system was criticized for its inability to include individuals who do not fit phase descriptions. Condemning the static nature of the phase system, McKern and Stewart (1957) introduced component analysis of pubic symphseal age assessment, which also formed the basis of the later female standards (Gilbert and McKern 1973). Component systems focus the observer's attention on particular details that are scored progressively. Each stage of a feature is given a number. Features are examined independently with the resultant stage scores for each feature added together to produce a final value that equates to a particular age range. Component scoring is not dependent on archetypes, making it possible to evaluate atypical individuals. In 1990, Suchey and Brooks introduced an alternative version of the phase system that is flexible and holistic in its application. Along with descriptions, observers utilize casts depicting early and late stages of each phase. Users are guided to seek patterns, with the casts explicitly demonstrating the dynamic range of possibilities for each phase. By observing the trajectory of change that occurs within a phase, the observer is able to assign atypical individuals appropriately.

Proponents of component scoring argue that it is a flexible alternative to phases that permits correct age assessment of "atypical" individuals (Gilbert and McKern 1973; McKern and Stewart 1957). Components capture the changes inherent to complex biological structures better than phases and facilitate statistical analyses do (Boldsen et al. 2002). Those opposing component scoring are concerned about interobserver error and complexity of application, particularly in the field (İşcan, Loth, and Wright 1984; Suchey 1979; Suchey, Wiseley, and Katz 1986). Advocates of a holistic approach stress the importance of patterns in revealing true age, simplifying methodology, and reducing interobserver error (Suchey and Brooks 1990; Suchey, Wiseley, and Katz 1986).

Kemkes-Grottenthaler (2002) suggests the modal phase, or holistic approach, may conform best to the human neurobiological basis of object recognition, which includes feature extraction, solving correspondence problems, and comparison to a reference.

Acknowledging the role of intra- and interpopulation variation was another hallmark of 1980s' skeletal age research. Although Todd observed differences between male and female pubic symphyses and noted the rate of metamorphosis varied among populations, he did not consider the distinctions to be significant (İşcan and Loth 1989). He did, however, produce separate sex- and population-based methods for the cranial sutures. By the 1950s, the need for distinct male and female pubic symphseal age criteria was apparent (Stewart 1957). Gilbert and McKern (1973) offered a solution, but problems quickly became evident (Suchey 1979). Tactics for coping with inter- and intrapopulation variation fell into two camps: (1) establish separate methods for each sex and population; or (2) devise a technique that is not sex or population dependent, either because of its nature or by using a sufficiently diverse sample.

Age indicators have not been examined in the same fashion by the same people, and the results are often contradictory. It appears there are significant sex differences in the aging process, making it necessary to devise independent scoring criteria and age indicator stages for most regions of the skeleton (Igarashi et al. 2005; İşcan, Loth, and Wright 1984, 1985; Katz and Suchey 1986; Todd and Lyon, Jr., 1925a, 1925b, 1925c). A few techniques are not sex specific (Kunos et al. 1999; Lamendin et al. 1992), and some bones demonstrate sex differences depending on how they are scored (Buckberry and Chamberlain 2002; Igarashi et al. 2005; Lovejoy et al. 1985b).

Population differences are less well understood. Sample limitations and lack of funding to travel make it difficult for a single researcher to conduct comparative studies of collections worldwide. Instead, techniques are proposed by one research group and are independently tested on other populations by different teams of investigators, often incorporating slight modifications. Although independent blind testing is desirable, a coherent program of research devoted to the analysis of population differences would make it easier to tease out the variables that are contributing to these mixed results. Suchey and colleagues are among the few who have been able to examine a diverse sample. They found it necessary to produce separate casts and descriptions for males and females, but addressed population differences by using slightly altered phase values for each ancestral group (Katz and Suchey 1989). The dearth of large-scale population studies begs the question: is it merely rate of change that differs, as indicated by Katz and Suchey (1989), or are there detectable differences in the pattern of aging?

Research in the 1980s demonstrated the variable nature of aging. Bone loss with age is highly site specific, each bone behaving as an individual organ (Walker and Lovejoy 1985). Radiographic analysis demonstrated differences in adjacent anatomical sites (for example, humerus and clavicle), differences unassociated with locomotor habits or activity levels (for instance, femur and calcaneus exhibited different patterns of change), and sex-specific differences between individual bones (Walker and Lovejoy 1985). Skeletal aging was shown to occur at different rates in different populations (Katz and Suchey 1989). The link between skeletal metamorphosis and years lived became more tenuous as factors such as health, mechanical wear, and nutrition assumed a predominant role.

Current Trends

Throughout the 1980s, Meindl, Lovejoy, and colleagues laid the foundation for a change in approach to skeletal age estimation, initiating research to address the problem from several perspectives. Suchey and colleagues were at the forefront of change, introducing 95% confidence intervals to age ranges (Brooks and Suchey 1990; Katz and Suchey 1986, 1989), anticipating future developments in forensic science that initiated a re-evaluation of best practice policy in the United States following the *Daubert* ruling on the admissibility of expert testimony in 1993 (*United States Supreme Court in Daubert v. Merrell Dow Pharmaceuticals* 1993).

On reviewing the state of age estimation in 1999, Ritz-Timme and colleagues made an explicit demand for accurate and precise techniques of age estimation to meet the requirements of forensic practice. They insisted that to qualify for use in forensic practice, techniques should be (1) transparent, provable, and published in a peer-reviewed journal; (2) tested using appropriate statistical procedures; (3) sufficiently accurate to fulfill the demands of a single case, meaning that 95% ranges must be considered; and (4) in cases of age estimation of living individuals, practitioners must abide by medical ethics and legal regulations (Ritz-Timme et al. 2000). Ritz-Timme and colleagues (2000) advocate the use of dental methods, bone histology, and multifactorial methods for all

adult ages. Pubic symphyseal techniques and rib morphology are recommended for use on adults under 40 years of age to achieve precise estimates. Their conclusions foreshadow a recent effort on the part of forensic anthropologists to improve and standardize their science in accordance with medico-legal requirements (Christensen 2005; Rogers 2005; Rogers and Allard 2004).

The 1990s saw a shift toward increased involvement of forensic anthropology in casework, teaching, publication, and research. Greater emphasis on the forensic aspects of forensic anthropology—in particular, admissibility—has fostered increased testing of existing indicators, the use of innovative technology to capture data—for example, 3-dimensional imaging and computed tomography (CT) scanning (Pasquier et al. 1999)—and validation of results, including Bayesian statistics (Lucy et al. 1996). A similar need for standardization in the subfield of paleodemography resulted in the "Rostock Manifesto," an outline of paleodemography's goals and expectations with respect to skeletal age. Two of the key concerns were to develop and validate age indicator stages through improved osteological methods, better reference samples, and the use of Bayesian statistics (Hoppa and Vaupel 2002). Although the need to improve skeletal age estimation was initiated in response to issues particular to each subfield, the resultant theoretical and practical convergence benefits both forensic anthropology and paleodemography.

Future Directions and New Interpretive Paradigms

According to İşcan and Loth (1989), the study of age-at-death estimation suffers from two primary oversights: (1) the inability of researchers to recognize that individual bones are part of a larger functional system; and (2) specialization leading to a methodological division among morphological, histological, and radiological techniques. They suggest future research focus on age-related changes in different parts of a single skeleton using a combination of analytical techniques (İşcan and Loth 1989). The goal is to develop better methods of age estimation by identifying (1) regions of the skeleton that best reflect chronological age and (2) approaches capable of capturing age-related changes in a meaningful manner. They recommend establishing modern skeletal collections of documented age, sex, and ancestry in order to clarify the biological and cultural factors influencing the aging process (İşcan and Loth 1989).

A review of the literature since 1989 reveals some progress in fulfilling İşcan and Loth's recommendations, but the tendency toward overspecialization continues to plague age estimation. Progress has not been uniformly achieved. Functional approaches that address biomechanical concerns (Stout 1996) and developmental processes (FitzGerald 1998; Ohtani and Yamamoto 1991) are more frequently incorporated into histological and dental techniques of age estimation than traditional skeletal morphology. Functional analyses of skeletal age indictors, such as cranial sutures (Hershkovitz et al. 1997) and cortical bone loss (Mensforth and Lovejoy 1985), are overshadowed by tests and revisions of existing methods. Emphasis is on improving existing criteria rather than on examining new sites and developing novel indicators.

Large-scale testing has produced innovative approaches to data analysis (Hoppa and Vaupel 2002). Attempts to resolve the "attraction to the middle" bias have revitalized efforts to assimilate age criteria from different skeletal elements. Combining indicators is becoming common practice, but specialization has limited the nature of those combinations. There are collective dental analyses (Gustafsen 1950; Lamendin et al. 1992), techniques that blend skeletal morphology (Hoppa and Vaupel 2002; Schmitt et al. 2002), and those that amalgamate histological characteristics (Thomas et al. 2000). Research that integrates dental, skeletal, radiological, and histological indicators, or combinations thereof, are less common (Kunos et al. 1999; Lovejoy et al. 1985a).

Subspecialization has divided the focus of physical anthropology along methodological lines (histology, gross morphology, biochemistry, radiology and other imaging technologies) and created anatomical divisions in the literature (skeletal versus dental). Each specialization has addressed age assessment of human remains within the framework of their larger concerns, but together they are only loosely integrated. Dental anthropology incorporates many of the fields outside clinical dentistry that are involved with odontological questions (Alt, Rösing, and Teschler-Nicola 1998). Similar concerns of intra- and interpopulation variation, accuracy, bias, and consolidating evidence from several age criteria have been addressed by dental anthropologists, but differences in the development and wear/degeneration between teeth and bones seem to encourage specialization in one or the other, producing a distinct body of literature (Alt, Rösing, and Teschler-Nicola 1998; Smith 1991). Depending on the cost, availability, and applicability of the methodology, new modalities and technologies may become part of the mainstream literature—for example, radiology—or produce their own specialized research interests—for instance, histology.

Armelagos and Van Gervan (2003) mourn the failure of the "New Physical Anthropology" to take hold in osteology. They question the relevance of applying innovative methods to old questions. Similarly, Buikstra and colleagues (2003) caution that advanced methods of analysis are "far outstripping our ability to generate contextually sensitive research designs in which to ground anthropologically significant questions," and they express a concern that forensic anthropology and bioarchaeology are becoming so specialized they are losing relevance to anthropology as a whole. The strength of anthropology, they argue, is in its broad perspective on humankind. Anthropology will benefit from a shared discourse on issues of concern to all subdisciplines (for example, warfare [Buikstra, King, and Nystrom 2003]). The special knowledge required to master new technology and analytical approaches encourages researchers to limit themselves to histological, morphological, biochemical, or diagnostic imaging when age is seen as a means to an end—that is, understanding evolution, ontogeny, past populations, or identification. It is only by viewing the process of aging as an end in itself, that a fully integrated approach to skeletal aging will be developed and the best methods of assessing the age of human remains will be defined. Engaging in a dialogue on the functional correlates of aging and the manner in which senescence is experienced by the individual and the population through time and cross-culturally offers an additional forum for integrating anthropological thought.

Conclusion

The historical-descriptive approach of early anthropology engendered descriptive anatomical analyses that produced static techniques of assessing skeletal age (Todd 1920; Todd and Lyon 1925a, 1925b, 1925c). The dependence on a single criterion for age estimation was established prior to Todd and continued for the next 30 years (Brooks 1955). Following the inception of the "New Physical Anthropology" (Washburn 1951) with its emphasis on function, theory, and processual methodology, independent testing of age indicators became commonplace (Brooks 1955; Hanihara 1952). Newly introduced techniques emphasized variability, scored through a dynamic component analysis of each feature (Gilbert and McKern 1973; McKern and Stewart 1957). Analytical approaches, such as bioarchaeology, combined with Bouquet-Appel and Masset's

(1982) critique of paleodemography and its raw data, prompted physical anthropologists to look at age estimation in a new light. A new era of critical analysis, with an emphasis on populations, testing/triangulating data, and a broader theoretical perspective introduced the faint glimmer of a functional approach to skeletal age assessment.

Understanding the physiology of aging is essential to devising meaningful skeletal age indicators. Examination of large skeletal samples revealed the non-linear nature of aging, with its significant inter-bone (Walker and Lovejoy 1985), sex specific (Katz and Suchey 1986; Suchey 1979), and inter-population variability (İşcan et al. 1984, 1985; Katz and Suchey 1989). Biomechanical factors did not become an explicit consideration in the literature of skeletal age estimation until histomorphometric analyses began to receive greater attention (Stout 1986, 1989; see also Crowder, this volume). Previous researchers had examined sites other than the traditional pubic symphysis, and cranial sutures, but did so in an effort to increase the number of available age indicators (Acsádi and Nemeskéri 1970; İşcan et al. 1984, 1985), for reasons of preservation (Lovejoy et al. 1985b), and to develop methods capable of assessing older adults (İşcan et al. 1984, 1985; Lovejoy et al. 1985a, 1985b).

The 1990s to the present day have seen a greater emphasis on validation studies relating to admissibility issues in forensic anthropology, which incorporate Bayesian statistics introduced by paleodemography. New technologies, such as 3-D imaging and micro CT scans, are becoming commonplace in an effort to refine and potentially replace traditional methods of skeletal age estimation. The problems inherent to skeletal age assessment have turned some researchers toward dental age estimation, including macroscopic techniques (e.g., Lamendin et al. 1992), examination of enamel microstructure (FitzGerald 1998), cementum annulation (Wittwer-Backofen, Gampe, and Vaupel 2004), and amino acid racemization in dentin (Ohtani and Yamamoto 1991).

Physical anthropology, in particular paleodemography and forensic anthropology, has made valuable contributions to our understanding of skeletal aging and age evaluation, addressing significant methodological and theoretical concerns relating to various themes: subadult versus adult aging and age estimation; chronological versus physiological age, including intra- and interpopulation variability; statistical analysis; and scoring and combining age indicators. Although age estimates are ultimately put to different purposes in paleodemography than in forensic anthropology,

and the level of analysis—that is, population versus individual—often differs, we share the goals of increased accuracy, reliability, and reduced bias in skeletal age assessment. Improving the validity of our techniques produces more realistic representations of past populations and defensible biological profiles of modern human remains.

Notes

1. Black and Scheuer 1996; Hoppa and FitzGerald 1999; Johnston and Zimmer 1989; Lampl and Johnston 1996; Saunders 2000; Smith 1991.

2. Deutsch, Tam, and Stach 1985; Greulich and Pyle 1959; Maresh 1955; Moorrees, Fanning, and Hunt 1963.

3. Acsádi and Nemeskéri 1970; Brooks 1955; Brooks and Suchey 1990; Gilbert and McKern 1973; Hanihara and Suzuki 1978; Katz and Suchey 1986; Kemkes-Grottenthaler 1996; McKern and Stewart 1957; Meindl et al. 1985; Pasquier et al. 1999; Saunders et al. 1992; Schmitt et al. 2002; Suchey 1979; Suchey, Wiseley, and Katz 1986; Workshop of European Anthropologists 1980.

4. Bedford et al. 1993; Buckberry and Chamberlain 2002; Igarashi et al. 2005; Lovejoy et al. 1985a; Murray and Murray 1991; Saunders et al. 1992; Schmitt et al. 2002.

5. Brooks 1955; Mann et al. 1991; Masset 1989; McKern and Stewart 1957; Meindl and Lovejoy 1985; Singer 1953; Todd and Lyon, Jr., 1924, 1925a, 1925b, 1925c.

6. Dudar 1993; İşcan et al. 1984, 1985; Kunos et al. 1999; Kurki 2005; Loth, İşcan, and Scheuerman 1994; Russell et al. 1993; Yoder, Ubelaker, and Powell 2001.

7. FitzGerald 1998; Gustafson 1950; Kim, Kho, and Lee 2000; Lamendin et al. 1992; Ohtani and Yamamoto 1991; Rösing and Kvaal 1999; Walker, Dean, and Shapiro 1991.

8. Hoppa and Vaupel (2002) for explanations and examples.

References

Acsádi, G., and Nemeskéri, J. 1970. *History of the Human Lifespan and Mortality*. Budapest: Akadémiai Kiadó.

Aiello, L. C., and Molleson, T. 1993. Are microscopic ageing techniques more accurate than macroscopic ageing techniques? *Journal of Archaeological Science* 20: 689–704.

Alt, K. W., Rösing, F. W., and Teschler-Nicola, M. 1998. *Dental Anthropology*. New York: Springer.

Anderson, D. L., Thompson, G. W., and Popovich, F. 1976. Age of attainment of mineralization stages of the permanent dentition. *Journal of Forensic Sciences* 21: 191–200.

Armelagos, G. J., and Van Gerven, D. P. 2003. A century of skeletal biology and paleopathology: Contrasts, contradictions, and conflicts. *American Anthropologist* 105(1): 53–64.

Ayd, P. M., and Troeger, M. M. 1999. Are jurors smart enough to understand scientific evidence?, in C. Meyer (ed.), *Expert Witnessing: Explaining and Understanding Science*, pp. 31–32. New York: CRC Press.

Aykroyd, R. G., Ludy, D., Pollard, A. M., and Solheim, T. 1997. Technical note: Regression analysis in adult age estimation. *American Journal of Physical Anthropology* 104: 259–265.

Baccino, E., Ubelaker, D. H., Hayek, L. C., and Zerilli, A. 1999. Evaluation of seven methods of estimating age at death from mature human skeletal remains. *Journal of Forensic Sciences* 44: 931–936.

Bass, W. M. 1995. *Human Osteology*. Columbia: Missouri Archaeological Society.

Bedford, M. E., Russell, K. F., Lovejoy, C. O., Meindl, R. S., Simpson, S. W., and Stuart-Macadam, P. L. 1993. A test of the multifactorial aging method using skeletons with known ages at death from the Grant Collection. *American Journal of Physical Anthropology* 91: 287–297.

Black, S., and Scheuer, L. 1996. Age changes in the clavicle: from the early neonatal period to skeletal maturity. *International Journal of Osteoarchaeology* 6: 425–434.

Boldsen, J. L., Milner, G. R., Konigsberg, L. W., and Wood, J. W. 2002. Transitional analysis: A new method for estimating age from skeletons, in R. D. Hoppa and J. W. Vaupel (eds.), *Paleodemography*, pp. 73–106. Cambridge: Cambridge University Press.

Bouquet-Appel, J-P., and Masset, C. 1982. Farewell to paleodemography. *Journal of Human Evolution* 11: 321–333.

Brooks, S. T. 1955. Skeletal age at death: The reliability of cranial and pubic age indicators. *American Journal of Physical Anthropology* 13: 567–597.

Brooks, S. T., and Suchey, J. M. 1990. Skeletal age determination based on the os pubis: A comparison of the Acsádi-Nemeskéri and Suchey-Brooks methods. *Human Evolution* 5: 227–238.

Buckberry, J. L., and Chamberlain, A. T. 2002. Age estimation from the auricular surface of the ilium: A revised method. *American Journal of Physical Anthropology* 119: 231–239.

Buikstra, J. E. 1977. Biocultural dimensions of archaeological study: A regional perspective, in R. L. Blakley (ed.), *Biocultural Adaptation in Prehistoric America*, pp. 67–84. Athens: University of Georgia Press.

Buikstra, J. E., King, J. L., and Nystrom, K. C. 2003. Forensic anthropology and bioarchaeology in the American Anthropologist: Rare by exquisite gems. *American Anthropologist* 105(1): 38–52.

Buikstra, J. E., and Ubelaker, D. H. 1994. *Standards for Data Collection from Human Skeletal Remains*. Fayetteville, AS: Archaeological Survey Research Series No. 44.

Byers, S. N. 2005. *Introduction to Forensic Anthropology*. New York: Pearson.

Christensen, A. M. 2005. Testing the reliability of frontal sinuses in positive identification. *Journal of Forensic Sciences* 50: 18–22.

Cox, M., and Mays, S. 2000. *Human Osteology in Archaeology and Forensic Science*. London: Greenwich Medical Media.

Crowder, C., and Austin, D. 2005. Age ranges of epiphyseal fusion in the distal tibia and fibula of contemporary males and females. *Journal of Forensic Sciences* 50: 1001–1007.

Demirjian, A. 1986. Dentition, in F. Falkner and J. M. Tanner (eds.), *Human Growth*, pp. 269–298. New York: Plenum.

Deutsch, D., Tam, O., and Stach, M. V. 1985. Postnatal changes in size, morphology and weight of developing postnatal deciduous anterior teeth. *Growth* 49: 202–217.

Dudar, J. C. 1993. Identification of rib number and assessment of intercostal variation at the sternal rib end. *Journal of Forensic Sciences* 38: 788–797.

Fazekas, I. G., and Kósa, F. 1978. *Forensic Fetal Osteology*. Budapest: Akadémiai Kiadó.

FitzGerald, C. M. 1998. Do enamel microstructures have regular time dependency? Conclusions from the literature and a large-scale study. *Journal of Human Evolution* 35: 371–386.

Giannelli, P., and Imwinkelried, E. J. 1999. *Scientific Evidence* (3rd ed.). Charlottesville, VA: Lexis Law Publishing.

Gilbert, B. M., and McKern, T. W. 1973. A method for aging the female os pubis. *American Journal of Physical Anthropology* 38: 31–38.

Greulich, W. W., and Pyle, S. I. 1959. *Radiographic Atlas of Skeletal Development of the Hand and Wrist* (2nd ed.). Palo Alto, CA: Stanford University Press.

Gustafson, G. 1950. Age determination on teeth. *Journal of the American Dental Association* 41: 45–54.

Hanihara, K. 1952. On the age changes in the male Japanese pubic bone. *Journal of the Anthropological Society of Nippon* 62: 245–260.

Hanihara, K., and Suzuki, T. 1978. Estimation of age from the pubic symphysis by means of multiple regression analysis. *American Journal of Physical Anthropology* 48: 233–240.

Hershkovitz, I., Latimer, B., Dutour, O., Jellema, L. M., Wish-Baratz, S., Rothschild, C., and Rothschild,

B. 1997. Why do we fail in aging the skull from the sagittal sutures? *American Journal of Physical Anthropology* 103: 393–399.

Hoppa, R. D., and Fitzgerald, C. M. 1999. *Human Growth in the Past*. Cambridge: Cambridge University Press.

Hoppa, R. D., and Vaupel, J. W. 2002. *Paleodemography: Age Distributions from Skeletal Samples*. Cambridge: Cambridge University Press.

Igarashi, Y., Uesu, K., Wakebe, T., and Kanazawa, E. 2005. A new method for estimation of adult skeletal age at death from the morphology of the auricular surface of the ilium. *American Journal of Physical Anthropology* 128: 324–339.

İşcan, M. Y. 1988. Rise of forensic anthropology. *American Journal of Physical Anthropology* 31: 203–229.

———. 1989. *Age Markers in the Human Skeleton*. Springfield IL: Charles C. Thomas.

İşcan, M. Y., and Loth, S. R. 1989. Osteological manifestations of age in the adult, in M. Y. İşcan and K. A. R. Kennedy (eds.), *Reconstruction of Life from the Skeleton*, pp. 23–40. New York: Wiley-Liss.

İşcan, M. Y., Loth, S. R., and Wright, R. K. 1984. Age estimation from the rib by phase analysis: White males. *Journal of Forensic Sciences* 29: 1094–1104.

———. 1985. Age estimation from the rib by phase analysis: white females. *Journal of Forensic Sciences* 30: 853–863.

Jackes, M. K. 1985. Pubic symphysis age distributions. *American Journal of Physical Anthropology* 68: 281–299.

———. 1992. Paleodemography: Problems and techniques, in S. R. Saunders and M. A. Katzenberg (eds.), *Skeletal Biology of Past Peoples: Research and Methods*, pp. 189–224. New York: Wiley-Liss.

———. 2000. Building the bases for paleodemographic analysis: Adult age determination, in M. A. Katzenberg and S. R. Saunders (eds.), *Biological Anthropology of the Human Skeleton*, pp. 417–466. New York: Wiley-Liss.

Johnston, F. E., and Zimmer, L. O. 1989. Assessment of growth and age in the immature skeleton, in M. Y. Işcan and K. A. R. Kennedy (eds.), *Reconstruction of Life from the Skeleton*, pp. 11–21. New York: Wiley-Liss.

Katz, D., and Suchey, J. M. 1986. Age determination of the male os pubis. *American Journal of Physical Anthropology* 69: 427–435.

———. 1989. Race differences in pubic symphyseal aging patterns in the male. *American Journal of Physical Anthropology* 80: 167–172.

Katzenberg, M. A., and Saunders, S. R. 2000. *Biological Anthropology of the Human Skeleton*. New York: Wiley-Liss.

Kemkes-Grottenthaler, A. 1996. Critical evaluation of osteomorphognostic methods to estimate adult age at death: A test of the "complex method." *Homo* 46: 280–292.

———. 2002. Aging through the ages: Historical perspectives on age indicator methods, in R. D. Hoppa and J. W. Vaupel (eds.), *Paleodemography*, pp. 48–72. Cambridge: Cambridge University Press.

Kim, Y.-K., Kho, H.-S., and Lee, K.-H. 2000. Age estimation by occlusal tooth wear. *Journal of Forensic Science* 45: 303–309.

Konigsberg, L., and Holman, D. 1999. Estimation of age at death from dental emergence and implications for studies of prehistoric somatic growth, in R. D. Hoppa and C. M. Fitzgerald (eds.), *Human Growth in the Past*, pp. 264–289. Cambridge: Cambridge University Press.

Kunos, C. A., Simpson, S. W., Russell, K. F., and Hershkovitz, I. 1999. First rib metamorphosis: Its possible utility for human age-at-death estimation. *American Journal of Physical Anthropology* 110: 303–323.

Kurki, H. 2005. Use of the first rib for adult age estimation: A test of one method. *International Journal of Osteoarchaeology* 15: 342–350.

Lamendin, H., Baccino, E., Humbert, J. F., Tavernier, J. C., Nossintchouk, R. M., and Zerilia, A. 1992. A simple technique for age estimation in adult corpses: The two criteria dental method. *Journal of Forensic Sciences* 37:1373–1379.

Lampl, M., and Johnston, F. E. 1996. Problems in the aging of skeletal juveniles: Perspectives from maturation assessments of living children. *American Journal of Physical Anthropology* 101(3): 345–355.

Liversidge, H. M., Herdeg, B., and Rösing, F. W. 1998. Dental age estimation of non-adults: A review of methods and principles, in K. W. Alt, F. W. Rösing, and M. Teschler-Nicola (eds.), *Dental Anthropology*, pp. 419–442. New York: Springer.

Loth, S. R., İşcan, M. Y., and Scheuerman, E. H. 1994. Intercostal variation at the sternal end of the rib. *Forensic Science International* 65: 135–143.

Lovejoy, C. O., Meindl, R. S., Mensforth, R. P., and Barton, T. J. 1985a. Multifactorial determination of skeletal age at death: A method and blind tests of its accuracy. *American Journal of Physical Anthropology* 68: 1–14.

Lovejoy, C. O., Meindl, R. S., Pryzbeck, T. R., and Mensforth, R. P. 1985b. Chronological metamorphosis of the auricular surface of the ilium: A new method for the determination of adult skeletal age at death. *American Journal of Physical Anthropology* 68: 16–28.

Lovejoy, C. O., Mensforth, R. P., and Armelagos, G. J. 1982. Five decades of skeletal biology as reflected in the American Journal of Physical Anthropology, in F. Spencer (ed.), *A History of American Physical Anthropology, 1930–1980*, pp. 329–336. New York: Academic Press.

Lucy, D., Aykroyd, R. G., Pollard, A. M., and Solheim, T. 1996. A Bayesian approach to adult human age estimation from dental observations by Johanson's age changes. *Journal of Forensic Sciences* 41: 189–194.

Mann, R. W., Jantz, R. L., Bass, W. M., and Willey, P. S. 1991. Maxillary suture obliteration: A visual method for estimating skeletal age. *Journal of Forensic Sciences* 36: 781–791.

Maresh, M. 1955. Linear growth of long bones of extremities from infancy through adolescence. *American Journal of Diseases of Children* 89: 725–742.

Masset, C. 1989. Age estimation on the basis of cranial sutures, in M. Y. İşcan (ed.), *Age Markers in the Human Skeleton*, pp. 71–103. Springfield IL: Charles C. Thomas.

Mays, S. 1998. *The Archaeology of Human Bones.* London: Routledge.

McKern, T. W. 1957. Estimation of skeletal age from combined maturational activity. *American Journal of Physical Anthropology* 15: 399–408.

McKern, T. W., and Stewart, T. D. 1957. *Skeletal Age Changes in Young American Males. Technical Report EP45.* Natick, MA: U.S. Army Quartermaster Research and Development Center.

Meindl, R. S., and Lovejoy, C. O. 1985. Ectocranial suture closure: A revised method for the determination of skeletal age at death and blind tests of its accuracy. *American Journal of Physical Anthropology* 68: 57–66.

Meindl, R. S., Lovejoy, C. O., Mensforth, R. P., and Walker, R. A. 1985. A revised method of age determination using the os pubis, with a review and tests of accuracy of other current methods of pubis symphyseal ageing. *American Journal of Physical Anthropology* 68: 29–45.

Mensforth, R. P., and Lovejoy, C. O. 1985. Anatomical, physicological, and epidemiological correlates of the aging process: A confirmation of multifactorial age determination in the Libben skeletal population. *American Journal of Physical Anthropology* 68: 87–106.

Moorrees, C. F. A., Fanning, E. A., and Hunt, E. E. 1963. Age variation of formation stages for ten permanent teeth. *Journal of Dental Research* 42: 1490–1502.

Murray, K. A., and Murray, T. M. 1991. A test of the auricular surface aging technique. *Journal of Forensic Sciences* 36: 1162–1169.

Ohtani, S., and Yamamoto, K. 1991. Age estimation using the racemization of amino acid in human dentin. *Journal of Forensic Sciences* 36: 792–800.

Pasquier, E., Pernot, L. D. S. M., Burdin, V., Mounayer, C., Le Rest, C., Colin, D., Mottier, D., Roux, C., and Baccino, E. 1999. Determination of age at death: Assessment of an algorithm of age prediction using numerical three-dimensional CT data

from pubic bones. *American Journal of Physical Anthropology* 108: 261–268.

Pfau, R. O. 1991. *A Method for Establishing the Chronological Age of Subadults Based upon the Covariance of Dental and Skeletal Development.* Ann Arbor, MI: UMI Dissertation Services.

Prince, D. A., and Ubelaker, D. 2002. Application of Lamendin's adult dental aging technique to a diverse skeletal sample. *Journal of Forensic Sciences* 47: 107–116.

Ritz-Timme, S., Cattaneo, C., Collins, M. J., Waite, E. R., Schütz, H. W., Kaatsch, H.-J., and Borrman, H. I. M. 2000. Age estimation: The state of the art in relation to the specific demands of forensic practise. *International Journal of Legal Medicine* 113: 129–136.

Rogers, T. L. 2005. Determining the sex of human remains through cranial morphology. *Journal of Forensic Sciences* 50: 493–500.

Rogers, T. L., and Allard, T. T. 2004. Expert testimony and positive identification of human remains through cranial suture patterns. *Journal of Forensic Sciences* 49: 203–207.

Rösing, F. W., and Kvaal, S. 1998. Dental age in adults: A review of estimation methods, in K. W. Alt, F. W. Rösing, and M. Teschler-Nicola (eds.), *Dental Anthropology*, pp. 443–468. New York: Springer.

Russell, K. F., Simpson, S. W., Genovese, J., Kinkel, M. D., Meindl, R. S., and Lovejoy, C. O. 1993. Independent test of the fourth rib aging technique. *American Journal of Physical Anthropology* 92: 53–62.

Saunders, S. R. 2000. Subadult skeletons and growth-related studies, in M. A. Katzenberg and S. R. Saunders (eds.), *Biological Anthropology of the Human Skeleton*, pp. 135–161. New York: Wiley-Liss.

Saunders, S. R., Fitzgerald. C., Rogers, T., Dudar, J. C., and McKillop, H. 1992. A test of several methods of skeletal age estimation using a documented archaeological sample. *Canadian Society of Forensic Science* 25: 97–118.

Scheuer, L., and Black, S. 2000. *Developmental Juvenile Osteology.* New York: Academic Press.

———. 2004. *The Juvenile Skeleton.* London: Elsevier.

Schmitt, A., Murail, P., Cunha, E., and Rougé, D. 2002. Variability of the pattern of aging on the human skeleton: Evidence from bone indicators and implications on age at death estimation. *Journal of Forensic Sciences* 47: 1203–1209.

Schwartz, J. H. 1995. *Skeleton Keys.* New York: Oxford University Press.

Singer, R. 1953. Estimation of age from cranial suture closure: A report on its unreliability. *Journal of Forensic Medicine* 1: 52–59.

Smith, B. H. 1991. Standards of human tooth formation and dental age assessment, in M. A. Kelley and

C. S. Larsen (eds.), *Advances in Dental Anthropology*, pp. 143–168. New York: Wiley-Liss.

Solheim, T., and Sundnes, P. K. 1980. Dental age estimation of Norwegian adults: A comparison of different methods. *Forensic Science International* 16: 7–17.

Stewart, T. D. 1957. Distortion of the pubic symphyseal surface in females and its effect on age determination. *American Journal of Physical Anthropology* 15: 9–18.

Stinson, S. 2000. Growth variation: Biological and cultural factors, in S. Stinson, B. Bogin, R. Huss-Ashmore, and D. H. O'Rourke (eds.), *Human Biology*, pp. 425–463. New York: Wiley-Liss.

Stojanowski, C. M., and Buikstra, J. E.. 2005. Research trends in human osteology: A content analysis of papers published in the American Journal of Physical Anthropology. *American Journal of Physical Anthropology* 128: 98–109.

Stout, S. D. 1986. The use of bone histomorphology in skeletal identification: The case of Francisco Pizarro. *Journal of Forensic Sciences* 31: 296–300.

———. 1989. Histomorphometric analysis of human skeletal remains, in M. Y. Işcan and K. A. R. Kennedy (eds.), *Reconstruction of Life from the Skeleton*, pp. 41–52. New York: Wiley-Liss.

Suchey, J. M. 1979. Problems in the aging of females using the os pubis. *American Journal of Physical Anthropology* 51: 467–470.

Suchey, J. M., Wiseley, D. V., and Katz, D. 1986. Evaluation of the Todd and McKern-Stewart method for aging the male os pubis, in K. J. Reichs (ed.), *Forensic Osteology*, pp. 33–67. Springfield, IL: Charles C. Thomas.

Thomas, C. D. L., Stein, M. S., Feik, S. A., Wark, J. D., and Clement, J. G. 2000. Determination of age at death using combined morphology and histology of the femur. *Journal of Anatomy* 196: 463–471.

Todd, T. W. 1920. Age changes in the pubic bone. *American Journal of Physical Anthropology* 33: 285–334.

Todd, T. W., and Lyon, Jr., D. W. 1924. Endocranial suture closure, its progress and age relationship: Part I. Adult males of white stock. *American Journal of Physical Anthropology* 7: 325–384.

———. 1925a. Cranial suture closure, its progress and age relationship: Part II. Ectocranial closure in adult males of white stock. *American Journal of Physical Anthropology* 8: 23–45.

———. 1925b. Cranial suture closure: its progress and age relationship: Part III. Endocranial closure in adult males of Negro stock. *American Journal of Physical Anthropology* 8: 47–71.

———. 1925c. Cranial suture closure: Its progress and age relationship: Part IV. Ectocranial closure in adult males of Negro stock. *American Journal of Physical Anthropology* 8: 149–168.

Ubelaker, D. H. 1999. *Human Skeletal Remains: Excavation, Analysis, Interpretation* (3rd ed.). Washington, D. C.: Taraxacum.

United States Supreme Court in Daubert v. Merrell Dow Pharmaceuticals, Inc., 509 U.S. 579 (1993).

Walker, P. L., Dean, G., and Shapiro, P. 1991. Estimating age from tooth wear in archaeological populations, in M. A. Kelley and C. S. Larsen (eds.), *Advances in Dental Anthropology*, pp. 169–178. New York: Wiley-Liss.

Walker, R. A., and Lovejoy, C. O. 1985. Radiographic changes in the clavicle and proximal femur and their use in the determination of skeletal age at death. *American Journal of Physical Anthropology* 68: 1–14.

Washburn, S. L. 1951. The new physical anthropology. *Transcript of the New York Academy of Science* 13: 298–304.

Webb, P. A. O., and Suchey, J. M. 1985. Epiphyseal union of the anterior iliac crest and medial clavicle in a modern sample of American males and females. *American Journal of Physical Anthropology* 68: 457–466.

White, T. D. 2000. *Human Osteology*. New York: Academic Press.

Wittwer-Backofen, U., Gampe, J., and Vaupel, J. W. 2004. Tooth cementum annulation for age estimation: Results from a large known-age validation study. *American Journal of Physical Anthropology* 123: 119–29.

Workshop of European Anthropologists. 1980. Recommendations for age and sex diagnosis of skeletons. *Journal of Human Evolution* 9: 517–549.

Yoder, C., Ubelaker, D. H., and Powell, J. F. 2001. Examination of variation in sternal rib end morphology relevant to age assessment. *Journal of Forensic Sciences* 46: 223–227.

HISTOLOGICAL AGE ESTIMATION

Christian M. Crowder

Since the introduction of the first histological method of age estimation by Ellis Kerley in 1965, numerous methods by various researchers have followed. Despite the attention histological age estimation has received in the literature, histological methods tend to be used when no other methods can be applied or for the sole purpose of distinguishing human bone fragments from nonhuman. This chapter reviews well-established histological methods of age estimation and explores the tribulations in the acceptance of these methods as a conventional tool for the estimation of age at death. Furthermore, it describes the biological factors that one must consider when developing and applying microscopic methods of age estimation. Finally, this chapter discusses contemporary research and future directions in cortical bone histomorphometry.

The Dynamics of Bone and Histological Age Estimation

Bone is a dynamic, metabolically and mechanically active tissue that varies in composition and structure throughout an organism's life. As cortical bone remodeling occurs over time, the relative density of secondary osteons in the cortex increases (Wu, Jett, and Frost 1967; Wu et al. 1970). In other words, as chronological age increases, the cortex

becomes crowded with intact and fragmentary osteons (Figure 19.1). Histological age estimation is based on the assumption that the replacement of primary bone with secondary bone and a continual turnover of osteons will occur at a predictable rate (Pfeiffer 1992). The development and interpretation of histological methods for age estimation, therefore, requires an extensive understanding of the microstructure and physiology of skeletal tissue. Because the information provided in this chapter focuses on methods and not the biological basis for histological age estimation, I recommend that those who wish to apply or to develop such methods take time to appreciate the nuances of bone microstructure.

Methodology is strongly emphasized in this chapter primarily because methods of age estimation used in the forensic context must meet specific demands owing to the evidentiary nature of analytical results. In the United States, the legal requirements for the evaluation of scientific evidence are set forth in *Daubert v. Merrel Dow Pharmaceuticals*, 113 S.Ct. 2786 (1993). According to the *Daubert* criteria, a trial judge must determine if a method has been adequately tested, subjected to peer review in a published journal, provided with potential error rates, and enjoys general acceptance within the relevant scientific community. Currently, methods of histological

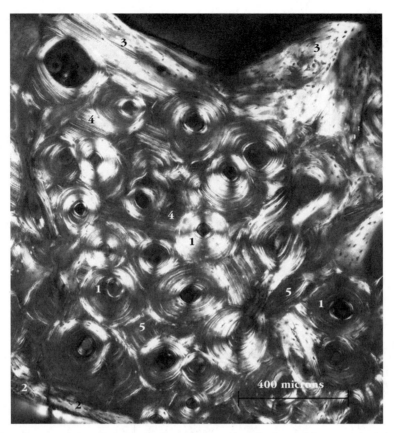

Figure 19.1 Rib cross-section depicting the five patterns of lamellar bone: (1) concentric, (2) outer (peri-osteal) circumferential, (3) inner (endosteal) circumferential, (4) primary interstitial, (5) osteonal interstitial lamellae. Examples of intact and fragmentary osteons are noted by numbers 1 and 5, respectively.

age estimation may not meet these standards. Very few large validation studies have been performed; thus error rates are unclear. Owing to the nature of biological variation, large age intervals are acceptable for the estimation of adult age at death in the anthropological community regardless of the method. Therefore, the level of accuracy in adult age estimation often consents to intervals greater than ten years. Crowder (2005) determined that the Thompson (1979) and the Cho and colleagues (2002) histological methods of age estimation demonstrate levels of inaccuracy and bias comparable to traditional morphological methods (Table 19.1). Therefore, the combination of gross morphological methods with these histological methods might produce more accurate results. One point of contention, however, is the high observer error associated with histological analysis despite the low levels reported in the literature. Often, precision analysis is performed using inadequate statistical methods, such as student t-tests and correlation coefficients, that do not provide for a clear assessment of method precision.

Methods and Comparison Studies

Early Studies and Their Evaluations

Ellis Kerley (1965) applied the first quantitative histological approach to the estimation of age at death. Kerley evaluated the absolute counts of intact and fragmentary secondary osteons, the percentage of circumferential lamellar bone, and the number of non-Haversian canals in 88 males, 29 females, and 9 of indeterminate sex. This method involves the evaluation of these variables from complete transverse cross-sections of the femur, tibia, and fibula. One circular microscopic field from the outer third of the anterior, posterior, medial, and lateral aspects of the bone's cross-section is evaluated. Regression equations for each variable and bone are then used to develop an age estimate profile chart, in which an age interval is

Table 19.1 Inaccuracy and bias values (in years) for methods of adult age estimation compared to selected histological methods.

Known Age (years)		4th Rib[1]	4th Rib[2]		Pubic Sym.[1]	Revised Pubic Sym.[3]	Auricular Surface[1]	Revised Auric. Surface[3]	Revised Auric. Surface[4]	Ectocranial Suture[1]	Multi-factorial[5]	Rib Histology[6]	Femur Histology[7]
			M	F									
< 29	Inaccuracy	5.0	0.8	4.3	12.7	3.1	3.9	3.2	12.6	11.1	5.2	7.0	9.3
	Bias	0.8	−0.8	0.3	10.3	1.9	3.4	2.6	12.4	11.1	4.9	−1.7	0.4
30–39	Inaccuracy	11.1	5.0	6.3	4.4	5.5	9.1	7.2	12.4	7.1	8.9	9.6	15.9
	Bias	11.1	−4.0	−1.8	−2.7	3.5	7.8	1.6	10.7	5.1	7.4	5.0	10.4
40–49	Inaccuracy	7.1	6.3	17.0	13.0	6.1	4.4	7.7	10.8	9.5	8.2	9.2	13.9
	Bias	−2.5	−2.8	−4.5	−13.0	0.2	−4.4	−2.9	9.0	−6.3	5.1	−3.3	4.8
50–59	Inaccuracy	9.1	9.2	8.4	20.1	7.5	9.1	11.1	8.6	12.9	8.3	10.4	10.6
	Bias	−9.1	−0.9	−8.2	−18.5	1.7	−7.6	1.9	3.9	−12.9	−4.9	−4.8	6.8
60–69	Inaccuracy	16.6	6.0	6.5	22.4	10.5	16.6	7.2	5.9	24.6	11.9	9.2	6.6
	Bias	−15.7	−4.6	−5.6	−22.4	−9.2	−16.6	−5.8	−3.0	−24.6	−10.4	−7.6	1.0
70–79	Inaccuracy	-	-	-	-	-	-	-	11.2	-	-	17.2	6.7
	Bias	-	-	-	-	-	-	-	−11.2	-	-	−16.2	−6.5

80+												
Inaccuracy	-	-	-	-	-	-	-	20.1	-	-	19.6	15.5
Bias	-	-	-	-	-	-	-	-20.1	-.	-	-19.6	-15.5
All Ages												
Inaccuracy	11.0	5.4	8.4	17.8	5.8	10.3	7.0	10.1	15.9	8.7	11.8 (**11.1**)	10.1 (**10.5**)
Bias	-5.6	-2.9	-4.0	-11.8	1.3	-6.3	0.0	0.1	-8.4	0.0	-6.7 (**-3.8**)	0.7 (**4.3**)
N	27	36	38	35	109	53	108	180	33	55	215 (**155**)	184 (**134**)

1. Saunders et al. 1992.
2. Loth (1995); used the Spitalfields sample.
3. Lovejoy et al. 1985.
4. Mulhern and Jones 2005. Test of the revised Buckberry and Chamberlain (2002) method using the Spitalfields sample.
5. Bedford et al. 1993. Represent mean values for 3 independent observers.
6. Data from this research using the Cho et al. (2002) method. The parentheses contain the total values if the sample is truncated at 70 years of age.
7. Data from this research using the Thompson (1979) method. The parentheses contain the total values if the sample is truncated at 70 years of age.
8. Inaccuracy and bias for the average histological age estimates of the rib and femur. The paired boxed columns compare sternal rib end to rib histology and auricular surface to femur histology age estimates using the Spitalfields known sample.

developed. Kerley and Ubelaker (1978) revised the original method to rectify an incorrectly published microscopic field size through the introduction of a correction factor to offset microscope field size differences. Stout and Gehlert (1982) suggest that the use of the correction factor to adjust osteon counts may be of limited value due to the spatial variation of microstructures within the cortex, thus resulting in method inaccuracy if the original Kerley field size is not applied.

Ahlqvist and Damsten (1969) reported difficulties in discerning between intact and fragmentary osteons using Kerley's definition, which defines an intact osteon as having 80% or more of its area intact with a complete Haversian canal. Instead of recording absolute osteon counts, they suggest using a square eyepiece grid to determine the percentage of remodeled and primary bone per field. The percentages are then averaged for four microscopic field locations. Recognizing the greater variation in remodeling at the linea aspera, they avoided this area for analysis by rotating the location of the fields to where they fall between the original Kerley fields. Regression equations to predict age at death were generated from only 20 femoral samples.

Debate over the methods introduced by Kerley and Ahlqvist and Damsten continued over several decades. Bouvier and Ubelaker (1977) compared the accuracy and the precision of the Kerley and Ahlqvist and Damsten methods using 40 femoral sections taken from the original Kerley sample.[1] They found that precision was similar, but the Kerley method was more accurate for the younger individuals and less accurate than the Ahlqvist and Damsten method for the older individuals. These results were attributed to the skew toward older individuals in the reference sample from which the method was derived. Stout and Gehlert (1980) questioned results from the Bouvier and Ubelaker study, noting the methodological flaw in testing the accuracy of a method using a sample from which the method was derived. Despite the use of an independent test sample, Stout and Gehlert reported similar results in the accuracy of the two methods. In another study, Stout and Stanley (1991) compared Kerley's method, which uses absolute osteon counts, to Ahlqvist and Damsten's method, which employs the percentage of osteonal bone. Evaluating a small sample of 35 long bones, excluding the femur, they determined that the best predictor of age was absolute osteon counts from the fibula.

Aiello and Molleson (1993) sampled 20 individuals from the Spitalfields (England) collection to test the accuracy of the Kerley method. However, instead of evaluating the Kerley field locations, they employed those developed by Ahlqvist and Damsten (1969). Furthermore, Singh and Gunberg's (1970) definition for intact osteons was adopted in place of the Kerley definition. Another evaluation of the Kerley method by Walker (1990) poses similar problems. A large portion of Walker's test sample consisted of anterior bone cores instead of entire cross-sections. Two anterior fields were evaluated in these samples, and the results were doubled to compensate for the missing fields. Given the numerous changes to the sampling technique that were introduced into these validation studies, the reliability of the Kerley method cannot be determined.

Singh and Gunberg (1970) evaluated histological age-related changes in a sample of 59 mandibles and 40 femora and tibiae anterior midshafts. For analysis of the long bones, two microscopic fields were selected at random within the anterior periosteal region, and the following variables were collected: the sum of the intact osteons counted in both fields; the average number of lamellae per osteon; and the average Haversian canal diameter. They attempted to avoid the potential error in discerning the number of osteon fragments among the interstitial bone; however, osteons that were partially obscured by the periphery of the microscopic field, cut obliquely, or seen only as fragments were included if they represented a complete Haversian canal. Regression analysis indicated that nonlinearities occurred at the later ages with all three variables. Regardless of this observation, a linear model was assumed for the remainder of the analyses.

Crowder (2005) evaluated the reliability of the Singh and Gunberg method with a sample of 184 individuals from the Spitalfields' skeletal collection. Results indicate that the method grossly overestimated age. Although a strong correlation between the number of intact osteons and chronological age exists, the inaccuracy of the method indicates a problem with the technique or the prediction equation. Crowder (2005) further noted that the method produced high observer error, likely associated with counting microstructures using an open microscopic field technique (one without a counting reticule).

Further Development and Testing of Methods

Ribs and Clavicles. Stout (1986) introduced a histological method using cross-sections from the middle third of the 6th rib based on research performed by Harold Frost and various colleagues spanning several decades (Frost 1969; Jett, Wu, and Frost 1967; Pirok et al. 1966; Santoro and Frost 1967; Wu et al. 1970). This method sought to eliminate issues such as sampling error due to field location and the influence of biomechanical factors on weight-bearing bones. Intact and fragmentary osteon counts per grid area are summed producing a variable referred to as osteon population density (OPD), solving the problem of differentiating between intact and fragmentary osteons. Background information pertaining to the creation of the regression equation, sample descriptive statistics, and the accuracy and precision of the method was not presented.

Pursuing the use of non-weight-bearing skeletal elements, Stout and Paine (1992) introduced a revision of the Stout (1986) 6th-rib-method and explored the use of the clavicle for histological age estimation. Equations were generated from a sample of 40 individuals derived from a forensic context. The sample age distribution differs from those of previous studies, in that it is skewed toward younger ages. No sex differences among the histological variables were noted, although only 8 of the 40 individuals were female. In a validation sample of 12 ribs and 7 clavicles, differences between the known and predicted mean ages were not significant. Stout and colleagues (1996) applied the clavicle equation to a sample of 83 individuals of known age from a 19th-century Swiss cemetery, producing inaccurate age estimates for subjects older than 40 years of age. There were no differences noted in OPD between sexes, indicating that the inclusion of 42 females in the test sample is most likely not the cause of the inaccuracy. The researchers hypothesized that the inaccuracy in age estimates was due to disparity in sample age distributions and the occurrence of the OPD asymptote (see section below on Remodeling Variation). A new prediction equation for the clavicle was generated through the combination of the original sample and the Swiss cemetery sample.

Dudar and colleagues (1993) assessed the accuracy of the rib-age prediction equations from the Stout (1986) and Stout and Paine (1992) studies on an independent sample of 55 individuals derived from cadavers and archaeological remains of known age. Results indicate that the Stout and Paine method significantly underestimates age, whereas the Stout (1986) method produced fairly accurate age estimates. The tendency of the Stout and Paine method to underestimate age was also reported in Pratte and Pfeiffer's (1999) study on 62 individuals of mixed ancestry. In contrast to Dudar and colleagues' results, the Stout method did not produce accurate age estimates. Pratte and Pfeiffer

noted a weak association between OPD and known age and hypothesized that extrinsic factors affecting bone remodeling (for example, alcoholism or malnutrition) may be the cause. Neither validation study produced sex-related differences.

In an attempt to combine histological methods with morphological methods, Stout and colleagues (1994) analyzed rib cross-sections and sternal rib end morphology from the 4th rib of 60 individuals between 11 to 88 years of age (mean age = 39.2) taken at autopsy. Histological methods from Stout and Paine (1992) and gross morphological methods from İşcan and colleagues (1984; 1985) were followed. The authors concluded that because the correlation between histological and morphological age estimates is lower than desired, the methods reflect different age-associated factors. They concluded that combining the two methods using multiple regressions might improve accuracy. Dudar and colleagues (1993) had reported similar results in their analysis of histological age estimates from the 6th rib and morphological age estimates from the 4th rib.

In 2002, Cho and colleagues presented a modification to the Stout (1986) and Stout and Paine (1992) rib methods. Rib cross-sections from 69 African-Americans and 34 European-Americans were used as a developmental set, with 34 African-Americans and 17 European-Americans forming the validation sample. In addition to the variables described by Stout and Paine (1992), mean osteonal cross-sectional areas were calculated. Results indicate that age-related changes in histological structures, namely osteon area and relative cortical area, differ among ancestral groups, whereas sex differences within the groups are negligible. Ancestry-specific equations were developed, as well as general equations that can be used if ancestry is unknown or indeterminate. The parameters for the equations can be adjusted if the proportions of African- and European-Americans from the region of origin are known. The validation sample produced results that were not significantly different from the developmental sample.

Crowder (2005) compared the reliability of the 6th-rib methods using 215 individuals from the Spitalfields collection. The Stout (1986) and Cho and colleagues (2002) equations performed similarly in all statistical tests, but the Stout and Paine (1992) equation grossly underestimated age. This bias has been noted in several of the aforementioned studies and indicates a possible problem with the regression equation. Analysis of observer error (all three methods employ the same data-collection technique) indicates that the OPD variable significantly reduces observer error compared to evaluating the OPD constituent variables separately.

Upper and Lower Extremities. Thompson (1979) developed a method designed to minimize the amount of destructive sampling and explore the utility of both the lower and the upper extremities for age estimation. Thompson sampled bone cores (0.4 cm in diameter) from the femora and tibiae of 116 cadavers and the humeri and ulnae of 31 cadavers. Various histomorphometric measurements were recorded through point counting using a 10 x 10 grid eyepiece disk micrometer. Overall, Thompson explored 19 variables, including a number of gross measurements (for example, core weight, cortical thickness, and cortical density). One variable, referred to as the percentage of osteonal area, was determined to be the single best indicator of age. Histological structures were recorded in four contiguous microscopic fields along the core's anterior periosteal surface. Both sex- and side-specific regression equations were developed.

Thompson (1981) tested the accuracy of the core method on 54 forensic cases consisting of different ancestral groups. The results indicated that the femur produces the most accurate age estimates with a trend for increased accuracy in individuals of European descent.[2] The other skeletal elements produced age estimates that were determined to be too inaccurate for forensic science application. Further analysis of the tibia by Thompson and Galvin (1983) indicated that the tibia is less accurate than the femur owing to a higher correlation with osteon area (size) and age at death. Osteon area was removed from the equation, and age estimates comparable to those from the femur were then obtained for individuals younger than 55 years. Thompson and Galvin proposed that two regression equations may be needed for the tibia: one to estimate age in individuals younger than 55 and one to estimate age for individuals over 55 years.

The method proposed by Thompson in 1979 has been evaluated by a number of researchers. Narasaki (1990) concluded that the Thompson method is less accurate than previously reported, especially among males, when applied to a sample of 52 modern Japanese cadavers. Proper method validation was not performed, in that Narasaki introduced two new variables into the method prior to evaluation. Furthermore, the test sample was heavily skewed with over half of the sample older than 80 years. The geriatric nature of the sample increases the susceptibility for altered cortical bone remodeling by factors associated with advanced age and chronic diseases. Pfeiffer (1992) estimated age at death for 29 individuals from historical

cemeteries, concluding that the Thompson method could be applied with reasonably high repeatability despite variations in bone preservation. Age estimates were accurate in only half of the cases; however, subperiosteal erosion may have caused the overestimation of age. Crowder's (2005) test of the reliability of the Thompson method resulted in age estimates with deviations from chronological age that were not significantly different from zero, but age estimates for individuals younger than 50 years generated larger inaccuracy values. The lack of younger individuals in Thompson's reference sample may explain the difference in inaccuracy for the younger age cohorts. Crowder notes that the Thompson method generates low observer error, likely attributed to the use of the point count grid method and more objective variable definitions.

Femur. Continuing with the exploration of the anterior femur as a histological age indicator, Ericksen (1991) introduced a method using the largest and most diverse sample compared to all the aforementioned studies. Cortical bone samples were removed from 328 individuals (154 males and 174 females) collected from George Washington University Medical School cadavers, cemeteries from the Dominican Republic, and autopsy specimens from Chilé. Much like the Thompson (1979) method, Ericksen's method recorded histological structures from the periosteal region of an anterior wedge using an eyepiece grid. The method evaluated five fields both microscopically and through photographs. Histological variables include counts of secondary osteons, type II osteons, osteon fragments, resorption spaces, and non-Haversian canals. The sum of the variables for the five fields is divided by the total area to determine the count per square millimeter. The remaining variables are collected using a 100-space grid superimposed on the field photographs to count the predominant microstructure per grid-square. These variables include unremodeled circumferential bone, osteonal bone, and fragmentary osteonal bone. Sex differences were prevalent within the sample; thus, sex-specific equations were developed in addition to a pooled sex equation.

Although the heterogeneous nature of the Ericksen sample may produce more widely applicable equations, Crowder (2005) suggests that the method introduces higher levels of observer error than does the Thompson (1979) method. The Ericksen variable definitions are extremely detailed, yet it is difficult to identify the nuances of certain bone microstructures, especially when diagenesis is present. This can be most problematic when discerning osteon fragments from crowded interstitial bone and resorption spaces from diagenetic destruction. Furthermore, higher error levels can be expected as result of the subjectivity in determining the predominant microstructure per square in a 100-squared grid. Interestingly, the Ericksen method produced significantly high observer error values for the individual variables, whereas the calculated ages did not. This suggests that the combination of the variables in the predictive equations reduces the individual variable error. Despite observer error issues, the accuracy of the Ericksen (1991) method is similar to the Thompson (1979) method (Crowder 2005).

Humerus. Yoshino and colleagues (1994) analyzed histological thin-sections from the diaphysis of the humerus of 40 Japanese males at a location near the surgical neck. Following the Ericksen (1991) method, Yoshino and colleagues evaluated histological structures using micrographs and direct observation in cases of doubtful interpretation. Results demonstrated a high multiple correlation coefficient and a standard error of estimate similar to Thompson's (1979) humeral samples. The authors validated the method with samples from the reference population, which produced a mean absolute difference of 5.1 years between known and estimated ages. Note that testing the method on the reference sample from which the method and equations were derived might result in a false impression of accuracy.

Skull. In an attempt to improve age estimation methods for the skull, Cool and colleagues (1995) investigated occipital bone histomorphometry using Australian cadavers. Occipital cores were extracted from a small sample of 17 male crania. Fractional volumes of primary, secondary, and fragmentary osteons and lamellar bone were recorded for the outer and the inner cortical table. Results indicate that although the occipital micromorphology exhibits age-related changes, the amount of variation around the variables is too great for accurate age estimation. Clarke (1987) had reported similar results in an earlier study evaluating the parietal bone. Curtis (2004) analyzed the microstructure of the left and the right frontal bone from a sample of 92 European-American cadavers, concluding that the histological structure does not appear to be as influenced by age-related changes compared to the postcranial elements.

Factors Affecting Histological Age Estimation

Microscopic age changes in cortical bone are a universal phenomenon, yet biological variability in bone remodeling rates owing to intrinsic and extrinsic factors affects histological age estimates. The following sections briefly discuss these factors as they relate to nonpathological bone.

Remodeling Variance

The onset and magnitude of bone turnover varies at different anatomical locations throughout the skeleton. Significant sampling error can occur within (spatial variance) and between (incoherence) cross-sections, with the latter's sampling error increasing dramatically as the amount of cortical area evaluated decreases (Frost 1969). Frost (1969) recommends that a minimum of 50 mm^2 of cross-sectional bone in nonpathological individuals should be evaluated to minimize sampling error. Crowder (2005) notes that incoherence between rib cross-sections is more pronounced in older individuals owing to the higher fragmentary OPD values. Pfeiffer and colleagues (1995) demonstrated the relation of spatial variance in bone remodeling to mechanical loading: the anatomical axes (the anatomical planes of a bone [for example, anterior, posterior, lateral, medial]) of the femur midshaft exhibited greater variability in bone remodeling than did the mechanical axes (the locations of mechanical loading owing to the mechanical environment of the bone). In an attempt to control for spatial variance, Iwaniec and colleagues (1998) determined the smallest amount of the anterior femur that should be evaluated to accurately predict the variation in the entire anterior wedge of the femoral midshaft. The study produced a promising sampling strategy that has yet to be developed into a method for the estimation of age at death.

Chan and colleagues (2007) and Tersigni (2005) evaluated sampling error in long-bone diaphyses using age estimates from two histological methods (Thompson 1979 and Kerley 1965, respectively). According to Chan and colleagues, the inter- and intrasection variation that occurs in bone remodeling within the femoral cortex has the potential to produce significant differences among age estimates taken from various femoral diaphyseal locations compared to the age estimated from the anterior midshaft. However, the sampling location is not necessarily confined to the anterior midshaft but can be applied with similar accuracy to locations along the anterior diaphysis. Tersigni (2005) determined that the variation in age estimates between cross-sections along the femur, tibia, and radius diaphyses using the Kerley (1965) method introduces significant error into the age estimates, whereas the humerus, ulna, and fibula demonstrate less within-bone microstructure variation. Tersigni suggests that the Kerley method should be used only for estimating age at midshaft, cautioning the application of the method on fragmentary bone in which the midshaft cannot be identified.

A larger obstacle than sampling error is an OPD asymptote[3] that occurs when new osteon creations remove all evidence of older ones (Wu et al. 1970). This phenomenon is predicted to occur around the 6th decade of life in the ribs; however, this age is not static. It is unclear if the onset of the asymptote varies between skeletal elements that remodel more slowly or that have larger cortical areas. Jackes (2000: 429) takes a more general stance regarding the onset of the age asymptote, stating that "at some stage in the aging process, unknown for each population, indeed for each individual, histological age assessment cannot be applied."

Population Variation

The literature has produced conflicting reports regarding variation in bone remodeling among ancestral groups. Although bone mass, quality and turnover rates have been shown to differ among ancestral groups, it is unclear how age estimates are affected. If bone turnover is increased in a specific region (for example, the endosteal surface), then current methods of histological age estimation that evaluate fields at the perisoteal surface may not demonstrate significant remodeling differences. For example, Kerley (1965) determined that ancestry has no effect on histological age changes, whereas Pratte and Pfeiffer (1999) and Cho and colleagues (2002), evaluating entire rib cross-sections, note differences in bone microstructure between groups. Differences may or may not be revealed, depending on the histological variables, sample size, and sample demographics. Comparisons using archaeological remains of unknown ages of death often demonstrate population differences in bone remodeling (Ericksen 1973; Mulhern 2000; Mulhern and Van Gerven, 1997; Richman, Ortner, and Schulter-Ellis 1979). The unknown age and sex distributions of the archaeological populations being compared may differ significantly, producing variations in bone microstructure that can be mistaken as population differences. For example, it has been suggested that osteon area exhibits population differences (Cho et al. 2002; Curtis 2004; Pfeiffer 1998; Pfeiffer et al. 2006; Wantanabe et al. 1998), albeit in most cases, these differences are not statistically significant. Furthermore, it has been postulated that age and sex differences exist in osteon area (Burr, Ruff, and Thompson 1990; Landeros and Frost 1964; Mulhern and Van Gerven 1997; Ortner 1975; Stout and Simmons 1979; Takahashi, Epker,

and Frost 1965). These perceived differences in osteon area may be an artifact of the sample age and sex distributions or dependent on the histomorphometric technique.

Sex-Specific Variation

It is well documented that bone density and the rate of bone remodeling differ between adult males and females (Agarwal et al. 2004, Ericksen 1991; Kerley 1965; Robling and Stout 2000; Thompson 1979). Pregnancy, parity, lactation, and menopause are biological factors that affect bone turnover in the female skeleton (Agarwal and Stuart-Macadam 2003). Although sex-specific equations for histological age estimation have been developed (Ericksen 1991; Thompson 1979), most of the aforementioned studies did not demonstrate sex differences in histomorphometric variables. This could be the result of small samples producing skewed sex and age distributions, the intracortical location of the microscopic field, or choice of statistical models. Sex differences in histomorphometric variables observed in archaeological populations could be the result of bone's response to mechanical loading due to a gender division of labor. As previously mentioned, sex differences have been suggested to manifest in osteon area; however, other studies disregard sex as a factor (Cho et al. 2002; Dupras and Pfeiffer 1996; Pfeiffer 1998). Although sample size and distribution should be a concern, these discrepancies suggest that other factors affect osteon area, such as differences in bone-formation rates, physical activity, and age at death.

Physical Activity

Biomechanical strain levels may vary within and between populations depending on the general patterns of physical activity. Strain-related differences in bone mass have also been documented within paired skeletal elements of an individual (Daley et al. 2004). Lack of activity on weight-bearing elements, such as that which occurs with prolonged bed rest, has been shown to alter bone resorption and formation rates (Inque et al. 2000). Controlled experiments using non-human mammals have demonstrated the effects of loading history on cortical bone modeling and remodeling (Skedros et al. 2003; Skedros, Hunt, and Bloebaum 2004). Research indicates that responses to weight-bearing exercise are specific to the loaded bone and do not appear to produce systemic effects (Robling 1998; Tommerup et al. 1993). The question remains: how do levels of activity affect the accuracy of histological age estimations in humans? The magnitude or duration of physical activity that is needed to produce significant differences in microstructures and, in turn, age estimates remains unknown. More research is needed comparing multiple skeletal elements from the same individual of a known sample.

Diagenesis

Taphonomic factors, namely, diagenesis, affect the microstructural integrity or appearance of bone and must be considered when estimating age at death. Diagenesis refers to the postdepositional changes that may affect both chemical and structural integrity of the bone sample (Pfeiffer 2000) (Figure 19.2). Diagenetic agents, such as water intrusion, bacteria, and fungi, can structurally alter bone micromorphology, sometimes without noticeable effects to the gross morphology (Jackes et al. 2001; Jans et al. 2004). This, in turn, may affect the reliability of both gross morphological and histological age estimates. Avoidance of cortical bone fields affected by diagenetic agents is possible during histological analysis; however, it has been demonstrated that cortical remodeling data are affected by sampling location owing to the nonuniformity in the distribution of histological structures (Drusini 1996; Iwaniec et al. 1998; Lazenby 1984; Pfeiffer, Lazenby, and Chiang 1995). It is possible to limit the effect of diagenesis through the use of an ultrasonic cleaner, acetic acid bath, or the application of stains. Nevertheless, one must adhere to the sampling protocol outlined by the method being applied.

Methodological Issues

While the intrinsic and extrinsic variables affecting bone histomorphometry are not controllable in the forensic context, methodological error can be limited. The evaluation technique determines the amount of subjectivity introduced. To improve histological methods, more objective variable definitions are needed. Definitions that require one to visually assess a percentage of bone present, absent, or remodeled are more subjective and would produce higher levels of observer error. Parfitt and colleagues (1987) standardized the nomenclature for hard-tissue histologists to relieve confusion and to reduce the semantic barriers that they must cross within the field; however, few researchers in anthropology have adhered to the protocol.

Sampling procedures are needed to adequately evaluate skeletal elements that have larger cortical areas (for example, femur, humerus) to limit the effect of spatial variance and to reduce observer error. In a recent histological method developed by Maat and colleagues (2006), only three 1-mm² fields were evaluated from the anterior femoral

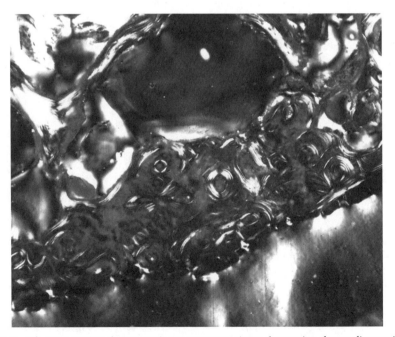

Figure 19.2   Rib cross-section demonstrating postmortem tissue destruction due to diagenetic agents.

midshaft. Although the inherently "destructive" nature of histological sampling is a concern for archaeological remains and museum skeletal collections, this trepidation in removing larger sections of bone should not exist in forensic analyses. The importance in evaluating an adequate amount of cortical bone is paramount in reducing remodeling variance error, which will improve the accuracy of the age estimate and assist with the overall identification process. To further reduce observer error, open microscopic field evaluations should not be performed. In older individuals, with large numbers of fragmentary osteons, one can easily lose one's place in the open microscopic field. Using a reticule or other eyepiece grid provides reference points for counting structures.

The choice of statistical model is an important consideration when developing an age predictive equation. By far, least squares linear regression is the most common model applied. Predicted age defined from the regression of chronological age produces a regression of the mean effect (Krøll and Saxtrup 2000). This generates a systematic bias in age estimates, resulting in the overestimation of age in younger individuals and the underestimation of age in older individuals. All the histological methods evaluated in this chapter demonstrate this bias, as do most gross morphological methods of adult age estimation. The over- and underestimation of age can be reduced by regressing y on x when considering the statistical model, a technique referred to as *classic calibration* (Aykroyd et al. 1999). Overall, linear regression may be a poor model for use in adult age estimation. Histological age indicators do not always exhibit a strong linear relationship throughout the human lifespan; thus polynomial or quadratic regression techniques should be considered. The estimation of adult age at death, using a single skeletal age indicator, will be inherently inaccurate, considering the amount of biological variability at any given age. It is for this reason that nonparametric and semiparametric models using probability theory to estimate age at death should be considered for future research.

Conclusion

The advancement of microscopy technology has enormous potential to significantly enhance histological analyses. Relatively simple to use are firewire digital-feed cameras, capturing software, and analytical programs. Viewing microscopic structures on a large monitor with software that can improve visualization can greatly decrease observer error and assist with multiperson analysis. The ability to mark structures that have been counted or to measure features on a screen with a digitizing tablet improves histomorphometric data collection; however, the budding forensic anthropologist or seasoned professional deciding to perform histological age estimation should be warned that digital imaging does not replace direct microscopic analysis through the eyepiece. The nature of a 2-D evaluation of a 3-D structure requires the observer to continuously focus up and down and adjust polarization and lighting. More technical advances include the use of microcomputed tomography (μCT), which is the first nondestructive imaging technology for histological analysis (Cooper et al. 2003; 2004). Currently, this technology is capable only of resolving Haversian canals, making it mostly suitable for the analysis of cortical porosity and not appropriate for use with established methods of histological age estimation.

It is apparent that existing histological methods of age estimation differ from one another in regard to skeletal element, sample location, and histomorphometric variables. Despite the general consensus that age-related changes are reflected to some degree in the microstructure of bone, the numerous difficulties in reproducing and evaluating results from previous histological studies have been a deterrent in their use as a standard method for the estimation of adult age at death. Furthermore, the macro- and micromorphological age-related changes within the skeleton are a complex interaction of intrinsic biological factors, extrinsic environmental factors, and inherent method biases that must be systematically examined. Adapting more rigorous procedures for developing and evaluating histological methods will aid researchers in generating more reliable methods of age estimation.

Notes

1. N.B.: Kerley does not report the origin of the samples used.

2. The Thompson (1981) sample included only six individuals of non-European descent.

3. The asymptote refers to the point where one is unable to quantify the accumulation or the density of remodeling events over time, because preexisting events are being erased.

References

Agarwal, S. C., Dumitriu, M., Tomlinson, G. A., and Grynpas, M. D. 2004. Medieval trabecular bone architecture: The influence of age, sex, and lifestyle. *American Journal of Physical Anthropology* 124: 33–44.

Agarwal, S. C., and Stuart-Macadam, P. 2003. An evolutionary and biocultural approach to understanding the effects of reproductive factors on the female skeleton, in S. C. Agarwald and S. D. Stout (eds.), *Bone Loss and Osteoporosis: An Anthropological Perspective*, pp. 121–136. New York: Kluwer Academic Plenum Publishers.

Ahlqvist, J., and Damsten, O. 1969. A modification of Kerley's method for microscopic determination of age in human bone. *Journal of Forensic Sciences* 14: 205–212.

Aiello, L. C., and Molleson, T. 1993. Are microscopic ageing techniques more accurate then macroscopic ageing techniques? *Journal of Archaeological Science* 20: 689–704.

Aykroyd, R. G., Lucy, D., Pollard, M., and Roberts, C. A. 1999. Nasty, brutish, but not necessarily short: A reconsideration of the statistical methods used to calculate age at death from adult human skeletal and dental age indicators. *American Antiquity* 64(1): 55–70.

Bedford, M. E., Russell, K. F., Lovejoy, C. O., Meindl, R. S., Simpson, S. W., and Stuart-Macadam, P. L. 1993. Test of the multifactorial aging method using skeletons with known ages-at-death from the Grant Collection. *American Journal of Physical Anthropology* 91: 287–297.

Bouvier, M., and Ubelaker, D. H. 1977. A comparison of two methods for the microscopic determination of age at death. *American Journal of Physical Anthropology* 46: 391–394.

Buckberry, J. L., and Chamberlain, A. T. 2002. Age estimation from the auricular surface of the ilium: A revised method. *American Journal of Physical Anthropology* 119: 231–239.

Burr, D. B., Ruff, C. B., and Thompson, D. D. 1990. Patterns of skeletal histological change through time: Comparison of an Archaic Native American population with modern populations. *Anatomical Records* 226: 307–313.

Chan, A., Crowder, C., and Rogers, T. 2007. Variation in Cortical Bone Histology within the Human Femur and its Impact on Estimating Age at Death. *American Journal of Physical Anthropology* 132: 80–88.

Cho, H., Stout, S. D., Madsen, R. W., and Streeter, M. A. 2002. Population-specific histological age-estimating method: A model for known African-American and European-American skeletal remains. *Journal of Forensic Sciences* 47(1): 12–18.

Clarke, D. F. 1987. Histological and Radiographic Variation in the Parietal Bone in a Cadaveric Population. Ph.D. thesis, Anatomy Department, The University of Queensland.

Cool, S. M., Hendrikz, J. K., and Wood, W. B. 1995. Microscopic age changes in the human occipital bone. *Journal of Forensic Sciences* 40(5): 789–796.

Cooper, D. L., Matyas, J. R., Katzenberg, and Hallgrimsson, M. A. 2004. Comparison of microcomputed tomographic and microradiographic measurements of cortical bone porosity. *Calcified Tissue International* 74: 437–447.

Cooper, D. L., Turinsky, A. L., Sensen, C. W., and Hallgrimsson, B. 2003. Quantitative 3D analysis of the canal network in cortical bone by microcomputed tomography. *Anatomical Record* 274B: 169–179.

Crowder, C. M. 2005. *Evaluating the Use of Quantitative Bone Histology to Estimate Adult Age at Death*. Ph.D. dissertation, University of Toronto, Toronto (ON).

Curtis, J. 2004. Estimation of Age at Death from the Microscopic Appearance of the Frontal Bone. Masters thesis, University of Indianapolis, Indiana.

Daley, R. M., Saxon, L., Turner, C. H., Robling, A. G., and Bass, S. L. 2004. The relationship between muscle size and bone geometry during growth and in response to exercise. *Bone* 3: 281–287.

Drusini, A. G. 1996. Sampling location in cortical bone histology. *American Journal of Physical Anthropology*. 100: 609–610.

Dudar, J. C., Pfeiffer, S., and Saunders, S. R. 1993. Evaluation of morphological and histological adult skeletal age-at-death estimation techniques using ribs. *Journal of Forensic Sciences* 38(3): 677–685.

Dupras, T. L., and Pfeiffer, S. K. 1996. Determination of sex from adult human ribs. *Canadian Society of Forensic Science* 29(4): 221–231.

Ericksen, M. F. 1973. *Age-Related Bone Remodeling in Three Aboriginal American Populations*. Ph.D. dissertation. George Washington University, Washington, D.C.

———. 1991. Histological estimation of age at death using the anterior cortex of the femur. *American Journal of Physical Anthropology* 84: 171–179.

Frost, H. M. 1969. Tetracycline based histological analysis of bone remodeling. *Calcified Tissue Research* 3: 211–237.

Inque, M., Tanaka, H., Moriwake, T., Oka, M., Sekiguchi, C., and Seino, Y. 2000. Altered biochemical markers of bone turnover in humans during 120 days of bed rest. *Bone* 26(3): 281–286.

İşcan, M. Y., Loth, S. R., and Wright, R. K. 1984. Age estimation from the rib by phase analysis: White males. *Journal of Forensic Sciences* 29: 1094–1104.

———. 1985. Age estimation from the rib by phase analysis: White females. *Journal of Forensic Sciences* 30: 853–863.

Iwaniec, U. T., Crenshaw, T .D., Scheninger, M. J., Stout, S. D., and Ericksen, M. F. 1998. Methods for improving the efficiency of estimating total osteon density in the human anterior mid-diaphyseal femur. *American Journal of Physical Anthropology* 107: 13–24.

Jackes, M. 2000. Building the basis for paleodemo-graphic analysis: Adult age determination, in M. A. Katzenberg and S. R. Saunders (eds.), *Biological Anthropology of the Human Skeleton*, pp. 417–466. New York: Wiley-Liss, Inc.

Jackes, M., Sherburne, R., Lubell, D., Barker, C., and Wayman, M. 2001. Destruction of microstructure in archaeological bone: A case study from Portugal. *International Journal of Osteoarchaeology* 11: 415–432.

Jans, M. M. E., Nielsen-Marsh, C. M., Smith, C. I., Collins, M. J., and Kars, H. 2004. Characterisation of microbial attack on archaeological bone. *Journal of Archaeological Science* 31: 87–95.

Jett, S., Wu, K., and Frost, H. 1967. Tetracycline-based histological measurement of cortical-endosteal bone formation in normal and osteoporotic rib. *Henry Ford Hospital Medical Bulletin* 15(4): 325–344.

Kerley, E. R. 1965. The microscopic determination of age in human bone. *American Journal of Physical Anthropology*. 23: 149–164.

Kerley, E. R., and Ubelaker, D. H. 1978. Revisions in the microscopic method of estimating age at death in human cortical bone. *American Journal of Physical Anthropology*. 49: 545–546.

Krøll, J., and Saxtrup, O. 2000. On the use of regression for the estimation of human biological age. *Biogerontology* 1: 363–368.

Landeros, O., and Frost, H. M. 1964. The cross section size of the osteon. *Henry Ford Hospital Medical Bulletin* 12(2): 517–525.

Lazenby, R. A. 1984. Inherent deficiencies in cortical bone microstructural age estimation techniques. *International Journal of Skeletal Research* 9-11: 95–103.

Loth, S. R. 1995. Age assessment of the Spitalfields cemetery population by rib phase analysis. *American Journal of Human Biology* 7(4): 465–471.

Lovejoy, C. O., Meindl, R. S., Pryzbeck, T. R., and Mensforth, R. P. 1985. Chronological metamorphosis of the auricular surface of the ilium: A new method for the determination of age at death. *American Journal of Physical Anthropology* 68: 15–28.

Maat, G. J., Maes, A., Aarents, J., and Nagelkerke, N. 2006. Histological age prediction from the femur in a contemporary Dutch sample. *Journal of Forensic Sciences* 51: 230–237.

Mulhern, D. M. 2000. Rib remodeling dynamics in a skeletal population from Kulubnarti, Nubia. *American Journal of Physical Anthropology* 111: 519–530.

Mulhern, D. M., and Jones, E. B. 2005. Test of revised method of age estimation from the auricular surface of the ilium. *American Journal of Physical Anthropology* 126: 61–65.

Mulhern, D., and Van Gerven, D. P. 1997. Patterns of femoral bone remodeling dynamics in a medieval Nubian population. *American Journal of Physical Anthropology* 104: 133–146.

Narasaki, S. 1990. Estimation of age at death by femoral osteon remodeling: Application of Thompson's core technique to modern Japanese. *Journal of the Anthropological Society of Nippon* 98(1): 29–38.

Ortner, D. J. 1975. Aging effects on osteon remodeling. *Calcified Tissue Research* 18: 27–36.

Parfitt, A. M., Drezner, M. K., Glorieux, F. H., Kanis, J. H., Malluche, H., Meunier, P. J., Ott, S. M., and Recker, R. R. 1987. Bone histomorphometry: standardization of nomenclature, symbols, and units. *Journal of Bone Mineral Research* 2: 595–610.

Pfeiffer, S. 1992. Cortical bone age estimates from historically known adults. *Zeitschrift für Morphologie und Anthropologie* 79(1): 1–10.

———. 1998. Variability in osteon size in recent human populations. *American Journal of Physical Anthropology* 106: 219–227.

———. 2000. Palaeohistology: Health and disease, in M. A. Katzenberg and S. R. Saunders (eds.), *Biological Anthropology of the Human Skeleton*, pp. 287–302. New York: Wiley-Liss, Inc.

Pfeiffer, S., Crowder, C., Harrington, L., and Brown, M. 2006. Secondary osteons and Haversian canal dimensions as behavioral indicators. *American Journal of Physical Anthropology* 131: 460–468.

Pfeiffer, S., Lazenby, R., and Chiang, J. 1995. Cortical remodeling data are affected by sampling location. *American Journal of Physical Anthropology* 96: 89–92.

Pirok, D., Ramser, J., Takahashi, H., Villanueva, A. R., and Frost, H. 1966. Normal histological, tetracycline and dynamic parameters in human, mineralized bone sections. *Henry Ford Hospital Medical Bulletin* 14: 195–218.

Pratte, D. G., and Pfeiffer, S. 1999. Histological age estimation of a cadaveral sample of diverse origins. *Canadian Society Forensic Science* 32(4): 155–167.

Richman, E. A., Ortner, D. J., and Schulter-Ellis, F. P. 1979. Differences in intracortical bone remodeling in three aboriginal American populations: Possible dietary factors. *Calcified Tissue International* 28: 209–214.

Robling, A. 1998. Histomorphometric Assessment of Mechanical Loading History from Human Skeletal Remains: The Relation between Micromorphology and Macromorphology at the Femoral Midshaft. Ph.D. dissertation, University of Missouri, Columbia.

Robling, A., and Stout, S. 2000. Histomorphometry of human cortical bone: Applications to age estimation, in M. A. Katzenberg and S. R. Saunders (eds.),

Biological Anthropology of the Human Skeleton, pp. 187–213. New York: Wiley-Liss, Inc.

Santoro, F., and Frost, H. 1967. Osteoid seams and resorption spaces in standard samples of human 6th and 11th ribs. *Henry Ford Hospital Medical Bulletin* 15(6): 241–246.

Saunders, S. R., Fitzgerald, C., Rogers, T., Dudar, C., and McKillop, H. 1992. A test of several methods of skeletal age estimation using a documented archaeological sample. *Canadian Society of Forensic Science* 25(2): 97–118.

Singh, I. J., and Gunberg, D. L. 1970. Estimation of age at death in human males from quantitative histology of bone fragments. *American Journal of Physical Anthropology* 33: 373–382.

Skedros, J. G., Hunt, K. J., and Bloebaum, R. D. 2004. Relationships of loading history and structural and material characteristics of bone: Development of the mule deer calcaneus. *Journal of Morphology* 259: 281–307.

Skedros, J. G., Sybrowsky, C. L., Parry, T. R., and Bloebaum, R. D. 2003. Regional differences in cortical bone organization and microdamage prevalence in Rocky Mountain Mule Deer. *Anatomical Record* Part A 274A: 837–850.

Stout, S. D. 1986. The use of bone histomorphometry in skeletal identification: The case of Francisco Pizarro. *Journal of Forensic Sciences* 31(1): 296–300.

Stout, S. D., Dietz, W. H., İşcan, M. Y., and Loth, S. R. 1994. Estimation of age at death using cortical histomorphometry of the sternal end of the fourth rib. *Journal of Forensic Sciences* 39(3): 778–784.

Stout, S. D., and Gehlert, S. J. 1980. The relative accuracy and reliability of histological aging methods. *Forensic Science International* 15: 181–190.

———. 1982. Effects of field size when using Kerley's histological method for determination of age at death. *American Journal of Physical Anthropology* 58: 123–125.

Stout, S. D., Marcello, A. P., and Perotti, B. 1996. Brief communication: A test and correction of the clavicle method of Stout and Paine for histological age estimation of skeletal remains. *American Journal of Physical Anthropology* 100: 139–142.

Stout, S. D., and Paine, P. R. 1992. Brief communication: Histological age estimation using rib and clavicle. *American Journal of Physical Anthropology* 87: 111–115.

Stout, S. D., and Simmons, D. J. 1979. Use of histology in ancient bone research. *Yearbook of Physical Anthropology* 44: 263–270.

Stout, S. D., and Stanley, S. C. 1991. Percent osteonal bone verses osteon counts: The variable of choice for estimating age at death. *American Journal of Physical Anthropology* 86: 515–519.

Takahashi, H., Epker, B., and Frost, H. M. 1965. Relation between age and size of osteons in man. *Henry Ford Hospital Medical Bulletin* 13: 25–31.

Tersigni, M. T. 2005. Serial Long Bone Histology: Inter- and Intra- Bone Age Estimation. Ph.D. dissertation, University of Tennessee.

Thompson, D. D. 1979. The core technique in the determination of age at death in skeletons. *Journal of Forensic Sciences* 24(4): 902–915.

———. 1981. Microscopic determination of age at death in an autopsy series. *Journal of Forensic Sciences* 26: 470–475.

Thompson, D. D., and Galvin, C. A. 1983. Estimation of age at death by tibial osteon remodeling in an autopsy series. *Forensic Science International* 22: 203–211.

Tommerup, L., Raab, D., Crenshaw, T., and Smith, E. 1993. Does weight-bearing exercise affect non-weight-bearing bone? *Journal of Bone Mineral Research* 8(9): 1053–1058.

United States Supreme Court in Daubert v. Merrell Dow Pharmaceuticals, Inc., 509 US. 579. 1993.

Walker, R. A. 1990. *Assessments of Human Cortical Bone Dynamics and Skeletal Age at Death from Femoral Cortical Histology.* Ph.D. dissertation, Kent state University, Ohio.

Watanabe, Y., Konishi, M., Shimada, M., Ohara, H., and Iwamoto, S. 1998. Estimation of age from the femur of Japanese cadavers. *Forensic Science International* 98: 55–65.

Wu, K., Jett, S., and Frost, H. 1967. Bone resorption rates in physiological, senile and postmenopausal osteoporoses. *Journal of Laboratory and Clinical Medicine* 69: 810–818.

Wu, K., Schubeck, H., Frost, M., and Villanueva, A. 1970. Haversian bone formation rates determined by a new method in a mastodon, and in human diabetes mellitus and osteoporosis. *Calcified Tissue Research* 6: 204–219.

Yoshino, M., Imaizumi, K., Miyasaka, S., and Sueshige, S. 1994. Histological estimation of age at death using microradiographs of humeral compact bone. *Forensic Science International* 64: 191–198.

20

STATURE ESTIMATION

P. Willey

An individual's stature is a frequently measured and readily observable biological trait. Along with age, sex, ancestry, and weight, stature is one of the first things we notice when meeting a person, and it is frequently included in antemortem medical, civilian, and military records. Because stature results from the accumulative interaction of genetics and environmental influences during growth and development, contemporary and past populations' statures have been examined by biological anthropologists as indicative of subadult well-being. In addition, height has been employed to assess the health of individuals and used as an indicator of population stress. Among other useful information, stature of skeletal remains or bodies assists authorities' efforts to identify remains of unknown individuals. With other biological parameters, including those mentioned above, stature of the deceased is one of the biological assessments that may prove critical in including or excluding the possible identity of remains.

The purpose of this chapter is to describe the process of estimating adult stature from skeletal remains and comparing that estimation with antemortem height. Stature is estimated in two ways: (1) measuring all bones constituting the components of stature, summing those measurements and adding a soft-tissue component; and (2) employing regression formulae with the measurement of a complete bone or a bone fragment. Several issues affect

the accuracy of stature comparisons; these issues include decreasing stature with adult aging and the reliability of antemortem records. This chapter also discusses topics needing additional research.

Complete Skeletons

The method requiring a complete skeleton, promoted by Dwight (1894), employs all skeletal elements constituting height and is sometimes called the "anatomical" method. Current applications of this approach usually employ the techniques of Fully (1956) or Fully and Pineau (1960). Using these techniques has been supported in recent decades by several studies (for example, Berg, Casey, and Raasch 1985; Bidmos 2005; Lundy 1985, 1988a), although Raxter, Auerbach, and Ruff (2006) recently revised this method.

The Fully method of stature estimation from the skeleton is more intuitive and obvious than the other principal approach. When using the entire skeleton, one measures all the skeletal elements constituting stature and sums those measurements; to that sum, a soft tissue "correction" is added.

First, measurements are taken. The measurements (Figure 20.1) consist of cranial height (basion-bregma), heights of the anterior vertebrae bodies (Cervical 3 through Lumbar 5), anterior height of the first sacral segment, bicondylar femoral length, physiological tibia length (excluding

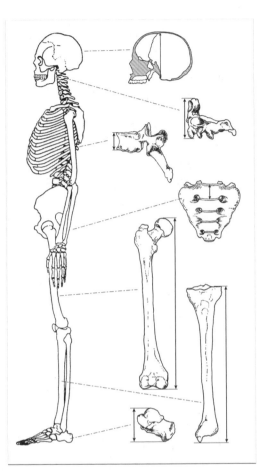

Figure 20.1 Measurements involved in estimating stature using the whole skeleton.

the superior tibial spines and including the medial malleous), and height of the articulated talus-calcaneus (oriented to include the angle of the foot's longitudinal arch). One deviation from this straightforward procedure concerns the atlas and the axis (C1 and C2) measurements; the atlas is omitted, and the axis's body, including the dens epistrophis (odontoid process), is measured.

All these measurements are summed, and based on that sum, a soft-tissue correction figure is added (Table 20.1 on the next page). The additional soft-

Whole skeleton-stature estimation for remains identified as Vincent Charley, 7th Cavalry Trooper. Summed measurements in parentheses indicate estimations of some vertebral body heights.	
Segment	*Length (cm)*
Skull height (bregma-basion)	13.0
Cervical body heights (summed)	(10.7)
Thoracic body heights (summed)	(24.8)
Lumbar body heights (summed)	14.2
Sacral segment 1 height	3.1
Bicondylar femur length	48.2
Physiological tibia length	40.9
Talus and calcaneous height	<u>7.2</u>
Total skeletal element heights	162.1
Soft tissue addition (from Table 20.1)	<u>10.5</u>
Stature estimation	172.6

Estimating Stature Using the Whole Skeleton

Stature was estimated using the entire skeleton of remains identified as those of Farrier Vincent Charley, a 7th Cavalry trooper who died during the Battle of the Little Bighorn (in Montana, United States) in June 1876. The skeleton was excavated and measured in the 1990s, and those measurements are presented in the table above. Making the estimation more challenging, five of the vertebrae are either missing or have incomplete anterior bodies; those measurements were estimated by interpolation (indicated in parentheses in the table). Once the elements and estimations constituting skeletal stature were summed (skeletal total = 162.1 cm), a soft-tissue figure (11.5 cm for this skeletal sum; see Table 20.1) was added to the total, yielding an estimated stature of 172.6 cm (67.9 in).

Farrier Charley's reenlistment information, recorded three months before his death at the age of 27 years, indicates that he was 5 feet 10¼ in (178.4 cm) tall (Nichols 2000: 55). The skeletal estimation of 172.6 cm is 6 cm (2.3 in) shorter than Charley's recorded stature—a surprising discrepancy for a technique that should be the most accurate. Although unlikely based on the precise stature recorded at reenlistment (noted to a quarter of an inch), the antemortem stature possibly is incorrect.

Table 20.1 Soft-tissue additions for skeletal-element sum used in whole-skeleton approach (from Fully and Pineau 1960: 145).

Skeletal Sum	Soft-Tissue Addition
≤153.5 cm	10.0 cm
153.6–165.5 cm	10.5 cm
≥165.5 cm	11.5 cm

tissue figure differs depending on the sum of skeletal element height measurements.

There are advantages and disadvantages using the full-skeleton technique to estimate stature. Advantageously, it can be employed regardless of the ancestry or sex of the individual. In addition, whole-skeleton stature estimation should be more accurate than other techniques, even when there are anomalous numbers of vertebrae (Lundy 1988b). If the individual is unusually proportioned (for example, long trunk and short limbs), the whole-skeleton technique should still provide an accurate estimation of stature.

Disadvantages of the technique include requiring complete elements and a complete skeleton—unless the analyst is prepared to estimate or to interpolate heights of missing elements. In addition, taking the 29 measurements required to estimate stature of the normal skeleton is tedious and time consuming. Many of these disadvantages are overcome by using an alternate approach.

Complete Limb Bones

Estimating stature using a limb-bone length measurement in regression formula was developed by Pearson (1899) and was among the earliest—if not the earliest—use of regression in anthropology. It is sometimes called the "mathematical" method of estimating height and is widely used today with a variety of bones.

The method is simple. It requires measuring the length of a limb bone, selecting the appropriate regression formula by sex and ancestry, inserting the measurement into the formula, and calculating the estimated stature. The standard formula follows the format:

$$\text{stature} = a + bx + \text{SE},$$

where a is the line's Y axis intercept,
b is the line's slope,
x is the limb bone length, and
SE is the standard error.

Estimating Stature Using the Regression Method

Using measurements of the same skeleton for which stature was estimated in the previous example (Farrier Vincent Charley, a 27-year-old who died in the Battle of the Little Bighorn), stature is estimated with a regression formula and limb-bone length. Trotter and Gleser's (1958: 84, Tab. 3) widely used stature estimation formula for White males for a single limb bone includes a formula for the left fibula, the limb bone with the smallest standard error and thus the most accurate stature estimator. The formula and calculations follow:

stature = 2.59 x (maximum left fibula length in cm) + 75.37 with a standard error of + 3.83.

Inserting the measurement of the left fibula from the skeleton identified as Farrier Charley's, the equation is as follows:

stature = 2.59 (40.2) + 75.37 = 179.488 cm (70.66 in).

The resulting estimation (179.488 cm, 70.66 in) is 1 cm (about ½ in) larger than Farrier Charley's recorded reenlistment height of 5 feet 10¼ in (Nichols 2000: 55). Especially when the estimation distribution is considered (95% confidence interval of + 7.51 cm [+ 2.96 in], following Giles and Klepinger 1988), the estimation fits Charley's antemortem record well.

Yet another technique with a different regression formula can be applied. Inserting the left fibula length measurement in FORDISC's (Ousley and Jantz 2005) stature function for 19th-century White males, the resulting stature estimation is 71.1 in (180.59 cm, with a 95% prediction interval of + 7.11 cm [2.8 in]). That result is similar to the one calculated using Trotter and Gleser's formula, as well as Farrier Charley's reenlistment stature, but both differ from the stature estimation based on the whole skeleton that was presented previously.

Limb-bone measurements are usually maximum lengths; the tibia measurement, however, is more complicated and is discussed below.

In addition to formulae for individual limb bones, there are also regression formulae for multiple limb bones. In multiple-regression applications, two or more limb-bone lengths are multiplied by coefficients, and a scalar (*a* in the formula above) is added to estimate stature. Whether univariate or multiple variate formulae are used, the formula with the smallest standard error is the most accurate and should be employed (see below).

Formulae are available by sex for a number of populations. In the United States, Trotter and Gleser's (1952; 1958; Trotter 1970) formulae are most often employed. They include large samples of U.S. Black and White males, and smaller samples of U.S. Mongoloid, Mexican, and Puerto Rican males as well as U.S. Black and White females.

An innovative approach using regression formulae is the stature estimation function in the software package FORDISC (Ousley and Jantz 2005). After one enters a limb-bone length in a screen and selects the stature option, FORDISC calculates statures for Blacks and Whites based on Trotter and Gleser's (1952) World War II sample. FORDISC also estimates Forensic Stature (antemortem stature based on driver's license, booking records, or medical documents) for Black and White females and males, and Hispanic males.

Statistical Fundamentals

Regression formulae are based on statistical calculations and assumptions. Assumptions and mistakes associated with employing regression formulae include using the single-best formula, estimating the confidence interval, and misuse of "range."

After one controls for sex and ancestry, the most accurate formula is the one with the smallest standard error. The formula with the smallest standard error usually employs an element of the lower limb or combined elements including the lower limb bones (Trotter and Gleser 1958), but whatever the element or elements—lower limb bones or not—the formula with the smallest standard error is the most accurate. Unfortunately, some practitioners are seduced into calculating several formulae and then averaging those estimations, thus reducing the accuracy of their estimation. This erroneous practice of averaging should be avoided; the formula with the smallest standard error should be used.

Another frequent and erroneous practice is using the standard error to provide a confidence

interval as if a confidence interval and a standard deviation were identical. It has been noted (Giles and Klepinger 1988) that the standard error is not the same as the standard deviation and therefore should not be employed as such. The prediction interval associated with a regression is a curvilinear, double parabolic distribution, not linear, as simply doubling the standard error implies. If an accurate confidence interval is required, then a confidence interval should be calculated and appropriately applied.[1] From a practical perspective, however, the confidence interval increases little within three standard deviations of the mean bone length (Ousley 1995; Ousley and Jantz 1996: 12).

An additional issue must be considered when presenting variation around a regression estimation. Using confidence intervals assumes that the regression parameters are known and similar to those employed in establishing the regression formula. But the origins of many unknown remains are not yet determined, let alone whether they were from the same population the regression formulae portray. A different assessment stature estimation variation is more appropriate: prediction intervals. As a consequence, FORDISC software provides 90% and 95% prediction intervals for its stature estimations (Ousley and Jantz 2005). Because prediction intervals do not assume that the same parameters employed to establish the formulae are appropriate for the estimation, prediction intervals are necessarily larger than confidence intervals.

As a final statistical warning: whether standard errors or confidence intervals are employed, the estimations are intervals not the misused term *range*. In statistics, a range is the difference between the maximum and the minimum observations—for example, the range of the interval with a maximum value of 12 and a minimum value of 5 is (12 − 5 =) 7.

Corrections

Limb-bone measurements are straightforward; in most standards they are the maximum lengths. There is an exception, however: Trotter's tibia measurements appear to be in error. Jantz, Hunt, and Meadows (1994, 1995) concluded that Trotter misreported tibiae measurements in most of her samples. The standard practice (and Trotter's description of how she measured tibia length) is from the lateral portion of the lateral condyle to the most distal end, *including* the medial malleous. However, when her measurements of the Terry Collection tibiae were remeasured, Trotter's measurements averaged 13 mm shorter than the remeasurements. Jantz, Hunt, and Meadows (1994, 1995) concluded that the difference was because Trotter's measurements *excluded* the medial malleolus. In addition to the Terry Collection specimens, Trotter and Gleser's World War II and their Korean War tibia measurements appear to be too short. As a consequence of these apparent errors, the resulting stature estimations based on Trotter and Gleser's 1952 tibiae formulae are 2.5–3.0 cm too short, depending on the ancestry, sex, and formula involved.

Considering these mismeasurements, Jantz, Hunt, and Meadows (1994, 1995) recommend either measuring the tibia as Trotter apparently did (that is, excluding the medial malleolus) or using the femur instead of the tibia. Finally, they recommend avoiding the Trotter and Gleser (1958) tibia and tibia-involved formulae altogether.

Advantages and Disadvantages

There are advantages as well as disadvantages to using regression formulae. The major advantages are that only one or at most several bones are needed, and measurements are simple. The calculations are easy and quick.

There are also disadvantages to the regression approach. Accuracy of the regression formulae estimations relies on consistent proportionality of limb-bone lengths to stature. Because body proportions may vary by sex, ancestry, and temporal period, accurate stature estimation requires correctly determining those parameters beforehand and having appropriate regression formulae for that sex, ancestry, and time period. Fortunately, there are regression formulae available for both sexes of many different populations and temporal periods. Individual proportional peculiarities, however, are an issue that is difficult to overcome with these formulae. A final disadvantage is that a complete limb bone is required.

There are two strategies to overcome the requirement for complete limb bones: estimating limb-bone length from fragmentary bones or using non-limb bones to estimate stature. Those approaches are presented next.

Fragmentary Limb Bones

One problem with both whole-skeleton and whole-limb-bone methods is that the requisite complete limb bones may not be available. This issue was anticipated by Seitz (1923) and later documented by other researchers, most notably Steele (1970). The solution to the problem is to estimate the length of a limb bone using the fragment that is available

and to apply a regression formula. Then, that estimated limb-bone length is used as if the bone were complete in another regression formula, as described previously. Because this approach relies on two estimations (limb-bone length and stature), it is less accurate than the previous approaches and should be avoided if possible.

Elements Other Than Limb Bones

As an additional problem, whole limb bones or even fragmentary limb bones are not always present. To overcome this obstacle, elements other than limb bones have been employed to estimate stature. The present discussion is limited to regression approaches with alternative approaches considered later.

During the past several decades, regression formulae have been calculated for estimating stature from measurements of the cranium (Chiba and Terazawa 1998), vertebrae (Tibbetts 1981), clavicle, scapula, innominate (Peng and Zhu 1983), metacarpals (Meadows and Jantz 1992), hand phalanges (Zhu 1983), tarsals (Holland 1995) and metatarsals (Byers, Akoshima, and Curran 1989). These techniques may prove useful in cases involving skeletons lacking limb bones or limb-bone fragments. A problem with their application, however, is that their stature prediction intervals are greater than that typically associated with estimations from limb bones; thus stature estimation is less accurate with these elements than with the use of limb bones.

Additional Statistical Approaches

Some researchers have utilized both regression and whole-skeleton approaches to estimate stature. This combination of approaches has been applied, for example, to the spine. Segments of the spine were measured on corpses or cadavers, and those segments regressed on stature (Jason and Taylor 1995; Terazawa et al. 1985; Terazawa et al. 1990), or individual vertebral bodies were measured then summed, and then that sum was regressed on stature (Tibbetts 1981).

Another approach, the stature-estimation method requiring the fewest arithmetic steps, is using ratio. The ratio between stature and an element length (for example, femur) is calculated to establish a coefficient (for example, Feldesman, Kleckner, and Lundy 1990). To estimate stature, then, a limb-length measurement is employed in the ratio.

There are several advantages associated with the ratio approach, which has been said by some to be superior to regression formulae. In addition to the simplicity of calculations, Feldesman and coauthors (1990; Feldesman and Fountain 1996) write that there are small, if any differences, by sex or ancestry, for at least some of the ratios. Thus, according to these authorities, there is no need to determine either sex or ancestry before applying certain ratios for the estimation of stature.

Yet the approach applied by Feldesman and colleagues has been criticized. The femur/stature ratio overestimates statures, especially that of taller individuals. It has a greater prediction interval and therefore is less accurate than those associated with regression estimations (Meadows and Jantz 1995: 765–766). The femur/stature ratio is a poorer estimator of stature than the more widely used regression approach (Konigsberg et al. 1998).

Age-Related Stature Decrease

Regardless of which stature-estimation method is employed, the age of the individual may affect the individual's living stature. As adults age, their statures decrease from their young-adult maximum. Although research supports the existence of age-related stature decrease, there are questions concerning the age of onset, rate of loss, and whether sex or ancestry influence the decrease.

The results of early work by Trotter and Gleser (1951) using Terry's Anatomical Collection (cadavers of females and males, Blacks and Whites from the early 20th-century Midwestern United States) indicated that stature decrease begins around 30 years of age. However, more recent analyses using self-reported maximum statures in a sample of White U.S. retirees (Galloway 1988) and a longitudinal study among Southwest U.S. Anglo-White females and Boston veteran males (Giles 1991) found that age-related stature decrease begins 15 years later than Trotter and Gleser claim, commencing at about 45 years of age (Figure 20.2).

The pioneering work of Trotter and Gleser (1951) determined that once stature decrease begins, it proceeds in a linear fashion at 0.6 mm per year (see Figure 20.2). A more recent study, however, found that the rate of loss is more than twice as fast as that Trotter and Gleser reported, or 1.6 mm per year (Galloway 1988). Giles (1991), in a longitudinal study, determined that once stature decrease begins, it occurs at a variable rate, not a constant linear decrease.

The pioneering study found stature decrease to be homogeneous by sex (Trotter and Gleser 1951), at least in proportion to stature (Galloway 1988). However, the longitudinal study reported sex differences (Giles 1991: 900, Tab. 1; Klepinger and Giles 1998: 435, Tab. 4), showing that males lose stature more rapidly than females do until about 75 years, when the trend reverses (see Figure 20.2).

Finally, the pioneering work determined that age-related stature loss is similar for both Blacks and Whites (Trotter and Gleser 1951). More recent studies (Galloway 1988; Giles 1991) employed only Whites, and no other forensic-related tests of ancestry differences in stature loss have been conducted.

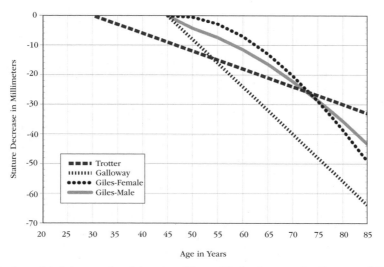

Figure 20.2 Age-related decrease in adult stature. "Trotter" is the decrease that Trotter and Gleser (1951) derived; "Galloway" the decrease Galloway (1988) calculated; "Giles-Fe" the decrease Giles (1991) found for females and "Giles-Ma" the male decrease.

How is age-related decrease applied when one is estimating the stature from the remains of middle-aged and older adults? It depends on the goal of the estimation, which may in turn depend on the kind of antemortem stature records available for comparisons with postmortem stature estimations. In practical terms, Galloway (1988) recommends reporting both maximum height (stature before commencement of age-related decrease) and height following age-related height loss. Thus, whatever antemortem stature record is available, both statures have been estimated and are available for comparison.

Antemortem Stature Records

Another variable that affects the reliability of comparisons between antemortem records and stature estimations is the accuracy of antemortem stature information. Accurate antemortem stature records are critical for comparing stature estimations. The problems associated with measuring antemortem stature, such as time of day, measuring technique, and interobserver error, have frequently been addressed (for example, Giles and Hutchinson 1991: 766–767). The subject of this section is a related matter; it considers the nature of antemortem records and how accurately they reflect actual height.

As a warning of the *in*accuracy of antemortem stature records, Snow and Williams (1971) noted the differences in stature measurements of one adult male. He was measured 19 times by medical and legal authorities during a 20-year period. The measurements varied from 62 to 67 inches, a five-inch range. These differences were not attributable to age-related decrease alone and are indicative of the inaccuracy of antemortem stature records, even those measured by authorities who should have an interest in accuracy.

Aside from differences in official measurements, there are distortions of self-reported heights. Employing the often-used driver's license (DL) and comparing its recorded statures with the living person's measured stature, Willey and Falsetti (1991) found a tendency for college students' DLs to overreport their statures (average overreporting of 0.965 cm). Males' DLs overreport their statures to a greater degree (average overreporting of 1.321 cm) than females' do (average overreporting of 0.574 cm). The distortions vary tremendously, from one male whose DL underreported his stature by 26.6 cm to another whose DL overreported his stature by 14.7 cm.

The problems of self-reported statures were investigated using a large U.S. Army personnel sample that was compared to U.S. Health and Nutrition Examination surveys. Examining self-reported statures of older individuals as well as those of shorter and taller groups, older individuals (>45 years) tended to exaggerate stature, most likely compounded with age-related stature decrease (Giles and Hutchinson 1991). The investigators also found that taller individuals do not tend to overestimate their statures, instead reporting their stature more accurately than do medium and shorter individuals. It may be noteworthy, however, that short (<60 in) and tall (>78 in) individuals are excluded from military induction and thus excluded from the sample (Giles and Hutchinson 1991: 771).

To quantify the degree of distortion associated with self-reporting and other antemortem stature records, Ousley (1995) developed the term *forensic stature*. Forensic stature is the antemortem stature information available for a missing person, which in his sample was usually obtained from DL, booking, or medical records. Ousley concludes that forensic statures are less precise than Trotter and Gleser's formulae indicate, and he recommends using a broad estimation interval in casework.

Based on these studies, forensic anthropologists should present a broad stature-estimation interval (for example, 90% prediction or confidence interval). Forensic anthropologists should also consider the measuring context, the measurer, and the reporting agency. Additionally, the source of the antemortem stature record should be identified and considered when one is making comparisons to estimated stature based on skeletal remains.

Topics for Future Research

There have been recent great strides and innovative approaches to estimating stature from bones. The frequency of publication during the past decade indicates the importance of stature estimation in forensic anthropology, and if the trend continues, much will be learned in future decades.

First and perhaps foremost, there must be continued development and enhancement of current techniques. Research in stature estimation during the next decade will improve statistical sophistication, employ additional elements, document age-related stature decrease, and employ imaging technologies, thus expanding many of the classic studies. In addition, forensic interest in population groups is changing, and additional research will be needed to estimate accurately their statures. In particular, subgroups from Central and South America, Eastern Europe, Southwest Asia, and Africa will require attention.

There are two additional areas ripe for stature-estimation research. One area that has been largely overlooked is estimating stature from soft-tissue-covered remains. In mass disasters, tissue-covered bodies often dominate the recovered portions, and accurate stature estimation may be possible without time-consuming maceration. It is also applicable to other recently deceased individuals, especially body segments with surviving soft tissue.

A number of recent studies have used body segments to estimate stature. Most emphasize vertebral column components (for example, Jason and Taylor 1995), limb segments (for instance, Nath, Garg, and Krishan 1991), hands (for example, Abdel-Malek et al. 1990), and feet (for instance, Giles and Vallandigham 1991). These few studies are but the tip of the potential body-segment iceberg, however. There are a great number of anthropometric surveys for many different populations, and many stature-correlated dimensions have the potential to provide useful formulae. In a preliminary assessment, Adams and Herrmann (2006) found lower correlations between body segments and stature than between limb-bone lengths and stature, suggesting that body fat obscures anthropometric landmarks. They conclude, nevertheless, that body segments may be employed to estimate stature but with less accuracy than whole bones.

Another area demanding attention concerns growth-related stature estimations. The vast majority of current stature estimation techniques are for adults. Yet in many forensic contexts, infants, children, and adolescents (subadults) are recovered, and they, too, require identification.

Little work on subadult stature estimation has been performed. Techniques are available for estimating subadult stature using diaphyseal lengths of Finnish and U.S. samples (Telkka, Palkama, and Virtama 1962; Visser 1998), fleshed tibia of Britains (Zorab, Prime, and Harrison 1963, 1964), and metacarpal X rays for Japanese and Guatemalan subadults (Himes, Yarborough, and Martorell 1977; Kimura 1992). Most of these studies, with few exceptions, are based on cross-sectional data.

One of the challenges of estimating subadult stature is obvious from this brief list. Few subadult stature-estimation techniques have been developed, and those that do exist are applicable only to a limited number of populations and a limited number of elements. Growth allometry (including proportional changes among limbs and limbs-trunk ratios during growth) is an additional variable beyond the secular, ancestry, and sex effects that influence adult stature estimation. Nevertheless, applying *adult* stature-estimation regressions to estimate subadult height is inadvisable (Imrie and Wyburn

1958), although some authorities apparently have made such estimations (Giles and Klepinger 1988: 1220–1221; Snow and Luke 1984: 272).

The previously described whole-skeleton technique might be applied to subadult skeletons if they are complete, including epiphyses, and if an accurate soft-tissue figure can be established. A more productive approach would probably be employing limb-bone diaphyseal lengths in regression formulae to estimate stature, such as in Smith's (2006) preliminary work.

Conclusion

Stature estimation of remains is an important component in forensic identification. The approaches used most often are the whole-skeleton and regression formulae involving limb bones. Both approaches provide relatively accurate estimations, although there are issues involving secular trends and the effects of age, sex, and ancestry in regression formulae. For less complete remains, less accurate techniques, including those that rely on fragmentary limb bones and non-limb-bone elements, may be employed. The future holds great promise for continued improvements of traditional approaches to stature estimation and wonderful potential for new ones.

Acknowledgments

I appreciate Soren Blau and Douglas Ubelaker's invitation to write this chapter and their editorial suggestions. Preliminary research in stature estimation was made possible by a California State University Research Mini-Grant during fall 1999; it involved preparation of a paper presented that year at the Smithsonian Institution–Central Identification Laboratory, Hawai'i, Conference on Advances in Personal Identification in Mass Disasters, Honolulu. George Thompson, then of Chico State's Merriam Library Interlibrary Loan/Reference Library sections, ably provided many of the hard-to-find articles. Gil Huston read the manuscript and made valuable suggestions. Figures 20.1 and 20.2 were rendered by Judy Stolen.

Note

1. See Giles and Klepinger (1988: 1220) for steps in calculating the confidence interval.

References

Abdel-Malek, A. K., Ahmed, A. M., El, S. A., El Sharkawi, A., El, M. A., and El Hamid, N. A. 1990.

Prediction of stature from hand measurements. *Forensic Science International* 46: 181–187.

Adams, B. J., and Herrmann, N. P. 2006. Estimating living stature from selected anthropometric (soft tissue) measurements: How do these compare with osteometric (skeletal) measurements? *Proceedings of the American Academy of Forensic Sciences* 12: 279–280.

Berg, S., Casey, M., and Raasch, F. 1985. The mathematical versus anatomical methods of stature estimate from long bones. *American Journal of Forensic Medicine and Pathology* 6: 73–76.

Bidmos, M. A. 2005. On the non-equivalence of documented cadaver lengths to living stature estimates based on Fully's method on bones in the Raymond A. Dart collection. *Journal of Forensic Sciences* 50: 501–506.

Byers, S., Akoshima, K., and Curran, B. 1989. Determination of adult stature from metatarsal length. *American Journal of Physical Anthropology* 79: 275–279.

Chiba, M., and Terazawa, T. 1998. Estimation of stature from somatometry of skull. *Forensic Science International* 97: 87–92.

Dwight, T. 1894. Methods of estimating the height from parts of the skeleton. *Medical Record of New York* 46: 293–296.

Feldesman, M. R., and Fountain, R. L. 1996. "Race" specificity and the femur/stature ratio. *American Journal of Physical Anthropology* 100: 207–224.

Feldesman, M. R., Kleckner, J. G., and Lundy, J. K. 1990. Femur/stature ratio and estimates of stature in mid- and late-Pleistocene fossil hominids. *American Journal of Physical Anthropology* 83: 359–372.

Fully, G. 1956. Une nouvelle methode de determination de la taille. *Annales de Médecine Légale* 35: 266–273.

Fully, G., and Pineau, H. 1960. Determination de la stature au moyen de squelette. *Annales de Médecine Légale* 40: 145–154.

Galloway, A. 1988. Estimating actual height in the older individual. *Journal of Forensic Sciences* 33: 126–136.

Giles, E. 1991. Corrections for age in estimating older adults' stature from long bones. *Journal of Forensic Sciences* 36: 898–901.

Giles, E., and Hutchinson, D. L. 1991. Stature and age-related bias in self-reported stature. *Journal of Forensic Sciences* 36: 765–780.

Giles, E., and Klepinger, L. 1988. Confidence intervals for estimates based on linear regression in forensic anthropology. *Journal of Forensic Sciences* 33: 1218–1222.

Giles, E., and Vallandigham., P. H. 1991. Height estimation from foot and shoeprint length. *Journal of Forensic Sciences* 36: 1134–1151.

Himes, J. H., Yarbourgh, C., and Martorell, R. 1977. Estimation of stature in children from radiographically determined metacarpal length. *Journal of Forensic Sciences* 22: 452–456.

Holland, T. D. 1995. Estimation of adult stature from the calcaneus and talus. *American Journal of Physical Anthropology* 96: 315–320.

Imrie, J. A., and Wyburn, G. M. 1958. Assessment of age, sex and height from immature human bones. *British Medical Journal* 1: 128–131.

Jantz, R. L., Hunt, D. R., and Meadows, L. 1994. Maximum length of the tibia: How did Trotter measure it? *American Journal of Physical Anthropology* 93: 525–528.

———. 1995. The measure and mismeasure of the tibia: Implications for stature estimation. *Journal of Forensic Sciences* 40: 758–761.

Jason, D. R., and Taylor, K. 1995. Estimation of stature from the length of the cervical, thoracic, and lumbar segments of the spine in American Whites and Blacks. *Journal of Forensic Sciences* 40: 59–62.

Kimura, K. 1992. Estimation of stature from second metacarpal length in Japanese children. *Annals of Human Biology* 19: 267–275.

Klepinger, L., and Giles, E. 1998. Clarification or confusion: Statistical interpretation in forensic anthropology, in K. J. Reichs (ed.), *Forensic Anthropology: Advances in the Identification of Human Remains*, pp. 427–440. Springfield, IL: Charles C. Thomas.

Konigsberg, L. W., Hens, S. M., Jantz, L. M., and Jungers, W. L. 1998. Stature estimation and calibration: Bayesian and maximum likelihood perspectives in physical anthropology. *Yearbook of Physical Anthropology* 41: 65–92.

Lundy, J. K. 1985. The mathematical versus anatomical methods of stature estimate from long bones. *American Journal of Forensic Medicine and Pathology* 6: 73–76.

———. 1988a. A report on the use of Fully's anatomical method to estimate stature in military skeletal remains. *Journal of Forensic Sciences* 33: 534–539.

———. 1988b. Sacralization of a sixth lumbar vertebra and its effect upon the estimation of living stature. *Journal of Forensic Sciences* 33: 1045–1049.

Meadows, L., and Jantz, R. L. 1992. Estimation of stature from metacarpal lengths. *Journal of Forensic Sciences* 37: 147–154.

———.1995. Allometric secular change in the long bones from the 1800s to the present. *Journal of Forensic Sciences* 40: 762–767.

Nath, S., Garg, R., and Krishan, G. 1991. Estimation of stature through percutaneous measurements of upper and lower limbs among male Rajputs of Dehradun. *Journal of the Indian Anthropological Society* 26: 245–249.

Nichols, R. H. 2000. *Men with Custer: Biographies of the 7th Cavalry.* Hardin, MT: Custer Battlefield Historical and Museum Association.

Ousley, S. 1995. Should we estimate biological or forensic stature? *Journal of Forensic Sciences* 40: 768–773.

Ousley, S. D., and Jantz, R. L. 1996. *FORDISC 2.0: Personal Computer Forensic Discriminant Functions User's Guide.* Knoxville: Forensic Data Bank, University of Tennessee.

———. 2005. *FORDISC 3.0: Personal Computer Forensic Discriminant Functions User's Guide.* Knoxville: Forensic Data Bank, University of Tennessee.

Pearson, K. 1899. Mathematical contributions to the theory of evolution. V. On the reconstruction of the stature of prehistoric races. *Philosophical Transactions of the Royal Society of London* 192: 169–244.

Peng, S., and Zhu, F. 1983. Estimation of stature from skull, clavicle, scapula and os coxa of male adult of southern Chinese. *Acta Anthropologica Sinica* 2: 253–259.

Raxter, M. H., Auerbach, B. M., and Ruff, C. B. 2006. Revision of the Fully technique for estimating statures. *American Journal of Physical Anthropology* 130: 374–384.

Seitz, R. P. 1923. Relations of epiphyseal length to bone length. *American Journal of Physical Anthropology* 6: 37–49.

Smith, S. L. 2006. Juvenile stature estimation using long bone lengths. *American Journal of Physical Anthropology* Supplement 42: 167.

Snow, C. C., and Luke, J. L. 1984. The Oklahoma City child disappearances of 1967: Forensic anthropology in the identification of skeletal remains, in T. A. Rathbun and J. E. Buikstra (eds.), *Human Identification: Case Studies in Forensic Anthropology*, pp. 253–271. Springfield, IL: Charles C. Thomas.

Snow, C. C., and Williams, J. 1971. Variation in premortem statural measurements compared to statural estimates of skeletal remains. *Journal of Forensic Sciences* 16: 455–464.

Steele, D. G. 1970. Estimation of stature from fragments of long limb bones, in T. D. Stewart (ed.), *Personal Identification in Mass Disasters*, pp. 85–97. Washington, D.C.: Smithsonian Institution, National Museum of Natural History.

Telkka, A., Palkama, A., and Virtama, P. 1962. Prediction of stature from radiographs of long bones in children. *Journal of Forensic Sciences* 7: 474–479.

Terazawa, K., Akabane, H., Gotouda, H., Mizukami, K., Nagao, M., and Takatori, T. 1990. Estimating stature from the length of the lumbar part of the spine in Japanese. *Medicine, Science, and the Law* 30: 354–357.

Terazawa, K., Takatori, T., Mizukami, K., and Tomii, S. 1985. Estimation of stature from somatometry of vertebral column in Japanese. *Japanese Journal of Legal Medicine* 39: 35–40.

Tibbetts, G. L. 1981. Estimation of stature from the vertebral column in American Blacks. *Journal of Forensic Sciences* 26: 715–723.

Trotter, M. 1970. Estimation of stature from intact long limb bones, in T. D. Stewart (ed.), *Personal Identification in Mass Disasters*, pp. 71–83. Washington, D.C.: Smithsonian Institution, National Museum of Natural History.

Trotter, M., and Gleser, G. 1951. The effect of aging on stature. *American Journal of Physical Anthropology* 9: 311–324.

———. 1952. Estimation of stature from long bones of American Whites and Negroes. *American Journal of Physical Anthropology* 10: 463–514.

———. 1958. A re-evaluation of estimation of stature based on measurements of stature taken during life and of long bones after death. *American Journal of Physical Anthropology* 16: 79–123.

Visser, E. P. 1998. Little waifs: Estimating child body size from historic skeletal material. *International Journal of Osteoarchaeology* 8: 413–423.

Willey, P., and Falsetti, T. 1991. Inaccuracy of height information on driver's licenses. *Journal of Forensic Sciences* 36: 813–819.

Zhu, F. 1983. Study on the estimation of stature from phalanges of middle finger. *Acta Anthropologica Sinica* 2: 375–379.

Zorab, P. A., Prime, F. J., and Harrison, A. 1963. Estimation of height from tibial length. *Lancet* 7274: 195–196.

———. 1964. Estimation of height from tibial length. *Lancet* 7368: 1063.

21

ANTEMORTEM TRAUMA

Eugénia Cunha and João Pinheiro

A traumatic injury requires the action of an external agent on the body. There are many possible agents of trauma, although mechanical forces are those most commonly seen by the forensic anthropologist. Antemortem traumatic injuries are those lesions produced before death, in opposition to postmortem wounds. Although antemortem lesions might be understood as synonymous with vital lesions, this is not totally true, because the concept "vital" includes not only the antemortem injuries but also the injuries that occurred immediately before death or that caused the death. Yet in forensic terminology, the designation "vital" is more commonly associated with the last two situations than with antemortem trauma. In effect, the anthropologic concept of antemortem is quite different from the medical and medico-legal ones. As explained later in this chapter, it has much more to do with old lesions than with lesions related to the moment of death, the so-called perimortem injuries.

The benefits of the forensic anthropologist's assessment of antemortem traumatic lesions are many; analysis of antemortem trauma can be particularly informative to the reconstruction of life episodes and thus work as excellent factors of individualization (Cattaneo et al. 2006; Cunha 2006; Cunha and Cattaneo 2006; Cunha and Pinheiro 2007; Komar 2003; Maples 1984; Steyn and İşcan 2005). The more antemortem injuries a skeleton has the more distinctive it will be, and thus the greater the chances are of achieving a positive identification.

Child abuse is an important forensic syndrome that has been extensively researched during the last decades. Diagnosis of child abuse may be made by assessing antemortem fractures, particularly those affecting the ribs, in the absence of other major trauma (Saukko and Knight 2006; Vigorita 1999). More recently, skeletal traumatic injuries have been an important tool in elucidating whether human rights violations have occurred: bones often hold the key to the evaluation of the injuries' chronology (Rodríguez-Martín 2006).

Note also that although cause of death may not directly relate to an antemortem lesion whose signs of bone repair mean that the injury was not lethal, sometimes the complications caused by that injury can result in the subsequent death of an individual. In other words, some antemortem trauma might be viewed, in general terms, as an indirect cause of death, although this qualification has other medico-legal implications. In fact, this type of antemortem trauma cannot be discarded as the cause of death. A classic example is the fracture of the neck of the femur in the elderly. Although rarely fatal, it may be followed by a subsequent complication such as bronchopneumonia or a pulmonary thromboembolism that results in death. From a forensic point of view, the original fracture will be considered in most jurisdictions as the cause of death, complicated by one of the factors above mentioned (Pinheiro 2006).

This chapter examines differential diagnoses among pathological and true traumatic injuries. In addition, it discusses the mechanisms and chronology of bone remodelling and outlines a method for categorizing traumatic injuries. Some practical cases that illustrate the benefits and the medicolegal value of assessing antemortem traumatic injuries are also provided.

Bone Injury

Bone injury is, for most people, synonymous with fracture. However, there are a variety of other conditions that can result in injury to the bone tissue, including tumours, infection, and genetic disorders. Because antemortem trauma is the subject of the present chapter, specific attention is given to fractures, although the other conditions are also discussed.

Pathogenesis of Fractures

"A fracture is a discontinuity of or crack in skeletal tissue, with or without injury to overlying soft tissues" (Aufderheide and Rodríguez-Martín 1998: 20). Fractures may result from the application of repeated forces of low magnitude over a certain period of time—the so-called stress or fatigue fractures—or from a single impact of a force with the capacity to overcome the elasticity and anisometric properties of the bone tissue—the "normal" fractures as they are considered in the common sense.

Specific and unusual stress over a certain length of time, say, some weeks, might result in a fatigue fracture (Ortner 2003). In these cases, the fracture does not occur immediately after the application of stress but with the repetition of that stress over the bone. Gymnasts, athletes (long-distance runners, baseball pitchers), ballet dancers, and military infantry recruits increasingly display such fractures as a result of repetitive and continuous activities (Ortner 2003; Vigorita 1999). Such fractures may act as good factors of individualization and thus contribute to positive identification.

Spondylolysis is one of the best-known examples of a stress fracture. It consists of a partial to complete separation between the vertebral body and the arch of the corresponding vertebra (Merbs 1989; Ortner 2003). Congenital predisposition to

such a defect has been proposed for specific populations (e.g., Barnes 1994).

Concerning "normal" fractures, that is, when the trauma is direct, the associated injury of soft tissue and comminuted fracture is related to the loading rate. When the force is applied distant from the fracture site, strong muscle contractions across a joint with a fixed distal segment (such as joints at the elbow and the knee) may result in separated fracture fragments (Day et al. 2004). These forces will act over the three principal planes of stress of a bone: compression, tension, and shear. Such forces may act independently or in association, determining different patterns of long-bone fractures (Day et al. 2004).

The vulnerability of bone to trauma is also related to its capacity to absorb energy, following the classic formula of kinetic energy as $1\backslash2mv^2$, where m is mass and v the velocity of the impacting object. This explains the higher degree of comminution and displacement observed on impacts with high-velocity objects. The same law is applied to gunshot wounds, whereby high-velocity projectiles determine a higher destruction, comminution, and soft-tissue injury than do low velocity munitions.

Pathological Fractures

Normal fractures such as those outlined above occur in normal, healthy bone. However, some conditions might produce abnormal, pathological bone, which will break easily with minor trauma, or even with the normal use of the bone. These are known as *pathological fractures*. In these cases, even when the trauma involved is of great magnitude, they are still considered pathological fractures. Distinguishing the basic disorders that favour these fractures is mandatory in the anthropological analysis.

The pathological conditions more often involved are osteogenesis imperfecta; osteoporosis related to many causes; rickets; osteomalacia; scurvy; osteomyelitis (hematogenic, secondary to injuries, tuberculosis); rheumatoid arthritis; avascular posttraumatic necrosis and post-irradiation necrosis, and tumors/neoplasms (bone, cartilage, connective tissue, angiogenic and mielogenic, and metastatic) (Aufderheide and Rodriguez-Martín 1998; Ortner 2003; Salter 2000). In the majority of these diseases, ageing can be considered a paramount predisposing factor, since bone loss is generally associated with age. Furthermore, it is well known that the specific setting of fractures within the skeleton depends on the age and the sex of the individual.

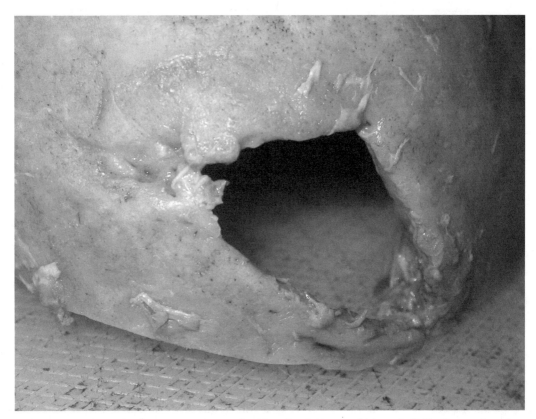

Figure 21.1 Example of antemortem trauma (accidental and therapeutic) in an individual approximately 50 years of age: a craniotomy detected during the autopsy of a fresh cadaver victim of a traffic accident, with clear signs of healing (note the smooth aspect of the edges), indicating that the individual survived. Observe on the right top the detail of a skull fracture consolidated, irradiating from the posterior corner of the craniotomy, quite different from long-bones pattern of repair (courtesy Instituto Nacional de Medicina Legal).

Types of Antemortem Trauma

There are several ways to classify trauma, depending on the way it is inflicted. Classification may be according to the mechanism/instrument employed (see Pinheiro 2006) or whether it was intentional or not (Table 21.1). Strict categorization of antemortem trauma is, however, difficult to achieve.

Trauma can occur either intentionally or accidentally as a result of actions against another person or be self-inflicted. Traumatic injuries can also result from cultural habits that can lead to bone deformation and surgical interventions or other therapies for pathological conditions (Figures 21.1 and 21.2). The categorization of trauma according to presence or absence of intention is stated in Table 21.1. However, the examples given can

Table 21.1 Attempt to classify antemortem trauma.

Type of Trauma	Examples
Accidental trauma	Many types of fractures, dislocations
Intentional trauma	Gunshot, stab, hammer or axe wounds
Cultural trauma	Chinese foot-binding
Therapeutic trauma	Surgical intervention

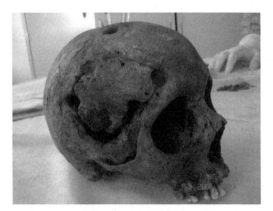

Figure 21.2 Human skull found on a beach in 2006, most probably that of a female Caucasoid individual aged older than 45 years (forensic anthropology case). It displays exuberant antemortem lesions on the right portion of the skull, affecting frontal, parietal, and temporal bones of that side, derived from a craniotomy, with the typical trepan holes (courtesy Instituto Nacional de Medicina Legal).

never exclusively describe the type of trauma, since, for instance, a dislocation and a fracture or a gunshot wound can obviously occur both accidentally or intentionally.

Ortner (2003) emphasizes that distinguishing between an accidental fracture (for example, resulting from a fall) and a fracture resulting from intentional violence might be virtually impossible. Although some authors (Grauer and Roberts 1996 in Ortner 2003: 136) consider that intentional violence is more likely to result in transverse fractures, whereas accidental fractures will more often result in oblique breaks. Based on our experience, we agree with Ortner's statement: when dealing with traumatic injuries, distinguishing between intentional and accidental trauma is, almost always, impossible. Another classic example is vertebral fractures. Although some authors argue that compression fractures of the spine tend to occur as a result of an accidental fall, in most cases, in our opinion, again based on our practice, it is virtually impossible to find exclusion arguments to preclude one of the two hypotheses.

In some cases of skull trauma, however, several clues may be available: a localised vault fracture with a depressed fragment and little or no radiating fractures is normally due to a local impact and, depending on the region, possibly produced by an aggressive act involving an object; a wide pattern of complex fractures, sometimes in spider-net pattern and/or reaching the base of the cranium, is more common in falls, traffic, and other type of accidents. Because of the potential legal effect of a

forensic anthropologist's findings, their interpretations must have an objective and well-supported argument in support of their conclusions (see Table 21.1). Furthermore, in a medico-legal context it is always dangerous to evaluate intentionality solely on the objective analysis of the bones.

On the contrary, the identification of cultural and therapeutic trauma is much easier. For the former, prior knowledge of the context—namely, ancestry—will be very helpful, since it is well known that certain traumatic injuries are particular to certain populations, such as feet deformation of Chinese females and cranial deformation as practiced by some communities in Chile (Aufderheide and Rodríguez-Martín 1998). In the interpretation of trauma resulting from therapeutic cases, the marks of surgical intervention (see Figures 21.1 and 21.2) and/or fracture treatment will be fundamental. A further importance of assessing the presence or absence of surgical devices is noted by Ubelaker (2003: 38): a strongly misaligned femur, with limited evidence of treatment, will most probably be an archaeological case and therefore, of no forensic significance.

However, when the mechanism causing the lesions is accounted for and trauma associated with specific pathological conditions and fatigue fractures are discarded, it is possible to define another way to classify trauma (Table 21.2). Usually, each of these types of trauma displays specific attributes that are well discussed in the chapter dealing with perimortem trauma (see Loe this volume). The difference here is that when those injuries are not lethal, they will show some kind of osteogenic response along the fractures lines and borders (see Figures 21.1 and 21.2). As in the interpretation of perimortem trauma, radiographs are mandatory to improve the interpretation of the fracture. Furthermore, it may also be possible to find evidence of some pieces of metal from the instrument that caused the damage to the bone. Scanning-electron microscopy may also provide helpful details to the mechanism diagnostic. Determining the type of weapon responsible for the injuries is also useful for the reconstruction of the traumatic event.

Mechanisms of trauma can, broadly speaking, result from the application of blunt, sharp, and perforating forces or a mixture of these (Pinheiro 2006). In any of these cases, the natural elasticity of the osseous tissue is exceeded as a consequence of the application of direct or indirect forces. Depending on the severity and the position of the force to the bone, fractures can be categorized as stated in Table 21.2. Although this is the same classification as that used for perimortem

Table 21.2 Classical classification of trauma according to the mechanisms of production (adapted from Aufderheide and Rodríguez-Martín 1998; Black 2005).

Type of Fractures	How It Is Caused
Tension or traction	Violent muscle contraction
Compression	Force applied in the axial direction
Twisting, rotation or torsion	Like shearing, but in the same plane as the diaphysis
Bending	Force is applied perpendicular to the long axis of the bone
Shearing	Two opposite forces perpendicular

fractures, it is obvious that in antemortem injuries, knowledge of the mechanism involved in producing them might be less important. However, in cases of human rights violation, when one is interpreting whether injuries occurred immediately before death, knowledge of the mechanism becomes much more important, particularly if the case under study will be subject to a trial.

A further aspect that should never be forgotten whenever bone lesions, of any type, are involved, is the absence of pathognomonic reactions. No matter how diverse the traumatic injuries might be, there are no pathognomonic traumatic reactions: "In other words, different causes can produce the same lesions and different lesions might have been caused by the same weapon/mechanism. This is indeed a complexity factor when dealing with the decodification of antemortem traumatic injuries" (Rodríguez-Martín 2006: 201).

Analysis of the distribution of traumatic injuries on a body may provide information about the nature of the event that caused the injury. Whether the lesions are limited to specific anatomic sites or can be found throughout the body, it is essential to ascertain what type of event was involved. Trauma interpretation is also aided by the separation of cranial and postcranial lesions, mainly because of the different nature of bones involved and the frequency of occurrence. Furthermore, because of the different pattern of reaction among the postcranial lesions, it is worthwhile to separate appendicular from axial bones, since, for instance, a long bone will display a distinct reaction from a rib. The type of bone (cancellous versus compact bone) also partially explains the different reaction pattern. Further, consideration of the different functions of bones (that is, to protect organs, support weight, and so forth), provides a more detailed interpretation of the consequences of trauma to that region; it becomes obvious that some bones, once severely injured, are more likely to be lethal.

Traumatic wounds of the head are the most common in forensic pathology. However, since severe injury to the skull often results in death, it is not common to fine huge associated antemortem lesions, unless there was a certain period of survival. Yet, as noted by Ortner (2003: 135), "the extent of injuries to the skull that an individual can survive is often remarkable." It is therefore paramount that the forensic anthropologist thoroughly examines the cranium for evidence of antemortem injury. The skull is a particularly valuable tool in forensic anthropology, since it is a "closed bony box" with an increased possibility of having marks or signs imprinted on it, if compared with thorax and abdomen, both with less bone and plenty of soft tissues. Healed incised wounds, small blunt traumatic injuries, with the typical bone depression, surrounded or not by infectious signs, are commonly found. The callus osseous in the skull has a different appearance, being smaller and less developed than that displayed on long bones (see Figure 21.1).

Gunshot wounds, if not lethal, will be observed as holes, maybe smaller than the initial lesions, bordered with smooth margins, occasionally with a thin layer of new bone closing the orifice. The size of the hole and the potential for closure as a result of healing are directly related to the type and the calibre of the ammunition. The anthropologist should look for discrete and often almost imperceptible signs of consolidated fractures radiating from the entrance wound. The classic appearance of internal bevelling on the entry hole and external bevelling on the exit wound will eventually be unapparent, depending on the time of the injury. Furthermore, it might be difficult to distinguish between the entrance and the exit wounds. To accomplish this objective, it is essential to open the vault with a saw in order to observe the inner aspect of the skull, a procedure often forgotten in anthropologic settings (Pinheiro and Cunha 2006).

years before death. These types of injuries have been helpful in the identification of old people, which are some of the most frequent cases involving a forensic anthropologist in Portugal (Cunha and Pinheiro 2007; Cunha, Pinheiro, and Corte-Real 2005).

Bone Reactions to Trauma

This section reviews the different reactions that bone has when traumatised.

Normal Consolidation

In comparison with other tissues, bone has a unique form of repair: a fracture is not repaired replacing the necrotic bone by fibrous tissue or a scar but by the bone tissue itself (Salter 2000). Bone repair can be divided in two main processes, the primary and the secondary consolidation (Hoppenfeld and Vasantha 2000; Salter 2000), although other authors consider more phases (six by Vigorita 1999). The first phase occurs when there is direct and straight contact between the bone ends, possible when the fracture reduction is done with rigid fixation using plates and screws. The callus will be formed in approximately two weeks. The process results essentially from the osteoclastic reabsorption followed by the osteoblastic formation of new bone. There is no radiographic evidence of a bone callus when this form of consolidation occurs, because the repair is done directly trough the compressed ends of the bone (Hoppenfeld and Vasantha 2000).

The secondary consolidation, the most common type, will show mineralization and replacement of the bone by a cartilaginous matrix that will have correspondence in a radiological callus. The higher the mobility of the fracture, the larger the callus will be. This consolidation is favoured by external fixation, casts and intramedullary nails. Classically, this consolidation can be divided in three phases: inflammatory; reparative, and remodelling (ibid.). The first one takes one to two weeks and begins with the increasing of the vascularization and the formation of a haematoma, with diverse cells and osteoclasts that will remove the bone necrotic tissue. The X ray will show an increased fracture line.

The reparative phase will last several months: the haematoma will be invaded by fibroblasts and condroblasts, which will synthesise connective tissue and cartilage that constitute the matrix to the soft callus. The callus will then mineralize resulting in a hard callus, which will stabilize the fracture. The third phase of remodelling will happen over a much longer period of time (months to years)

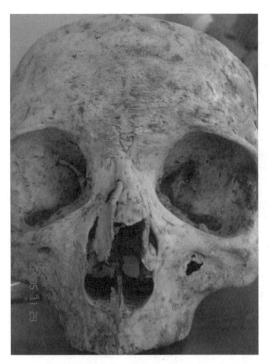

Figure 21.3 Noticeable and misaligned antemortem trauma on the nasal bones of an adult individual (unsolved forensic anthropology case performed 20 years ago; Manuel et al. 2004). Although these fractures might have been clearly noticeable by relatives, the person was never identified, perhaps because of the lack of medical files and the limitations of missing-persons data at the time (courtesy Instituto Nacional de Medicina Legal).

Healing can also be observed on fractures of the nasal bones (Figure 21.3) and of the zygomatic arch. Much less common, yet still possible to find, is the irregular external surface of the outer table of the skull bones as a response to scalping (Ortner 2003). We argue that this situation should always be verified when dealing with a suspicion of human rights violation. Injuries to the thorax, ribs, and vertebrae are of extreme importance, in particular for identification purposes, because often they are not lethal. Subsequently, they will consolidate and last until the victim dies, later, of another cause. If, eventually, that body is subjected to an anthropological examination, the callus osseous will survive to tell the story of this individual.

This was the situation of a case involving an elderly female whose body was identified by the authors (Figure 21.4). The contiguous and severe antemortem traumatic fractures affecting several ribs were later confirmed by her family, who stated that she suffered from a severe fall some

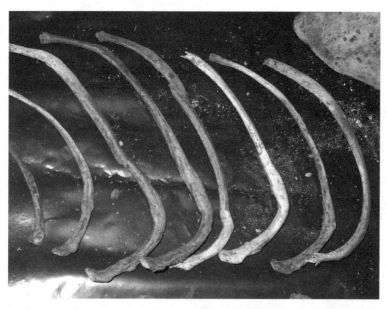

Figure 21.4 Contiguous and misaligned old fractures affecting several ribs of an elderly female, which were a valid and extremely useful factor of individualization, latter confirmed by her family (forensic anthropology case performed by the authors in 2005). The pattern of consecutive ribs fractured in two parts could correspond (when it determines a detached fragment of the rib cage) to the most dangerous surgical complication of rib fractures—the flail chest, potentially lethal. However, this was not the case (courtesy Instituto Nacional de Medicina Legal).

and consists of the replacement of the immature reticular bone by lamellar mature bone, owing to osteoblastic and osteoclastic activity.

The role of the periosteum is crucial in bone repair (Hoppenfeld and Vasantha 2000; Salter 2000). Its integrity, responsible for the vascularization and the degree of injury of the soft tissues surrounding the fracture, is essential for a rapid fracture repair. That is why a comminuted fracture takes longer to consolidate. The periosteum is thicker in the bone parts surrounded by muscles (for example, femoral diaphysis) than in subcutaneous bones (for instance, the antero-medial aspect of the tibia or the intra-articular portions of bone) (Salter 2000). The periosteum is also stronger, larger and more osteogenic during childhood (ibid.). As a consequence, age is an important factor in bone response; children will consolidate quicker than older people. For rib fractures in childhood, two weeks are enough to consolidate, a classic sign for the battered child syndrome.

Abnormal Consolidation and Secondary Reactions of Bone

Apart from a delay in consolidation (average of six months), two other main problems with anthropological consequences might arise when a fracture does not have a normal evolution: vicious consolidation (the repair is done at the right time but in a bad position), and the absence of union and the formation of a soft fibrous union of bones, called *pseudoarthrosis*, indicating lack of immobility and wrong or absent treatment (Rodríguez-Martín 2006).

Pseudoarthrosis, so-called because a synovial-like cavity develops between the un-united fractured fragments (Vigorita 1999), occurs when the ends of the affected bone are surrounded by connective tissue and callus but do not consolidate. It is the most common complication when a fracture does not consolidate. Misalignment can also occur. And when the overlying muscles are affected and respond with the production of bone directly in the muscle tissue, accompanied by hematoma, *myositis ossificans traumatica* can result. Such a result involves the formation of irregular calcified bone masses, in most instances related with calcified crushed muscles (DiMaio and Francis 2001).

Other reactions of abnormal bone are osteomyelitis in open fractures, posttraumatic osteoporosis, refracture, and avascular necrosis. The last, also known as aseptic necrosis, would be better called osteonecrosis (Day et al. 2004), because this term is closer to the histopathological process observed and does not relate to any specific etiology. Osteonecrosis means the death of a segment of bone from a lack of circulation, not from disease. The condition is not avascular, since the vessels are present, although compromised in their function by mechanical disruptions (fractures), occlusion of arterial vessels, pressure on the arterial wall, and occlusion of the venous outflow. The most frequent osteonecrosis associated with trauma are femoral neck fractures; dislocation of femoral head; displaced fracture of scaphoid; displaced fracture of talar neck; and four-part fracture of the femoral head (Day et al. 2004).

Posttraumatic osteoarthritis and arthritis in the nearby bone joints should also be considered, particularly in relation to their effect on different postures or gait after a fracture. Since open fractures have a much greater risk of infection, when open intra-articular fractures occur, they may result in septic arthritis. In extreme cases, situations such as gangrene, pus-forming followed by septicemia, sequestrum may also occur.

All these reactions are part of fracture complications and are of paramount importance clinically and well discussed in every orthopaedic textbook. Anthropologists should never forget that behind a bone reaction many, often vital, consequences for the individual might have happened (Pinheiro 2005). This includes haemorrhages, neurological injuries, vascular lesions, muscle sections, and visceral (thoracic or abdominal) wounds, among many others, depending on the bone fractured. It is vital to consider the body as a whole and bear in mind that bone is, in many instances, the last body system to respond to an "aggression."

Analysis of Antemortem Trauma

In many anthropological cases, the basic factors of the biological profile are not enough for positive identification, obliging the expert to look for the so-called factors of individualization. Antemortem fractures are among the most valid features to enable individualization (Cattaneo et al. 2006; Cunha 2006; Roberts 1996). However, the interpretation of these injuries is not always straightforward. Many questions can be addressed in any case of trauma analysis, where discrimination of ante-, peri-, and postmortem alterations has to be done, which is, indeed, the great challenge in every forensic anthropology examination. To achieve the main objectives of a forensic examination and overall to answer the question—*Did the traumatic event occur before death?*—the interpretation of traumatic injuries to the skeleton should always pursue a five-step schema whenever a bone alteration, presumably traumatic, is detected:

1. Is it a postmortem artefact or a true alteration?

2. Accepted as a true alteration, is it an ante-, peri-, or postmortem defect?

3. If it is antemortem, is the aetiology morphological or pathological?

4. Within the pathological alterations, is the aetiology traumatic?

5. When the aetiology is traumatic, is it possible to comment on when the fracture occurred—that is, a long time before death or immediately before?

The first step to perform is to discard all the taphonomical alterations that can mimic and/or be confounded by true lesions. Animal bites, roots effects, microfauna action are examples of taphonomical alterations that can lead to erroneous interpretations. They can both hide and mimic not only peri- and postmortem wounds but also antemortem traumatic injuries. Several examples can be found in literature (Cunha and Pinheiro 2007; Cunha, Umbelino, and Tavares 2001; Etxeberria 2003; Ubelaker 1998).

When there is no evidence of osteogenic reaction, the pattern of injury is crucial—namely, the discrimination among green-bone response, determining a perimortem wound and a dry-bone one, characteristic of a postmortem injury. Despite the existence of some clues extensively discussed in the literature (e.g., Sauer 1998), the determination remains difficult, often based on one's experience, sometimes being virtually impossible to distinguish between perimortem and postmortem fractures (see Loe this volume and Nawrocki this volume).

Once postmortem alterations have been identified, one must then distinguish between peri- and antemortem trauma. Antemortem lesions will be recognized when a callus or any type of bone reaction, such as porotic appearance of the periosteum, new bone formation, smooth surfaces, and/or misalignment, can be identified. Signs of bone remodelling can be used to discriminate between peri- and antemortem trauma, in particular, when the period of time elapsed since the traumatic injury was longer than two weeks.

Remaining then solely with antemortem alterations, one should next verify whether they are morphological or pathological. Actually, within antemortem alterations it is important to take into consideration that some morphological alterations or anatomical variations can be confounded with lesions; in other words, morphological variants can occasionally mimic trauma. Some of the most well-known morphological alterations to mimic

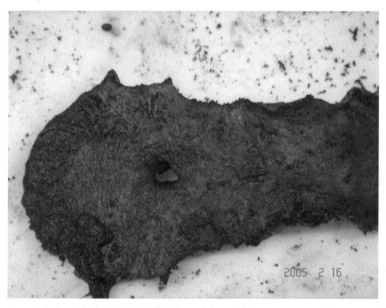

Figure 21.5   A morphological variation—perforation of the adult human sternum (courtesy of the authors).

antemortem trauma is os acromiale, the sternal perforation and the septal aperture on the lower epiphysis of the humerus. Although nonfusion of the end of the acromial process might be confused with an ancient cutting wound, not considering the anatomical variants on the lower epiphysis of the humerus and on the corpus of the sternum can lead to misdiagnosis. In what concerns possible confusion is a perforation of the sternum (Figure 21.5). With rounded and smooth edges, such an alteration could be erroneously mistaken for a thoracic firearm injury by inexperienced practitioners. Further complications can derive from the existence of two 1st or 12th ribs or double/bifid ribs (Moore and Dalley 2004), which can cause problems in analysing the rib cage, a known difficult task in anthropological examinations. Occasionally, these variations are associated with vertebral malformation (Moore and Dalley 2004), which will increase the complexity of the interpretation of the supposed injuries. All these arguments justify the reason to have a solid background in anatomical variation.

It is then necessary to determine whether the lesion has a traumatic aetiology. In most cases, this differential diagnosis is not difficult to achieve; in others, it is quite complex: the aspect of a vicious callus can be confounded with a tumour or other type of bone illness. Congenital defects such as the ones affecting vertebrae can also enhance these difficulties; even spina bifida can be misdiagnosed as a traumatic injury (Figure 21.6). This condition involves the failure of the normal fusion of the

midline in the posterior neural arches and is frequently found affecting the sacrum or the lumbosacral region of the spine. In the case illustrated here (an unsolved forensic case dating back to the 1980s) (see Figure 21.6), however, the adult individual shows three thoracic vertebrae with incomplete fusion of the posterior arches. The margins

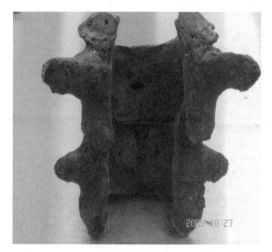

Figure 21.6   Failure of the fusion of the posterior neural arch on a thoracic vertebra of an adult male individual (forensic anthropology case dating back to the 1980s). The smooth aspect of the margins might be confounded with the ones of antemortem trauma (courtesy Instituto Nacional de Medicina Legal).

are so smooth that confusion with a remodelled trauma might be possible. Yet, an injury on that location most probably might have produced serious effects on locomotion/gait. When information about the circumstances of death is not available to confirm a possible accident or traumatic event, or when the medical files are insufficient, this task of determining traumatic aetiology will be even harder.

In the final case report, one must separate observation from inference, to keep description distinct from speculation and to state clearly whether bone lesions are detected. In the case of absence, the inference should never be that the victim did not suffer from any aggression and /or disease. Many violent episodes do not leave any trace on the skeleton (Cunha 2006).

The final stage of assessing antemortem trauma is attempting to determine the chronology of injuries. This determination involves the identification of antemortem injuries that occurred so close to death that the healing process was not yet recorded, or are poorly recorded on the skeleton—the so-called perimortem trauma (Sauer 1998: 323). Obviously, these injuries are much more difficult to detect than those with clear signs of remodelling/response. The very early stages of healing, such as the ones of porous nature detected by means of microscopy, can be the key clues. In some criminal circumstances, they might be the only evidence of torture immediately before death. It is worthwhile emphasizing the difficulty in distinguishing between perimortem and antemortem trauma occurring immediately (some hours or a few days) before death. Yet, we still have to consider that the traumatic injuries occurred immediately after death. Although the dried-bone response to trauma is known to be quite distinctive from that of fresh-bone fractures (Sauer 1998)—since the different patterns are dependent on the quantity and the quality of both the bone moisture and bone organic part—the length of time required for moisture and organic loss is obviously paramount. In turn, because this time depends on the environment where decomposition takes place (for example, heat accelerates collagen deterioration), the time period becomes a multifactorial phenomena. Fitzgerald's report (1975: 325), cited by Sauer (1998), well documents this statement: at room temperature, bone loses measurable elasticity, which lasts about five hours after death. Furthermore, Maples (1986 in Sauer 1998) suggests that the typical attributes of green-bone response may persist for several weeks after death, which has direct implications on the concepts of ante-, peri-, and postmortem.

As previously stated, these concepts do not have exactly the same meaning for forensic pathologists and anthropologists. For the former, and consequently for a trial, it is absolutely essential to determine whether a lesion was vital (produced during life) or postmortem. For anthropologists, it is relative, as described above, given a green-bone response, which can last for hours, days, or more after death. This leads to obvious and important legal consequences. In a case of a victim of a serial killer found in a river and autopsied by the authors, an undoubtedly perimortem fracture of the 4th rib was diagnosed. However, we could not confirm to the police whether it had resulted from aggression to the still-live victim or after death, during the disposal of the body into the river.

Interpreting Evidence of Bone Remodelling and Its Relation to Chronology

The amount and type of trauma displayed in the skeleton are dependent on a series of factors that are well systematized by Black (2005). We also have tried to systematize some consequences of those factors (Table 21.3). Their knowledge might be particularly helpful in estimating the chronology of the event.

It is well known that evidence for remodelling associated with a skeletal lesion indicates that the injury occurred antemortem. However, the question remains as to how much time before. Sauer (1998) says that when remodelling occurs, it means that the injury happened at least one week before. However, as outlined by Black (2005), antemortem trauma, as any other pathological condition, is not a static event. It is therefore quite complex to infer, on the basis of the alterations on the dry bone, whether the lesions were in their early stages, active or non-active, healed or unhealed, particularly in a forensic context. This means that the same pathology can express itself in the skeleton in various ways.

The osteogenic response depends on several factors, such as the type of fracture (severity, location, type of bone, apposition of the ends, stability) and the age, sex, nutritional status, and state of the individual's health (Hoppenfeld and Vasantha 2000; Ortner 2003; Salter 2000). Obviously, there are too many variables to permit any kind of reliable prediction. Ortner (2003) cites the general guidelines given by Paton (1992 in Ortner 2003: 128): "cortical bone in adults heals in about three months, cancellous bone takes about six weeks, and children repair fracture about twice as quickly

Table 21.3 Factors affecting the amount and type of trauma displayed in the skeleton and its general relation with chronology.

Factors	Eventual Meaning/Effect
Nature and severity of trauma	The more severe the lesion is, the more evident it might be
Time since trauma	The larger the time interval, the higher the chances of resorption of fractures lines and the more evident callus formation will appear*
Amount, degree, and type of healing	The less healing, the lower the post-mortem interval**
Existence/inexistence of infection	The greater the infection, the more exuberant the lesion might be*
The presence/absence of signs of treatment	Absence of treatment: not a forensic case?

* If no treatment had occurred
** Until the end of consolidation, after which the callus will stabilize.

as adults." Thus, a general rule is that the length of time needed to heal increases with age. Some key features/signs can be very helpful: the formation of layers of woven bone is a sign of rapid bone formation.

Although empiric data on times of reaction are difficult to achieve, some research in this field has been undertaken. Using skeletons with traumatic injuries and showing evidence of having been autopsied (the autopsy reports were found at the Archives of the National Institute of Legal Medicine in Portugal) from the Lisbon Identified Skeletal Collection, Macedo (2006) undertook research to try to confront the forensic anthropological expertise performed today with the data displayed at the autopsy report at the time of death, about 50 years ago. Because information was available for some individuals indicating whether they stayed at the hospital before death, it was a unique opportunity to document reaction times/chronology for bone remodelling and traumatic events. As expected, physical condition at the time of death, as well as age of death, influenced the bone response. In a significant number of cases, the anthropological findings about traumatic injuries concurred with the cause of death stated on the autopsy reports.

The first signs of reactions are visible only microscopically, the inflammatory cells by 48 hours and the haematoma even earlier (<12 h) (Vigorita 1999). The initial bone reaction is known to start, more consistently, after one week with osteoclastic reabsorbing of necrotic bone tissue, at a structural level (Hoppenfeld and Vasantha 2000; Rodríguez-Martín 2006). New bone formation is

usually said to begin by the same first week and has been described as happening in rabbits by 24 hours and in osteoporotic human bones by 48 hours (Vigorita 1999). However, the skill is to recognize the physical evidence of this reaction in anthropological sets. Rodríguez-Martín (2006) suggests that the margins of the lesions where one expects to verify the first signs of healing show a smooth and rounded reaction observable under a dissecting microscope, which is not usually available in normal forensic anthropologic sets.

To evaluate a fracture consolidation, orthopaedists use the clinical symptoms (pain, sensibility, and mobility), the historical background, and, above all, radiological criteria. Obviously, this is useless for the objectives of a forensic anthropologist, apart from the degree of subjectivity always present in such an evaluation. The requirement is to determine, solely on the basis of a dry bone, when the response began and in what phase it was occurring. Macroscopic evidence of bone reaction is needed, yet descriptions in literature are limited.

Microscopically, the first signs of osteogenic response can be identified. At about the same time as the beginning of the above-mentioned osteoclastic reabsorbing (one to two weeks after the traumatic event occurred), the first radiological signs will appear (Salter 2000). Sometimes the formation of new bone is the confirmation of a fracture only suspected on the initial X ray. When X rays translate a white opacity for dense tissues (bone, cartilage, haematoma), by the same time some type of bone reaction might already be seen morphologically by the naked eye, depending logically on some factors discussed below. Subsequently, we can establish that the first signs of bone repair might be seen by the first to second weeks.

As previously stated, the time of repair depends on the specific bone: for a radial distal fracture, six–eight weeks are usually enough, although for a diaphyseal tibia fracture, three months will be necessary (Table 21.4), because there is minimal soft-tissue support for this bone. Metaphyseal fractures generate small callus, because there is less periosteum and good cooption of the bone tops. The same happens with intra-articular fractures—a small callus—caused by the small amount of periosteum and the presence of synovial fluid. The type of treatment will also influence the time of consolidation, depending on the proximity or separation they will proportionate.

For orthopaedic specialists, a fracture is consolidated when they no longer observe on X ray the fracture line, the bone callus is present, and the patient has no pain, good mobility, and the capacity to support height. For anthropologists, these things are not helpful. Nonetheless, some orthopaedic specialists' concepts about consolidation and time of repair may be useful to the forensic anthropologist.

Taking all these factors into consideration, we can say, in general, for the entire skeleton, that a normal fracture in a healthy, medium individual, with a normal evolution and with no complications, will consolidate between four weeks and three months (Hoppenfeld and Vasantha 2000; Salter 2000). Taking this as rule of thumb, we felt the need during our practice in forensic anthropology, for a guide to assist in the normal time previewed for specific consolidation of a bone. In an attempt to fill this gap, we provide a list of the normal time of consolidation for the majority of the human skeleton (see Table 21.4). This list should be used merely as a tool in helping to determine the chronology of a certain injury and never considered as a strict law of time of bone repair.

Need for Documentation on Trauma

Depending on the type and the severity of the lesion, trauma can significantly affect the individual's lifestyle. Specific peculiarities such as gait, handedness, mobility/immobility, and/or particular posture of the head are easily remembered by the victim's relatives and friends, becoming, therefore, key clues to identification. A misaligned fracture of the femur will most probably result in an abnormal gait that will be a fundamental osteobiographical

sign of identification. The context of the detected traumatic injuries is also important. Whether the lesions are accompanied by osteoarthritis lesions, enthesopathies (reactive bone on sites for bone tendons, ligaments, and articular capsule attachments [Ortner 2003: 561]), or other reactions is crucial to the final interpretation.

In the majority of cases, antemortem bone traumatic injuries are useful only for identification when antemortem records are available for comparison. The quality of these records is thus fundamental. The need for documentation of injuries is well discussed by Payne-James (2005). The author calls attention to the limitations of the documentation of injuries provided by medical practitioners: "In many cases documentation is appropriate for the therapeutic management of the injured person, but is rarely of the quality required subsequently to assist in issues such as causation or timing of an injury" (Payne-James 2005: 80). Furthermore, he emphasizes the importance for all forensic practitioners to be aware of the definitions of terms such as *injury*, *assault*, and *wound* in the jurisdiction in which they work, since they might have specific applications. The lack of good and precise descriptions of injuries and incompleteness of medical files constitute a common problem in the medico-legal activity wherever it is practiced.

An objective description of the lesions should permit another expert to do his or her own diagnostic assessment; in other words, one must always keep in mind that if the description of the lesions is not separate from the interpretation of the lesions, a second opinion can be precluded. Moreover, if a complete medical file is available, with which we can compare the data displayed in the skeleton, the chances of achieving a positive identification will be significantly increased. Such was the situation in a case of an elderly woman whose good medical records permitted the confirmation of the venous exuberant bone pathology of the lower leg bones, found at the autopsy by Pinheiro and associates (2004), and subsequently her positive identification. Some factors that may be relevant for the necessary reconciliation between ante- and postmortem data are given by Payne-James (2005) as follows: time of injury or injuries; the existence or absence of injury treatment; whether there was pre-existing illness; whether the individual practiced regular physical activity; occupation; regular medication; and handedness. The availability of these data is potentially extremely useful to forensic investigations.

Table 21.4 Normal periods for postcranial adult bones consolidation (weeks) (Hoppenfeld and Vasantha 2000).

Clavicle	6–12
Upper limb	
Humerus: proximal end	6–8
Diaphysis and distal end	8–12
Olecraneon	10–12
Radius head	6–8
Forearm	8–12
Wrist (Colles)	6–8
Scaphoid	4–20
Metacarpals	4–6
Phalanges	3–6*
Lower limb	
Femur: neck, subtrochanter, supracondilar, diaphysis	12–16
Inter-trochanter	12–15
Patela	8–12
Tibia: plate, diaphysis	10–12
Horizontal base	6–8
Ankle extra-articular	6–10
Intra-articular	8–12
Talus	6–10
Calcaneous	8–12
Middle foot	6–10**
Anterior foot (Metatarsal and toes)	4–8**
Vertebral column	
Cervical column	6–12
C1	8–16
C2	8–12
Dens	12–16
Thoraco-lumbar column	8–16

* Clinical consolidation; radiological consolidation will take 10–12 weeks
** Depending on bones

Value of Antemortem Trauma for Forensic Anthropology

The value of antemortem trauma for forensic anthropology is mainly identification, the diagnosis of battered-child syndrome, a means to document human rights violation, and a possible contribution to the determination of the cause of death (Sauer and Simson 1984). As previously mentioned, when identification is the main concern, healed traumatic injuries are among the most helpful factors of individualization (Cattaneo et al. 2006; Cunha 2006; Cunha and Cattaneo 2006; Cunha and Pinheiro 2007; Komar 2003; Maples 1984; Steyn and İşcan 2005). Furthermore, the way those injuries had been treated will also be very valuable to identification, in particular, when marks of surgical interventions are detected. Various types of prostheses and other devices, such as implants, can be found within human remains. Such devices can be traced back to their manufacturer and are often issued with a unique serial or production lot number (Bennett and Benedix 1999). For example, a case examined in 2006 by one of the authors involved an adult skull that exhibited exuberant signs of a therapeutic craniotomy (see Figure 21.2). The individual survived for many months after operation, as indicated by the well-rounded edges of the holes. In this case, the type of suture allowed the supposition that the craniotomy was performed some decades ago. Most probably the skull was stolen from a cemetery and thrown out to the beach (remaining soil in the skull may have been able to prove this). Therefore, most probably it was not truly a forensic case (Rogers 2005). In Portugal, the time limit for forensic significance is 15 years.

The two examples of craniotomies provided in Figures 21.1 and 21.2 are, in a way, the opposite of each other. In the forensic anthropology case (see Figure 21.2), where only the skull was present and in the absence of any medical files and/or further data, it was the type of craniotomy displayed—namely, the type of suture—that lead to the supposition that we were dealing with a particularly ancient case. In the other case (see Figure 21.1), the autopsy provided the cause of death (traumatic injuries of the chest and pneumothorax) and excluded the cranial lesion as the cause of death. Yet, the poor medical documentation in this case—namely, the lack of medical data on that surgery—prevented any further conclusions. Furthermore, if this skull had been found much later, completely dry and isolated as the other one, the data to infer on this basis would have been much more restricted. However, some

weeks after the autopsy, the husband confirmed a serious traffic accident with a motorcycle, whose handlebar had penetrated into the skull when the victim was 4 years old.

In a child younger than 1 year—when rib fractures are not explained by major trauma, skull fractures result from short falls or metaphyseal long-bone fractures, and femoral fractures are observed—regardless of the cause of death ascertained, one must suspect child abuse (Saukko and Knight 2006; Vigorita 1999). This diagnosis is also suspected or reinforced when other fractures of different chronologies are found. Antemortem trauma can play an extraordinary role in the detection of a typical forensic syndrome.

The forensic analysis of skeletal remains of illegal immigrants or individuals who die under arrest is a relatively new area of intervention for forensic anthropologists (e.g., Rodríguez-Martín 2006). Antemortem traumatic injuries can be used as a means to document the violation of human rights. Rodríguez-Martín (2006) argues that the forensic anthropologist skills in palaeopathology—namely, on the interpretation of antemortem traumatic injuries—can significantly contribute to the resolution of many cases of human rights violation. Therefore, antemortem trauma can be considered a very powerful tool in the investigation of violence (ibid.). For this reason, it is vital to have a detailed knowledge of the types of bone reaction and the mechanism of healing in order to document what happened. Rodríguez-Martín (2006) gives a detailed description of bone response, accompanied by the lesions related to the several methods of punishment or torture. He calls attention to the interest in detecting fractures involving bones of the hands and feet, which can be evidence of the application of torture methods such as *falaka* or *falanga* (repeated beats on the sole or the palm).

The identification of slightly healed defence fractures—namely, the classical Parry fracture, on the forearm bones—will be a chief element to the reconstruction of the events surrounding the dead, when dealing not only with human rights violations but also in cases of attempted and/or true homicides. In fresh bodies, however, parallel cuts on wrists are almost always synonymous of suicide tentative. However, it is very improbable that these cuts, classified usually as superficial, may go as deep as the bone. Thus, injuries with the same location might have, according to the type and depth, different meanings in forensic anthropology and pathology.

The detection of an amputation with survival will also constitute a key element regarding whether criminal consequences are involved. As pointed out by Rodríguez-Martín (2006), intentional amputation is a well-known method of torture, although the difficulty is to discriminate between intentional and accidental amputations. Affected typical areas are the upper-limb bones. The osteogenic response (bone-tissue formation) will indicate whether the individual survived the traumatic event. The criteria to follow for a chronological diagnosis of amputation are given by Aufderheide and Rodríguez-Martín (1998).

Finally, antemortem trauma has the potential to contribute to the knowledge of events prior to death. As previously discussed, if the bone displays signs of remodelling, the injuries underneath it did not cause the death. However, the complications derived from the traumatic injuries can cause the subsequent death. Thus correct interpretation of the lesions displayed within a skeleton, not only traumatic but also others, such as infectious ones, can provide clues to the understanding of the cause of death (Pinheiro 2006). For example, an open fracture of the femur may not result in immediate death but may lead to later serious complications—namely, a severe infection that ultimately results in death. Nonetheless, as stated before, this type of analysis must always be cautious, totally avoiding any type of over-interpretation.

Conclusion

The analysis of antemortem trauma is an important part of the forensic anthropologist's overall assessment. Signs of physiological response, healed wounds, callus formation, smooth edges, and thickly rounded surfaces are some of the classical features to verify that the injury was antemortem. Trauma that occurred antemortem may be useful for identification purposes. In addition, antemortem trauma may also be useful in diagnosing battered-child syndrome, documenting human rights violation, and contributing to the determination of the cause of death (Sauer and Simson 1984).

The examples of craniotomies and many others studied in this chapter illustrate the differences between having expertise in dry bone compared to fresh bone. Differences in expertise promote the need for effective cooperation between the forensic anthropologist and the forensic pathologist (Cunha and Cattaneo 2006; Cunha and Pinheiro 2007; Pinheiro and Cunha 2006). Without such concepts, some key clues might be imperceptible; this chapter provides a clear example of the value of a multidisciplinary approach. For a complete interpretation of

the lesions displayed on dry bone, one should acquire experience with fresh bone and keep in mind the several phases through which the bone will go, as well as the limitations and dangers of deriving assumptions on cause of death on the basis of dry bone. This is indeed an area that requires more research.

Reading pathology from bare bones has its limitations that must be taken into account, especially when they involve antemortem trauma. Even when a bony injury is identified, one cannot speculate about the consequences for the victim, that is, cause of death (Pinheiro 2005). Nonetheless, although a skeleton is always less informative than a fresh cadaver, in most instances, the skeleton is the ultimate body system to respond to an aggression. Once the bones are affected, the signs of the traumatic injuries will remain on the bones long after death, significantly contributing to the osteobiographies of their owners. These are valuable elements for forensic anthropology in the various situations involved, from a routine case to mass disasters and crimes against humanity.

References

Aufderheide, A., and Rodríguez-Martín, C. 1998. *The Cambridge Encyclopedia of Human Paleopathology*. Cambridge: Cambridge University Press.

Barnes, E. 1994. *Developmental Defects of the Axial Skeleton in Paleopathology*. Boulder, CO: University of Colorado Press.

Bennett, J. L., and Benedix, D. C. 1999. Positive identification of remains recovered from an automobile based on presence of an internal fixation device. *Journal of Forensic Sciences* 44(6): 1296–1298.

Black, S. M. 2005. Bone pathology and antemortem trauma, in J. Payne-James, R. Byard, T. S. Corey, and C. Henderson (eds.), *Encyclopedia of Forensic and Legal Medicine*, pp. 105–112. Amsterdam: Elsevier/Academic Press.

Cattaneo, C., Porta, D., Angelis, D., and Grandi, M. 2006. Personal identification of cadavers and human remains, in A. Schmitt, E. Cunha, and J. Pinheiro (eds.), *Forensic Anthropology and Medicine: Complementary Sciences from Recovery to Cause of Death*, pp. 359–379. Totowa, NJ: Humana Press.

Cunha, E. 2006. Pathology as a factor of personal identity in forensic anthropology, in A. Schmitt, E. Cunha, and J. Pinheiro (eds.), *Forensic Anthropology and Medicine: Complementary Sciences from Recovery to Cause of Death*, pp. 333–358. Totowa, NJ: Humana Press.

Cunha, E., and Cattaneo, C. 2006. Forensic anthropology and forensic pathology: The state of the art, in A. Schmitt, E. Cunha, and J. Pinheiro (eds.), *Forensic Anthropology and Medicine: Complementary Sciences from Recovery to Cause of Death*, pp. 39–53. Totowa, NJ: Humana Press.

Cunha, E., and Pinheiro, J. 2007. Forensic anthropology in Portugal: From current practice to future challenges, in M. Brickley and R. Ferllin (eds.), *Forensic Anthropology: Case Studies from Europe*, pp. 38–57. Springfield, IL: Charles C Thomas.

Cunha, E., Pinheiro, J., and Corte-Real, F. 2005. When old people get lost: The identification of their bodies. 17th Meeting of the International Association of Forensic Sciences. Hong Kong.

Cunha, E., Umbelino, C., and Tavares, T. 2001. Necrópole de São Pedro de Marialva. Dados antropológicos. *Património Estudos* 1: 139–143.

Day, S., Ostrum, R. F., Chao, E. Y. S., Rubin, C. T., Aro, H. T., and Einhorn, T. A. 2004. Bone injury, regeneration and repair, in J. A. Buckwalter, T.A., Einhorn, and S. R. Simon (eds.), *Orthopaedic Basic Science. Biology and Biomechanics of the Musculoskeletal System* (2nd ed.). Rosemont, IL: American Academy of Orthopaedic Surgeons.

DiMaio, V. J., and Francis, J. R. 2001. Heterotopic ossification in unidentified remains. *American Journal of Forensic Pathology* 22(2): 160–164.

Etxeberria, F. 2003. Patología traumática, in A. Isidro, and A. Malgosa (eds.), *Paleopatología. La Enfermedad no Escrita*, pp. 195–204. Barcelona: Masson.

Hoppenfeld, S., and Vasantha, L. M. 2000. *Treatment and Rehabilitation of Fractures*. Philadelphia: Lippincott Williams & Wilkins.

Komar, D. 2003. Lessons from Srebrenica: The contributions and limitations of physical anthropology in identifying victims of war crimes. *Journal of Forensic Sciences* 48(4): 713–716.

Macedo, M. 2006. Os casos forenses da Colecção de Esqueletos do Museu Nacional de História Natural de Lisboa. Unpublished Masters' thesis. University of Lisbon. Faculty of Medicine.

Manuel, R., Cunha, E., Pinheiro, J., Ribeiro, I., and Santos, J. C. 2004. Revisiting old forensic cases from Lisbon: Two interesting cases. Poster presented at the 1st meeting of Forensic Anthropology Society of Europe. Frankfurt.

Maples, W. 1984. The identifying pathology, in T. A. Ratbhurn and J. E. Buikstra (eds.), *Human Identification: Case Studies in Forensic Anthropology*, pp. 363–370. Springfield, IL: Charles C. Thomas.

Merbs, C. 1989. Trauma, in M. Y. İşcan and K. A. R. Kennedy (eds.), *Reconstruction of Life from the Skeleton*, pp. 161–189. New York: A. R. Liss.

Moore, K. L., and Dalley, A. F. 2004. *Clinically Oriented Anatomy*. Philadelphia: Lippincott Williams and Wilkins.

Ortner, D. 2003. *Identification of Pathological Conditions in Human Skeletal Remains* (2nd ed.). San Diego: Academic Press.

Payne-James, J. 2005. Injury, fatal and nonfatal, in J. Payne-James, R. Byard, T. S. Corey, and C. Henderson (eds.), *Encyclopedia of Forensic and Legal Medicine*, pp. 80–94. Amsterdam: Elsevier: Academic Press.

Pinheiro, J. 2005. Traumatic lesions and cause of death: A forensic anthropology challenge. 1st Paleopathology Association South American Meeting. Rio de Janeiro.

———. 2006. Introduction to forensic medicine and pathology, in A. Schmitt, E. Cunha, and J. Pinheiro (eds.), *Forensic Anthropology and Medicine: Complementary Sciences from Recovery to Cause of Death*, pp. 13–37. Totowa, NJ: Humana Press.

Pinheiro J., and Cunha, E. 2006. Forensic investigation of corpses in various states of decomposition: A multi-disciplinary approach, in A. Schmitt, E. Cunha, and J. Pinheiro (eds.), *Forensic Anthropology and Medicine: Complementary Sciences from Recovery to Cause of Death*, pp. 159–195. Totowa, NJ: Humana Press.

Pinheiro, J., Cunha, E., Cordeiro, C., and Vieira, D. N. 2004. Bridging the gap between forensic anthropology and osteoarchaeology: A case of vascular pathology. *International Journal of Osteoarchaeology* 14(2): 137–144.

Roberts, C. A. 1996. Forensic anthropology 2: Positive identification of the individual: Cause and manner of death, in J. Hunter, C. Roberts, and A. Martín (eds.), *Studies in Crime: An Introduction to Forensic Archaeology*, pp. 122–137. London: Berttler and Tanner.

Rodríguez-Martín, C. 2006. Identification and differential diagnosis of traumatic lesions of the skeleton, in A. Schmitt, E. Cunha, and J. Pinheiro (eds.), *Forensic Anthropology and Medicine: Complementary Sciences from Recovery to Cause of Death*, pp. 197–221. Totowa, NJ: Humana Press.

Rogers, T. 2005. Recognition of cemetery remains in a Forensic context. *Journal Forensic Sciences* 50(1): 5–11.

Salter, R. B. 2000. *Textbook of Disorders and Injuries of the Musculoskeletal System* (3rd ed.). Philadelphia: Lippincott Williams and Wilkins.

Sauer, N. 1998. The timing of injuries and manner of death: Distinguishing among antemortem, perimortem and postmortem trauma, in K. Reichs (ed.), *Forensic Osteology*: 321–332. Springfield, IL: Charles C. Thomas.

Sauer, N. J., and Simson, L. R. 1984. Clarifying the role of forensic anthropologists in death investigations. *Journal Forensic Sciences* 29(4): 1081–1086.

Saukko, P., and Knight, B. 2006. *Forensic Pathology*. London: Arnold.

Steyn, M., and İşcan, M. Y. 2000. Bone pathology and antemortem trauma in forensic cases, in J. A. Siegel, P. J. Saukko, and G. C. Knufer (eds.), *Encyclopedia of Forensic Sciences*, pp. 217–227. San Diego: Academic Press.

Ubelaker, D. 1998. Taphonomic applications in forensic anthropology, in W. Haglund and M. Sorg (eds.), *Forensic Taphonomy: The Post-Mortem Fate of Human Remains*, pp. 77–88. Boca Raton, FL: CRC Press.

———. 2003. Interpretación de las anomalías esqueléticas y su contribución a la investigación forense. *Cuadernos de Medicina Forense* 33: 35–42.

Vigorita, V. J. 1999. *Orthopaedic Pathology*. Philadelphia: Lippincott Williams and Wilkins.

22

PERIMORTEM TRAUMA

Louise Loe

Perimortem trauma refers to any injury or wound to the body, occurring around the time of death, that may affect the bone and/or soft tissues (Roberts 1991: 226). In a forensic pathology examination, the identification of any such lesions may indicate the cause and manner of death, suggest how the body was treated during the perimortem interval, and provide insight into its disposal (Galloway 1999). When injuries involve the skeleton, the forensic anthropologist plays an important role, often being better placed than the medical examiner and forensic pathologist to identify and interpret skeletal changes (Roberts 1996). Skeletally, perimortem trauma may be identified as fractures or breaks in the continuity of a bone that may pierce, divide, crush, or penetrate the skeletal tissues. Careful study of these changes may assist interpretations made by the forensic pathologist; it can serve to corroborate soft-tissue evidence that may be used in court and, at the same time, may highlight discrepancies in a case that may not be indicated by soft-tissue change alone (Galloway 1999).

The aim of this chapter is to synthesise the current theoretical and practical issues associated with perimortem trauma analysis of skeletal remains recovered from forensic contexts. Such synthesis cannot be successfully undertaken without understanding the biomechanics of bone; therefore,

this is reviewed first, followed by a review of the criteria that may be employed to distinguish perimortem from antemortem and postmortem trauma. Projectile, sharp, and blunt trauma are then reviewed, with particular emphasis on fracture patterns and the information that may be potentially gained from fracture pattern analysis. The circumstances of fracture patterns are then discussed, including those factors that may mimic perimortem trauma. Limitations are discussed and methodologies considered.

Principles of Perimortem Trauma

To interpret perimortem trauma, one must have an understanding of the biomechanics of bone fracture, including the extrinsic and intrinsic variables that influence fracture patterns.

Biomechanics of Bone Fracture

Some of the earliest studies to explore the biomechanics of bone fracture date back to the early 19th century. Such studies experimented with autopsy specimens, living animals, and both human and nonhuman skeletal remains to explore fracture dynamics in the skull. An important study is that of Gurdjian, Webster, and Lissner (1950), who applied a strain-sensitive lacquer to skulls (the

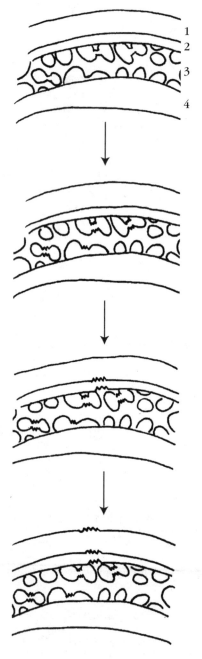

A) Section through skull showing different structures

   1 = External compact bone
   2 = Junctional zone between external compact
       bone and diplöe
   3 = Diplöe
   4 = Internal compact bone

B) Fracture of the trabeculae of the diplöe
   (indicated by zig-zag lines)

C) Fracture of the junctional zone between the
   external compact bone and the diplöe
   (fracture indicated by zig-zag lines)

D) Fracture of the external compact bone
   (fracture indicated by zig-zag lines)

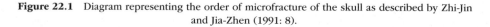

Figure 22.1   Diagram representing the order of microfracture of the skull as described by Zhi-Jin
and Jia-Zhen (1991: 8).

"stresscoat" technique) to explore fracture mechanisms and introduced several key principles that are still employed today. There are numerous publications that provide reviews of the biomechanics of bone fracture (e.g., Berryman and Haun 1996; Frankel and Nordin 1980; Galloway 1999; Hipp and Hayes 2003; Mascie-Taylor and Bogin 1995). Some of these relate specifically to bone fracture, whereas others concern bone biomechanics at a more general level.

Bone is anisotrophic—that is to say, it has the ability to respond differently, depending on the direction of the loading force. It is governed by the interaction of collagen fibres that afford it tensile strength and hydroxyapatite crystals that afford it compressive strength (Frankel and Nordin 1980). A fracture will occur in bone only if sufficient force allows it to travel through the interface of collagen fibres, from crystal to crystal (Berryman and Haun 1996).

In response to an extreme load, bone responds in an elastic then plastic manner before failing (Mascie-Taylor and Bogin 1995). This means that bone can recover its shape and dimensions after loading (elastic phase). However, when elastic qualities reach their maximum capacity, the outer fibres begin to yield, and increased loading beyond this point results in deformation (plastic phase), even after the loading has ceased (Frankel and Nordin 1980). Bone fracture occurs when the ultimate strength of a particular region of bone is exceeded (Hipp and Hayes 2003). At the microscopic level, the trabeculae are the first structures to break, followed by the interface between compact bone and trabecular bone and ending with fracture of the outer compact bone (Zhi-Jin and Jia-Zhen 1991) (Figure 22.1).

Fractures may result at the point of impact (direct force), or they may occur at a different site to the point of impact (indirect force). They are traditionally described in response to four main types of force: tension, compression, bending, and torsion. These forces typically result in transverse, oblique, butterfly, and spiral fracture patterns, respectively (Crawford 1983). These patterns are not mutually exclusive, and the majority of fractures seen in a clinical setting are a complex combination of several loading forces and fracture patterns (Hipp and Hayes 2003).

Fracture Propagation, Extent, and Morphology

Fracture propagation, extent, and morphology are determined by a complex interaction of extrinsic and intrinsic variables (Harkess, Ramsey, and Ahmadi 1984). Extrinsic variables relate to the physics of the applied force, such as its magnitude and direction (Tomezak and Buikstra 1999). Intrinsic variables relate to the properties of the bone, including its morphology, elasticity, and structural buttressing (Berryman and Haun 1996). For example, three main types of fracture are seen in the facial skeleton that are determined in relation to the structural buttressing of the orbits, maxilla, and nasal bone. These fractures have been classified as Le Fort I, Le Fort II, and Le Fort III, after Rene Le Fort, who first described them (Berryman and Symes 1995a; Rogers 1992) (Figure 22.2).

Another example concerns the decrease in rib restraint and the changes in disc size and shape at the thoracicolumbar junction. These morphological traits mean that this region of the spine is more susceptible to fracture than others are (Tomezak and Buikstra 1999). Furthermore, bones that have a large surface area will resist forces more successfully than those that have a small surface area, because there is greater area in which to dissipate the force.

Adult bones fail sooner than child bones do, because the former are brittle and the latter, elastic (Currey and Butler 1975). Brown and associates (2005) examined blunt trauma and demonstrated that skeletal involvement also varies for obese and non-obese individuals, mortality being a more likely outcome among the former. Bones may also be predisposed to fracture because of pathology that may require surprisingly little force (Fenton, de Jong, and Haut 2003).

Finally, fractures will propagate along the lines of least resistance. Therefore, they will usually extend toward foramina, regions of weakness where blood vessels merge (Zhi-Jin and Jia-Zhen 1991). The concentration of foramina on the base of the cranium means that this is a common site for fractures to occur (Gurdjian, Webster, and Lissner 1950). Often, but not always, they are interrupted by the suture lines and the epiphyses (Bonnichsen 1979; Kanz and Grossschmidt 2005: 210).

Cranial Fracture Patterns

Several texts describe the mechanisms of fracture in the cranial vault (Berryman and Haun 1996; Gurdjian, Webster, and Lissner 1950; Hart 2005; Smith, Berryman, and Lahren 1987). Bone is weaker under tension than it is under compression and will therefore break on the tension side first (Berryman and Haun 1996). If the energy of the insult is of sufficient force, secondary and tertiary fractures may develop in the area surrounding the impact site. Secondary fractures (also known as

This classification is an oversimplification of fractures involving the face. Actual fractures may be a combination of these Le Fort types.

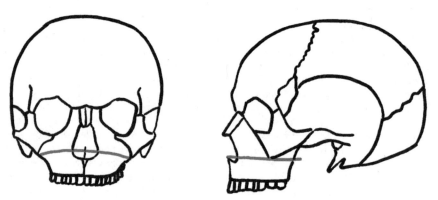

LE FORT I
Horizontal fracture through the nasal aperture and maxilla. Results in separation of the alveolar portion of the maxilla and may occur when the lower face receives a blow from the front or from the side.

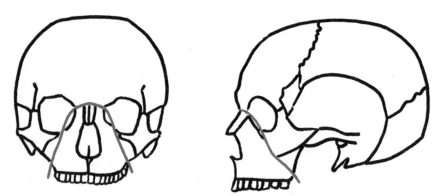

LE FORT II
Pyramidal fracture through the maxilla, lower orbits and upper nasal bones. Results in separation of the mid-face and may occur when the mid-face is impacted from the front.

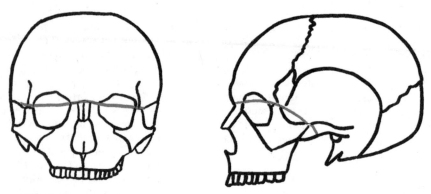

LE FORT III
Transverse fracture through the upper orbits and region of the nasal bone. Results in separation of entire face from the braincase and may occur when the nasal bridge or upper maxilla is impacted with a centrally focused blow.

Figure 22.2 Le Fort fractures of the facial skeleton (modified from Byers [2005: 325] and Galloway [1999: 74].

radiating fractures or fissures) are linear; tertiary fractures are curvilinear and form perpendicular to these. Secondary and tertiary fractures vary depending on the direction of the force and the type of weapon. For example, wide, split fissures are associated with an oblique force and multiple fissures are associated with broad blunt weapons (Berryman and Haun 1996; Gurdjian, Webster, and Lissner 1950). Concentric fractures may form in the absence of linear fractures, and, depending on the energy of the insult, more than one may be present in concentric bands (Hart 2005).

Pattern and shape of injury relates to the velocity of the blow: the higher the velocity the more distinct the pattern and the less likely there will be associated deformations (Gurdjian, Webster, and Lissner 1950). For example, large depressed lesions with satellite patterns are caused by slow-loading blunt instruments, whereas neat holes are determined by high-velocity bullets. However, discrete patterns are not always associated with high-velocity weapons: shattering will occur when the velocity of a missile is considerable.

The number of linear fractures is determined by the amount of energy of the force, with fewer being associated with less force (Gurdjian, Webster, and Lissner 1950). Further, linear fractures occur in locations that are weakest in relation to the initial impact area. Thus, an impact in a certain location will have a predictive influence over the location of the linear fracture. For example, a blow to the posterior parietal region has three related areas that are most likely to come under stress, these being (in order of susceptibility) the temporal bone, the superior parietal region, and the parietal mastoid region. Linear fractures can involve all three if the energy of the force is severe, or just the most susceptible if it is adequate. Further patterns are described by Lovell (1997: 155) and are useful for exploring the point of impact and mechanism of the injury.

The relationship between radiating fractures may be examined to determine the sequence of injuries where more than one occurs. This is based on the principle that secondary fractures terminate in primary ones and on observations of fracture patterns in broken glass (Madea and Staak 1988). When radiating fractures are not present, it is not usually possible to sequence multiple injuries.

Also associated with fracture production is bevelling, or cratering, which refers to the removal of a cone of bone. If the cone is removed as a result of a right-angled strike, the bevel has a symmetrical appearance (Kanz and Grossschmidt 2005). It arises as the fracture propagates and encounters shear forces causing angulation in its direction and

it may be present ecto- or endocranially (Berryman and Haun 1996).

General Characteristics of Perimortem Trauma

The identification of perimortem trauma rests on the principle that bone that has an intact organic matrix ("green bone") will respond differently to bone that has partial organic matrix ("dry bone"). Criteria relating to perimortem fracture identification primarily focus on the cranium and the long bones.

Typical characteristics of green-bone fractures include fracture margins that are sharp and smooth, radiating fracture lines and fracture lines that are straight. Irregular fracture margins (or splintering); fragments that tend to stay attached to one another (or hinging); peeling or lifting of fracture margins; bending; margins that are usually discoloured or the same colour as the surrounding bone; and trabeculae that are stained from the haematoma may also indicate perimortem trauma (Berryman and Haun 1996; Brothwell 1981; Kanz and Grossschmidt 2005). Knüsel and Outram (2006: 255) describe "spalling," or the removal of chips of cortical bone in association with a perimortem parry fracture. Additionally, Galloway (1999) argues that maggots and larvae may be observed in trabeculae that have been exposed as a result of fractures occurring during the perimortem or early postmortem periods. Dry-bone fractures result in smaller and more regular fragments, have margins that are rough and uneven, and (often) have discontinuous fracture lines (Kanz and Grossschmidt 2005; Sauer 1998).

Fracture margin texture, fracture angle (created by the fracture surface and the cortical surface) and fracture outline (in relation to the longitudinal axis) distinguish green fractures from dry fractures in long bones (Villa and Mahieu 1991). Fractures with smooth textures, an obtuse or acute fracture angle, and a curved outline are associated with green bone, whereas those that have jagged textures, have a right angle, and are transverse in outline are associated with dry-bone fractures (Villa and Mahieu 1991: 34–35) (see Figures 22.3a and 22.3b).

Knüsel and Outram (2006) further divide dry-bone fractures into those that show a mineralised response and those that show a dry response. Dry fractures occur in bone that has still retained some of its organic properties; it is not mineralised, but it is not "green" either. Stepped fracture outlines and a rough, corrugated surface texture are features of this type of fracture (Knüsel and Outram 2006: 262). In a forensic context, the identification

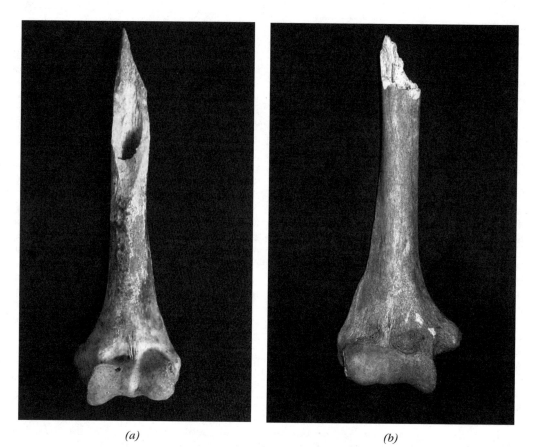

(a)   *(b)*

Figure 22.3 *(a)* Perimortem helical fracture involving the mid-shaft of a left humerus from a Bronze Age deposit at Charterhouse Warren Farm swallet, Somerset, England (courtesy Wells Museum). *(b)* Postmortem fracture involving the mid-shaft of a right humerus from one of the Medieval or post-Medieval burials from Oxford Castle (courtesy Oxford Archaeology).

of dry fractures may facilitate the assessment of secondary burial in cases where, for example, remains have been exhumed and reburied to conceal a crime.

At the microscopic level, Shipman (1981: 371–372) distinguishes between two types of change: (1) when the fracture plane lies between two adjacent collagen bundles exposing a smooth laminar surface and (2) when the fracture plane lies perpendicular to the dominant bundle direction, exposing a roughened and stepped surface as the result of sudden rupture. The first type refers to horizontal tension failure (dry-bone fracture) and the second refers to spiral tension failure (green-bone fracture). Houck's (1998) experimental study contrasts the microscopic appearance of knife cut marks made to fresh bone that was subsequently air dried, with further knife cut marks made to bone after it was dry. In the wet bone, the line of the periosteum is located apart from the line of cut, whereas in the

dried bone, the location of the line of both is the same (Houck: 420).

Biologically, there is considerable overlap between the perimortem and the antemortem and postmortem periods. For example, injuries can occur well before death but show no signs of healing, even though they are classified as perimortem. Under controlled laboratory conditions maintained at room temperature, the elastic properties of bone decrease after approximately five hours following death (Kanz and Grossschmidt 2005). However, in some burial environments the moisture content of bone may be retained several weeks after death (Maples 1999), and, therefore, fractures can occur that bear the characteristics of fresh breaks.

There is enormous variation in the amount of lapsed time before macroscopic signs of healing, seen as new bone formation, can be detected on bone. This takes at least a week or as long as three weeks, depending on extrinsic and intrinsic variables such as the nature and the extent of the injury, the health status of the individual, and genetic variations (Buikstra and Ubelaker 1994; Sauer 1998: 332). For these reasons, observations relating to the type, severity, and location of the injury, the victim's age, the likelihood of secondary infection, and the forensic pathologist's opinion regarding survivability in relation to these factors should also be considered when attempting to distinguish antemortem from perimortem lesions (Galloway 1999).

If soft tissue survives, healing may be detected histologically between five and seven days following an injury, whereas radiologically, it cannot be identified until between 10 and 14 days have lapsed. Most beneficial is the application of high-powered microscopy, which enables healing to be detected as areas of osteoclastic activity (bone resorption) after about one week following the insult. This is followed by osteoblastic activity, or new bone deposition (Boylston 2000).

Classification

Perimortem trauma is usually described in terms of the injury that caused it and is thus divided into projectile, sharp-force, and blunt-force injuries.

Projectile Trauma

Projectile trauma broadly refers to the characteristic changes that result from objects that travel through the air with enough velocity to impact bone (Byers 2005). Such projectiles include those from a range of devices, in particular, firearms, crossbows and other bows, muskets, catapults, and spear/javelin-type weapons (e.g., Bowman, MacLaughlin, and Scheuer 1992; Byers 2005; Downs et al. 1994; Liston and Baker 1996; Novak 2000; Roberts 2003; White 1988). Given the rise in terrorist bombings over recent years, it is surprising that few studies have looked at projectile injuries caused by missile fragments, despite the fact that they cause more deaths than do the actual blast effects (Knight 1996).

Devices. One cannot analyse projectile injuries without prior knowledge of the devices themselves. Firearms and ammunition are the most complex and sophisticated of these, and they receive the most attention in the literature. This literature broadly relates to single and multiple projectiles, internal and external bullet construction, and the size of the firearm (handguns and rifles). A comprehensive review of these key issues is provided by DiMaio (1999), Dodd (2005), Mahoney (2005), and Walter (2000). Adam (1989),

Chamberlain and Gander (1974), and Quertermous and Quertermous (1994a, 1994b) discuss details of manufactured gun models used today.

Mechanics of Projectile Injury. The velocity with which a projectile contacts the body characterises the resultant wound. Thus, a high-velocity projectile that travels at least 610 m/sec has a more explosive effect on its target than does a low-velocity projectile travelling at 305 m/sec or less (Gellman, Wiss, and Moldawer 2003). However, the nature of the target is also a variable. For example, bullets must travel at greater velocity to penetrate thicker bones (DiMaio 1999). The amount of kinetic energy required by a projectile to cause damage to humans is not great: a projectile fired at bone by, for example, a catapult or a gas canister with as little as 66 foot-pounds of kinetic energy (5.58×10^{20} electron volts) can be deadly (Byers 2005: 311).

Tissue damage occurs when the kinetic energy of the projectile is either entirely or partly absorbed. A projectile, therefore, may not necessarily result in trauma if it fails to transfer its kinetic energy, but the more that is transferred, the greater the tissue damage (Knight 1996). If missile mass is doubled, kinetic energy is also doubled. However, if velocity is doubled, the kinetic energy is quadrupled. Therefore, both mass and velocity are important determinants of tissue damage, but velocity has more influence (Gellman, Wiss, and Moldawer 2003).

Missiles may pass completely through soft tissues retaining their kinetic energy and leave a missile track. Some missiles are designed to slow or stop inside the body so as to ensure that as much kinetic energy is transferred as possible and that maximum damage is caused. Thus, a bullet may pass straight through the body (a "through and through" injury); it may deviate from the original trajectory, split into distinct parts in the body, and produce more than one exit wound; or it (particularly pellets) may remain in the body. Bullets may also be deflected off hard tissue, causing fragments of bone to be dispelled in many directions, leaving multiple secondary exit wounds (Knight 1996: 243).

The dynamics of projectiles as they travel through the air also influence the amount of kinetic energy. For example, the trajectory of a projectile may take on various forms, depending on the projectile's weight, design, and distance from the target. Projectiles may tumble end over end and enter on their side; wag and yaw from side to side on their axial trajectory; process (yaw in a circular pattern about the centre of gravity in the form of a decreasing spiral) and nutate (rotate in a small circle forming a rosette pattern, as would a spinning top) with complex spiral or circular movements about the axis; or the base may rotate around the axis, the tip remaining on a straight path (Owen-Smith 1981: 18).

Mechanism of Injury. Missiles may penetrate bone, depending on a variety of factors. As outlined above, variables include velocity, kinetic energy, bullet construction, and bullet weight. Other factors are the angle of interaction between the bullet and the bone (in turn, influenced by the trajectory of the bullet) and the type of bone (for example, long or flat).

Laceration and crushing, shock waves, and cavitation (a cavity that is formed in the wake of the bullet and causes the bullet track to be stretched outward) are the primary mechanisms of injury in shotgun trauma and are described by Knight (1996) and Owen-Smith (1981). Firm tissue (for instance, muscle) may be lacerated and crushed as the bullet forces a track, or a permanent cavity, through it; this occurs when a low-velocity bullet penetrates the body. Studies of gelatin blocks show that, despite similar missile velocities, the profile of the permanent cavity varies considerably depending on the dynamics of the bullet and whether, for example, the bullet fragments (Fackler, Bellamy, and Malinowski 1988). High-velocity bullets generate spherical shock waves ahead of them, causing injuries in locations other than those immediately in the bullet track. High-velocity bullets also produce temporary fusiform cavities that form around the bullet track in the wake of the bullet and may damage surrounding structures (Owen-Smith 1981). Secondary missiles are another mechanism and include fragments of fractured bone or fragments of bullet that may be expelled in a number of different directions, causing injury to surrounding soft tissues (Gilman, Wiss, and Moldawer 2003).

When a gun is fired, a number of by-products, such as carbon, gasses, grains of powder, and abrasion from heat and friction, will result in soft-tissue wounds. Examples include soot soiling, powder tattooing, and a grease ring. Soft-tissue wounds vary, depending on the type of missile fired (for example, hand gun or shot gun), intermediary artefacts (for example, clothing), and whether the firearm is in contact or at close, intermediate, or long range. Detailed accounts of the different by-products of a firearm are provided by Knight (1996: 247–261) and DiMaio (1999) and are summarised in Table 22.1.

Firearm Wounds in Bone. Firearm wounds in bone are primarily described in the literature in relation to the cranium and concern entrance and exit wounds, radiating fractures, and concentric heaving fractures. Entrance wounds have sharp, internally bevelled margins and are round or conical in plan, depending on the angle of the impact, the stability of the bullet, and the morphology of the bone. Hence, wounds most commonly occur on the parietal or occipital bones, on the frontal bone less so. Exit wounds tend to be larger than entrance wounds and have a bevelled margin externally. On penetration of the outer table, the projectile forces a cone-shaped path through the bone, creating a wider girth on the inner table compared to the outer table. On exiting the cranium, the same process occurs, but this time in reverse, so that the wound on the outer table is wider than it is on the inner table.

Entrance and exit wounds are difficult to identify on the thin bones of juvenile crania, in particular, the temporal bone. Such wounds may also not be visible on any victim, juvenile or adult, if surgical debridement has been performed, bones are inadequately recovered from site, or taphonomic alteration (especially animal scavenging) obscures the wound margins. This is particularly difficult if remains are highly fragmentary (either as a result of postmortem damage or in the case of comminutions), such as in contact gunshot wounds (Fenton et al. 2005). Thus maximum recovery from site and reconstruction are essential. Entrance and exit wounds have been studied to estimate bullet calibre, but this effort has achieved limited success (Berryman and Symes 1995b; Ross 1996).

It is now a widely accepted (but still imperfectly understood) phenomenon that a bevelled margin may be produced on the surface opposite to the direction of the bullet. This situation is believed to occur if a bullet enters perpendicularly or tangentially to the surface of the bone. Where this occurs, the reverse bevel is usually smaller than the bevel it opposes (Coe 1982). Bones may also present two entrance wounds and one exit wound if a bullet is deflected back into the body when it hits an intermediary target on exiting.

The shape of a firearm wound in bone can vary, depending not just on whether it is an entry or an exit wound but also on impact velocity, trajectory of the projectile, tissue density, type of bullet, and whether or not the bullet deforms. Different firearm wound shapes in relation to these variables are summarised by Byers (2005: 300–302).

Smith, Berryman, and Lahren (1987) summarise the sequence of fracture development in gunshot trauma. Radiating fractures first initiate around the impact site, and concentric heaving fractures are produced as intracranial pressure causes out bending of the plates of bone. Radiating fractures may

Table 22.1 Summary of the different by-products of a gun having been fired (after Knight 1996: 247–261).

	Explanation
Soiling and burning/blistering Singeing of hair	As a result of products of explosion (if greater distance, hair may be "clubbed" as a result of the keratin melting and solidifying).
Soot soiling	Carbon deposition that stains the skin and exposed tissues; easily washed off.
Powder tattooing	Small burns from specks of propellant; will not wash off.
Peppering	From unburned flakes and grains of powder; more disparate the greater the distance from the weapon.
Grease ring	Black, dirty mark made by the end of the gun barrel from heat, grease, and metal particles from bullet and lubricating oil. Occurs if held against the skin when fired.
Abrasion collar	Abrasion from heat and friction as missile enters and causes the skin to invert around the missile. Leaves discoloured skin around the wound. Also, damage to subcutaneous blood vessels results in bruising around the wound.
Everted and split skin	Characteristic of exit wounds that are also stellate and quite clean.
"Rat hole" or "rat nibbling"	Edges of wound crenated and scalloped. Occurs in short- to mid-range gunshot discharge.
Carbon monoxide	Cherry pink colour on interior of bullet track and surrounding tissues; may be present on exit wound. Is the result of carbon monoxide combined with haemoglobin and myoglobin.
Muzzle impression	When muzzle pressed hard against the skin or the skin is drawn up against the muzzle when discharge gases are deflected off bone, temporarily raising the skin and subcutaneous tissue into a dome.
Bullet wipe	Fragments or streaks of metal adhere to bone and reflect the direction of the bullet.

also accompany exit wounds. However, these are not to be confused with entrance-wound radiating fractures, which travel faster than the speed of a bullet and, therefore, advance to the other side of the vault before the bullet. Radiating fractures associated with an exit wound may terminate in a radiating fracture associated with an entrance wound and can be useful for determining the direction of a bullet when the entrance and exit wounds are themselves missing (Smith, Berryman, and Lahren 1987).

Postcranial Projectile Trauma. Reference to projectile trauma to the postcranial skeleton is negligible in the forensic literature, and presently most knowledge derives from medical texts. Unlike cranial fractures, postcranial fractures resulting from direct impact tend to leave fewer prescribed patterns other than considerable comminution, bone loss, and perhaps nicks and depressions from metal fragments. Bone fractures resulting from indirect shock waves tend to show a linear pattern with little displacement (Ryan 1997).

Eismont and Lattuga (2003) review gunshot injuries to the spine. They report that associated secondary fractures involving the vertebral body are common in gunshot injuries to the posterior arch or pedicles. However, secondary changes to posterior elements are unlikely when the vertebral body is the primary site of injury presumably because, owing to its cancellous structure, it transmits less energy to surrounding structures (Ryan 1997: 989).

The same conclusion was reached by Heulke and Darling (1964), who observed that fragmentation was greater in green bone than in dry bone, and in diaphyses than in epiphyses. Radiating fracture lines travelled at right angles to the point of impact and resulted in the detachment of a triangular fragment of bone, a pattern that is consistent with a butterfly fracture. A more recent study undertaken by Ubelaker and Adams (1994) indicates that butterfly fractures are not solely related to perimortem trauma but may also be identified in dry-bone fractures. Based on experiments that yielded similar results, Ragsdale and Sohn's study (1988) describes how diaphyses fragment into larger pieces and act as secondary projectiles.

As in the cranium, a tangential entrance wound in tubular bones can also result in a keyhole lesion (Berryman and Gunther 2000), although interpretation would benefit from additional experimentation. Bevelling has been described on flat bones, such as ribs and the pelvis, and may be used to explore directionality (Besant-Matthews 2000; Spitz 1980), although this bevelling is somewhat harder to observe than in the cranium (Galloway and Zephro 2005).

Sharp-Force Trauma

Injuries that cut and divide tissue are classified as sharp trauma and are caused by instruments that produce cut/incision, stab, or cleft/notch wounds. These are caused by a compression force that is both dynamic and acutely focused and may result in lesions that penetrate through to the endocranial or medullary surface of bone, skip or glance off bone, or slice, chop, or scrape bone, depending on the angle and the impact of the instrument.

Diagnostic features of each type of wound (cut, stab, or cleft) relate to its shape, length, and width and the morphological appearance of the wall of the lesion and associated secondary lesions. Primary characteristics broadly relate to the fact that cuts are longer than they are wide and have parallel margins, one hinged and one polished. Stab wounds may be identified as punctures that are shorter than they are wide, and cleft wounds are linear and broad. Secondary characteristics include fractures that radiate from the point of impact, hinge fractures, and separation of bone fragments from the main lesion (bone wastage, or chipping). Hinge fractures and bone wastage will vary in extent, depending on the instrument (Table 22.2). Note that with reference to puncture wounds made with knives of a certain size, the length of the wound corresponds to the width of the blade (Williams et al. 1998).

Literature is limited in terms of information on individual tool-mark characteristics, with most focusing on class characteristics (e.g., Blumenschine, Maren, and Capaldo 1996; Greenfield 2000; Houck 1998; Shipman 1981). Tool marks are difficult and often impossible to identify (Reichs 1998). Studies that have explored individual characteristics include Andahl (1978), Bonte (1975), Olsen (1988), and Symes, Berryman, and Smith (1998) on saw marks; Humphrey and Hutchinson (2001) on the macroscopic characteristics of machetes, cleavers, and axes; Alunni-Perret and associates (2005) on

Table 22.2 Firearm wound shapes and their likely associated variables (based on Byers 2005: 300–302).

Shape	Bullet Type Most Commonly Associated with	Associated Variables
Round	Jacketed; nondeforming	Trajectory and angle of bullet perpendicular to target; common in entry wounds.
Oval	Jacketed	Trajectory not perpendicular to target; bullet tumbling when it strikes; common in entry wounds.
Keyhole	Any	Trajectory of bullet very acute; limited penetration of bullet; seen in entry and exit.
Irregular	Deforming bullets more common	Usually caused by shattering; common in exit.

microscopic features of wounds made by a hatchet; Walker and Long (1977) on cut marks made by a steel hand axe, a steel knife, and stone tools; Sivaram (1977) on wound characteristics made by a serrated sickle; and Rao and Hart (1983) on cut marks made by a marine survival knife in cartilage. Sharp-trauma injuries have also been reported in association with cuts made by mower blades (Walsh-Haney 1999) and boat-propeller blades (Stubblefield 1999) and the likelihood that they are the result of accidental or homicidal trauma.

Microstriations and Directionality. Microstriations are faint lines that run along the longitudinal axis of the walls of a cut and reflect imperfections in the instrument as it is drawn across the bone (Figure 22.4). Their appearance may vary, depending on the instrument used. This observation has largely been developed in the zooarchaeological and archaeological literature, which contrasts the appearance of cut marks made by stone tools with those made by bladed tools (e.g., Greenfield 2000). Although the study of stone tools is not of great relevance to the forensic anthropologist, the associated literature makes a valuable contribution to present understandings of class characteristics, including general configuration, contour, and profile.

Another significant contribution is to the interpretation of directionality of cut marks. At the macroscopic level, angle and direction of an instrument may be indicated by the profile of the lesion and its location (Novak 2000). However, these may be expanded, through high-powered microscopic analysis, to include information on whether the cut was being made from left to right, or from right

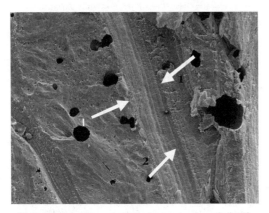

Figure 22.4 Scanning electron micrograph (x80) showing an experimental cut mark (arrow 1) with internal microstrictions (arrow 2). The cut was made on animal bone using a flint tool (photograph courtesy Dr. M Smith).

to left. In their experimental study that applied SEM analysis to cut marks made on bovine bone, Bromage and Boyde (1984) determined three criteria of directionality: morphological changes, including bone smears, oblique faulting, and oblique chipping, which may be observed on the floor and walls of the cut. Although these features were not the focus of their study, Bromage and Boyde (1984) observed that they were also useful for indicating handedness. Other factors, including the relative position of the victim and the assailant and variation in cutting edge, remain to be fully explored at this level (Bromage and Boyde 1984; Houck 1995).

Scanning Electron Microscopy. The application of scanning electron microscopy (SEM) to cut-mark analysis has, for a long time, occupied an ambivalent status in terms of its perceived usefulness among anthropologists (Blumenschine, Maren, and Capaldo 1996; Bunn 1981; Loe and Cox 2005; Shipman 1981). Microscopic analyses feature little in the literature, and very little research has explored methodological approaches for the quantitative analysis of cut marks using SEM. Exceptions include preliminary work by Bartelink, Wiersema, and Demaree (2001), who applied SEM analysis to explore quantitative methods for distinguishing cut marks on bone made by a scalpel blade, a paring knife, and a kitchen utility knife. The results highlighted the difficulty in identifying a particular implement, a concern that echoes that of Houck (1998) on macroscopic analysis, owing to the fact that cut-mark width tended to overlap for different knife types. However, combined with qualitative analyses, this approach was considered valuable (Houck 1998).

More recently, Alunni-Perret and associates (2005) reported on the benefits of applying SEM analysis to identify individual tool-mark characteristics. Microscopic criteria for distinguishing hacking trauma from knife trauma, or pure sharp trauma from sharp-blunt trauma, are presented. Interestingly, this is one of the few cut-mark studies to experiment on human bone, most to date having been undertaken on animal remains.

Blunt-Force Trauma

Trauma resulting from contact with a blunt instrument or a fall may be identified on dry bone as focal or penetrating injuries that have discrete patterns, which sometimes bear characteristic hallmarks of a particular type of weapon (for example, a pole axe), or as areas of crushing with few distinctive features. Severity, extent, and appearance of blunt-force trauma are mediated by a number of factors, including the nature of the impact, the area struck, the angle of the force, and the amount and duration of the force.

Most blunt trauma is described in the literature in terms of insults from weapons (e.g., Boylston 2000; Novak 2000). More recently, Tomezak and Buikstra (1999) have reviewed fracture patterns sustained as a result of falls (vertical deceleration injuries) and vehicular-pedestrian accidents (horizontal deceleration injuries). Fracture patterns for each are explored, including consideration of the different variables that may determine their outcome (for instance, body mass, speed and size of automobile acceleration, body position, height of fall, humidity, and air drag of clothes).

Fractures That Result from Local Deformations. Fracture production arising from blunt trauma is usually described in four stages: (1) inbending at the site of impact producing a compressive force on the outer table and tensile force on the inner table, peripheral outbending and initial fracture production on the inner table; (2) formation of radiating fractures; (3) inbending of plates of bone; and (4) concentric fracture formation in areas of tension produced on the outer table (Berryman and Haun 1996; Berryman and Symes 1995a).

The area directly below and around the impact site may rebound if the impact is not of a sufficient velocity or energy (Gurdjian, Webster, and Lissner 1950). Such rebounding may result in linear fractures that extend toward the impact area and in the opposite direction (a result of the impact area coming under tension as it immediately rebounds from compression). Otherwise, a depressed fracture will result. This fracture will vary, depending on the brittleness and the elasticity of the bone when the impact occurs (Berryman and Symes 1995a: 340):

1. A plug of bone is forced inward (brittle bone);

2. There is in-bending, and the fracture advances from the inner to the outer table (elastic bone);

3. The outer table and diploë are crushed, but no fracture occurs on the inner table (brittle diploë);

4. There is in-bending of the inner table with shattering of the inner table and diploë (brittle diploë).

The fracture is dependant on the magnitude of the blow, the instrument used, and the area struck. The main types of impact pattern are summarised by Boylston (2000: 363) after King (1992):

1. Linear fracture with radiating fissure fractures;

2. Depressed fracture;

3. Depressed fracture à la signature;

4. Depressed fracture produced by a sharp-edged weapon;

5. Depressed pond fracture (also comminuted);

6. Depressed satellite fracture;

7. Comminuted fracture.

These injuries are further classified as depressed, expressed diastatic, and gutter fractures. A depressed fracture results from bone fragments being pushed inward and is either comminuted (broken into many different fragments) or has a pond or satellite appearance. When bone fragments protrude outward from the cranium, they are described as expressed fractures. Fractures that involve the parting of sutures (common in children) are classified as diastatic, whereas those that arise as a result of an instrument grazing bone are referred to as gutter. Another classification system is described by Galloway (1999) and includes patterns relating to the cranium, axial skeleton, and upper and lower extremities. These are broadly categorised as complete fractures and incomplete fractures.

Other postcranial blunt trauma patterns include incomplete and buckle rib fractures and are described by Love and Symes (2004). In their study, incomplete fractures were observed in children and adults aged between 21 and 76 years with no significant bias toward a particular age group. This observation is contrary to the belief that such fractures are more common in children. Buckle fractures resulting from compressive force had not been described before.

Fractures That Result from Indirect Violence. Le Fort fractures and ring fractures are examples of those that occur away from the area of impact. Ring fractures partially or completely encircle the foramen magnum, depending on the force. They arise when the skull is driven down onto the vertebral column, usually as the result of a fall from a height. In severe cases, they may continue into the petrous portion of the temporal bone and terminate at the foramen of the middle fossa (Byers 2005: 324).

Blunt Trauma versus Gunshot Trauma. Berryman and Haun (1996) suggest that if skull fragments are impossible to reconstruct, they are more likely to have arisen as a result of a slow loading force (that is, blunt trauma) than a fast loading force (for example, projectile trauma). This is because, under a slow loading force applied over a large area, bone will fracture when it is in its plastic phase of deformation. A rapid loading force applied to a small area will result in a brittle response causing an explosive pattern of fracture with minimal or no plastic deformation (Berryman and Symes 1995a). Caveats to this rule include the fact that sediment pressure may act as a slow loading force and therefore, cause similar plastic deformation in remains that are still wet. Furthermore, these responses are mediated by numerous extrinsic and intrinsic variables, including the age of the individual (for instance, children's bones are more plastic than adult bones), the duration of the blow, and the density and the morphology of the bone, among other factors.

Although concentric fractures are observed in both blunt and projectile trauma, the ways these are produced are very different. In blunt trauma, the bevel is usually located internally, whereas in gunshot trauma, the bevel is usually external. However, reverse bevelling may occur in projectile trauma, and bevel direction may not always be apparent in blunt trauma, depending on buttressing of the vault, from the impact site and the spherical shape of the skull (Berryman and Haun 1996; Berryman and Symes 1995a). These factors have recently been tested by Hart (2005), who, using 211 forensic specimens, demonstrated a strong statistical relationship between mechanism of trauma and direction of concentric fracture, particularly in areas of the skull that are not buttressed. Under these circumstances, concentric fractures develop under tension on the inner table and advance to the outer table producing an external bevel as shear forces are encountered, unlike the concentric fractures seen in blunt trauma.

Perimortem Trauma Patterns in the Skeleton: Causes

Much of the literature on the circumstances of trauma is anecdotal. Gellman, Wiss, and Moldawer (2003) note in passing that gunshot trauma to the foot is more common under accidental circumstances, when a gun is being loaded or cleaned. Fractures that affect the hands and forearms are associated with defence injuries (Roberts 1996) and those involving the facial skeleton, an attack (Walker 1997). Injuries that predominantly affect one side of the skeleton more than the other may indicate handedness of the assailant, and fractures that occur on the back of the skull may be caused by an attack from behind (ibid.). Certain fractures

are associated with falls (for example, a Colles fracture of the wrist). The head and the neck are the most common areas to receive insults during an attack (Knight 1996), whereas fractures to the sternum, scapula, and ribs may be associated with direct blows (Roberts 1996). A useful summary of the most frequent areas to be affected by projectile trauma in various conflicts is presented in Ryan (1997).

More recent anthropological literature focuses on the identification of victims of child abuse, as evidenced in skeletal remains (e.g., Cattaneo et al. 2006; Lewis 2007; Lewis and Rutty 2003; Torwalt et al. 2002). Diagnostic features include peri- and postmortem lesions with multiple fractures being present in most cases (Cattaneo et al. 2006). Fractures involving the ribs are regarded as a strong indicator of child abuse (Cattaneo et al. 2006: 5; Kerley 1978) and tend to be bilateral (Walker, Cook, and Lambert 1997), with those involving the posterior portion of the rib being highly indicative of the victim having been squeezed around the torso (Lewis 2007; Lewis and Rutty 2003: 206). Fractures involving the skull tend to be linear, rather than comminuted or depressed, and are more likely to cross the sutures (Walker, Cook, and Lambert 1997). Other sites that are commonly involved include the facial skeleton, metaphyses, epiphyses, and diaphyses and are discussed by Lewis (2007), Walker, Cook, and Lambert (1997), and Williams and associates (1998), who also consider radiographic changes and antemortem lesions.

Fractures involving the hyoid are associated with manual and ligature strangulation, suffocation, a direct blow to the neck, and hanging. This is the same for fractures involving the cricoid and thyroid cartilages, provided they have ossified (usually in older adults). Fractures of the hyoid tend to occur on the posterior and middle portions of the greater horn (Pollanen et al. 1995).

A fracture involving the odontoid process of the second cervical vertebra (axis) is typical of hanging (that is, "Hangman's fracture"). However, absence of a fracture involving these structures cannot be regarded as reliable evidence that trauma has not occurred (Ubelaker 1992). Whether the hyoid bone fractures is highly dependent on whether the separate bony elements that make up this bone have fused, a process that does not normally occur until the third decade, that may occur into late adulthood, or that may not occur at all (O'Halloran and Lundy 1987; Pollanen and Chiasson 1996; Scheuer and Black 2000). Thus, younger individuals are less likely to sustain fractures to this bone, because it is more elastic in its unfused state. Even when fractures do occur, they are often difficult to distinguish from postmortem fractures in the absence of soft-tissue haemorrhaging.

Cut marks may be present on bone as the result of dismemberment, decapitation, cannibalism, defleshing, and deliberate disarticulation. These may be differentiated from one another based on their frequency, location, and orientation, as well as the type of cut mark and associated injuries. For example, cut, chop, and/or saw marks located at or near articulations and orientated perpendicular to the longitudinal axis of the bone are associated with disarticulation and dismemberment (Olsen and Shipman 1994; Reichs 1998). These activities are discussed in more detail by Reichs (1998), including how dismemberment patterns may inform about the motives, state of mind, and knowledge of the perpetrators, as well as link victims from different murder scenes to the same perpetrator if lesions share similarities in their distribution, appearance, and location.

Superficial cut marks that are randomly located are associated with defleshing. If these marks occur on the skull and tend to follow the crown, they are indicative of scalping, whereas if they are multi-directional and involve the face and basicranium, they are indicative of defleshing (Mays and Steele 1996; Olsen and Shipman 1994).

Decapitation is indicated by the presence of cut marks on the cervical vertebrae, clavicles, basiocciptal, and mandible. However, microscopic analysis may be required to determine whether the decapitation occurred at, or after, death (that is, skull removal). It is also important to assess the context of the finds. For example, cut marks on a clavicle from the Neolithic burial chamber at West Tump, Gloucestershire, England, are described by Smith and Brickley (2004) and interpreted as evidence for decapitation. This was probably performed after death as a part of the practice of disarticulating body parts and moving them between locations, a practice that was widespread at that time.

Certain perimortem sharp-force trauma patterns are associated with the surgical removal of a piece of bone from the cranium. This practice, also known as trepanation, may be performed by scraping, grooving, bawing-and-cutting, or creating rectangular intersecting incisions (Lisowski 1967). Several examples have been identified in the archaeological record (Arnot, Finger, and Smith 2003); problems with this study include the fact that it is usually impossible to distinguish unsuccessful trepanation (that is, performed before death) from exploratory surgery (performed shortly after death) and identify the motives behind such intervention, unless there is an associated trauma (Roberts and McKinley 2003).

Other circumstances that may be reflected in perimortem trauma patterns relate to falls in which the height of a fall influences the orientation of the body when it lands and thus the parts of the skeleton affected. For example, individuals falling from low heights (up to about 12 m) are more likely to sustain fractures to their skull, forearm, and cervical vertebrae. Injuries to the chest, pelvis, and thoracic vertebrae are more common among individuals who have fallen from greater heights (over approximately 12 m). Fractures involving the lower extremities, the cervical spine, skull, and pelvis are common in vehicular pedestrian accidents, whereas fractures involving the skull and thoracico-lumbar junction are common in falls (Tomezak and Buikstra 1999).

In addition to trauma patterns, weathering and evidence for scavenging provide evidence about the nature of an assemblage exhibiting perimortal trauma. Remains that are weathered and scavenged suggest exposure following death; this situation is more likely to be encountered in the remains of victims of a massacre than of other events, such as accidental trauma (Hurlbut 2000).

Although patterns of perimortem trauma may indicate the circumstances that gave rise to them, one must remember that very rarely can such interpretations be extended to suggest the cause (for example, heart disease, cancer, haemorrhage) and manner (for instance, suicide, accident, murder) of death. It is not the legal obligation of forensic anthropologists to determine this, although they have a very important role in assisting the forensic pathologist or medical examiner in doing so (Byers 2005). Interpretations of trauma are particularly important given the fact that trauma accounts for most suspicious deaths, and skeletal trauma may provide the only information about the cause and manner of death if the body has decomposed (Byers 2005; Roberts 1996). The relationship between skeletal lesions and cause and manner of death is a very ephemeral one; a stab wound may have caused death, but it may also have been delivered following death by other means (Byers 2005: 276–277).

Pseudo-Trauma

Factors that may mimic perimortem trauma can be broadly classified as those relating to pathology and medical procedures, skeletal morphology, burning, or animal and environmental activity. Lewis and Rutty (2003) warn that there are numerous skeletal pathologies that may be mistaken for child abuse—birth trauma and accidental and self-afflicted trauma being among these. Further, Torwalt and associates (2002) describe spontaneous fractures secondary to osteopaenia (a lower than normal bone-mineral density) in a child who died at 4 years, a case of natural disease that could be mistaken for child abuse.

Anatomical features, for example, blood vessel markings, may have superficial similarities with cut marks. Naturally occurring apertures such as in the sternum (the sternal aperture) may, to the untrained eye, be mistaken for bullet wounds (see Cunha and Pinheiro this volume). However, such features are usually easy to distinguish from genuine perimortem trauma based on their smooth, biological, and often less well-defined margins, as well as familiarity with skeletal anatomy.

Sufficient exposure to fire may hinder identification of perimortem trauma, in particular, gunshot and blunt trauma (Herrmann and Bennett 1999; Pope and Smith 2004). In such cases, reconstruction and microscopic examination are essential, so that characteristic patterns of heat-induced trauma may be distinguished from genuine injuries. Heat-induced trauma patterns include longitudinal, curved transverse and straight transverse fractures as well as patina and delamination (Herrmann and Bennett 1999: 461).

Carnivore or rodent tooth marks may be confused with cut marks; several papers describe criteria for distinguishing these (Blumenschine 1988; Blumenschine, Maren, and Capaldo 1996; Haglund, Reay, and Swindler 1988; Laudet and Fosse 2001; Milner and Smith 1989). Carnivore and rodent tooth marks tend to follow the contour of the bone, frequently occur in broad parallel groups on prominent areas of bone, are perpendicular in orientation, and may accompany tooth pits and punctures (Binford 1981).

Carnivore scavenging activity, which involves static loading, results in crushing at the ends of bones and fracture (Villa and Mahieu 1991) and can be difficult to distinguish from fractures caused by human activity, which involve dynamic loading. In addition to understanding the presence of associated tooth marks, knowledge of scavenging patterns, such as those reviewed by Bonnichsen (1979), is essential. This was highlighted by Puskas and Rumney (2003) on bilateral fractures of the coronoid processes in relation to intra-oral gunshot trauma and canid scavenging. Besides scavenging, trampling and fluvial activity may also result in fresh breaks to bone (Behrensmeyer, Gordon, and Yanagi 1986; Brooks and Brooks 1997; Shipman and Rose 1983).

Striations may occur on bone that has come into contact with sharp stones or substrate through being trampled or transported in water and may be mistaken for cut marks. These tend to be multidirectional, faint, intersect with one another, lack meaningful anatomical locations, and be of uneven thickness and depth (Blumenschine and Slevaggio 1988: 765; Cook 1986: 282–283; Olsen and Shipman 1988: 543; Shipman and Rose 1983).

Some limitations of the data illustrate the extent to which the present understanding of the biomechanics of perimortem trauma is inadequate, particularly in relation to the postcranial skeleton. This lack is exemplified in Love and Symes's (2004) study of rib fractures, which found that, contrary to experimental and observational biomechanic studies, ribs failed first under compressive rather than tensile force. Further, chronological age was not found to influence the presence or absence of incomplete fractures, suggesting that plasticity versus brittleness may not have such an influence over fracture mechanics as has been assumed. This situation requires further testing, particularly, as Love and Symes argue, through studies that consider biomechanics at the gross rather than at the tissue level.

At the root of these problems is the uniformitarian assumption that all bones will respond to trauma and/or modification in a universal manner (Reichs 1998; Young 1989). Further, the problem of "equifinality," which means that some trauma-related features reflect nothing more than the interaction between bone and an instrument, results in enormous cross-over between criteria for distinguishing different events (Cook 1986: 284; Oliver 1989: 91). Thus, marks made on bone may relate to the same mechanical movements but quite different events (for example, a human drawing a sharp stone across bone or a sharp stone being drawn across bone in the context of trampling).

Complete recovery of bone fragments is a challenge, because they may be lost in maggot masses, be transported away by insects, or surrounded by soft tissue in varying stages of decomposition (Galloway 1999). Further, the characteristics of a perimortem-induced injury may be modified (and hence obscured or erased) by factors such as weathering, soil abrasion, and animal scavenging, a process referred to by Shipman and Rose (1983: 60) as "taphonomic overprinting."

Regarding sharp-force trauma, the anthropologist is unlikely to observe the true frequency of this trauma in any given case, owing to the fact that many injuries, such as those to the chest area, will perforate the soft tissues without marking the bone. Further, the appearance of a sharp-force injury on bone will vary depending on the thickness of the soft tissue covering it. Thus, cuts to fingers are often small and extremely fine, owing to the fact that the overlying tissues absorb the energy of the cutting instrument (Alunni-Perret et al. 2005).

Last, sediment pressure may not only cause plastic deformation to bone but also cause fracture, particularly among bones with thin cortices relative to their large diameters (for example, femora and tibiae) (Trinkhaus 1985: 206–207). Where this situation involves relatively green bone, the characteristic features are, essentially, perimortem. Further, relatively fresh long bones will naturally break along the long axis of the bone, because of the orientation of the collagen fibre bundles and Haversian systems. Such breaks are known as longitudinal fractures or split line cracks and are discussed by Johnson (1985) and Bonnichsen (1979). This pattern is not necessarily, therefore, the result of human activity.

Limitations such as those mentioned require a cautious approach to analysis. To this end, several texts deal with methodologies from the recovery of human remains to court testimony. These include Galloway (1999) on blunt force trauma; Loe and Cox (2005) and Reichs (1998) on tool-mark analysis; Lovell (1997) on fracture mechanisms; and DiMaio on gunshot wounds (1999).

Important points include the fact that perimortem trauma should be classified according to the predominant characteristics of the wound, not the mechanism or weapon that may have been responsible (Galloway 1999; Lovell 1997). Further, interpretations that attempt to explain the circumstances in which injuries arose should be avoided (Galloway 1999). Instead, the anthropologist's goal should be to identify the forces that may have been applied and the specific causes that they may or may not be consistent with.

Other key points include the fact that the anthropologist should be involved from the moment human remains are discovered, and a multidisciplinary approach (e.g., Cattaneo et al. 2006 on diagnosing child abuse) is essential.

Conclusion

Perimortem trauma is perhaps one of the most challenging areas of forensic anthropology. Eliminating antemortem and postmortem lesions and distinguishing genuine perimortal injuries from normal anatomical variation, pathology, and taphonomic changes are the main issues. These

are compounded by the ever-increasing sophistication of weapons and by attempts made by perpetrators to cover up their crimes, factors that require experience and knowledge of skeletal anatomy to identify. Although some areas of the discipline, such as macroscopic estimation of age and sex, are being replaced by more advanced techniques (for example, DNA analysis), perimortem trauma, once ignored in forensic textbooks (for example, El-Najjar and McWilliams 1978; Stewart 1979), is receiving increasing emphasis in courtroom testimonies. This situation has been influenced by mounting atrocities against humanity worldwide, from domestic stabbings and firearm-related deaths to mass genocide and terrorist attacks. Perimortem trauma analysis has, therefore, become a critical aspect of the forensic anthropologist's role, and thus future work should aim to develop present understanding of fracture biomechanics, their modification by taphonomic agents, and epidemiological trends.

Acknowledgments

The author is grateful to the referees and Dr. Mary Lewis for their valuable comments on the text. Christopher Hawkes of Wells museum is also thanked for his permission to use the specimen photographed in Figure 22.3a.

References

Adam, R. 1989. *Modern Handguns: The Complete Illustrated Guide to Military and Civilian Handguns in Production Today.* Edison, NJ: Chartwell Books.

Alunni-Perret, V., Muller-Bolla, M., Laugier, J-P., Lupi-Pégurier, L., Bertrand, M-F., Staccini, P., Bolla, M., and Quatrehomme, G. 2005. Scanning electron microscopy analysis of experimental bone hacking trauma. *Journal of Forensic Sciences* 50: 796–801.

Andahl, R. O. 1978. The examination of saw marks. *Journal of Forensic Sciences* 18: 31–46.

Arnot, R., Finger, S., and Smith, C. U. M. (eds.). 2003. *Trepanation. History, Discovery, Theory.* Lisse, The Netherlands: Swets and Zeitlinger.

Bartelink, E. J., Wiersema, J. M., and Demaree, R. S. 2001. Quantitative analysis of sharp-force trauma: An application of scanning electron microscopy in forensic anthropology. *Journal of Forensic Sciences* 46: 1288–1293.

Behrensmeyer, A. K., Gordon, K. D., and Yanagi, G. T. 1986. Trampling as a cause of bone surface damage and pseudo-cutmarks. *Nature* 319: 768–771.

Berryman, H. E., and Gunther, W. M. 2000. Keyhole defect production in tubular bone. *Journal of Forensic Sciences* 45: 483–487.

Berryman, H. E., and Haun, S. J. 1996. Applying forensic techniques to interpret cranial fracture patterns in archaeological specimens. *International Journal of Osteoarchaeology* 6: 2–9.

Berryman, H. E., and Symes, S. A. 1995a. Recognising gunshot and blunt cranial trauma through fracture interpretation, in K. Reichs (ed.), *Forensic Osteology: Advances in the Identification of Human Remains* (2nd ed.), pp. 333–352. Springfield, IL: Charles C. Thomas.

———. 1995b. Diameter of cranial gunshot wounds as a function of bullet caliber. *Journal of Forensic Sciences* 40: 751–754.

Besant-Matthews, P. E. 2000. Examination and interpretation of rifled firearm injuries, in J. K. Mason (ed.), *The Pathology of Trauma*, pp. 42–60. New York: Oxford University Press.

Binford, L. 1981. *Bones: Ancient Men and Modern Myths*. New York: Academic Press.

Blumenschine, R. J. 1988. An experimental model of the timing of hominid and carnivore influence on archaeological bone assemblages. *Journal of Archaeological Science* 15: 483–502.

Blumenschine, R. J., Maren, C. W., and Capaldo, S. D. 1996. Blind tests of inter-analyst correspondence and accuracy in the identification of cut marks, percussion marks, and carnivore tooth marks on bone surfaces. *Journal of Archaeological Science* 23: 493–507.

Bonnichsen, R. 1979. *Pelistocene Bone Technology in the Beringian Refugium*. Ottawa: Archaeology Survey of Canada, National Museum of Man Mercury Series, Paper No. 89.

Bonte, W. 1975. Tool marks in bones and cartilage. *Journal of Forensic Sciences* 20: 315–325.

Bowman, J. E., MacLaughlin, S. M., and Scheuer, J. L. 1992. Burial of an early 19th-century suicide in the crypt of St Bride's Church, Fleet Street. *International Journal of Osteoarchaeology* 2: 91–94.

Boylston, A. 2000. Evidence for weapon-related trauma in British archaeological samples, in M. Cox and S. Mays (eds.), *Human Osteology in Archaeology and Forensic Science*, pp. 357–379. London: Greenwich Medical Media Ltd.

Brooks, S., and Brooks, R. H. 1997. The taphonomic effects of flood waters on bone, in H. Haglund and M. H. Sorg (eds.), *Forensic Taphonomy: The Postmortem Fate of Human Remains*, pp. 553–558. Boca Raton, FL: CRC Press.

Bromage, T. G., and Boyde, A. 1984. Microscopic criteria of the determination of directionality of cutmarks on bone. *American Journal of Physical Anthropology* 65: 359–366.

Brothwell, D. R. 1981. *Digging up Bones* (3rd ed.). London: British Museum (Natural History).

Brown, C. V. R., Neville, A. L., Rhee, P., Salim, A., Velmahos, G. C., and Demetriades, D. 2005. The impact of obesity on the outcome of 1,153 critically injured blunt trauma patients. *Journal of Trauma* 59: 1048–1051.

Bunn, H. T. 1981. Archaeological evidence for meat eating by plio-pleistocene hominids from Koobi Fora and Olduvai Gorge. *Nature* 291: 574–577.

Byers, S. N. 2005. *Introduction to Forensic Anthropology* (2nd ed.). Upper Saddle River, NJ: Pearson Education, Inc.

Cattaneo, C., Marinelli, E., Di Giancamillo, A., Di Giancamillo, M., Travetti, O., Vigano, L., Poppa, P., Porta, D., Gentilomo, A., and Grandi, M. 2006. Sensitivity of autopsy and radiological examination in detecting bone fractures in an animal model: Implications for the assessment of fatal child physical abuse. *Forensic Science International* 164: 131–137.

Chamberlain, P., and Gander, T. 1974. *Machine Guns*. London: MacDonald and Jane's.

Christ, T. A. J., Washburn, A., Park, H., Hood, I., and Hickey, M. A. 1997. Cranial bone displacement as a taphonomic process in potential child abuse cases, in W. D. Haglund and M. H. Sorg (eds.), *Forensic Taphonomy: The Postmortem Fate of Human Remains*, pp. 319–336. Boca Raton, FL: CRC Press.

Coe, J. I. 1982. External beveling of entrance wounds by handguns. *American Journal of Forensic Medicine and Pathology* 3: 215–219.

Courville, C. B., and Kade, H. 1964. Split fractures of the skull produced by edged weapons and their accompanying brain wounds. *Bulletin of the Los Angeles Neurological Society* 29: 32–39.

Crawford, A. J. 1983. *Outline of Fractures* (8th ed.). New York: Churchill Livingstone.

Currey, J. D., and Butler, G. 1975. The mechanical properties of bone tissue in children. *Journal of Bone and Joint Surgery* 57: 810–814.

De la Grandmaison, G. L., Brion, F., and Durigon, M. 2001. Frequency of bone lesions: An inadequate criterion for gunshot wound diagnosis in skeletal remains. *Journal of Forensic Sciences* 46: 593–595.

de Gruchy, S., and Rogers, T. L. 2002. Identifying chop marks on cremated bone: A preliminary study. *Journal of Forensic Sciences* 47: 933–936.

DiMaio, V. J. M. 1999. *Gunshot Wounds: Practical Aspects of Firearms, Ballistics, and Forensic Techniques* (2nd ed.). Boca Raton, FL: CRC Press.

Dodd, M. 2005. *Terminal Ballistics: A Text and Atlas of Gunshot Wounds*. Boca Raton, FL: CRC Press.

Downs, J. C. U., Nichols, C. A., Scala-Barnett, D., and Lif-schultz, B. D. 1994. Handling and interpretation of crossbow injuries. *Journal of Forensic Sciences* 39: 428–445.

Eismont, F. J., and Lattuga, S. 2003. Gunshot wounds of the spine, in B. D. Browner, J. E. Jupiter, A. M. Levine, and P. G. Trafton (eds.), *Skeletal Trauma* (3rd ed.), pp. 983–1003. Philadelphia: W. B. Saunders Co.

El-Najjar, M. Y., and McWilliams, K. R. 1978. *Forensic Anthropology: The Structure, Morphology, and Variation of Human Bone and Dentition.* Springfield, IL: Charles C. Thomas.

Fackler, M. L., Bellamy, R. F., and Malinowski, J. A. 1988. The wound profile: Illustration of the missile tissue interaction. *Journal of Trauma* 28 (Supp1): S21–S29.

Fenton, T. W., de Jong, D. O., and Haut, R. C. 2003. Punched with a fist: The etiology of a fatal depressed cranial fracture. *Journal of Forensic Sciences* 48: 277–281.

Fenton, T. W., Stefan, V. H., Wood, L. A., and Sauer, N. J. 2005. Symmetrical fracturing of the skull from midline contact gunshot wounds: Reconstruction of individual death histories from skeletonised human remains. *Journal of Forensic Sciences* 50: 274–285.

Frankel, V. H., and Nordin, M. 1980. *Basic Biomechanics of the Skeletal System.* Philadelphia: Lea and Febiger.

Galloway, A. 1999. *Broken Bones: Anthropological Analysis of Blunt Force Trauma.* Springfield, IL: Charles C. Thomas.

Galloway, A., and Zephro, L. 2005. Skeletal trauma analysis of the lower extremity, in J. Rich (ed.), *Forensic Medicine of the Lower Extremity: Human Identity and Trauma Analysis of the Thigh, Leg and Foot*: 253–277. Totowa, NJ: Humana Press.

Gellman, H., Wiss, D. A., and Moldawer, T. D. 2003. Gunshot Wounds to the musculoskeletal system, in B. D. Browner, J. E. Jupiter, A. M. Levine, and G. Trafton (eds.), *Skeletal Trauma* (3rd ed.), pp. 90–119. Philadelphia: W. B. Saunders Co.

Gilbert, W. H., and Richards, G. D. 2000. Digital imaging of bone and tooth modification. *The Anatomical Record* (New Anat.) 261: 237–246.

Greenfield, H. J. 2000. The origins of metallurgy in the central Balkans based on the analysis of cut marks on animal bones. *Environmental Archaeology* 5: 93–106.

Gurdjian, E. S., Webster, J. E., and Lis sner, H. R.1950. The mechanism of skull fracture. *Journal of Neurosurgery* 7: 106–114.

Haglund, W. B., Reay, D. T., and Swindler, D. R. 1988. Tooth mark artefacts and survival of bones in animal scavenged human remains. *Journal of Forensic Sciences* 33: 985–997.

Harkess, J. W., Ramsey, W. C., and Ahmadi, B. 1984. Principles of fractures and dislocations, in C. A. Rockwood, Jr., and D. P. Green (eds.), *Fractures in Adults* Vol. 1, pp. 1–146. Philadelphia: J. B. Lippincott Company.

Hart, G. O. 2005. Fracture pattern interpretation in the skull: Differentiating blunt force from ballistics trauma using concentric fractures. *Journal of Forensic Sciences* 50: 1276–1281.

Herrmann, N. P., and Bennett, J. L. 1999. The differentiation of traumatic and heat-related fractures in burned bone. *Journal of Forensic Sciences* 44: 461–469.

Heulke, D. F., and Darling, J. H. 1964. Bone fractures produced by bullets. *Journal of Forensic Sciences* 9: 461–469.

Hipp, J. A., and Hayes, W. C. 2003. Biomechanics of fractures, in B. D. Browner, J. E. Jupiter, A. M. Levine, and P. G. Trafton (eds.), *Skeletal Trauma* (3rd ed.), pp. 90–119. Philadelphia: W. B. Saunders Co.

Houck, M. M. 1998. Skeletal trauma and the individualization of knife marks in bones, in K. Reichs (ed.), *Forensic Osteology: Advances in the Identification of Human Remains*, pp. 410–424. Springfield, IL: Charles C. Thomas Publishers.

Humphrey, J. H., and Hutchinson, D. L. 2001. Macroscopic characteristics of hacking trauma. *Journal of Forensic Sciences* 46: 228–233.

Hurlbut, S. A. 2000. The taphonomy of cannibalism: A review of anthropogenic bone modification in the American Southwest. *International Journal of Osteoarchaeology* 10: 4–26.

Johnston, E. 1985. Current developments in bone technology, in M. B. Schiffer (ed.), *Advances in Archaeological Method and Theory*, pp. 157–235. London: Academic Press, Inc.

Kanz, F., and Grossschmidt, K. 2005. Head injuries of Roman gladiators. *Forensic Science International* 160: 207–216.

Kerley, E. R. 1978. The identification of battered-infant skeletons. *Journal of Forensic Sciences* 23: 163–168.

King, S. 1992. Violence and Death during the Fall of the Roman Empire: Interpretations of a Late 4th-Century/Early 5th-Century AD Charnel Deposit from Arras, France. Unpublished M.Sc. dissertation, University of Bradford.

Knight, B. 1996. *Forensic Pathology* (2nd ed.). London: Arnold.

Knüsel, C. J., and Outram, A. K. 2006. Fragmentation of the body: Comestibles, compost, or customary rite?, in R. Gowland and C. Knüsel (eds.), *Social Archaeology of Funerary Remains*, pp. 253–278. Oxford: Oxbow Books.

Laudet, F., and Fosse, P. 2001. Un assemblage d'os grignoté par les rongeurs au Paléogène (Oligocène supérieur, phosphorites du Quercy). *Sciences de la Terre et des Planètes* 333: 195–200.

Lewis, M. E. 2007. *The Bioarchaeology of Children: Perspectives from Biological and Forensic Anthropology.* Cambridge: Cambridge University Press.

Lewis, M. E., and Rutty, G. 2003. The endangered child: The personal identification of children in forensic anthropology. *Science and Justice* 43: 201–209.

Lisowski, F. P. 1967. Prehistoric and early historic trepanations, in D. R. Brothwell and A. T. Sandison (eds.), *Diseases in Antiquity*, pp. 651–672. Springfield, IL: Charles C. Thomas.

Liston, M. A., and Baker, B. J. 1996. Reconstructing the massacre at Fort William Henry, New York. *International Journal of Osteoarchaeology* 6: 28–41.

Loe, L., and Cox, M. 2005. Perimortem and post-mortem surface features on archaeological human bone: Why they should not be ignored and a protocol for their identification and interpretation, in S. R. Zakrzewski and M. Clegg (eds.), *Proceedings of the Fifth Annual Conference of the British Association for Biological Anthropology and Osteoarchaeology*. BAR International Series 1383. Oxford: Archaeopress.

Love, J. C., and Symes, S. A. 2004. Understanding rib fracture patterns: Incomplete and buckle fractures. *Journal of Forensic Sciences* 49: 1153–1158.

Lovell, N. C. 1997. Trauma analysis in palaeopathology. *Yearbook of Physical Anthropology* 40: 139–170.

Madea, B., and Staak, M. 1988. Determination of the sequence of gunshot wounds to the skull. *Journal of the Forensic Science Society* 28: 321–328.

Mahoney, P. F. 2005. *Ballistic Trauma: A Practical Guide* (2nd ed.). London: Springer.

Maples, W. R. 1999. Trauma analysis by the forensic anthropologist, in K. J. Reichs (ed.), *Forensic Osteology: Advances in the Identification of Human Remains* (2nd ed.), pp. 218–228. Springfield, IL: Charles C. Thomas.

Mascie-Taylor, C. G. N., and Bogin, B. (eds.). 1995. *Human Variability and Plasticity*. Cambridge: Cambridge University Press.

Mays, S., and Steele, J. 1996. A mutilated human skull from Roman St Albans, Hertfordshire, England. *Antiquity* 70: 155–161.

Meel, B. E. 2004. Incidence and patterns of violent and/or traumatic deaths between 1993 and 1999 in the Transkei Region of South Africa. *Journal of Trauma-Injury Infection & Critical Care* 57: 125–129.

Milner, G. R., and Smith, V. G. 1989. Carnivore alteration of human bone from a late prehistoric site. *American Journal of Physical Anthropology* 79: 43–49.

Nichols, R. G. 2003. Firearm and toolmark identification criteria: A review of the literature, part II. *Journal of Forensic Sciences* 48: 318–327.

Novak, S. 2000. Battle-related trauma, in F. Fiorato, A. Boylston, and C. Knüsel (eds.), *Blood Red Roses. The Archaeology of a Mass Grave from the Battle of Towton AD 1461*, pp. 90–102. Oxford: Oxbow Books.

O'Halloran, R. L., and Lundy, J. K. 1987. Age and ossification of the hyoid bone: Forensic implications. *Journal of Forensic Sciences* 32: 1655–1659.

Oh, S. 1983. Clinical and experimental morphological study of depressed skull fracture. *Acta Neurochirurgica* 68: 111–121.

Olsen, S. L., and Shipman, P. 1994. Cut marks and perimortem treatment of skeletal remains on the Northern Plains, in D. W. Owsley and R. L. Jantz (eds.), *Skeletal Biology in the Great Plains: Migration, Warfare, Health and Subsistence*, pp. 377–387. Washington, D.C.: Smithsonian Institution Press.

Owen-Smith, M. S. 1981. *High Velocity Missile Wounds*. London: Edward Arnold.

Owsley, D. W., Ubelaker, D. H., Houck, M. M., Sandness, K. L, Grant, W. E., Craig, E. A., Woltanski, T. J., and Peerwani, N. 1995. The role of forensic anthropology in the recovery and analysis of Branch Davidson Compound victims: Techniques of analysis. *Journal of Forensic Sciences* 40: 341–348.

Pollanen, M. S., Bulger, B., and Chiasson, D. A. 1995. The location of hyoid fractures in strangulation revealed by xeroradiography. *Journal of Forensic Sciences* 40: 303–305.

Pollanen, M. S., and Chiasson, D. A. 1996. Fracture of the hyoid bone in strangulation: Comparison of fractured and unfractured hyoids from victims of strangulation. *Journal of Forensic Sciences* 41: 110–113.

Pope, E. J., and Smith, O. C. 2004. Identification of traumatic injury in burned cranial bone: An experimental approach. *Journal of Forensic Sciences* 49: 431–440.

Puskas, C. M. , and Rumney, D. T. 2003. Differential diagnosis of intra-oral gunshot trauma and scavenging using a sheep crania model. *Journal of Forensic Sciences* 48: 1219–1225.

Quertermous, R., and Quertermous, S. 1994a. *Pocket Guide to Handguns: Identification and Values 1900 to Present*. Paducah, KY: Collector Books.

———. 1994b. *Pocket Guide to Rifles: Identification and Values 1900 to Present*. Paducah, KY: Collector Books.

Ragsdale, B. D., and Sohn, S. S. 1988. Experimental gunshot fractures. *Journal of Trauma* 28: S109–S115.

Rao, V. J., and Hart, R. 1983. Tool mark determination in cartilage of stabbing victim, *Journal of Forensic Sciences* 28: 794–799.

Reichs, K. J. 1998. Postmortem dismemberment: Recovery, analysis and interpretation, in K. J. Reichs (ed.), *Forensic Osteology. Advances in the Identification of Human Remains* (2nd ed.), pp. 353–388. Springfield, IL: Charles C. Thomas.

Roberts, C. A. 1996. Forensic anthropology 2: Positive identification of the individual; cause and manner of death, in J. C. Hunter, C. Roberts, and A. Martin (eds.), *Studies in Crime: An Introduction to Forensic Anthropology*, pp. 122–138. London: Batsford.

Roberts, C. A., and McKinley, J. 2003. Review of trepanations in British antiquity focusing on funerary context to explain their occurrence, in R. Arnot, S. Finger, and C. U. M. Smith (eds.), *Trepanation: History, Discovery, Theory*, pp. 55–78. Lisse, The Netherlands: Swets & Zeitlinger.

Roberts, G. 2003. Bayonets: Their Design, Manufacture and Use and the Subsequent Injuries to the Human Skeletal System. Unpublished M.Sc. thesis. Bournemouth University.

Rogers, L. F. 1992. *Radiology of Skeletal Trauma* (2nd ed.). New York: Churchill Livingstone.

Ross, A. H. 1996. Caliber estimation from cranial entrance defect measurements. *Journal of Forensic Sciences* 41: 629–633.

Ryan, J. M. 1997. *Ballistics Trauma: A Clinical Relevance in Peace and War.* New York: Oxford University Press.

Sauer, N. J. 1998. The timing of injuries and manner of death: Distinguishing among antemortem, perimortem, and postmortem trauma, in K. J. Reichs (ed.), *Forensic Osteology: Advances in the Identification of Human Remains* (2nd ed.), pp. 321–332. Springfield, IL: Charles C. Thomas.

Scheuer, L., and Black, S. 2000. *Developmental Juvenile Osteology.* London: Academic Press.

Shipman, P. 1981. Applications of scanning electron microscopy to taphonomic problems, in A. E. Cantwell, J. B. Griffin, and N. A. Rothschild (eds.), *The Research Potential of Anthropological Museum Collections*, pp. 357–385. New York: Annals of the New York Academy of Science.

Shipman, P., and Rose, J. 1983. Early hominid hunting, butchering and carcass-processing behaviours: Approaches to the fossil record. *Journal of Anthropological Archaeology* 2: 57–98.

Sivaram, S. 1977. Unusual instrument marks on bones. *Journal of Forensic Sciences* 9: 109–110.

Smith, M. J., and Brickley, M. B. 2004. Analysis and interpretation of flint toolmarks found on bones from West Tump long barrow, Gloucestershire. *International Journal of Osteoarchaeology* 14: 18–33.

Smith, O. C., Berryman, H. E., and Lahren, C. H. 1987. Cranial fracture patterns and estimate of direction from low velocity gunshot wounds. *Journal of Forensic Sciences* 32: 1416–1421.

Spitz, W. U. 1980. Injury by gunshot: Part I: Gunshot wounds, in W. U. Spitz and R. S. Fisher (eds.), *Medicolegal Investigation of Death: Guidelines for the Application of Pathology to Crime Investigation*, pp. 216–274. Springfield, IL: Charles C. Thomas.

Stewart, T. D. 1979. *Essentials of Forensic Anthropology.* Springfield, IL: Charles C. Thomas.

Stubblefield, P. R. 1999. Homicide or accident off the coast of Florida: Trauma analysis of mutilated human remains. *Journal of Forensic Sciences* 44: 716–719.

Symes, S. A., Berryman, H. E., and Smith, O. C. 1998. Saw marks in bone: Introduction and examination of residual kerf contour, in K. Reichs (ed.), *Forensic Osteology Advances in the Identification of Human Remains* (2nd ed.), pp. 389–409. Springfield, IL: Charles C. Thomas.

Tomezak, P. D., and Buikstra, J. E. 1999. Analysis of blunt trauma injuries: Vertical deceleration versus horizontal deceleration injuries. *Journal of Forensic Sciences* 44: 253–262.

Torwalt, C., Balachandra, A. T., Youngson, C., and de Nanassay, J. 2002. Spontaneous fractures in the differential diagnosis of fractures in children. *Journal of Forensic Sciences* 47: 1340–1344.

Tucker, B. K., Hutchinson, D. L., Gilliland, M. F. G., Charles, T. M., Daniel, H. J., and Wolfe, L. D. 2001. Microscopic characteristics of hacking trauma. *Journal of Forensic Sciences* 46: 234–240.

Ubelaker, D. H. 1992. Hyoid fracture and strangulation. *Journal of Forensic Sciences* 37: 1216–1222.

Ubelaker, D. H., and Adams, B. J. 1994. Differentiation of perimortem and postmortem trauma using taphonomic indicators. *Journal of Forensic Sciences* 40: 509–512.

VanRooyen, M. J., Sloan, E. P., Radvany, A. E., Peric, T., Kulis, B., and Tabak, V. 1995. The incidence and outcome of penetrating and blunt trauma in central Bosnia: The Nova Bila hospital for war wounded. *Journal of Trauma-Injury Infection and Critical Care* 38: 863–866.

Villa, P., and Mahieu, E. 1991. Breakage patterns of human long bones. *Journal of Human Evolution* 21: 27–48.

Walker, P. L. 1997. Wife beating, boxing, and broken noses: Skeletal evidence for the cultural patterning of violence, in D. L. Martin and D. W. Frayer (eds.), *Troubled Times: Violence and Warfare in the Past*, pp. 145–179. Amsterdam: Gordon and Breach Publishers.

Walker, P. L., Cook, D. C., and Lambert, P. M. 1997. Skeletal evidence for child abuse: A physical anthropological perspective. *Journal of Forensic Sciences* 42: 196–207.

Walker, P. L., and Long, J. C. 1977. An experimental study of the morphological characteristics of tool marks. *American Antiquity* 42: 605–616.

Walsh-Haney, H. A. 1999. Sharp-force trauma analysis and the forensic anthropologist: Techniques advocated by William R. Maples, Ph.D. *Journal of Forensic Sciences.* 44: 720–723.

Walter, J. 2000. *Modern Military Guns.* London: Greenhill Books, Military Manuals.

Weber, J., and Czarnetzki, A. 2001. Brief communication: Neurotraumatological aspects of head injuries resulting from sharp and blunt force in the early Medieval period of Southwestern Germany. *American Journal of Physical Anthropology* 114: 352–356.

White, W. J. 1988. *The Cemetery of St. Nicholas Shambles*. Special Paper 9. London: London & Middlesex Archaeological Society.

Williams, D. J., Ansford, A. J., Priday, D. S., and Forrest, A. S. 1998. *Forensic Pathology*. London: Churchill Livingstone.

Zhi-Jin, Z., and Jia-Zhen, Z. 1991. Study on the microstructures of skull fracture. *Forensic Science International* 50: 1–14.

23

FORENSIC TAPHONOMY

Stephen P. Nawrocki

Taphonomy is defined as the study of the phenomena that affect the remains of biological organisms at the time of and after death. The field was originally developed in the 1930s by palaeontologists attempting to explain the distribution of plant and animal fossils in the geological record (Efremov 1940). By the 1970s, taphonomy was being applied to the study of prehistoric human remains, and more recently to human remains recovered in historic and forensic contexts (Behrensmeyer and Hill 1980; Bonnichsen and Sorg 1989; Brain 1981; Galloway 1999; Haglund and Sorg 1997, 2002; Lyman 1994; Micozzi 1991; Nawrocki 1995; Shipman 1981; Stewart 1979; White 1992). This chapter discusses the effects of environmental, individual, and behavioral factors on the preservation of human skeletal remains. Because of the complex relationship between these variables, the importance of a holistic approach in the interpretation of taphonomic processes is stressed.

The Scope of Taphonomy

The scope of taphonomy is broad, encompassing both perimortem and postmortem processes, as well as soft and hard tissues. As such, taphonomy as practiced in the forensic context frequently involves a number of different forensic experts. For example, the changes that occur to the body in the immediate postmortem period (intraocular fluid pressure, algor mortis, rigor mortis, livor mortis, skin slippage, autolysis, and putrefaction) are generally recorded by the forensic pathologist during an autopsy. The insects that colonize a decaying body are analyzed by the forensic entomologist. Later postmortem changes to the soft tissues (mummification, adipocere formation, and skeletonization), as well as changes to the bones themselves, are generally studied by the forensic anthropologist. Perimortem trauma may be analyzed either by the pathologist and/or the anthropologist, depending on the circumstances. The common thread linking these diverse and seemingly disparate areas is the focus on the processes and forces that alter the body from its living, vital condition and the resulting modifications of the tissues that must be interpreted by the forensic expert.

In general, taphonomic processes result in the loss of biological information available to the analyst. For example, algor mortis, or the process of cooling after death, makes it difficult and eventually impossible for the scientist to determine the original body temperature of the animal. A carnivore that gnaws the end of a long bone is removing morphological details that otherwise might be measured or observed. A tractor may plow over a skeleton, dispersing the individual bones and making them difficult to recover. In some circumstances, taphonomic processes may actually help to preserve information by slowing down decomposition, such as when a body is buried or frozen, or when it mummifies. In addition, taphonomic processes leave their imprints on the remains, helping the analyst to reconstruct the broader ecological system of which the remains had once been a part. Even the process of algor mortis can be used to help estimate the time since death of the individual. However, in most situations encountered by the forensic analyst, the net effect of taphonomic processes is the loss of biologically meaningful information that otherwise would have been used to establish the identity of the decedent or the cause of death. It is useful then to view the remains as having passed through a number of ecological filters or screens, each of which has removed some proportion of the data that was once available.

Nawrocki (1995) identified three broad classes or categories of taphonomic processes and variables. *Environmental factors* are aspects of the environment that affect the remains. Temperature, ultraviolet radiation from the sun, and rainfall would all be classified as *abiotic* (nonliving) environmental factors. Carnivores, rodents, and plant roots can be classified as *biotic* (living) environmental factors. *Individual factors* are those intrinsic traits that the decedent brings to the decomposition process, such as body weight, age at death, and sex. *Behavioral* or *cultural* factors are the actions of humans that affect the remains, such as burial, embalming, and autopsy. Behavioral factors can be introduced by an assailant, by authorized funerary or medico-legal officials, and, in the case of suicide, by the decedent him- or herself.

The taphonomic literature lists dozens if not hundreds of specific taphonomic factors that must be taken into account when one is analyzing human remains. However, experience suggests that three factors in particular tend to have the greatest effect on remains in a forensic setting: water, temperature, and exposure. The absence, presence, and quantity of water at the recovery scene can affect the remains at both the macroscopic and microscopic levels. Flowing water scatters remains and other evidence. The presence of excess water fosters the formation of adipocere ("grave wax"), an alkaline substance that eventually degrades bone surfaces. Too little water fosters mummification, preserving soft tissues and inhibiting necrophagous insect activity. Periodic wetting and drying encourage fracture formation as the bone expands and contracts. At the molecular level, water breaks down the protein-mineral bonds in the bone, increasing its fragility.

Temperature significantly affects biological and chemical reactions. As temperatures increase, insects and bacteria become more active, eating, growing, and reproducing more quickly. As temperatures dip to freezing, ice crystals form in soft tissues, bone, and soils, destroying cell structure, fostering the propagation of microfractures, and disrupting natural soil layering. However, biological processes slow as temperatures drop, and thus the decomposition process can grind to a near halt.

Remains exposed on the ground surface decompose and erode more quickly than do those that are buried. Burial tends to shelter the remains from animals, water, and climatic extremes (such as freezing). In addition, buried remains and evidence are not as susceptible to scattering and thus are more likely to be recovered and available for analysis. However, burial makes remains more difficult to locate at the outset, and so more time may pass before recovery, allowing subsurface factors (such as erosion of bone from soil acids) more opportunity to occur.

Taphonomy and the Crime Scene

The outdoor forensic scene is a dynamic microecosystem in which the three major categories of taphonomic factors interact in significant ways. Figure 23.1 presents a simple schematic of these interactions. On the one hand, the assailant affects the remains by introducing trauma, initiating burial, and positioning the body within the grave. In return, the victim's characteristics affect how the assailant processes the body; if the decedent is large or very heavy, the assailant may not be able to dispose of the body in a remote area or as quickly or as deeply as a small and light decedent. This two-way interaction is labeled pathway "A" in Figure 23.1. Pathway "B" illustrates the interaction between the assailant and the environment. The assailant alters the natural soil stratigraphy when excavating the grave, tramples vegetation, and leaves compacted footprints. In return, the environment influences where the assailant chooses to place the body, with plants (for example, poison ivy) and/or animals/insects (for example, mosquitoes) potentially affecting the assailant. Pathway "C" illustrates the interaction between the environment and the remains. The environment (soil, plants, animals, climate) affects the way and rate that the remains (flesh, bone) decompose. In return, the decomposing remains give off fluids that change soil pH, moisture content, and nutrient availability.

In a forensic context, two broad subfields of taphonomy have emerged in the past decade.

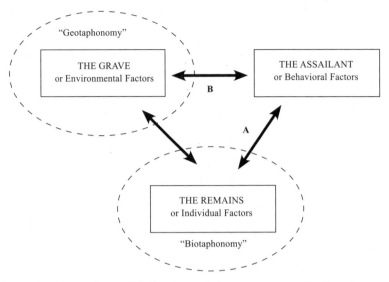

Figure 23.1 Interaction model of taphonomic factors encountered at forensic scenes.

The more traditional application is *biotaphonomy*, which examines modifications to the remains themselves. The scope of biotaphonomy centers on the remains in Figure 23.1. A more recent addition is *geotaphomomy*, which is concerned with the effects of the assailant and the decomposing remains on the surrounding geological and sedimentological environment (Hochrein 1997a, 1997b, 2002). The scope of geotaphonomy is therefore centered on the environment in Figure 23.1. Issues of interest in geotaphonomy include the differential aeration, compaction, and mixing of the soil within a graveshaft, staining and chemical alteration of the soil by decomposition fluids, the production and identification of toolmarks, footprints, and handprints in the soil, and the disruption (acceleration or retardation) of plant growth in the vicinity of the body. The immediate practical applications of geotaphonomy lie in the ability to locate buried remains, to identify graves that have had the remains removed from them, and to help reveal the actions of the assailant.

Clearly, careful geotaphonomic analysis requires detailed observation at the crime scene, and most geotaphonomists would identify themselves primarily as field archeologists rather than osteologists. Biotaphonomy has traditionally fallen within the confines of the osteology laboratory, although most practitioners have also come to realize that a detailed understanding of the context of the recovery scene is crucial to an accurate biotaphonomic reconstruction. It is much more difficult to envision the range and diversity of forces and factors that could have affected a skeleton if one has not examined the specific microenvironment of the recovery scene first hand.

The Circumstances of Death

By applying both biotaphonomic and geotaphonomic approaches, and by taking into account the environment of the recovery scene, the taphonomist may hope to reconstruct what may be broadly described as the "circumstances of death," including:

1. time or season of death (postmortem interval);

2. original location of death;

3. final resting spot of the decedent prior to being subjected to environmental forces that may have dispersed the remains;

4. relevant perimortem and postmortem behaviors of the assailant and the victim, such as interpersonal violence, ritual preparation of the body, and concealment or burial of the remains;

5. actual physical trauma inflicted on the remains near the time of death.

Unfortunately, it can be difficult to discern exactly when a traumatic injury to a bone actually occurred (see Loe this volume). Fracture characteristics are dependent not only on the forces and objects that produce them but also on the physical state of the bone at the moment of impact. Living bone contains significant moisture, fats, and collagen protein, all of which affect how fractures propagate. Dry, dead bone reacts differently in the absence of these intrinsic soft tissues. Fractures in living bone tend to be smooth edged and spiraling, whereas fractures in dry bone tend to be jagged, friable, and transversely oriented. However, bone does not immediately acquire its postmortem characteristics, and it may take quite some time for a skeleton to begin reacting as if it really were dead. In other words, a gunshot wound acquired at the moment of death can look the same as one inflicted minutes, hours, and even days afterward, if not longer. The "perimortem" period, therefore, is quite broad and defined not by the physiological death event or the passage of a fixed unit measure of time, but rather by the highly variable process of decomposition. Working under these limitations, anthropologists must be extremely cautious when interpreting trauma. Ethically, it can be argued that the anthropologist should not make pronouncements regarding the cause or manner of death, because the data rarely allow one to reconstruct the exact timing of the injury. Instead, the anthropologist should simply describe instances of perimortem injury and allow the appropriate medico-legal officials to make their interpretations of the trauma within the broader context of the investigation.

Failure to reconstruct the circumstances of death properly can derail a death investigation. For example, natural processes frequently move a skull away from the body after decomposition of the neck tissues has occurred. Police at the scene or prosecutors interpreting the scene photographs may erroneously infer that the head was "severed" from the body by an assailant. Such an inference would clearly guide the medico-legal system's classification and pursuit of the case; "decapitation" would tend to implicate another individual in the death, turning what would otherwise be a suicide or drug overdose into a homicide.

In addition to elucidating the circumstances of death, the forensic taphonomist may be asked to assess competing explanations of the evidence by:

6. clarifying instances of postmortem "pseudotrauma" (such as animal gnawing) that could be misinterpreted as perimortem trauma;

7. verifying or excluding the statements of witnesses or potential suspects regarding the perimortem treatment and postmortem history of the remains;

8. verifying or excluding the recovery account provided by civilians when the source of the remains is in question.

For example, during the course of a serial homicide investigation in central Indiana in the 1990s (Baker Bontrager and Nawrocki 2005; Nawrocki and Baker 2001; Nawrocki et al. 1998), the wife of the suspect revealed that a few years earlier, her teenage son had discovered a human skeleton in the woods behind their house. Her initial impression was that it was an historic pioneer burial that had eroded from an embankment. When she later asked her husband about the skeleton, he explained that it had been an anatomical specimen once owned by his father, a physician, and that he had recently placed it in the woods, thinking that it would disintegrate. The next day the husband collected and disposed of this skeleton (one of his victims), and the matter was at least temporarily resolved to his family's satisfaction. If the wife had called the police immediately and the skeleton had been collected and sent out for analysis, would the forensic scientist in charge have been able to verify or reject the husband's claim? Commercially prepared anatomical specimens tend to display a specific pattern of modifications, including chemical bleaching, drilling, grinding, and repairs. Those that have been used for teaching anatomy may show "handling wear" and polishing, and those that have been hanging in display cabinets for years will display accumulated grime and dust in predictable locations. The remains of recently deceased homicide victims, in contrast, are expected to display a very different set of characteristics, depending on the postmortem interval and the nature of the recovery location. The taphonomist sorts through the traits displayed by the remains and would reject the suspect's claim if too many features were found to be inconsistent with the proposed story.

The Taphonomic Profile

An anthropologist assists in the identification of the decedent by constructing a *biological profile*. This profile is a summary of the decedent's biological characteristics, including ancestry, (see Sauer and Wankmiller this volume), sex (see Braz this volume), age at death (see Rogers; see Crowder this volume), body size (see Willey this volume), and distinguishing characteristics. In essence, the biological profile is a set of hypotheses that are tested when the decedent is eventually identified. The specific hypotheses (for example, "sex = male") are generated by referring to the body of anthropological research on the human skeleton.

The taphonomist works in a similar fashion. The first step in determining the circumstances of death is the construction of the *taphonomic profile*

(Nawrocki et al. 1997; Schultz et al. 2003). This profile is a set of hypotheses regarding the perimortem and postmortem history of the remains, drawn from a detailed description of the condition of the bones, soft tissues, and the immediate recovery site. These hypotheses specifically address the sources, sequencing, and timing of any modifications to the remains and soil. The profile can also include a reconstruction of the ecosystem(s) in which the perimortem and postmortem histories occurred if no information on the original recovery site is available, as might happen when bones are turned in to the local authorities anonymously or when they have been curated (stored) for many years in private collections. As with the biological profile, the hypotheses are generated from comparisons of the remains to specimens with known postmortem histories and by referencing the taphonomic literature. These hypotheses can be tested when the decedent is identified and the actual circumstances of death become known via witness or suspect testimony, or when they are verified with other, independent scientific evidence.

To illustrate the process of taphonomic analysis in general and the creation of taphonomic profiles in particular, the following sections examine two different ecosystems and the pattern of basic postmortem modifications that are likely to be encountered in each one. The discussions use examples drawn primarily from the northeastern and midwestern United States, although with some thought the scenarios can be adjusted to fit specific conditions encountered in other parts of the world. Although certain modifications (such as carnivore damage) can occur in many ecosystems, the overall pattern encountered in each environment is unlikely to be duplicated exactly in the others. It is the overall constellation of traits, rather than the presence or absence of any particular trait, that defines the profile.

Location of Remains

To appreciate the potential impact the environment has on human skeletal remains, two different environmental settings, forested landscapes and agricultural fields, are discussed.

Forested Environments

By definition, wooded areas tend to provide cover that conceals illicit activities and prohibits easy identification or location of evidence owing to reduced sight lines. Therefore, bodies that are deposited in woodland settings are generally found by accident by hunters and hikers long after skeletonization and dispersal of the bones has commenced. Recoveries usually occur during the cooler months when the foliage is at a low point and the ground surface can be seen. Forests are very active in a biotic sense, with extensive animal, plant, and bacterial activity ranging from the soil all the way up through the canopy. This activity can change dramatically from season to season and even over short distances, with local variations in elevation, moisture, and plant cover. Thus human remains found in woods can display a wide range of overlapping and time-sequential postmortem modifications, making them a challenge to interpret.

The forest floor accumulates leaf litter and plant debris that decomposes slowly to form the topsoil. Bones on the surface can be partially or completely covered by this debris, which when wet will stain the bones dark brown or even black as tannins leach onto their surfaces. Fungus, mold, and algae can produce exotic colors (oranges, reds, greens, and blues). Sunlight penetrates intermittently and seasonally, gently bleaching exposed portions of the bones. Minerals in the topsoil stain the bones on their dependent (downward) surfaces. The end result is a patchwork of different shades and shapes on all surfaces (Figure 23.2).

Roots from trees, shrubs, and vines are frequently found growing across and through bones and clothing (see Figure 23.2). Because plant roots secrete acids, where they contact the bone they can leave small, sinuous, rounded channels that should not be mistaken for cutmarks. These channels are often lighter in color than the surrounding bone surfaces, because they remove cortex that has already been stained by minerals in the soil,

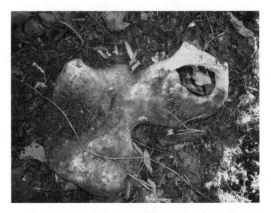

Figure 23.2 Human coxa on an active forest floor. Note the patchwork of light and dark areas caused by leaves, sun bleaching, algae, and soil. Roots have grown across and into the bone (courtesy of the author).

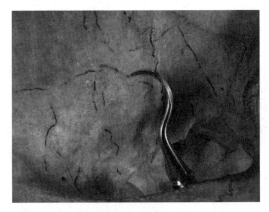

Figure 23.3 Root staining on a human cranium (courtesy of the author).

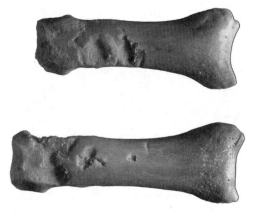

Figure 23.4 Typical carnivore damage to human hand phalanges. Note the crushed edges, deep gouges, punctures, and tooth scratches (bottom) (courtesy of the author).

leaving behind white, unstained bone below. In other circumstances, root masses may leave dark, sinuous stains rather than etchings (Figure 23.3).

In most parts of North America, medium- to large-bodied mammalian predators and scavengers can be found in woodland settings. These may include opossums, foxes, domesticated and feral dogs, coyotes, bobcats, mountain lions, and bears. Some of these animals (especially the canids) are known to scavenge and disperse human remains well after death, even past the point where the external soft tissues have completely decomposed (Haglund, Reay, and Swindler 1988, 1989). The throat and face, genital region, and internal organs of the central body cavity are favored soon after death. Ribs are frequently broken or gnawed at their sternal ends to open the thoracic cavity. Hands are especially vulnerable and are one of the first portions of the body to be disarticulated and removed, as are toes, if not protected by shoes. Later in the decomposition process, scavenging shifts to the remaining dried scraps of tissue surrounding the joints and to the more sheltered bone marrow. Marrow contains fats and proteins that can be accessed by chewing the ends off of long bones or by gnawing down the spongy flat bones (ribs, sternum, pelvis, vertebral bodies). Because it is protected, marrow can survive much longer than the external soft tissues, resulting in periodic episodes of carnivore scavenging that continue throughout the postmortem period.

Since odiferous remains are still likely to contain trapped fats, moisture, and collagen, carnivore fractures should, at least theoretically, be more similar to perimortem fractures rather than to dry, postmortem fractures. However, the unique morphology of carnivore teeth and jaws compared to typical death weaponry (guns, knives, blunt

objects) allows the taphonomist to distinguish carnivore damage from true death-related trauma (assuming, of course, that the predator was not the cause of death to begin with!). Carnivore damage can be identified by both the overall pattern or distribution of damage to the skeleton as well as by the specific modifications made by the teeth. Ragged crushing of edges, crests, and ends is the norm, generally accompanied by conical or triangular punctures, broad gnawing channels, and deep scratches or striations (Figure 23.4). Bone that has actually been swallowed and passed through the animal's digestive system will have smoothed edges and an acid-etched appearance (Figure 23.5). Of course, scat in the vicinity of the body should be collected and examined for missing bones and fragments.

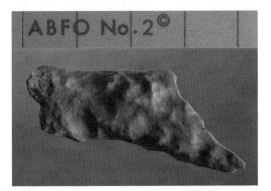

Figure 23.5 Fragment of animal cortical bone that has been digested by a domestic dog. Note pitting and smoothed edges resulting from exposure to stomach acids (courtesy of the author).

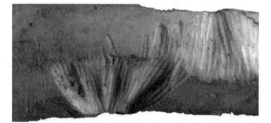

Figure 23.6 Rodent gnawing. Note the fan-shaped series of fine, parallel striations (courtesy of the author).

As bones lose their organic content (tissues, fats, collagen), other mammals may enter the picture. Small rodents begin to seek out and gnaw bone surfaces in order to obtain minerals (calcium, phosphate) during lean times and also to sharpen and shorten their continuously growing incisors. Rodent gnawing can take the appearances of small "fans" or triangles of fine, parallel striations (Figure 23.6). Usually, edges and projections are removed first, meaning that biologically diagnostic features of the bone (brows, muscle attachment points) may be lost, giving a false impression of gracility and thus femaleness. In the midwestern United States, we rarely encounter outdoor rodent gnawing during the first year of the postmortem period, presumably because the bones are not yet dry enough. Sometimes rodent gnawing can be found superimposed over carnivore gnawing or

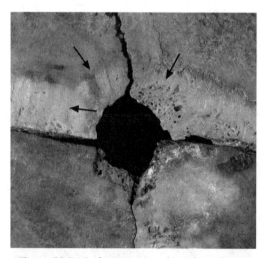

Figure 23.7 Rodent gnawing along the radiating fractures of a gunshot entrance wound. The beveling caused by the gnawing (arrows) gives the erroneous impression that the wound is an exit (courtesy of the author).

other modifications that occurred earlier in the perimortem or postmortem sequence (Figure 23.7).

The biotically active forest floor results in quick destruction of the decomposition fluid stain in the soil and rapid breakdown of hair and natural fibers (as in cotton and wool clothing). Plastics and human-made fibers (nylon, polyester) survive longer, particularly since they tend to be partially shielded from ultraviolet radiation by the overhanging tree and shrub canopies and by accumulated leaf litter. Dispersal of the remains in the forest depends primarily on the land contour and terrain features, drainage characteristics, and access by carnivores. Investigators are well advised to learn to recognize and follow game trails. Rodent burrows and bird nests should be examined carefully. Secondary, superficial burial of individual bones and smaller pieces of evidence that were originally deposited on the surface can occur as a result of multiple seasons of leaf litter buildup as well as by freeze-thaw cycles in the topsoil. Moist soil, when frozen, can develop deep fissures into which small elements can fall from the surface. During a rain or snowmelt, soil will be washed into the fissures, releveling the ground surface. This process (known as *cryoturbation*) can result in significant loss of evidence in just a few years, and the archeologist should therefore modify search and recovery strategies at the scene to find these concealed elements.

In summary, the taphonomic profile for remains found in forested settings reflects the complex interplay of biotic and abiotic factors across seasons and between varying pockets within the ecosystem. Mottled and complex bone staining patterns are to be expected, as is plant, carnivore, and rodent modification. Dispersal of remains will be dependent on the slope of the terrain and carnivore activity, although because of the presence of trees and brush, one would expect less transport than would normally be encountered in other ecological settings.

Remains in Agricultural Fields

In contrast to the biotically active, highly variable, and sheltered ecosystem of the forest, agricultural fields tend to be less biotically diverse, more spatially homogeneous, less sheltered, and more culturally modified. Farmers tend to work their fields at predictable times throughout the year, and human remains are found most frequently during cultivation (spring) and harvesting (fall).

Most large farm fields in the North America are strictly controlled with chemicals and fertilizers, producing efficient monocultures but reducing botanical diversity within. Broad-leaf killers and the shade produced by taller crops inhibit competitive plant growth between rows, leaving patches of the ground surface exposed for much of the year. Bones present on the surface will tend to show much less plant root invasion when compared to forested environments, although if the ground is sufficiently moist, algae will grow and stain the bones and soil green. The highly irregular patchwork pattern of colors and dark shapes produced by leaves and twigs on a forest floor is generally not seen in fields. However, because cultivation may partially bury bones, larger elements may display uneven or diffuse brownish-red staining from irons in the soil.

Grasses, weeds, and shrubs tend to accumulate at the boundaries of fields, providing a suitable nesting and foraging habitat for small rodents and their hunters. However, we tend to see much less rodent gnawing on remains found in fields, probably because loose, dry bones become buried by successive seasons of cultivation before they can be modified. The presence of carnivore damage is highly variable. If a coyote den or hunting trail is in the vicinity, or if farm dogs live nearby, then the remains may quickly attract these scavengers. However, the open exposure of cultivated fields may tend to discourage wild canids while attracting other types of scavengers. The soaring vultures, some of which locate dead carcasses with their highly developed sense of smell, are more likely to be seen feeding on human remains in fields than in forests. Although it is unlikely that vultures will be able to directly damage bone with their beaks or claws, they are certainly important in evisceration and damaging the soft tissues.

Bones in a field are generally exposed to high levels of ultraviolet radiation and become extensively sun-bleached. As water evaporates or freezes on the surface of the bone, small microfractures accumulate and converge to form larger networks of flaking and erosion, ultimately resulting in extensive damage (Figure 23.8). If these fractures form on a curved surface, a star-shaped pattern may occur that can be misinterpreted as perimortem blunt force trauma (Figure 23.9). After a few years of constant exposure, the bone may crumble from the accumulated erosion. Human-made fibers in clothing and plastics break down more quickly in fields because of higher exposure to ultraviolet radiation. Colors of personal belongings may fade rapidly.

Cultivation and harvesting practices that employ heavy machinery have two major effects on remains and evidence deposited in fields: extreme dispersal and damage. Plows, planters,

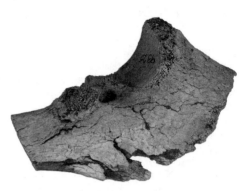

Figure 23.8 Proximal ulna of a cow illustrating extensive sun-bleaching and exposure-related fracturing (courtesy of the author).

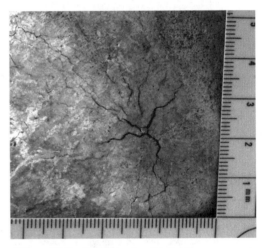

Figure 23.9 Star-shaped or "stellate" arrangement of postmortem fractures on the curving surface of a human parietal bone, resulting from sun-bleaching and freeze-thaw cycles. The keys to correct diagnosis are the rather wavy fracture lines and the presence of fractures that do not converge at the center of the defect (courtesy of the author).

and disking equipment drawn by tractors have numerous projecting elements that can easily capture and transport bodies, portions of bodies, and bones. Skulls in particular are readily impaled and can be dragged hundreds of yards before breaking or being pulled off. The degree of dispersal depends on a number of factors that are difficult to quantify. Loose clothing may catch easily. As the body decomposes, its vertical profile diminishes. Therefore, fresh remains may be more easily trapped than decomposed remains. However, fresh remains are generally heavier than isolated elements and may fall from the machinery more quickly. A "lo-till" tillage method, which leaves the previous year's crop residue on the surface rather than plowing it under in the spring, disturbs the soil much less than a "full-till" method. The type and configuration of the machinery, the tillage method employed, and the speed of the tractor will all affect dispersal rates.

In the end, one would expect significantly more dispersal of remains in cultivated fields than in forested environments, necessitating more human power and time during the recovery. Search strategies should take into account the type of crop, the cultivation patterns used by the farmer, and the presumed original point of deposition of the body. Remains will tend to disperse along the primary direction of plowing rather than perpendicular to it. Since farmers usually replicate their plowing patterns from year to year, it should not be difficult for the investigator to predict the most likely direction of movement of remains even if the postmortem interval is more than one or two growing seasons. However, bones that are picked up by the rotating barrel of a combine can be shot out laterally, perpendicular to the direction of plowing. Therefore, it is important to interview the farmer to learn what types of equipment have been used in recent years and whether there were any deviations from normal cultivation practices.

Locating the original position of the body can be extremely difficult in agricultural fields. If the individual decomposed since the last tillage, the investigator may be able to locate the decomposition stain. Otherwise, one will have to reconstruct the epicenter by carefully plotting the distribution of bones and evidence on a map. If the remains were struck soon after being deposited, the entire body could have been transported and the mapped epicenter may be far off of the original deposition point. If, however, the remains had decomposed significantly prior to being hit, a pocket or concentration of small bones, loose teeth, and hair fragments may indicate the location of deposition, if they can be found.

Farming equipment can inflict significant trauma to the remains, including blunt force fractures, crushing, gouging, scratching, puncturing, and cutting (Figure 23.10). Depending on when it occurs, farming damage can be very difficult to distinguish from perimortem trauma related to the cause of death. Incised wounds caused by disking equipment on fresh bones can look exactly like knife wounds. However, the distribution of the wounds on the skeleton will not necessarily conform to what would be expected for a typical attack by an assailant. In addition, if the disking unit hit

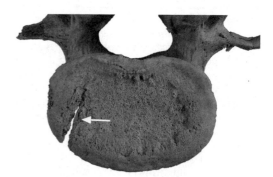

Figure 23.10   Sharp-force trauma to a lumbar vertebra caused by disking equipment (arrow). The margins of this incised wound show slight erosion due to continued surface exposure (courtesy of the author).

the remains after they had become at least partially disarticulated, the cuts may not make anatomical sense, crossing a joint on one side but not on the facing surface, or crossing areas that would normally be inaccessible to an assailant (such as the vertebral bodies).

In summary, the taphonomic profile of remains found in an agricultural setting differs in important ways from those found in a wooded setting. Bone staining patterns are likely to be simpler compared to those in forests, and plant modifications are less likely. Animal activity will be more variable and less easy to predict, although rodent gnawing tends to be less common. Dispersal of remains is likely to be greater by orders of magnitude compared to forests, and the chance of quick burial of evidence is higher, depending on the cultivation methods being used and the timing of deposition of the body around cyclical farming activities. However, the regularity of plowing at least makes it possible to come up with good predictions about the direction of dispersal. The investigator should expect significant trauma introduced by farming equipment, and it will be a challenge to differentiate this trauma from that inflicted at the time of death.

Conclusion

Forensic taphonomy is a broad and somewhat nebulously defined field that integrates methods and data from a number of disciplines, including anthropology, paleontology, geology, biology, entomology, chemistry, and pathology. By constructing a taphonomic profile for a set of remains, the analyst tries to answer important questions concerning the circumstances of death of the individual. A useful and accurate profile is dependent on:

1. Proper and thorough recovery methods at the scene: has everything been found?

2. Background research and interviewing of relevant individuals: can the landowner provide some insight regarding the recent history of the property?

3. Detailed description of the physical condition of the remains in the lab: have all modifications been identified?

4. Knowledge of relevant taphonomic factors that apply in various environments: how does this scene differ from others?

5. A comparative ecological approach.

In other words, taphonomy must be holistic as it is applied in forensic settings, and the analyst must be able to shift easily between laboratory analysis and fieldwork.

There is considerable research that can be conducted in the future to help guide the discipline. Because of the great variety of environmental factors and the unpredictable length of time that potentially passes prior to discovery of remains, it is difficult to design comprehensive experiments that can control for even the most important variables. To date, most forensic taphonomy studies have been largely·anecdotal, drawing primarily from casework rather than from experimental data obtained from rigorously controlled settings. The biggest drawback of such retrospective studies is that they may have significant gaps in the data, representing the cases that were NOT encountered during the study period. For example, Megyesi, Nawrocki, and Haskell (2005) attempted to generate a more precise method of estimating time since death from decomposing soft tissues using crime scene temperature data. The authors drew their study sample from real case files, but no deaths were recorded that had fallen between about 80 and 130 days postmortem. This gap in the data could have significantly affected their results, but given the research design, there was no way to overcome the problem short of waiting for more cases to come in.

Perhaps the most crucial issue facing future researchers is that of differentiating between perimortem and postmortem modifications, and particularly between death-related trauma and injuries that occur after death but still within the perimortem "fresh" interval. Of the issues that the anthropologist is likely to testify on in a court of law, the identification and the clarification of skeletal trauma are probably the most common. However, there are few detailed primers in the literature that cover the topic, and most practitioners must rely simply on their experience excavating and examining thousands of bones from diverse settings. Ironically, there are far more publications regarding the construction of the biological profile than of the taphonomic profile, yet few anthropologists actually testify on biological procedures, because final positive identification is generally the purview of other experts! Clearly, interdisciplinary efforts to identify trauma are sorely needed, including controlled experimentation as well as comprehensive case reviews.

Finally, anthropologists must themselves recognize that their training and expertise give them a much broader mandate to assist in medico-legal casework than has generally been acknowledged. The anthropology subsection of American Academy of Forensic Sciences is formally titled "Physical Anthropology," reflecting the emphasis that the earliest practitioners of the art placed on laboratory analysis of skeletal remains. However, archaeology, as a valid subfield of anthropology and one that is not taught by any other discipline, is clearly needed in medico-legal investigations throughout the world (Dirkmaat and Adovasio 1997). The unique position of anthropologists is such that they can offer expertise both in the laboratory and in the field, and this dual role gives them a unique perspective that should greatly assist in the guidance and development of the science of forensic taphonomy.

References

Baker Bontrager, A., and Nawrocki, S. 2005. A taphonomic analysis of burned remains from the Fox Hollow serial homicide site. *American Journal of Physical Anthropology.* Supplement 40: 68–69.

Behrensmeyer, A., and Hill, A. 1980. *Fossils in the Making: Vertebrate Taphonomy and Paleoecology.* Chicago: University of Chicago Press.

Bonnichsen, R., and Sorg, M. 1989. *Bone Modification.* Center for the Study of the First Americans. Orono, ME: University of Maine.

Brain, C. 1981. *The Hunters or the Hunted? An Introduction to African Cave Taphonomy.* Chicago: University of Chicago Press.

Dirkmaat, D., and Adovasio, J. 1997. The role of archaeology in the recovery and interpretation of human remains from an outdoor forensic setting, in W. Haglund and M. Sorg (eds.), *Forensic Taphonomy,* pp. 39–64. Boca Raton, FL: CRC Press.

Efremov, I. 1940. Taphonomy, a new branch of paleontology. *Pan-American Geologist* 74: 81–93.

Galloway, A. (ed.). 1999. *Broken Bones: Anthropological Analysis of Blunt Force Trauma.* Springfield, IL: Charles C. Thomas.

Haglund, W., Reay, D., and Swindler, D. 1988. Tooth mark artifacts and survival of bones in animal scavenged human skeletons. *Journal of Forensic Sciences* 33(4): 985–997.

———. 1989. Canid scavenging/disarticulation sequence of human remains in the Pacific Northwest. *Journal of Forensic Sciences* 34(3): 587–606.

Haglund, W., and Sorg, M. (eds.). 1997. *Forensic Taphonomy*. Boca Raton, FL: CRC Press.

———. 2002. *Advances in Forensic Taphonomy*. Boca Raton, FL: CRC Press.

Hochrein, M. 1997a. The dirty dozen: The recognition and collection of tool marks in the forensic geotaphonomic record. *Journal of Forensic Identification* 47: 171–198.

———. 1997b. Buried crime scene evidence: The application of forensic geotaphonomy in forensic archaeology, in P. Stimson and C. Mertz, C. (eds.), *Forensic Dentistry*, pp. 83–99. Boca Raton, FL: CRC Press.

———. 2002. An autopsy of the grave: Recognizing, collecting, and preserving forensic geotaphonomic evidence, in W. Haglund and M. Sorg (eds.), *Advances in Forensic Taphonomy*, pp. 45–70. Boca Raton, FL: CRC Press.

Lyman, L. 1994. *Vertebrate Taphonomy*. Cambridge: Cambridge University Press.

Megyesi, M., Nawrocki, S., and Haskell, N. 2005. Using accumulated degree-days to estimate the postmortem interval from decomposed human remains. *Journal of Forensic Sciences* 50(3): 618–626.

Micozzi, M. 1991. *Postmortem Changes in Human and Animal Remains*. Springfield, IL: Charles C. Thomas.

Nawrocki, S. 1995. Taphonomic processes in historic cemeteries, in A. Grauer (ed.), *Bodies of Evidence*, pp. 49–66. New York: Wiley-Liss.

Nawrocki, S., and Baker, A. 2001. Fluvial transport of human remains at the Fox Hollow serial homicide site. *Proceedings of the American Academy of Forensic Sciences* 7: 246–247.

Nawrocki, S., Pless, J., Hawley, D., and Wagner, S. 1997. Fluvial transport of human crania, in W. Haglund and M. Sorg (eds.), *Advances in Forensic Taphonomy*, pp. 529–552. Boca Raton, FL: CRC Press.

Nawrocki, S., Schmidt, C., Williamson, M., and Reinhardt, G. 1998. Excavation and analysis of human remains from the Fox Hollow serial homicide site, Hamilton County, Indiana. *Proceedings of the American Academy of Forensic Sciences* 4: 205–206.

Schultz, J., Williamson, M., Nawrocki, S., Falsetti, A., and Warren, M. 2003. A taphonomic profile to aid in the recognition of human remains from historic and/or cemetery contexts. *Florida Anthropologist* 56: 141–147.

Shipman, P. 1981. *Life History of a Fossil*. Cambridge, MA: Harvard University Press.

Stewart, T. 1979. *Essentials of Forensic Anthropology.* Springfield, IL: Charles C. Thomas.

White, T. 1992. *Prehistoric Cannibalism at Mancos 5MTUMR-2346*. Princeton, NJ: Princeton University Press.

24

BURNED HUMAN REMAINS

Tim Thompson

Burned human remains have been the focus of study by anthropologists and archaeologists for over 60 years.[1] The complexity of the heat-induced transformation process, in conjunction with the sheer range of contexts in which they are found, has allowed for an exciting range of studies to be undertaken. One might therefore surmise that we know a great deal about this subject: we do not. The nature of many of these studies has been preliminary in status, driven by incidental curiosity, and therefore lacking in coordination and cohesiveness. Thus we have snippets of information, which we have great difficulty integrating and subsequently applying to actual forensic or archaeological scenarios.

The purpose of this chapter is to provide a summary of the work conducted in this field to date. Initially, research and practice are placed within a social framework. This is followed by a consideration of the knowledge base as it currently stands, and finally the future developments of the subject are explored.

Much has already been made of the lack of integration concerning the study of burned remains (Thompson 2005). First, there is a lack of communication between the three main disciplines that study the subject (forensic anthropology, archaeology, and medicine), which manifests in a lack of cross-discipline publication, citation, and

collaborative research. Second, there is a disjunction between the study of the soft tissues and the hard tissues. Acknowledging this disjunction, however, this chapter focuses on the effects of burning on the hard tissues, mainly because of the fact that bone and teeth fall more within the remit of the anthropologist and archaeologist and because of the relative complexity of the transformations of the hard tissues compared to the soft tissues. Good summaries of the effects of burning on the soft tissues can be found in Payne-James, Busuttil, and Smock (2003) and Saukko and Knight (2004).

The Context of Burned Human Remains

The context of discovery is important for practicing forensic anthropologists and archaeologists, because the location, recovery, and examination of burned human remains are often extremely challenging, occurring in scenes that are often highly significant in a judicial context. Initial problems that must be overcome include the collection of highly fragmented material from among a mass of fire-damaged debris, together with the fragile nature of the material and the stabilisation and storage of this delicate source of evidence (Dirkmaat 2002; Mayne Correia and Beattie 2002; McKinley and Roberts 1993). Furthermore, the techniques that one must employ in order to create an accurate biological or osteological profile of an individual generally rely on unmodified bone dimensions. Unfortunately, heat-induced dimensional change to osseous elements has been shown to be highly significant and can result in a change to long-bone length of up to 30% (Thompson 2005).

The study of the remains associated with fire scenes can provide useful information beyond the establishment of a biological profile of the deceased. Information regarding the burning environment itself, the nature of the fuel and pyre, the state of the body prior to burning, and, potentially, the intensity of the fire can all be gleaned from a thorough examination of burned human remains.

An understanding of the heat-induced transformation of the human body is also important for forensic anthropologists and archaeologists, since the range of contexts from which burned bodies can be recovered is broad. For forensic practitioners, this can include dwelling fires, mass fatality incidents, and self-immolation (e.g., Eckert, James, and Katchis 1988; Fanton et al. 2006; Shkrum and Johnston 1992; Sledzik and Rodriguez 2002; Sukhai et al. 2002); for archaeologists, this can include funerary rites and the study of human-faunal relations (e.g., Baby 1954; Binford 1963; Bond 1996; Cain 2005; McKinley 1994; Nicholson 1995; Wells 1960); and for social anthropologists, this can include the study of modern rituals associated with death and communication with ancestors and the gods (e.g., Downes 1999; Murad 1998; Oestigaard 2000). Interpretations are further compounded by the fact that fire and burning are used in a variety of ways, including as a functional medium for transformation or as a potent symbol in its own right. In all these situations, however, the study of burned remains inevitably leads to the study of humans and their actions. In this respect, context is all important: burned human remains do not just simply occur in a vacuum but are, rather, mostly the result of human agency.

Many terms have sloppily been used interchangeably within the literature to describe burned human remains and their contexts—such examples include burned remains, cremations, cremains, and calcined remains. However, they do not all mean the same thing. To describe the remains themselves, we should limit ourselves to the use of *burned human remains* or simply *burned remains*. *Cremation* is a term that relates to the social aspect of burning human bodies, such as a funerary rite, as with the clinical approach to modern Western cremations, or the pyre-based Hindu and Iron Age cremation events. *Calcination* is a physical process of transformation within the

bones, and since it is unlikely to affect the entire skeleton or set of remains, use of the term *calcined remains* to describe the bones of interest inherently implies that the entire entity has progressed through this process. Finally, there is no need for the term *cremains*—the conjoining of *cremated* and *remains* and is unnecessary: we do not conjoin *dismembered remains, weathered remains,* or any other taphonomic process, so there is no need to do it in this instance.

Historical Themes and Prior Developments

Early analyses of burned bone tended to be isolated or preliminary studies (such as Binford 1963; Bradtmiller and Buikstra 1984; Buikstra and Swegle, 1989; Wells 1960). Interesting though they are, the result has been that a cohesive, coherent body of knowledge has been lacking. These early publications tended to focus on the more apparent heat-induced changes, those that could be seen by the naked eye, or at most, with scanning electron microscopy. Reliance on these publications is therefore unsatisfactory, and the piecemeal nature of this research has resulted in practitioners holding a rather erroneous view of both the information available from burned bone and the physico-chemical consequences of burning on bone.

However, one of the earliest studies has also turned out to be one of the more progressive. Van Vark (1974, 1975) appreciated that, owing to the occurrence of heat-induced changes in bone, multivariate statistical methods were needed to improve the precision and accuracy of anthropological techniques. However, Van Vark also noted that problems arise with the use of multivariate statistical methods owing to both the heat-induced changes in bony dimensions themselves and the incomplete recovery of the fragmentary skeleton. These issues will inhibit any techniques that rely on unmodified bone dimensions and many planes of measurement. Van Vark (1974) concluded that, despite these issues, multivariate statistical methods can still be used to successfully discriminate biological sex.

There are two methodological limitations, however, with Van Vark's work. First, his multivariate functions often cannot be applied to burned remains that have only a small amount of recovered hard tissue (Van Vark 1974). This is likely to be a common situation, especially when one is dealing with archaeological remains. Second, he states that often only proportional measures, that is, indices, can be used (Van Vark 1974). In theory, this is a sound principle, his rationale being that proportional measures will not be affected by shrinkage. However, more recently it has become clear that a bone does not shrink uniformly. This fact will therefore affect the outcome of indices owing to the changing relationship between the variables being measured (McKinley 2000; Thompson 2002). Unfortunately, subsequent studies moved away from this rigorous statistical methodology toward a more empirical approach, the consequences of which can still be seen.

The next series of enquiries tended to focus on the use of actualistic experimental studies for understanding the effects of burning on bone. Studies such as those undertaken by Thurman and Willmore (1981), Gilchrist and Mytum (1986), Buikstra and Swegle (1989), and Spennemann and Colley (1989) aimed to provide explanations of how and why burned bones looked as they did. It is important to appreciate that forensic anthropology and forensic archaeology were still very much in their infancy at this time, meaning that these early burned-bone studies derived from archaeological questioning. One of the key arguments in these early studies (Baby 1954; Binford 1963; Buikstra and Swegle 1989; Thurman and Willmore 1981) was that recognising specific fracture patterns will allow one to state whether the remains were fleshed, recently defleshed, or dry when burned, which has important medicolegal and archaeological implications. Thurman and Willmore's (1981) experimental study on dry bones recorded longitudinal and perpendicular fractures and the presence of gridded patterns. Buikstra and Swegle (1989) later noted that longitudinal fractures occur along the length of the bone but that transverse fractures are less frequent than in fleshed remains. This observation supports the observations of other publications (including more recent ones) that have argued that the fracture patterns of fleshed remains are less linear, less regular, and have frequent elliptical cracking (Baby 1954; Binford 1963; McKinley 2000; Mayne Correia 1997; Thurman and Willmore 1981).

Colour change was also examined in these early studies, and the conclusion was that bone altered from its natural colour of creamy white, through dark greys and black, and then, if burning continued, through light greys to white. Colour change has been suggested, with varying degrees of conviction, as a means of predicting the temperature of the fire in which the remains were burned (e.g., Chandler 1987, Grévin et al. 1998 and Shipman, Foster, and Schoeinger 1984). However, later work has shown this idea to be simplistic and likely to be seriously flawed due to the actions

of a vast number of other variables (Thompson 2004). Colour change is better described as the loss of carbon from the osteological matrix (Mayne Correia 1997).

Studies of burned bone subsequently evolved in two ways: (1) either they continued the theme of examining why bones looked as they did, but through the application of more revealing technologies, or (2) they began to examine the implications of the effects of burning for anthropological information. In Shipman, Foster, and Schoeinger's (1984) classic study of the effects of burning on bone and teeth, they examined the changing nature of the crystal structure of the inorganic matrix. Using X-ray diffraction (XRD), they noted that there was a gradual increase in hydroxyapatite crystal size, which was associated with an increase in temperature. Shipman, Foster, and Schoeinger (1984) explain this as a function of some crystals enlarging at the expense of others.[2] In addition, they argue that their data show that the degree of heat-induced shrinkage of the whole bone is directly correlated to the temperature of burning. This statement has subsequently been supported by many other workers (e.g., McKinley 2000). Gilchrist and Mytum (1986) and Shipman, Foster, and Schoeinger (1984) also noted large ranges (beginning at less than 5% and reaching as much as 45%) in the amount of shrinkage recorded. These results compare less favourably with the work of Buikstra and Swegle (1989), Holland (1989), and Spennemann and Colley (1989), who found that heat-induced shrinkage was never greater than 3%. These differences, however, are likely due to differences in experimental protocol.

Recent Themes and Current Developments

The focus of research into the effects of heating and burning on bone has shifted from interest in the macroscopic heat-induced changes to the microscopic changes. This is a function of a change in philosophy combined with a more imaginative and innovative approach to the use of experimental techniques within the subject. The understanding of the macroscopic changes to bone as presented by the earlier studies is extremely important and highlights the significant effect that burning can have on bones. However, these macroscopic alterations in themselves are not enough to explain the relationship between heating and bone change, since these macroscopic changes are actually caused by more fundamental dynamics. Thus, we can refer to these macroscopic changes (such as colour change or fracture patterns) as secondary-level changes, whereas those underlying microscopic changes can be termed primary-level changes (Thompson 2004). Added to this is the realisation and acknowledgment that both primary and secondary-level changes of bone are affecting the results of anthropological techniques, which in turn may affect our attempts at human identification.

The Adoption of Innovative Microscopic Investigative Techniques

As the focus moved toward looking more closely at primary-level heat-induced changes in bone, it became necessary to adopt an assemblage of new methods of study. This was achieved though the assimilation of techniques from other disciplines, such as physical chemistry and the soil sciences. The first issue of interest concerned the influence of burning on the elemental composition of bones. Changes in trace-element composition may result from heat-induced recrystallisation of the inorganic phase evicting elements from the bony matrix or uptake of elements from the firewood, soft tissues, or burning context (Grupe and Hummel 1991). Experimental analyses on pig femora allowed Grupe and Hummel (1991) to produce linear regression equations to describe the changes in certain trace elements. Changes in calcium, phosphorus, and strontium provided the most robust formulae. Changes in barium and lead were less robust, whereas the changes in copper, zinc, and magnesium appeared not to be related to temperature changes at all. However, Herrmann and Grupe (1988) warned, and this is also true for Grupe and Hummel (1991), that the recorded increases in trace elements may not simply be due to elemental uptake but to reductions in the organic component of the bone, thereby increasing element concentration relatively, not absolutely. Sillen and Hoering (1993) advanced these notions by attempting to use the concentrations of elements to state whether bone had been burned or not. Unfortunately, with regard to changes in the mineral component, heat-induced diagenesis is so similar to normal bone diagenesis (Herrmann and Grupe 1988; Koon, Nicholson, and Collins 2003) that trace element concentration alone can identify only whether bone has suffered some form of diagenesis, rather than the cause.

Following the examination of heat-induced elemental alteration, researchers began to focus on the issues surrounding the physical changes to the bone microstructure, specifically through studies of crystal structure and porosity. X-ray diffraction has been repeatedly used to examine the changes of the microscopic crystal architecture of bone due to burning (Holden, Phakey, and Clement 1995a; Newesely 1988; Rogers and Daniels 2002; Shipman, Foster, and Schoeinger. 1984; Stiner et al. 1995). The results of Rogers and Daniels's (2002) X-ray diffraction experiments suggest that there is an increase in crystal size associated with an increase in the burning temperature. Thus, crystals transform from their small but highly anisotropic state into one with a significantly larger equidimensionality (Rogers and Daniels 2002). They place the key transformation section point at around 800°C, which is consistent with Holden, Phakey, and Clement (1995a), whose experiments placed this key period between 600°C and 1,000°C. Furthermore, large highly ordered crystals (associated with higher burning temperatures) produce higher splitting factors than do small disordered crystals (Roberts et al. 2002; Stiner et al. 1995). However, the apparent crystal changes may actually be due to alterations in crystal size distribution rather than simply size (Rogers and Daniels 2002)—that is, the resorption of small crystals being interpreted as crystal growth.

In the last few years, small-angle X-ray scattering (SAXS), a new technique for discerning subtle changes to bone nanostructure, has been developed and been shown to accurately detect changes to crystal size, shape, and orientation within bone (Hiller et al. 2003). SAXS results show that bone crystallites begin to alter in the first 15 minutes of heating to 500°C or above. They then appear to stabilise to a temperature-specific thickness and shape with prolonged heating. While the samples heated to lower temperatures or for shorter periods produced XRD traces showing little alteration to the apatite, corresponding information obtained from SAXS showed an early, subtle change in crystal parameters. SAXS has also shown that burning causes the crystals to become more platelike, rather than needle-like as in unburned bone, progressing then toward a polydisperse crystal shape (Hiller et al. 2003).

The zenith of human identification is often argued to be DNA. However, the extraction of DNA from burned human remains brings with it unique challenges, mainly because DNA begins to denature at around 100°C. Because the average house fire reaches 700°C, if not more, there seems little chance of successfully recovering DNA for use in confirming the identity of the deceased in fire-death scenarios. However, several experimental studies have managed to tease out this biomolecular fingerprint. In 1991, Duffy, Waterfield, and Skinner successfully detected sex cromatin from the pulp of human teeth burned up to 700°C. Tsuchimochi and associates (2002) also managed to detect the Y-chromosome from burned teeth, although this was at a lower temperature and in isolated teeth. It must not be forgotten that in actual forensic scenarios, the surrounding soft tissues will have an important role to play in protecting the DNA within the hard tissues from heat penetration (Duffy, Waterfield, and Skinner 1991).

Sajantila and colleagues (1991) and Ye and associates (2004) have managed to successfully extract more complete profiles from burned remains using polymerase chain reaction (PCR). Although the former was successful in actual forensic applications, the DNA was extracted from the soft tissues rather than bone. DNA has even, although perhaps somewhat controversially, been extracted from burned remains recovered from archaeological contexts (Brown, O'Donoghue, and Brown 1995). What is clear from the literature is that, despite the few interesting studies presented here, little has been conducted into the field of DNA extraction and amplification from burned human remains. This is clearly a fundamental issue of critical importance and must be the focus of future research.

DNA is not the only biomolecular evidence of current interest to anthropologists and archaeologists investigating the potential of burned bone in human identification. Although burning will clearly destroy the components of blood, blood proteins such as albumin may still be detectable. Cattaneo and associates (1994) demonstrated this was true of both modern experimentally burned bone and cremated archaeological material. Exciting though this is, Cattaneo and associates (1995) themselves state that bone integrity is vital for protein survival, which is surely unlikely in burned remains. Cattaneo and colleagues (1994) present only a preliminary study here, and further work is obviously required to clarify this issue.

In a rare occurrence within burned bone research, Cattaneo and associates (1999) applied their innovative approach to actual situations by comparing the usefulness of histological, immunological, and DNA analysis for the differentiation of burned human and nonhuman bone. Interestingly, results of their experiments showed that the differentiation of human and nonhuman species was most reliable using quantitative histological methods rather than immunological or DNA analysis. However, immunological methods were found to be more useful than DNA analyses owing to the apparent resilience of albumin to heat relative to DNA (Cattaneo et al. 1999).

The Adoption of Novel Approaches to Visualising Heat-Induced Change

With the secondary-level changes to bone often being so clear and vivid, early studies relied on simple photography (and currently, digital photography) to aid examination of these changes. However, as researchers have begun to investigate the more primary-level changes, a suite of new imaging modalities has been introduced. The potential of scanning electron microscopy (SEM) has been appreciated for a number of years and has been used in studies examining the effects of burning on bone (e.g., Herrmann and Bennett 1999; Holden, Phakey, and Clement 1995a, 1995b; Quatrehomme et al. 1998) and teeth (e.g., Carr, Barsley, and Davenport 1986; Wilson and Massey 1987). Current developments are now focussing on using SEM to answer specific questions rather than to collect general, qualitative information. Transmission electron microscopy has only recently been employed, but Koon, Nicholson, and Collins (2003) have shown its potential in differentiating unburned bone from that heated to low temperatures.

The other main imaging modality to be utilised in current burned bone research is magnetic resonance imagery. Preliminary studies (Thompson and Chudek 2007) have shown that this technique has the potential to image the external and internal changes of the compact and cancellous bone simultaneously, with great resolution. Furthermore, since the technique is nondestructive it allows for the imaging of the same piece of bone before and after repeated cycles of burning. Although this technique has great potential, it has yet to provide a significant amount of quantitative data on heat-induced osseous change.

Counteracting the Impact of Heat-Induced Change on Human Identification

The undeniable and unavoidable conclusion of all these studies of burned bone is that bone can change dramatically as a result of burning and heating. Thus we must assume that heat-induced changes to bone will affect any and all anthropological techniques applied to the bone, although the influence will vary according to the direct and indirect effects of the heat-induced changes (Thompson 2004). Although the impact on identification techniques has been of general interest previously (Bradtmiller and Buikstra 1984; Van Vark 1974, 1975), it is only with current research that this is being specifically addressed.

In essence, the question is not whether burning will affect human identification, but to what extent. Current studies tend to focus on two areas: (1) the comparative usefulness of morphological and metric techniques and (2) whether antemortem features survive the burning environment. In the former, experimental studies combined with statistical analyses have shown that metric methods of sex determination are highly vulnerable to the effects of heat-induced changes (Thompson 2002, 2004, 2005), potentially resulting in the misclassification of sex. In the latter, experimental studies have shown that antemortem sharp- and blunt-force trauma are distinguishable from heat-induced features (de Gruchy and Rogers 2002; Herrmann and Bennett 1999), that gunshot trauma was not distinguishable (Herrmann and Bennett 1999), although this is not true in every case (Pope and Smith 2004), and that evidence for antemortem injuries present in the surrounding soft tissue can also be suggested from the skeletal evidence (Pope and Smith 2004). De Gruchy and Rogers (2002) note however, that the likelihood of finding antemortem trauma on burned remains is dependent on the anatomical region that was traumatised, with ribs being more likely to be completely destroyed by fire, thus taking their antemortem features with them. These studies also note the danger of neglecting heat-induced shrinkage in the interpretation of trauma from burned bones. Finally, recent research has also been able to scientifically explain and refute the myths surrounding both spontaneous human combustion (Christensen 2002; de Haan and Nurbakhsh 2001) and the perceived tendency for heads to explode in fires (Pope and Smith 2004).

Future Development

The future development of research into the effects of burning on the human body must focus on three areas. First, we must continue with the lines of research discussed above, but with larger studies, in order to collect more data and thus allow us to fully understand just what is happening within the hard tissues of the body, as well as the influence of other external factors (such as soft tissue, personal effects, and the nature of the fuel for the fire). Second, we must strive for better integration, and, third, we must begin to apply our new-found knowledge to the forensic arena. These last two areas are discussed below.

Integration

The lack of integration of burned bone research falls into two areas: the approach to studying the

human body and the multidisciplinary nature of the subject. The integration of the different systems and tissues of the human body into one conceptual framework has already been discussed above. The development of exciting and useful research depends on practitioners and researchers appreciating that there are three disciplines contributing data to this arena and that each discipline is specialising in a different area, the combination of which will provide the fullest understanding of the subject. The archaeological discipline has much to offer in terms of the effects on the hard tissues, the medical discipline in terms of the effects on the soft tissues and the living human body, and the forensic discipline in terms of the influence of external variables and the recovery of the remains. In addition to increasing collaborative research, each discipline must become much more aware of the publications and expertise in the other disciplines.

Application to Actual Forensic Contexts

For research to be meaningful, there must be some form of application of research findings. Although some burned-bone research has been applied to actual forensic anthropological and archaeological cases, this is still an area that requires significant development. In addition to building a body of publications demonstrating such things as the most effective methods of locating and safely recovering burned material (e.g., Mayne Correia and Beattie 2002), we need to be able to examine the actual effect of these heat-induced changes on the results of anthropological techniques and methods of human identification. Such examination will necessitate the devising of correction factors for existing techniques (Thompson 2004) and new predictive models to extrapolate data from small studies to the wider forensic arena (Thompson 2002). All of this will then require testing and reporting.

Conclusion

The analysis of burned human remains holds an important place within the remit of the forensic anthropologist and archaeologist. The remains themselves are complicated, requiring practitioners to take into consideration a range of heat-induced changes throughout the tissues of the body, changes that themselves are highly dependent on the relationship of the fire to the body, the type of tissues involved, and even the topographical region of the tissue. In addition, the forensic scenes in which burned remains are recovered are complex, fragile, and criminalistically significant.

Thus this aspect of forensic anthropology and archaeology is exciting to research, allowing for great scope in research projects and interdisciplinary collaborations. At all times, however, we must not lose track of the question that should be driving our research forward: how well do we fulfil our current and future context-based requirements and demands? A tremendous foundation has already been created within the study of burned human remains, and the future developments and direction predicted here will allow for this foundation to mature and become firmly established within the context of forensic anthropological and archaeological practice.

Acknowledgment

Many thanks to Dr. Becky Gowland (Durham University), who kindly read through and gave advice on early drafts of this chapter.

Notes

1. For earlier reviews, see McKinley (2000) and Mayne Correia (1997).

2. Incidentally, Shipman, Foster, and Schoeinger (1984) were the first group of anthropologists to use a standardised colour chart for defining colour in the examination of heat-induced change. Although this allows for a significant increase in the potential for interexperiment comparison, it is unfortunate that few other studies have adopted this approach.

References

Baby, R. S. 1954. Hopewell cremation practices. *The Ohio Historical Society Paper in Archaeology* 1: 1–7.

Binford, L. R. 1963. An analysis of cremations from three Michigan sites. *Wisconsin Archaeologist* 44: 98–110.

Bond, J. M. 1996. Burnt offerings: Animal bone in Anglo-Saxon cremations. *World Archaeology* 28(1): 76–78.

Bradtmiller, B., and Buikstra, J. E. 1984. Effects of burning on human bone microstructure: A preliminary study. *Journal of Forensic Sciences* 29(2): 535–540.

Brown, K. A., O'Donoghue, K., and Brown, T. A. 1995. DNA in cremated bones from an early Bronze Age cemetery cairn. *International Journal of Osteoarchaeology* 5: 181–187.

Buikstra, J. E., and Swegle, M. 1989. Bone modification due to burning: Experimental evidence, in R.

Bonnichsen and M. H. Sorg (eds.), *Peopling of the Americas*, pp. 247–258. Orono, ME: Center for the Studies of the First Americans.

Cain, C. R. 2005. Using burned animal bone to look at Middle Stone Age occupation and behaviour. *Journal of Archaeological Science* 32: 873–884.

Carr, R. F., Barsley, R. W., and Davenport, W. D. 1986. Postmortem examination of incinerated teeth with the scanning electron microscope. *Journal of Forensic Sciences* 31(1): 307–311.

Cattaneo, C., Di Martino, S., Scali, S., Craig, O. E., Grandi, M., and Sokol, R. J. 1999. Determining the human origin of fragments of burnt bone: A comparative study of histological, immunological and DNA techniques. *Forensic Science International* 102: 181–191.

Cattaneo, C., Gelsthorpe, K., Phillips, P., and Sokol, R. J. 1995. Differential survival of albumin in ancient bone. *Journal of Archaeological Science* 22: 271–276.

Cattaneo, C., Gelsthorpe, K., Sokol, R. J., and Philips, P. 1994. Immunological detection of albumin in ancient human cremations using ELISA and monoclonal antibodies. *Journal of Archaeological Science* 21: 565–571.

Chandler, N. P. 1987. Cremated teeth. *Archaeology Today* August: 41–45.

Christensen, A. M. 2002. Experiments in the combustibility of the human body. *Journal of Forensic Sciences* 47(3): 466–470.

De Gruchy, S., and Rogers, T. L. 2002. Identifying chop marks on cremated bone: A preliminary study. *Journal of Forensic Sciences* 47(5): 933–936.

De Haan, J. D., and Nurbakhsh, S. 2001. Sustained combustion of an animal carcass and its implications for the consumption of human bodies in fires. *Journal of Forensic Sciences* 46(5): 1076–1081.

Dirkmaat, D. C. 2002. Recovery and interpretation of the fatal fire victim: The role of forensic anthropology, in W. D. Haglund and M. H. Sorg (eds.), *Advances in Forensic Taphonomy: Method, Theory, and Archaeological Perspectives*, pp. 451–472. Boca Raton, FL: CRC Press.

Downes, J. 1999. Cremation: A spectacle and a journey, in J. Downes and T. Pollard (eds.), *The Loved Body's Corruption: Archaeological Contributions to the Study of Human Mortality*. Glasgow: Cruithne Press.

Duffy, J. B., Waterfield, J. D., and Skinner, M. F. 1991. Isolation of tooth pulp cells for sex chromatin studies in experimental dehydrated and cremated remains. *Forensic Science International* 49: 127–141.

Eckert, W. G., James, S., and Katchis, S. 1988. Investigation of cremations and severely burned bodies. *American Journal of Forensic Medicine and Pathology* 9(3): 188–200.

Fanton, L., Jdeed, K., Tilhet-Coartet, S., and Malicier, D. 2006. Criminal Burning. *Forensic Science International* 158: 87–93.

Gilchrist, R., and Mytum, M. C. 1986. Experimental archaeology and burnt animal bone from archaeological sites. *Circaea* 4(1): 29–38.

Grévin, G., Bailet, P., Quatrehomme, G., and Ollier, A. 1998. Anatomical reconstruction of fragments of burned human bones: A necessary means for forensic identification. *Forensic Science International* 96: 129–134.

Grupe, G., and Hummel, S. 1991. Trace element studies on experimentally cremated bone. I. Alteration of the chemical composition at high temperatures. *Journal of Archaeological Science* 18: 177–186.

Herrmann, B., and Grupe, G. 1988. Trace element content in prehistoric cremated human remains, in G. Grupe and B. Herrmann (eds.), *Trace Elements in Environmental History*. Proceedings of the Symposium held from June 24th to 26th, 1987, at Göttingen, pp. 91–101. Berlin: Springer-Verlag.

Herrmann, N. P., and Bennett, J. L. 1999. The differentiation of traumatic and heat-related fractures in burned bone. *Journal of Forensic Sciences* 44(3): 461–469.

Hiller, J., Thompson, T. J. U., Evison, M. P., Chamberlain, A. T., and Wess, T. J. 2003. Bone mineral change during experimental heating: An X-ray scattering investigation. *Biomaterials* 24(28): 5091–5097.

Holden, J. L., Phakey, P. P., and Clement, J. G. 1995a. Scanning electron microscope observations of incinerated human femoral bone: A case study. *Forensic Science International* 74: 17–28.

——. 1995b. Scanning electron microscope observations of heat-treated human bone. *Forensic Science International* 74: 29–45.

Holland, T. D. 1989. Use of the cranial base in the identification of fire victims. *Journal of Forensic Sciences* 34(2): 458–460.

Koon, H. E. C., Nicholson, R. A., and Collins, M. J. 2003. A practical approach to the identification of low temperature heated bone using TEM. *Journal of Archaeological Science* 30: 1393–1399.

Mayne Correia, P. 1997. Fire modification of bone: A review of the literature, in W. D. Haglund and M. H. Sorg (eds.), *Forensic Taphonomy: The Post-Mortem Fate of Human Remains:*, pp. 275–293. Boca Raton, FL: CRC Press.

Mayne Correia, P., and Beattie, O. 2002. A critical look at methods for recovering, evaluating, and interpreting cremated human remains, in W. D. Haglund and M. H. Sorg (eds.), *Advances in Forensic Taphonomy: Method, Theory, and Archaeological Perspectives:*, pp. 435–450. Boca Raton, FL: CRC Press.

McKinley, J. I. 1994. Bone fragment size in British cremation burials and its implications for pyre technology and ritual. *Journal of Archaeological Science* 21: 339–342.

——. 2000. The analysis of cremated bone, in M. Cox and S. Mays (eds.), *Human Osteology: In Archaeology and Forensic Science*, pp. 403–421. London: Greenwich Medical Media Ltd.

McKinley, J. I., and Roberts, C. 1993. Excavation and post-excavation treatment of cremated and inhumed human remains. Reading: *Institute of Field Archaeologists Technical Paper* Number 13.

Murad, T. A. 1998. The growing popularity of cremation versus inhumation: Some forensic implications, in K. J. Reichs (ed.), *Forensic Osteology: Advances in the Identification of Human Remains* (2nd ed.), pp. 86–105. Springfield, IL: Charles C. Thomas.

Newesely, H. 1988. Chemical stability of hydroxapatite under different conditions, in G. Grupe and B. Herrmann (eds.), *Trace Elements in Environmental History: Proceedings of the Symposium Held from June 24th to 26th, 1987, at Göttingen*: 1–16. Berlin: Springer-Verlag.

Nicholson, R. A. 1995. Out of the frying pan into the fire: What value are burnt fish bones to archaeology? *Archaeofauna* 4: 47–64.

Oestigaard, T. 2000. The deceased's life cycle rituals in Nepal: Present cremation burials for the interpretations of the past. *British Archaeological Reports International Series* 853.

Payne-James, J., Busuttil, A., and Smock, W. 2003. *Forensic Medicine: Clinical and Pathological Aspects*. London: Greenwich Medical Media Ltd.

Pope, E. J., and Smith, O. C. 2004. Identification of traumatic injury in burned cranial bone: An experimental approach. *Journal of Forensic Sciences* 49(3): 1–10.

Quatrehomme, G., Bolla, M., Muller, M., Rocca, J.-P., Grévin, G., Bailet, P., and Ollier, A. 1998. Experimental single controlled study of burned bones: Contribution of scanning electron microscopy. *Journal of Forensic Sciences* 43(2): 417–422.

Roberts, S. J., Smith, C. I., Millard, A., and Collins, M. J. 2002. The taphonomy of cooked bone: Characterizing boiling and its physio-chemical effects. *Archaeometry* 44(3): 485–494.

Rogers, K. D., and Daniels, P. 2002. An X-ray diffraction study of the effects of heat treatment on bone mineral microstructure. *Biomaterials* 23: 2577–2585.

Sajantila, A., Ström, M., Budowle, B., Karhunen, P. J., and Peltonen, L. 1991. The polymerase chain reaction and post-mortem forensic identity testing: Application of amplified D1S80 and HLA-DQo loci to the identification of fire victims. *Forensic Science International* 51: 23–34.

Saukko, P., and Knight, B. 2004. *Knight's Forensic Pathology* (3rd ed.). London: Arnold.

Shipman, P., Foster, G., and Schoeinger, M. 1984. Burnt bones and teeth: An experimental study of color, morphology, crystal structure and shrinkage. *Journal of Archaeological Science* 11: 307–325.

Shkrum, M. J., and Johnston, K. A. 1992. Fire and suicide: A three-year study of self-immolation deaths. *Journal of Forensic Sciences* 37(1): 208–221.

Sillen, A., and Hoering, T. 1993. Chemical characterization of burnt bones from Swartkrans, in C. K. Brain (ed.), *Swartkrans: A Cave's Chronicle of Early Man*, pp. 243–249. Pretoria: Transvaal Museum Monograph 8.

Sledzik, P. S., and Rodriguez III, W. C. 2002. Damnum Fatale: The taphonomic fate of human remains in mass disaster, in W. D. Haglund and M. H. Sorg (eds.), *Advances in Forensic Taphonomy: Method, Theory, and Archaeological Perspectives*, pp. 321–329. Boca Raton, FL: CRC Press, Inc.

Spennemann, D. H. R., and Colley, S. M. 1989. Fire in a pit: The effects of burning on Faunal remains. *Archaeozoologia* 3: 51–64.

Stiner, M. C., Kuhn, S. L., Weiner, S., and Bar-Yosef, O. 1995. Differential burning, recrystallization, and fragmentation of archaeological bone. *Journal of Archaeological Science* 22: 223–237.

Sukhai, A., Harris, C., Moorad, R. G. R., and Dada, M. A. 2002. Suicide by self-immolation in Durban, South Africa: A five-year retrospective review. *American Journal of Forensic Medicine and Pathology* 23(3): 295–298.

Thompson, T. J. U. 2002. The assessment of sex in cremated individuals: Some cautionary notes. *Canadian Society of Forensic Science Journal* 35(2): 49–56.

———. 2004. Recent advances in the study of burned bone and their implications for forensic anthropology. *Forensic Science International* 146S: S203–S205.

———. 2005. Heat-induced dimensional changes in bone and their consequences for forensic anthropology. *Journal of Forensic Sciences* 50(5): 1008–1015.

Thompson, T. J. U., and Chudek, J. A. 2007. A novel approach to the visualisation of heat-induced structural change in bone. *Science and Justice* 47: 99–104.

Thurman, M. D., and Willmore, L. J. 1981. A replicative cremation experiment. *North American Archaeologist* 2(4): 275–283.

Tsuchimochi, T., Iwasa, M., Maeno, Y., Koyama, H., Inoue, H., Isobe, I., Matoba, R., Yokoi, M., and Nagao, M. 2002. Chelating resin-based extraction of DNA from dental pulp and sex determination from incinerated teeth with Y-chromosomal alphoid repeat and short tandem repeats. *American Journal of Forensic Medicine and Pathology* 23(3): 268–271.

Van Vark, G. N. 1974. The investigation of human cremated skeletal material by multivariate statistical methods I. Methodology. *Ossa* 1: 63–95.

———. 1975. The investigation of human cremated skeletal material by multivariate statistical methods II. Measures. *Ossa* 2: 47–68.

Wells, C. 1960. A study of cremation. *Antiquity* 34: 29–37.

Wilson, D. F., and Massey, W. 1987. Scanning electron microscopy of incinerated teeth. *American Journal of Forensic Medicine and Pathology* 8(1): 32–38.

Ye, J., Ji, A., Parra, E. J., Zheng, X., Jiang, C., Zhao, X., Hu, L., and Tu, Z. 2004. A simple and efficient method for extracting DNA from old and burned bone. *Journal of Forensic Sciences* 49(4): 1–6.

25

CRANIOFACIAL IDENTIFICATION: TECHNIQUES OF FACIAL APPROXIMATION AND CRANIOFACIAL SUPERIMPOSITION

Carl N. Stephan

If the identity of a set of skeletal remains cannot be established through the usual anthropological methods, DNA, or dental record comparisons, craniofacial identification methods that couple the anatomy of the skull with the surface anatomy of the face may offer some assistance (Krogman and İşcan 1986; Stewart 1979). Such methods take two forms: comparison of skulls of unknown identity to antemortem faces of known identity (craniofacial superimposition) and prediction of faces of unknown identity from skulls of unknown identity (facial approximation). Both methods thus deal with the human face, a feature of the body that dominates the characterization of each person in everyday life (Bruce and Young 1998). It is this aspect that gives these investigative methods their power, but ultimately for different reasons. That is, the distinctiveness of the surface anatomy of the face holds clear roles in superimposition; however, the value of the face for facial approximation may also lie with the public appeal that accompanies a busy part of such high social importance (Stephan 2003a).

General Overview of Methods

The following section provides an overview of the methods used in craniofacial identification, including superimposition and facial approximation.

Superimposition

Superimposition methods are based on the comparison (through overlay/mix) of an image of a skull of unknown identity with an image of a known antemortem face to determine if there is an anatomical match of the two. These methods are, therefore, employed when the skeletal remains are suspected to represent an individual of whom an antemortem photograph(s) exists. Assuming that protocols of the method are correctly followed, a match of the skull to the antemortem face suggests that the remains belong to the person depicted in the image. If no match is made, strong support is given to the idea that the remains do not belong to the person represented in the image. Clearly, antemortem images of recent origin should be used so that differences resulting from age/growth do not complicate the comparisons.

Owing to technological advances, comparisons of a skull to a face are now being commonly achieved through video equipment; previously it was conducted using photographs or tracings of photographs. In the near future, the process likely will become completely digital and computerized (see, e.g., Lan 1992), but despite these technological advances, the fundamentals of the method remain unchanged: determining the anatomical fit of a face to a skull.

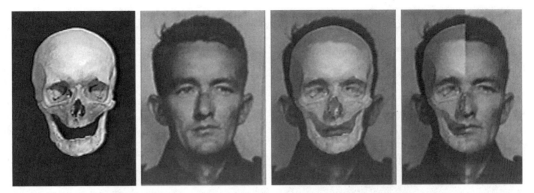

Figure 25.1 Video superimposition showing a possible match between the skull and the face. Essentially all 12 criteria reported by Austin-Smith and Maples (1994) are fulfilled. Worthy of mention is (1) the skull outline completely falls within that of the soft tissue (anterior cranium fits forehead, mandible fits jaw [note here that the border of the jaw is falling in heavy shadow as a result of the lighting on the antemortem face]); (2) anterior temporal line of skull fits that of the face; (3) eyebrows follow the supraorbital margin; (4) orbits encase eye and medial and lateral canthi align with relevant bony features; (5) breadth and height of nose fit dimensions of nasal aperture of skull; (6) general contours of face fit those of skull, for example, contouring of cheeks fit the zygomatic bones, and contouring of chin fits the mental eminence. Exhibited from left to right are (the skull, antemortem-face photograph to be compared, superimposition of face on skull, and superimposition of face on skull with a left-side half wipe.

To conduct a video superimposition, the skull is typically positioned in front of one video camera, while an antemortem photograph of the face of the person suspected to provide a match is positioned in front of another camera of identical make and model—note that, to reduce inconsistencies, the cameras should be ordered and bought as pairs (Helmer 1984; Taylor and Brown 1998). The two subsequent images are overlaid (superimposed) at varying opacities using a video mixer (Figure 25.1). In order to determine if the skull fits in the correct anatomical position "beneath" the face, the orientation of the skull is adjusted to match, as near as possible, the head orientation of the person in the photograph, and the magnification of the photograph is adjusted to fit the skull. Known soft-tissue depth distributions and anatomical face relationships (see below for examples) are used to assess if a match is demonstrated (Austin-Smith and Maples 1994; Helmer 1984; Taylor and Brown 1998).

Facial Approximation

The process of establishing a facial appearance from a skull (facial approximation) is conducted when there are no known individuals to whom the remains are suspected to belong, or recent photographs of such persons cannot be obtained/do not exist. The process has traditionally been accomplished using manual methods that require drawing or sculpture (Gatliff and Taylor 2001; Gerasimov 1971; Prag and Neave 1997; Taylor 2001). As with superimposition, recent technological improvements have enabled attempts to fully digitize facial approximation. However, although computer-generated/assisted techniques tend to be more objective, standardized, and repeatable, their abilities to represent realistic face morphology are currently limited in contrast to manual methods. Recent computerized approaches include warping a face to fit the skull with average soft-tissue depths in place (Vanezis et al. 2000) and warping faces in combination with skulls so that, after transforming the skull component of a craniofacial complex to match the known skull, the resulting face (which has also been warped) serves as the approximation (Nelson and Michael 1998; Quatrehomme et al. 1997; Tu et al. 2005; Turner et al. 2005). Regardless which facial approximation technique is used (manual or computerized), the process depends on taking an unknown skull, analyzing its morphology, and estimating the facial appearance from this information under blind conditions (Figure 25.2). The final constructed face is then advertised in the media, often with accompanying case findings/descriptions, in the hope that the person to whom the skull belongs is recognized.

Although the terminology used to describe the method of building faces from skulls has been subject to wide debate, the term *facial approximation*

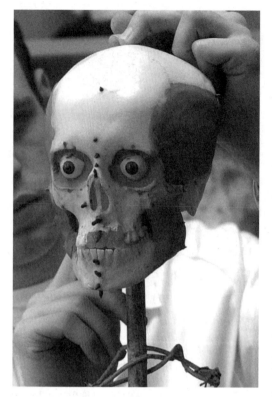

Figure 25.2 Partially completed facial approximation showing "in progress" construction of the face with average soft-tissue depths, eyeballs, and some muscles of mastication in place on a precision replica skull (photo Mark Brake, *The Advertiser*).

has received increasing support from a wide array of practitioners and authors since being first proposed by George in 1987 (e.g., Brown et al. 2004; De Greef et al. 2006; Evenhouse, Rasmussen, and Sadler 1990; Haglund 1998; Haglund and Reay 1991; Reichs and Craig 1998; Stephan and Henneberg 2001; Stephan et al. 2005; Taylor 2001; Turner et al. 2005). Thus, this term is used throughout this chapter.

Facial reconstruction has been another popular term, especially in the media, probably because the name draws attention ("reconstruction" implies technicality and exactness); however, this term has been criticized on a number of fronts:

1. The term has already been used to refer to other techniques (for example, the process of reassembling a shattered or broken skeletal element [Rhine 1990]) and surgical reconstruction of the tissue of the face in medicine (Converse 1977);

2. "reconstruction" implies that nothing is added, altered, or subtracted and is, thus, misleading with respect to the method (Rhine 1990);

3. "reconstruction" implies a perfect replication—something that cannot be achieved using current methods (George 1987).

Other names have also been suggested, such as "reproduction," "restoration," "reconstitution," and "forensic sculpture" but have been unpopular for reasons similar to those mentioned above (e.g., George 1987; Rhine 1990). The joint use of "facial approximation" and "facial reconstruction" has also recently been proposed so as to subclassify methods depending on whether they use average soft-tissue depths (Ryan and Wilkinson 2006). However, this use of such terms is also inappropriate for two primary reasons: (1) all facial approximation methods depend on the same fundamentals—combined use of soft-tissue averages and face anatomy (Stephan 2006); and, (2) as already highlighted, "reconstruction" (implying exact replication) is widely recognized to be impossible using established/current methods (George 1987).

Previously, it was common for methods of facial approximation to be classified into one of three theoretical frameworks: (1) methods that depended on average soft-tissue depths alone (called "American/morphometric/soft-tissue depth methods"); (2) methods that depended on skull anatomy alone (called "Russian/morphoscopic/anatomical methods"); and (3) methods that relied on a combination of both average soft-tissue depth information and skull anatomy (termed "combination methods"). However, evidence from the German and Russian literature (Ullrich 1958, 1966; Gerasimov 1955, respectively) show these frameworks to have little value (Stephan 2006). It is clear that Gerasimov, the founder of "Russian" methods, heavily relied on average soft-tissue depth information for his face constructions and built only a few of the facial muscles (Gerasimov 1955; Ullrich 1958, 1966; see also Figure 25.3). Furthermore, it has been reported (Taylor 2001) and illustrated (Stephan 2006) that so-called "American" or "soft-tissue depth" methods incorporate anatomical components for realistic face construction (for example, to represent soft tissue found between landmarks for averages), adding further contradiction to the traditional classificatory frameworks. These observations demonstrate that all facial approximation methods are of the same kind and should consequently be described as such (Stephan 2006).

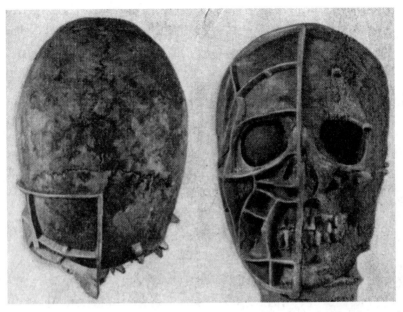

Figure 25.3 One of the images Gerasimov used to illustrate his method of facial approximation. Note that only the temporalis and masseter muscles are built; average soft-tissue depths (modified according to the underlying bony relief of the skull) are represented on the skull as wax pyramids (clearly evident on the left image). The soft-tissue depths are then connected to construct the face contour. (images reproduced from M. M. Gerasimov 1955. *Vosstanovlenie lica po čerepu*, p. 133 Moskva: Trudy Instituta Etnografiji).

Aims of Craniofacial Identification Methods

Both superimposition and facial approximation methods aim to contribute information helpful for the establishment of the identity of a set of skeletal remains, and it is under these broad terms that techniques can be referred to as "methods of identification." However, the ability of a method to *contribute* to an identification should not be confused with its ability to *provide an identification* (that is, positive identification). Although the ultimate judgment of the appropriateness and ability of a method rests with a court, facial approximation and superimposition are generally not considered to be methods used for positive identification (Ubelaker 2002). It is broadly acknowledged that the anatomy of skulls and faces, and the relationships between the two, seem not individualizing enough to enable precise determinations of the person to whom a set of skeletal remains belongs. Furthermore, errors inherent in the methods (for example, photographic distortions in superimposition and practitioner speculation in facial approximation) limit abilities for establishing an identity.

Superimposition methods are generally used as a measure of a match and are assigned heavier weight for exclusion but are not generally used for positive identification of individuals (there may be exceptions if corresponding dental characters are clearly evident on the skull and facial photograph). Facial approximation methods are given much less weight in regard to determining a match, since methods are largely untested and appear to stretch known anatomical boundaries. Facial approximation is widely regarded to be a method of "last resort" and is mainly used for initiating further investigative leads. The consensus is that facial approximation methods rarely produce reliable, correct, and purposeful facial recognitions. However, this starkly contrasts with claims by some practitioners, and the commonly held public perception, that purposeful face recognition is reliably achieved.

History and Development of Craniofacial Identification Methods

Modern craniofacial identification methods have developed out of early attempts to authenticate the identities of skeletons that were suspected to represent well-known historical figures—for example, Schiller (Welcker 1883, 1888) and Bach (His 1895). Superimposition (using skull outlines overlaid on portraits) developed before facial approximation (see, for example, Figure 25.4). Soon following superimposition development, anatomists built faces from skulls (notable here are His, and Kollmann and Büchly) (Figure 25.5).

Soft-tissue depth averages were often used by the above-mentioned authors, and much European-centered research continued the focus on soft-tissue depths in the years to follow (e.g., Birkner

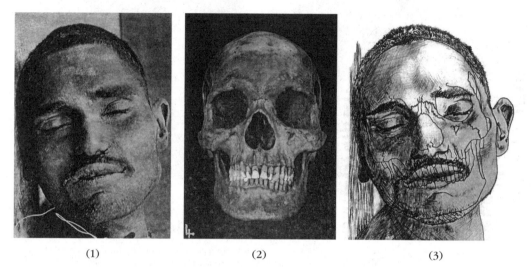

(1)   (2)   (3)

Figure 25.4 Pearson and Morant's superimposition of a face on a skull using a known specimen (note that the original authors pay significant acknowledgment to D. E. Derry for the results): (1) face soon after death; (2) skull with soft tissues removed; (3) superimposition of tracings from (1) and (2) (image from K. Pearson and G. M. Morant 1934; the Wilkinson head of Oliver Cromwell and its relationship to busts, masks, and painted portraits *Biometrika* 26, plates I and II).

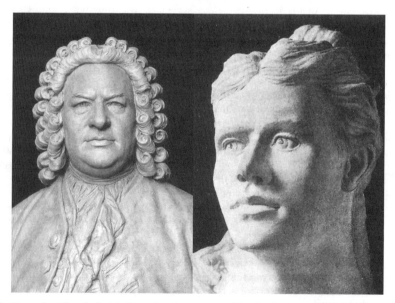

Figure 25.5 Examples of early facial approximations reported in the literature: (*left*) facial approximation of Bach produced by His (image reproduced from W. His 1895. *Johann Sebastian Bach: Forschungen über dessen Grabstätte, Gebeine und Antlitz. Bericht an den Rath der Stadt Leipzig*. Leipzig: F. C. W Vogel, plate VI); (*right*) facial approximation of a Neolithic woman produced by Kollmann and Büchly (image from J. Kollmann and W. Büchly. 1898. Die Persistenz der Rassen und die Reconstruction der Physiognomie prähistorischer Schädel. *Archives für Anthropologie* 25: 337).

1904 and Fischer 1905, cited in Stadtmuller 1922; Martin 1957; also Czekanowski 1907; Edelman 1938; Stadtmuller 1922; von Eggeling 1909). This has continued to be the pattern in more recent times with further reliance on mean soft-tissue depths and additional production of soft-tissue depth data (Table 25.1).

The first published report of superimposition methods used in forensic casework was by Glaister and Brash (Glaister and Brash 1937). These authors were able to corroborate the identity of two individuals using tracings derived from antemortem photographs (Figure 25.6). After this, methods progressed to recording superimpositions by photographs alone, whereby magnification effects were of primary concern up until the 1970s. With the development of video recording by Ginsburg's team in 1951 and the video revolution of the 1970s, new superimposition methods followed. Motion-picture cameras replaced the traditional still-frame camera, and video superimpositions were first introduced and implemented around 1976 (Helmer and Grüner 1977; Snow 1976), at about the time when VHS format had been introduced to compete with the soon-to-be abandoned Betamax format. Not surprisingly, many forensic practitioners from around the globe independently capitalized on the new technology for identical craniofacial identification purposes, and it was in the 1980s that the methods became widespread (Bastiaan, Dalitz, and Woodward 1986; Brown 1983; Delfino et al. 1986; Iten 1987; Koelmeyer 1982).

Although superimposition has attained a reputation of being a reliable anthropological method, especially for exclusion, few quantitative studies of method accuracy have been conducted. Perhaps the most comprehensive is that conducted by Austin-Smith and Maples (1994), who found that false positive matches were obtained for the comparison of three skulls to 97 lateral and 98 frontal images of nontarget individuals (note that anterior dentition was not evaluated as part of these tests). For lateral images alone, false-positive matches were found in 9.5% of cases. For frontal images alone, the false positive rate was 8.5%. Both these rates were reduced to 0.6% when frontal and lateral images were used in conjunction with each other. The Austin-Smith and Maples study thus demonstrated that without anterior dentition analysis craniofacial superimposition is reliable when two photographs of the subject (representing different angles) are used for comparison. With anterior dentition analysis, it is recognized that positive identifications can more readily be established (Austin-Smith and Maples 1994; McKenna, Jablonski, and Fearnhead 1984; Webster et al. 1986).

The first published reports of facial approximation casework predate those of superimposition. In 1913, von Eggeling commented on their consideration for forensic applications but was unconvinced of their benefit. Three years later, facial approximation produced its first recorded success in a New York forensic investigation (Wilder and Wenworth 1918). Since that time, facial approximation methods have been useful in many forensic cases (e.g., Gatliff and Snow 1979; Gerasimov 1971; Prag and Neave 1997; Suzuki 1973; Taylor 2001). However, the ability of methods to achieve correctly recognizable faces remains controversial (Brues 1958; Haglund 1998; Haglund and Reay 1991; Montagu 1947; Stephan 2002b, 2003b; Stephan and Henneberg 2001; Suk 1935). The driving factor of this controversy is that casework success may result from the inclusion of other case-specific factors in the media advertisement, not from face recognition alone (Haglund 1998; Haglund and Reay 1991; Stephan 2002a, 2003b; Stephan and Henneberg 2001). Crucial empirical tests remain to be conducted on the matter; however, the first-ever written report of forensic facial approximation (Wilder and Wenworth 1918) illustrates clearly the likelihood of confounding factors even when only a head is shown (that is, no case description provided). The constructed head (said to be correctly recognized as Dominick La Rosa) was displayed with a colored necktie retrieved from the remains of the body (Wilder and Wenworth 1918). On viewing the head, one of the assessors exclaimed "that's Dominick's necktie . . ." (Wilder and Wenworth 1918).

A popular method for determining the accuracy of a facial approximation has been the resemblance between a facial approximation and a target face (person to whom the skull belongs). Although commonly used in the past, such resemblance ratings are known to be limited because they are insensitive measures with poor discrimination power (Stephan and Arthur 2006), are unable to account for nontarget faces that may bear greater resemblance to the facial approximation (Stephan 2002a) and rely on exact face similarity as a measure of accuracy when recognition is the more relevant variable (Stephan 2002a). These limitations are perhaps not surprising, since resemblance ratings are comparable to "show up" tests in eyewitness identification, which are widely known to be biased (Gonzalez, Ellsworth, and Pembroke 1993; Malpass and Devine 1983; Wells 1993). Note also that practitioners have on occasion "touched up" their facial approximations (for example, added similar hair style and eyebrow shape) after the facial appearance of the person to

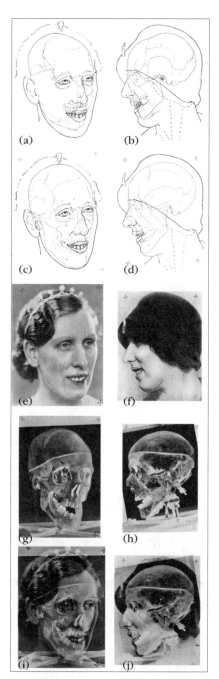

Figure 25.6 Craniofacial superimpositions by Glaister and Brash (1937) using images of Mrs. Ruxton. The left column concerns work done on a "three quarter" studio portrait (c); the right column concerns work done on a profile snapshot (h); (a) and (f) show superimposed outlines of skull 1 with Mrs. Ruxton's portraits, as used to draw conclusions that the two did not "correspond"; (b) and (g) show superimposed outlines of skull 2 with Mrs. Ruxton's portraits, as used to draw conclusions that the two "fit"; (e) and (j) show actual photographic superimpositions of each face and skull image, respectively [(e) = (c) + (d); (j) = (h) + (i)], which are provided by Glaister and Brash for purely illustrative purposes (these images were not used to draw any formal conclusions) (images reproduced from J. Glaister and J. C. Brash. 1937. *Medico-legal Aspects of the Ruxton Case,* pp. 153, 155, 162–163, 166–167. Baltimore: William Wood and Co.). .

Table 25.1 Methods of soft-tissue depth measurement: advantages, disadvantages, and examples of studies using methods (adapted from C. N. Stephan and E. K. Simpson 2008).

Method	Advantages	Disadvantages	Studies Employing Method
Needle Puncture	• Inexpensive equipment required (e.g., ruler and pin) • Participants do not move • Soft tissue directly measured • Any site on the head can be measured • No radiation exposure to subjects	• Used to measures decedents (invasive) and often embalmed cadavers • Landmark placement can be troublesome • Contact method. Skin may "dimple" upon needle insertion (complicated by rubber stoppers) • Participants usually in supine position ("unnatural" gravity effects on face)	• Domaracki and Stephan 2006 • Simpson and Henneberg 2002 • O'Grady et al. 1990 cited in Taylor and Angel 1998 • Rhine and Campbell 1980 • Suzuki 1948
Radiograph	• Can measure living participants (noninvasive) • Noncontact method • Images usually taken of participants in upright position	• Radiation exposure • Soft-tissue depth can be measured only in planes perpendicular to "line of sight" and at periphery of skull • Imaging artifacts may be present, e.g., magnification effects • Relatively expensive equipment required	• Williamson et al. 2002 • Smith and Buschang 2001 • Garlie and Saunders 1999 • Miyasaka et al. 1999 • Aulsebrook et al. 1996 • Ogawa 1960
Ultrasound	• Can measure living participants (noninvasive) • Can measure participants in an upright position • Can be used as a noncontact method • Any site on the head can be measured • Little radiation exposure	• Often used as contact method; instrument application may cause soft-tissue compression and inaccurate readings • When not used as a contact method, participants heads have not been in upright positions ("unnatural" gravity effects on face) • Imaging artifacts may be present, e.g., sound wave velocity may not closely approximate 1540 m/sec, depending on tissue structure/s. • Expensive equipment required	• De Greef et al. 2006 • Wilkinson 2002 • El-Mehallawi et al. 2001 • Manhein et al. 2000 • Aulsebrook et al. 1996 • Helmer 1984

Table 25.1 *Continued*

Method	Advantages	Disadvantages	Studies Employing Method
CT	• Can measure living participants (noninvasive) • Noncontact method • Any site on the head can be easily measured	• Large radiation exposure to subjects • Expensive equipment required • Imaging artifacts may be present • Participants usually in supine position ("unnatural" gravity effects on face)	• Phillips and Smuts 1996
MRI	• Can measure living participants (noninvasive) • Noncontact method • Any site on the head can be easily measured • Little radiation exposure	• Expensive equipment required • Imaging artifacts may be present • Participants usually in supine position ("unnatural" gravity effects on face)	• Sahni et al. 2002

whom the skeletal remains belong is known (e.g., Gerasimov 1955, 1971; Helmer et al. 1993); thus, resemblances to target individuals in these cases are probably misleading.

In contrast to casework success and resemblance ratings, recognition tests, whereby assessors must identify the target individual from a face array or their memory, appear to offer the most robust tests. These tests can be carried out in familiar and unfamiliar conditions. Familiar tests, when assessors closely know the target individual, are optimal, because this is the condition under which casework recognition normally occurs. Such studies are rare, however, since the next of kin may be placed in awkward emotional positions, or living people must be subjected to radiation exposure to capture information necessary for skull replication. Only one systematically structured familiar recognition study has been reported in the literature so far. The study examined two-dimensional (2-D) facial approximations constructed by warping average faces to fit exact antemortem representations of target individuals (Stephan et al. 2005).

Thus the face construction process did not require skulls and circumvented the concerns highlighted above (Stephan et al. 2005). Since 2-D face shapes were *exactly replicated* by warping average faces to *known* shapes rather than approximating skulls using traditional methods, this study tested accuracies of method not normally attainable in forensic casework. Successful recognition rates of the warped average faces were found to average 43%, but because exact face shapes were replicated, corresponding accuracy of real-life blind facial approximation can be expected to be considerably less (Stephan et al. 2005).

The remaining studies that have tested facial approximation recognition have employed unfamiliar recognition protocols. Snow and colleagues conducted the first such study in 1970, using 2 facial approximations and antemortem photographs displayed in face arrays that also included antemortem faces of nontarget individuals (known as distractor, or foil faces). Both facial approximations were recognized above chance rates, one at a success rate of 68%, the other 26%

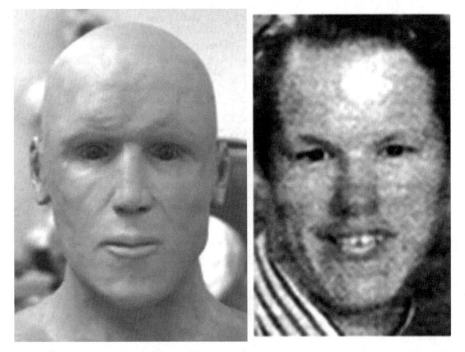

Figure 25.7 Example of a blindly constructed facial approximation that was judged to bear fairly high resemblance to the target but performed poorly on recognition tests (image from C. N. Stephan and M. Henneberg 2006. Recognition by facial approximation: Case-specific examples and empirical tests. *Forensic Science International* 156: 182–191. Note that the facial approximation displays narrow mouth width and deeply set eyes, because it was constructed using older published guidelines that have been more recently demonstrated as empirically inaccurate; see Stephan 2002b, 2003a; Wilkinson and Mautner 2003).

(chance rate = 14%, mean rate across both facial approximations = 47%). Stephan and Henneberg (2001) tested 16 facial approximations (4 methods on four skulls) built following published protocols. Only 1 of the 16 facial approximations was recognized above chance rates at a success rate of 24% (chance rate = 5%, mean success rate across all 16 facial approximations = 8%). Stephan and Henneberg (2006) also conducted recognition trials on a facial approximation (see Figure 25.7 on the previous page) that was judged to bear good resemblance to the target individual (~7 out of 10) and found that it was not recognized above chance rates (chance rate = 10%, mean success rate = 20%). Furthermore, these authors found that assessors did better when they did not use the facial approximation to guide their responses but rather guessed who the target individual was, even though the facial approximation was judged to have high resemblance to the target face. Van Rensburg (1993) conducted a face array study of 15 facial approximations using death masks rather than antemortem photographs and reported an average success rate of 26% (chance rate = 7%), although statistical significances went unreported. Wilkinson and Whittaker (2002; see also Wilkinson 2004) conducted recognition tests of facial approximations constructed from five "juvenile" skulls that received successful identification in 44% of cases (chance rate reported as 10%); however, the protocols employed for this test weaken results since (1) the face pool included individuals of disparate ages (8–18 years), which likely favored high recognition rates, and (2) the face pool was repeatedly used across all facial approximations (complicating the chance rate used for statistical analysis; for example, in the case of a correct identification for one facial approximation, subsequent chance of correct identification for other facial approximations would be increased).

Method Principles

Superimposition and facial approximation methods are both underpinned by knowledge of human anatomy, and, consequently, it is in this discipline that practitioners must have strong expertise, which includes knowledge and familiarity of soft-tissue guidelines that have been formulated to assist practitioners in their evaluations of the skull and predictions of the face (e.g., Austin-Smith and Maples 1994; Caldwell 1986; Fedosyutkin and Nainys 1993; Gerasimov 1971; Krogman and İşcan 1986; von Eggeling 1913). The soft-tissue prediction guidelines reported in superimposition circles have tended to be relatively more conservative (e.g., Austin-Smith

and Maples 1994; Taylor and Brown 1998) than those originating from within the realm of facial approximation (e.g., Fedosyutkin and Nainys 1993; Wilkinson 2004). Theoretically, the guidelines used in both methods should be constrained by real and verifiable anatomical relationships if they are to be employed under the umbrella of forensic science. In reality, however, facial approximation techniques often tend to be more flamboyant and, thus, move more toward the realms of speculation (the latter termed by other authors as "art") rather than science. A major causative factor for this situation is that facial approximation methods cannot be kept in check by comparisons to a known antemortem comparison face, as is the case for superimposition. Thus, facial approximation methods are less constrained than superimposition and provide opportunity for soft-tissue-relationship hungry practitioners to draw on "artistic license" and untested prediction methods. Arguably, the features for which no tested guidelines exist should be conservatively represented in facial approximation along the lines of typicality to maintain objectivity and repeatability, especially if methods are to be emphasized in any way as being scientific.

An extended review of the existing soft-tissue prediction/assessment guidelines is not possible here owing to space limits; however, the following section summarizes some of the prominent guidelines and classifies each depending on whether or not it has been empirically demonstrated. Well-established and conservative methods used in superimposition (for example, eyes within bony orbits; nasal aperture within dimensions of soft-tissue nose [Austin-Smith and Maples 1994]), are not discussed. Evidence-based guidelines are briefly discussed; untested guidelines are listed. Note that deviations from the stipulated guidelines are probably needed with changes in posture, pose, and facial expression (Taylor and Brown 1998). This aspect largely limits the usefulness of soft-tissue prediction guidelines in superimposition where antemortem comparison faces may not be obtainable in neutral expression (Taylor and Brown 1998).

Depth of Soft Tissue Covering the Skull

Tested Guidelines. Many soft-tissue depth studies have been published using a number of techniques, including ultrasound of living subjects and needle puncture of cadavers (for recent examples, see Table 25.1). These data are useful in predicting or assessing the relationship of the external surface anatomy of the face from/to the skull and are thus applicable to both facial approximation and superimposition. Typically, soft-tissue depths are classified by variables such as sex, age, fatness/mass, and population group and are described most commonly by the first moment statistic or mean. Since there are other ways that data can be summarized (for example, using medians and modes), careful consideration should be given to which methods are most appropriate (Domaracki and Stephan 2006).

Additionally, any categorization of the soft-tissue depth data and its consequential use according to these groups should be justified on (1) the results of statistical analyses *and* (2) the practicality/applicability of the findings (Maat 1998–1999; Smith and Throckmorton 2006; Stephan, Norris, and Henneberg 2005).

Eyes

Tested Guidelines. Multiple ophthalmology studies demonstrate that eyeball projection from the orbit averages 16 mm from the deepest portion of the lateral orbital wall (Barretto and Mathog 1999; Drews 1957; Dunsky 1992; Goldberg, Belan, and Hoenig 1999; Migliori and Gladstone 1984). This mean value (16 mm) has been demonstrated to perform well in contrast to other methods, such as Bertelsen's equation (Bertelsen 1954), which takes into account interpupillary distance (Swan and Stephan 2005). The mean projection from the lateral orbital wall also demonstrates the inaccuracy of the once commonly used guideline that the apex of the cornea falls on a tangent from the mid-antero-superior orbital rim to the mid-antero-inferior orbital rim (Stephan 2002b). Stewart (1983) provides detailed descriptions for the positioning of the endocanthus and ectocanthus (which were both found to lie close to the same vertical level) relative to the malar tubercle. If the malar tubercle is absent, as appears to be in about 4.5–24% of cases (Stewart 1983), the attachment of the lateral canthal ligament can be well approximated 11 mm below the frontozygomatic suture (Whitnall 1911), and the medial canthal ligament 10 mm inferior to the level of the frontozygomatic suture (Stewart 1983).

Untested Guidelines.

- The eyeball is centrally positioned in the orbit (Krogman and İşcan 1986; Wilkinson 2004). Note that data from Eisenfield and colleagues (1975) are applicable to the verification of this guideline, but sample sizes were small and findings inconclusive.

- The eyeball is positioned at the point formed by the crossing of two lines, one from maxillofrontale to the ectoconchion, the other bisecting the orbit between its

superior and inferior margins (Krogman and İşcan 1986).

- The length of the palpabral fissure is 60–80% of the width of the orbit (Fedosyutkin and Nainys 1993).

- A low nasal root plus strong anterior lacrimal crest suggest the presence of an epicanthic fold (Wilkinson 2004).

- The eyebrows are lower in individuals with strong supraorbital margins (Fedosyutkin and Nainys 1993).

Nose

Tested Guidelines. Nose width has been shown to be best determined by dividing the nasal aperture width by 60% in contrast to fixed quantitative additions to the breadth of the nasal aperture (Hoffman et al. 1991). Methods proposed by George (1987) have also been shown to perform well in predicting nose projection, with results being repeatable across practitioners (Ryan and Wilkinson 2006; Stephan, Henneberg, and Sampson 2003). Published directions for the tangential nose-tip positioning method of Gerasimov (1971), which uses the "last third of the nasal bone," has been shown to be highly inaccurate (Stephan, Henneberg, and Sampson 2003). However, adjustments to the published description (that is, by using the "most distal tip" of the nasal bones) have been reported to perform well (Ryan and Wilkinson 2006). Methods using the subnasal soft-tissue depth and the length of the nasal spine (e.g., Krogman 1962) have found little support from empirical tests (Ryan and Wilkinson 2006; Stephan, Henneberg, and Sampson 2003).

Untested Guidelines.

- A "spatulate" nasal spine indicates a wide or bulbous nose tip, and a bifid nasal spine indicates a cleft nasal tip (Wilkinson 2004).

Mouth

Tested Guidelines. The most useful guideline so far described for determining mouth width is that the distance between the canines represents 75% of the width of the mouth (Stephan and Henneberg 2003). The width between the medial aspects of the irises has also been shown to perform well (Stephan 2003a; Wilkinson et al. 2003); however, this method has limited application in facial approximation, owing to its reliance on soft-tissue structures that are not evident on skeletal remains. The guidelines suggesting that

mouth width is equal to intercanine width and distance between the pupils have been demonstrated to be inaccurate (Stephan 2003a). George (1987) found the stomion to fall within the lower third of the central incisor height for females and within the lower quarter for males; however, other authors report slight variations on this (e.g., Fedosyutkin and Nainys 1993). The height of the lips is also reported to be determinable based on the height of the enamel on the central incisors (Wilkinson, Motwani, and Chiang 2003).
Untested Guidelines.

- The width of the mouth equals the width between the mandibular second molars (Fedosyutkin and Nainys 1993).
- The width of the philtrum equals the width between the mid-points of the upper central incisors (Fedosyutkin and Nainys 1993).
- Mouth width equals "radiating" tangents from the junction of the canine and first premolar on either side (Wilkinson 2004).
- Strength of the nasolabial fold depends on the depth of the canine fossa (Wilkinson 2004).

Eyebrows

Tested Guidelines. On average, female superciliares fall close to the plane of the lateral iris, but this trend does not seem to hold well for males (Stephan 2002c). In general, it is noted that the eyebrows display considerable variation (Rozprym 1934; Stephan 2002c). Oestreicher and Hurwitz (1990) have shown that there is a slight trend for eyebrows to become more inferior with increasing age, but absolute differences are small (0.7 mm from <40 to >59 years). Females are also found to have eyebrows that are higher than males by approximately 2 mm (Oestreicher and Hurwitz 1990).
Untested Guidelines.

- The eyebrows are 3–5 mm above the supraorbital margin (Krogman and İşcan 1986).
- The eyebrows sit on or below the orbital margin (Fedosyutkin and Nainys 1993).

Ears

Tested Guidelines. Few guidelines exist for determining the morphology of the ear from the skull. Farkas and associates (2000) have shown that the height of the nose does not reliably represent the height of the ear; most people (95%) have ears

9–10 mm larger than their noses (range 1–21 mm). Likewise, the profile angle of the nose has been shown to poorly represent the angle at which the long axis of the ear is set, with this guideline being invalid for >90% of the population (Farkas, Forrest, and Litsas 2000; Farkas et al. 1985; Skiles and Randall 1983).
Untested Guidelines.

- Strongly developed supramastoid crests and roughened lateral aspects of mastoids indicate large ear protrusion (Fedosyutkin and Nainys 1993; Wilkinson 2004).
- If the mastoid process is directed downward when the skull is in the Frankfurt horizontal, the ear lobe is attached (Fedosyutkin and Nainys 1993).
- If the mastoid points forward, the ear lobe is free (Fedosyutkin and Nainys 1993).

Hair Line

Tested Guidelines. There are no tested guidelines for the determining the position of the hairline.
Untested Guidelines.

- The hairline is marked by a transition on the frontal bone from a smooth to roughened surface that can be seen under 4.8x magnification after coating the surface of the skull with glycerin (Fedosyutkin and Nainys 1993; Wilkinson 2004).

Conclusion

Under the right circumstances, methods of craniofacial superimposition and facial approximation can assist in the process of identifying skeletal remains. Superimpositions can be conducted when facial images, of potential matches, exist in addition to a skull. Ideally, at least two images of the subject taken from different angles should be used, and pictures with visible anterior dentition should be sought. When facial images of potential matches do not exist, attempts to predict the anatomy and the appearance of the face can be made. The constructed face can then be advertised in the media (usually along with a case description) with the hope that someone may recognize the person concerned.

Superimposition is recognized as being most useful for excluding individuals to whom the remains do not belong, but with a number of facial views (and visible dentition on both skull and face photo) confidence can be high in determining a match.

The reliability and accuracy of facial approximation are undisputedly lower, and the mechanism through which methods achieve success is unclear. A combination of contextual and case-specific information, chance, and purposeful face recognition is likely to be responsible, but the degree that each factor contributes is yet to be determined.

Acknowledgments

Special thanks are extended to the Discipline of Anatomical Sciences, University of Adelaide, for use of the skull and antemortem photograph in Figure 25.1; the Forensic Odontology Unit, University of Adelaide, for use of video superimposition equipment to help produce Figure 25.1; M. Brake for permission to use the image displayed in Figure 25.2; R. Taylor for the primary production of the skull cast used in Figure 25.2; and D. Ubelaker for useful comments on the manuscript.

References

Aulsebrook, W. A., Becker, B. J., and İşcan, M.Y. 1996. Facial soft-tissue thickness in the adult male Zulu. *Forensic Science International* 79: 83–102.

Aulsebrook, W. A., İşcan, M. Y., Slabbert, J. H., and Becker, P. 1995. Superimposition and reconstruction in forensic facial identification: A survey. *Forensic Science International* 75: 101–120.

Austin-Smith, D., and Maples, W. R. 1994. The reliability of skull/photograph superimposition in individual identification. *Journal of Forensic Sciences* 39: 446–455.

Barretto, R. L., and Mathog, R. H. 1999. Orbital measurement in black and white populations. *The Laryngoscope* 109: 1051–1054.

Bastiaan, R. J., Dalitz, G. D., and Woodward, C. 1986. Video superimposition of skulls and photographic portraits: A new aid to identification. *Journal of Forensic Sciences* 31: 1373–1379.

Bertelsen, T. 1954. On 720 measurements with Lueddes exophthalmometer. *Acta Opthalmologica* 32: 589–595.

Brown, K. A. 1983. Developments in cranio-facial superimposition for identification. *The Journal of Forensic Odonto-somatology* 1: 57–64.

Brown, R. E., Kelliher, T. P., Tu, P. H., Turner, W. D., Taister, M. A., and Miller, K. W. P. 2004. A survey of tissue-depth landmarks for facial approximation. *Forensic Science Communications* 6, www.fbi.gov/hq/lab/fsc/backissu/jan2004/index.htm.

Bruce, V., and Young, A. 1998. In the eye of the beholder. New York: Oxford University Press.

Brues, A. M. 1958. Identification of skeletal remains. *Journal of Criminal Law and Criminology and Police Science* 48: 551–556.

Caldwell, P. C. 1986. New questions (and some answers) on the facial reproduction techniques, in K. J. Reichs (ed.), *Forensic Osteology*, pp. 229–254. Springfield, IL: Charles C. Thomas.

Czekanowski, J. 1907. Untersuchungen über das Verhältnis der Kopfmässe zu den Schädelmässen. *Archiv fur Anthropologie* 6: 42–89.

De Greef, S., Claes, P., Vandermeulen, D., Mollemans, W., Suetens, P., and Willems, G. 2006. Large-scale in-vivo Caucasian soft tissue thickness database for craniofacial reconstruction. *Forensic Science International* 159S: S126–S146.

Delfino, V. P., Colonna, M., Potente, F., and Introna, F. J. 1986. Computer-aided skull/face superimposition. *The American Journal of Forensic Medicine and Pathology* 7: 201–212.

Domaracki, M., and Stephan, C. N. 2006. Facial soft tissue thicknesses in Australian adult cadavers. *Journal of Forensic Sciences* 51: 5–10.

Drews, L. C. 1957. Exophthalmology. *American Journal of Ophthalmology* 43: 37–58.

Dunsky, I. L. 1992. Normative data for Hertel exophthalmometry in a normal adult black population. *Optometry and Vision Science* 69: 562–564.

Edelman, H. 1938. Die profilanalyse: Eine studie an photographischen und rontgenographischen durchdringungsbildern. *Zeitschrift fur Morphololologie und Anthropologie* 37: 166–188.

Eisenfeld, J., Mishelevich, D. J., Dann, J. J., and Bell, W. H. 1975. Soft-hard tissue correlations and computer drawings for the frontal view. *The Angle Orthodontist* 45: 267–272.

El-Mehallawi, I. H., and Soliman, E. M. 2001. Ultrasonic assessment of facial soft tissue thickness in adult Egyptians. *Forensic Science International* 117: 99–107.

Evenhouse, R., Rasmussen, M., and Sadler, L. 1990. Computer aided forensic facial approximation. *Biostereometric Technology and Applications* 1380: 147–156.

Farkas, L. G., Forrest, C. R., and Litsas, L. 2000. Revision of neoclassical facial canons in young adult Afro-Americans. *Aesthetic Plastic Surgery* 24: 179–184.

Farkas, L. G., Hreczko, T. A., Kolar, J. C., and Munro, I. R. 1985. Vertical and horizontal proportions of the face in young adult North American Caucasians: Revision of Neoclassical canons. *Plastic and Reconstructive Surgery* 75: 328–337.

Fedosyutkin, B. A., and Nainys, J. V. 1993. The relationship of skull morphology to facial features, in M. Y. İşcan and R. P. Helmer (eds.), *Forensic Analysis of the Skull*, pp. 199–213. New York: Wiley-Liss.

Garlie, T. N., and Saunders, S. R. 1999. Midline facial tissue thicknesses of subadults from a longitudinal radiographic study. *Journal of Forensic Sciences* 44: 61–67.

Gatliff, B. P. 1984. Facial sculpture on the skull for identification. *The American Journal of Forensic Medicine and Pathology* 5: 327–332.

Gatliff, B. P., and Snow, C. C. 1979. From skull to visage. *The Journal of Biocommunication* 6: 27–30.

Gatliff, B. P., and Taylor, K. T. 2001. Three-dimensional facial reconstruction on the skull, in K. T. Taylor (ed.), *Forensic Art and Illustration*, pp. 419–475. Boca Raton, FL: CRC Press.

George, R. M. 1987. The lateral craniographic method of facial reconstruction. *Journal of Forensic Sciences* 32: 1305–1330.

Gerasimov, M. 1955. *Vosstanovlenie lica po cerepu*. Moskva: Izdat. Akademii Nauk SSSR.

———. 1971. *The Face Finder*. London: Hutchinson & Co.

Glaister, J., and Brash, J. C. 1937. *Medico-Legal Aspects of the Ruxton Case*. Baltimore: William Wood and Co.

Goldberg, R. A., Belan, A., and Hoenig, J. 1999. Relationship of the eye to the bony orbit, with clinical correlations. *Australian and New Zealand Journal of Ophthalmology* 27: 398–403.

Gonzalez, R., Ellsworth, P. C., and Pembroke, M. 1993. Response biases in lineups and showups. *Journal of Personality and Social Psychology* 64: 525–537.

Haglund, W. D. 1998. Forensic "art" in human identification, in J. G. Clement and D. L. Ranson (eds.), *Craniofacial Identification in Forensic Medicine*, pp. 235–243. London: Arnold.

Haglund, W. D., and Reay, D. T. 1991. Use of facial approximation techniques in identification of Green River serial murder victims. *The American Journal of Forensic Medicine and Pathology* 12: 132–142.

Helmer, R. 1984. *Schädelidentifizierung durch elektronische Bildmischung: Zugleich ein Beitrag zur Konstitutionsbiometrie und Dickenmessung der Gesichtsweichteile*. Heidelberg: Kriminalistik-Verlag.

Helmer, R. P., and Grüner, O. 1977. Schädelidentifizierung nach dem Superprojektionsverfahren mit Hilfe einer Videoanlage. *Zeitschrift für Rechtsmedizin* 80: 183–187.

Helmer, R. P., Rohricht, S., Petersen, D., and Mohr, F. 1993. Assessment of the reliability of facial reconstruction, in M. Y. İşcan and R. P. Helmer (eds.), *Forensic Analysis of the Skull*: 229–246. New York: Wiley-Liss.

His, W. 1895. Anatomische Forschungen über Johann Sebastian Bach's Gebeine und Antlitz nebst Bemerkungen über dessen Bilder. *Abhandlungen der mathematisch-physikalischen Klasse der Königlichen Sächsischen Gesellschaft der Wissenschaften* 22: 379–420.

Hoffman, B. E., McConathy, D. A., Coward, M., and Saddler, L. 1991. Relationship between the piriform aperture and interalar nasal widths in adult males. *Journal of Forensic Sciences* 36: 1152–1161.

Iten, P. X. 1987. Identification of skulls by video superimposition. *Journal of Forensic Sciences* 32: 173–188.

Koelmeyer, T. D. 1982. Videocamera superimposition and facial reconstruction as an aid to identification. *The American Journal of Forensic Medicine and Pathology* 3: 45–48.

Kollmann, J., and Büchly, W. 1898. Die Persistenz der Rassen und die Reconstruction der Physiognomie prähistorischer Schädel. *Archives fur Anthropologie* 25: 329–359.

Krogman, W. M. 1962. *The Human Skeleton in Forensic Medicine*. Springfield, IL: Charles C. Thomas.

Krogman, W. M., and İşcan, M. Y. 1986. *The Human Skeleton in Forensic Medicine*. Springfield, IL: Charles C. Thomas.

Lan, Y. 1992. Development and current status of skull-image superimposition: Methodology and instrumentation. *Forensic Science Review* 4: 126–136.

Maat, G. J. R. 1998–1999. Facial reconstruction: A review and comment. *TALANTA* 30–31: 247–253.

Malpass, R. S., and Devine, P. G. 1983. Measuring the fairness of eyewitness identification lineups, in S. M. A. Lloyd-Bostock and B. R. Clifford (eds.), *Evaluating Witness Evidence: Recent Psychological Research and New Perspectives*, pp. 81–102. New York: John Wiley and Sons.

Manhein, M. H., Listi, G. A., Barsley, R. E., Musselman, R., Barrow, N. E., and Ubelaker, D. H. 2000. In vivo facial tissue depth measurements for children and adults. *Journal of Forensic Sciences* 45: 48–60.

Martin, R. 1957. *Lehrbuch der Anthropologie*. Stuttgart: Gustav Fischer Verlag.

McKenna, J. J. I., Jablonski, N. G., and Fearnhead, R. W. 1984. A method of matching skulls with photographic portraits using landmarks and measurements of the dentition. *Journal of Forensic Sciences* 29: 787–797.

Migliori, M. E., and Gladstone, G. J. 1984. Determination of the normal range of exophthalmometric values for black and white adults. *American Journal of Ophthalmology* 988: 438–442.

Miyasaka, S. 1999. Progress in facial reconstruction technology. *Forensic Science Review* 11: 50–90.

Montagu, M. F. A. 1947. A study of man embracing error. *Technology Review* 49: 345–347.

Nelson, L. A., and Michael, S. D. 1998. The application of volume deformation to three-dimensional facial reconstruction: A comparison with previous techniques. *Forensic Science International* 94: 167–181.

Oestreicher, J. H., and Hurwitz, J. J. 1990. The position of the eyebrow. *Ophthalmic Surgery* 21: 245–249.

Ogawa, H. 1960. Anatomical study on the Japanese head by X-ray cephalometry. *The Journal of the Tokyo Dental College Society [Shika Gakuho]* 60: 17–34.

Phillips, V. M., and Smuts, N. A. 1996. Facial reconstruction: Utilization of computerized tomography to measure facial tissue thickness in a mixed racial population. *Forensic Science International* 83: 51–59.

Prag, J., and Neave, R. 1997. *Making Faces: Using Forensic and Archaeological Evidence*. London: British Museum Press.

Quatrehomme, G., Cotin, S., Subsol, G., Delingette, H., Garidel, Y., Grevin, G., Fidrich, M., Bailet, P., and Ollier, A. 1997. A fully three-dimensional method for facial reconstruction based on deformable models. *Journal of Forensic Sciences* 42: 649–652.

Reichs, K. J. and Craig, E. 1998. Facial approximation: Procedures and pitfalls, in K. J. Reichs (ed.), *Forensic Osteology: Advances in the Identification of Human Remains*, pp. 491–513. Springfield, IL: Charles C. Thomas.

Rhine, J. S. 1990. Coming to terms with facial reproduction. *Journal of Forensic Sciences* 35: 960–963.

Rhine, J. S., and Campbell, H. R. 1980. Thickness of facial tissues in American blacks. *Journal of Forensic Sciences* 25: 847–858.

Rozprym, F. 1934. Eyebrows and eyelashes in man: Their different forms, pigmentation and heredity. *The Journal of the Royal Anthropological Institute* 64: 353–395.

Ryan, C., and Wilkinson, C. M. 2006. Appraisal of traditional and recently proposed relationships between the hard and soft dimensions of the nose in profile. *American Journal of Physical Anthropology* 130: 364–373.

Sahni, D., Jit, I., Gupta, M., Singh, P., and Suri, S. 2002. Preliminary study on facial soft tissue thickness by magnetic resonance imaging in Northwest Indians. *Forensic Science Communications* 4, www.fbi. gov/hq/lab/fsc/backissu/jan2002/sahni.htm.

Simpson, E., and Henneberg, M. 2002. Variation in soft-tissue thicknesses on the human face and their relation to craniometric dimensions. *American Journal of Physical Anthropology* 118: 121–133.

Skiles, M. S., and Randall, P. 1983. The aesthetics of ear placement: An experimental study. *Plastic and Reconstructive Surgery* 72: 133–140.

Smith, S. L., and Buschang, P. H. 2001. Midsagittal facial tissue thickness of children and adolescents from the Montreal growth study. *Journal of Forensic Sciences* 46: 1294–1302.

Smith, S. L., and Throckmorton, G. S. 2006. Comparability of radiographic and 3D-ultrasound measurements of facial midline tissue depths. *Journal of Forensic Sciences* 51: 244–247.

Snow, C. C. 1976. A video technique for skull-face superimposition. 28th Annual Meeting of the American Academy of Forensic Sciences, Washington, D.C.

Stadtmuller, F. 1922. Zur Beurteilung der plastischen Rekonstruktionsmethode der Physiognomie auf dem Schädel. *Zeitschrift für Morpholologie und Anthropologie* 22: 337–372.

Stephan, C. N. 2002a. Do resemblance ratings measure the accuracy of facial approximations? *Journal of Forensic Sciences* 47: 239–243.

———. 2002b. Facial approximation: Falsification of globe projection guideline by exophthalmometry literature. *Journal of Forensic Sciences* 47: 1–6.

———. 2002c. Position of superciliare in relation to the lateral iris: Testing a suggested facial approximation guideline. *Forensic Science International* 130: 29–33.

———. 2003a. Facial approximation: An evaluation of mouth width determination. *American Journal of Physical Anthropology* 121: 48–57.

———. 2003b. Anthropological facial "reconstruction": Recognizing the fallacies, "unembracing" the error, and realizing method limits. *Science and Justice* 43: 193–199.

———. 2006. Beyond the sphere of the English facial approximation literature: Ramifications of German papers on Western method concepts. *Journal of Forensic Sciences* 51: 736–739.

Stephan, C. N., and Arthur, R. S. 2006. Assessing facial approximation accuracy: How do resemblance ratings of disparate faces compare to recognition tests? *Forensic Science International* 159S: S159–S163.

Stephan, C. N., and Henneberg, M. 2001. Building faces from dry skulls: Are they recognized above chance rates? *Journal of Forensic Sciences* 46: 432–440.

———. 2003. Predicting mouth width from intercanine width: A 75% rule. *Journal of Forensic Sciences* 48: 725–727.

———. 2006. Recognition by facial approximation: Case-specific examples and empirical tests. *Forensic Science International* 156: 182–191.

Stephan, C. N., Henneberg, M., and Sampson, W. 2003. Predicting nose projection and pronasale position in facial approximation: A test of published methods and proposal of new guidelines. *American Journal of Physical Anthropology* 122: 240–250.

Stephan, C. N., Norris, R. M., and Henneberg, M. 2005. Does sexual dimorphism in facial soft tissue depths justify sex distinction in craniofacial identification? *Journal of Forensic Sciences* 50: 513–518.

Stephan, C. N., Penton-Voak, I. S., Clement, J.G., and Henneberg, M. 2005. Ceiling recognition limits of two-dimensional facial approximations constructed using averages, in J. G. Clement and M. Marks (eds.), *Computer Graphic Facial Reconstruction*, pp. 199–219. Boston: Academic Press.

Stephan, C. N. and Simpson, E. K. 2008. Facial soft-tissue depths in craniofacial identification (part I): An analytical review of the published adult data, *Journal of Forensic Sciences* 53: 1264.

Stewart, T. D. 1979. *Essentials of Forensic Anthropology: Especially as Developed in the United States*. Springfield, IL: Charles C. Thomas.

———. 1983. The points of attachment of the palpebral ligaments: Their use in facial reconstructions on the skull. *Journal of Forensic Sciences* 28: 858–863.

Suk, V. 1935. Fallacies of anthropological identifications. *Publications de la Facultae des sciences de l'Universitae Masaryk* 207: 3–18.

Sutton, P. R. N. 1969. Bizygomatic diameter: The thickness of the soft tissues over the zygions. *American Journal of Physical Anthropology* 30: 303–310.

Suzuki, H. 1948. On the thickness of the soft parts of the Japanese face. *Journal of the Anthropology Society Nippon* 60: 7–11.

Suzuki, T. 1973. Reconstitution of a skull. *International Criminal Police Review* 264: 76–80.

Swan, L. K., and Stephan, C. N. 2005. Estimating eyeball protrusion from body height, interpupillary distance, and inter-orbital distance in adults. *Journal of Forensic Sciences* 50: 1–3.

Taylor, J. A., and Brown, K. A. 1998. Superimposition techniques, in J. G. Clement and D. L. Ranson (eds.), *Craniofacial Identification in Forensic Medicine:*, pp. 151–164. London: Arnold.

Taylor, K. T. 2001. *Forensic Art and Illustration*. Boca Raton, FL: CRC Press.

Taylor, R. G., and Angel, C. 1998. Facial reconstruction and approximation, in J. G. Clement and D. L. Ranson (eds.), *Craniofacial Identification in Forensic Medicine*, pp. 177–185. London: Arnold.

Tu, P., Hartley, R. I., Lorensen, W. E., Alyassin, A., Gupta, R., and Heier, L. 2005. Face reconstructions using flesh deformation modes, in J. G. Clement and M. K. Marks (eds.), *Computer-graphic Facial Reconstruction*, pp. 145–162. Boston: Elsevier Academic Press.

Turner, W. D., Brown, R. E. B., Kelliher, T. P., Tu, P. H., Taister, M. A., and Miller, W. P. 2005. A novel method of automated skull registration for forensic facial approximation. *Forensic Science International* 154: 149–158.

Ubelaker, D. H. 2002. Cranial photographic superimposition, in C. H. Wecht (ed.), *Forensic Sciences:*, pp. 3–38. New York: Matthew Bender, Inc.

Ullrich, H. 1958. Die methodischen Grundlagen des plastischen Rekonstruktionsverfahrens nach Gerasimov. *Zeitschrift für Morphologie und Anthropologie* 49: 245–258.

———. 1966. Kritische Bemerkungen zur plastischen Rekonstruktionsmethode nach Gerasimov auf Grund personlicher Erfahrugen. *Ethnographisch-archäologische Zeitschrift* 7: 111–123.

van Rensburg, J. 1993. Accuracy of recognition of 3-dimensional plastic reconstruction of faces from skulls, *Anatomical Society of Southern Africa*, p. 20. Krugersdorp: Game Reserve.

Vanezis, P., Vanezis, M., McCombe, G., and Niblett, T. 2000. Facial reconstruction using 3-D computer graphics. *Forensic Science International* 108: 81–95.

von Eggeling, H. 1909. Anatomische Untersuchungen an den Köpfen von vier Hereros, einem Herero und einem Hottentottenkind, in L. Schultze (ed.), *Zoologische und anthropologische Ergebnisse einer Forschungsreise im westlichen und zentralen Südafrika in den Jahren 1903–1905*, pp. 322–348. Jena: Gustav Fischer.

———. 1913. Die Leistungsfähigkeit physiognomischer Rekonstruktionsversuche auf Grundlage des Schädels. *Archiv für Anthropologie* 12: 44–47.

Webster, W. P., Murray, W. K., Brinkhous, W., and Hudson, P. 1986. Identification of human remains using photographic reconstruction, in K. J. Reichs (ed.), *Forensic Osteology: Advances in the Identification of Human Remains*, pp. 256–276. Springfield, IL: Charles C. Thomas.

Welcker, H. 1883. *Schiller's Schädel und Todtenmaske, nebst Mittheilungen über Schädel und Todtenmaske Kant's*. Braunschweig: Viehweg F. and Son.

Welcker, H. 1888. Zur Kritik des Schillerschädels. *Archives für Anthropologie* 17: 19–60.

Wells, G. L. 1993. What do we know about eyewitness identification? *American Psychologist* 48: 553–571.

Whitnall, S. E. 1911. On a tubercle on the malar bone, and on the lateral attachments of the tarsal plates. *Journal of Anatomy and Physiology, London* 45: 426–432.

Wilder, H. H., and Wenworth, B. 1918. *Personal Identification: Methods for the Identification of Individuals, Living or Dead*. Boston: Gorham Press.

Wilkinson, C. 2004. *Forensic Facial Reconstruction*. Cambridge: Cambridge University Press.

Wilkinson, C. M. 2002. In vivo facial tissue depth measurements for White British children. *Journal of Forensic Sciences* 47: 459–465.

Wilkinson, C. M., and Mautner, S. A. 2003. Measurement of eyeball protrusion and its application in facial reconstruction [Technical Note]. *Journal of Forensic Sciences* 48: 12–16.

Wilkinson, C. M., Motwani, M., and Chiang, E. 2003. The relationship between the soft tissues and the skeletal detail of the mouth. *Journal of Forensic Sciences* 48: 728–732.

Wilkinson, C. M., and Whittaker, D. K. 2002. Juvenile forensic facial reconstruction: A detailed accuracy study. Proceedings of the 10th Biennial Scientific Meeting of the International Association for Craniofacial Identification, Bari.

Williamson, M. A., Nawrocki, S. P., and Rathbun, T. A. 2002. Variation in midfacial tissue thickness of African-American children. *Journal of Forensic Sciences* 47: 25–31.

26

BIOMOLECULAR APPLICATIONS

Lori Baker

Molecular analysis is now a routine part of forensic investigations. Bones, teeth, blood and semen stains, debris from fingernails, muscle tissue, cigarette butts, fingerprints, dandruff, and hair are some of the potential sources of material for DNA analyses that could be encountered by forensic anthropologists and archaeologists. Although morphological skeletal analysis is essential for providing such information as the sex, age at death, and stature of the decedent, DNA analysis can discriminate individuals that share the same morphological characteristics.

There are two human genomes found in almost all cells in the human body: the nuclear genome found in the nucleus of the cell and mitochondrial genome, which is found in the mitochondrion located in the cytoplasm of the cell (Figure 26.1). Nuclear DNA is arranged along the 46 chromosomes, 23 contributed by each parent. Mitochondrial DNA is contained in a small circular genome and is contributed only by the mother. Both nuclear and mitochondrial DNA are examined from skeletal remains for forensic identification purposes, and both are discussed in this chapter. A comprehensive review of forensic DNA is provided by Butler (2005).

This chapter provides information regarding collection, preservation, and analysis of genetic samples as well as the types of questions that genetic analysis can answer in a forensic context. The importance of standardizing molecular techniques and nomenclature is discussed with specific reference to advisory boards. The focus is on DNA analysis from human skeletal remains; therefore, many of the same techniques described are applicable to ancient DNA studies.

Collection and Preservation

When anthropologists and archaeologists are called on to analyze skeletal remains, the process may include the selection and removal of a portion of bone and/or tooth samples for genetic testing. It is important to reiterate the importance of molecular-based identification procedures in both the forensic and archaeological context: principles, protocols, and procedures for selection, cutting, and packaging of skeletal remains are similar when one is pursuing either forensic or ancient DNA analysis. The most notable difference is the imperative chain of custody requirements for forensic specimens.

The prevalence of genetic testing in forensic and archeological environments dictates the assumption that molecular analysis will be performed on specimens of interest. Consequently, proper precautions should be employed at all times to prevent contamination of skeletal remains. To

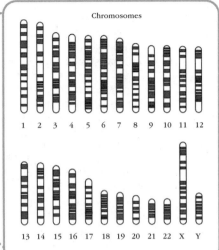

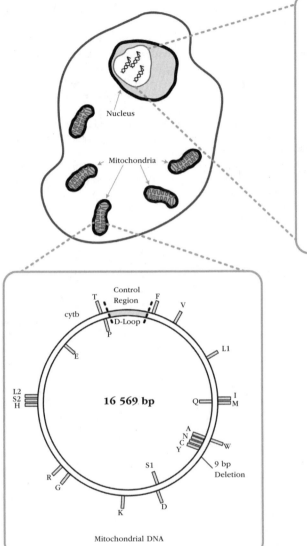

Figure 26.1 Diagram of a cell showing details of nuclear chromosomal DNA and the mitochondrial circular genome.

prevent the transfer of the examiner's DNA to the skeleton, the examiner should always wear gloves when excavating, collecting and analyzing skeletal remains. Molecular techniques have advanced enough that DNA from a single fingerprint or a flake of skin can severely compromise genetic testing during the process of molecular amplification (Lowe et al. 2002; van Oorschot and Jones 1997). This type of contamination can potentially lead to a mixture of DNA types in the analysis or the overwhelming of the sample DNA by the contaminate DNA resulting in an incorrect genetic profile. Proper sample preparation may limit the significance of surface contamination but does not guarantee its elimination altogether.

In addition to being vigilant about contamination, anthropologists and archaeologists must make critical decisions about which bones have the greatest potential to yield DNA and how large of a portion of bone must be collected. It is well recognized that cortical bone is a much better reservoir of DNA than is trabecular bone, and weight-bearing long bones, such as the femur and the tibia, provide the largest amount of cortical bone.

Alternatively, the petrous portion of the temporal bone is also a very hard, dense part of the skeleton and is typically a good bone for genetic testing.

A recent study illustrates the substantial impact of bone type on success rate. Andelinovic and associates (2005) report that over the 12 years of testing from the mass graves in Croatia, Bosnia, and Herzegovina, 92% of femora and 90% of teeth tested gave full genotypes. No genotypes were obtained from ribs, mandibles, or calcanei.

Just as the decomposition process of biological tissue begins immediately upon death, DNA immediately begins a process of degradation. Internal forces within cells begin the breakdown process. In addition, just as the environment plays a role in the rate of flesh decomposition, the environment also plays a significant role in the rate of DNA degradation. It has been shown that environmental conditions have more influence on DNA preservation than does time (Colson et al. 1997; Hoss et al. 1996; Poinar et al. 1996). DNA is best preserved under neutral or slightly alkaline conditions, in dry low temperatures, and in the absence of microorganisms (Burger et al. 1999; Iwamura, Soares-Vieira, and Muñoz 2004). Counterintuitively, several studies have shown that the general appearance of the bone is not a good indicator of successful analysis (Baker 2002; Burger et al. 1999; Faerman et al. 1995).

Taking a Sample

When possible, send a whole bone to the genetics laboratory, ensuring that bone samples can be taken in a controlled environment with contamination precautions. However, some simple precautions can facilitate clean field-site sampling. Gloves should be changed between each sample and should never touch unbleached surfaces. It is important to remember that touching one's face to wipe away perspiration or to scratch an itch will transfer DNA to the glove and potentially to the bone or tooth. Equipment, such as bone saws and blades, should be made free of extraneous DNA by being cleaned with bleach before and between each sample to avoid cross-contamination. Ideally, the surface of the bone should be washed with bleach, sanded, and then washed again before the bone is cut.

Bones should not be cut until all osteological measurements and analyses are completed. Care should be taken not to remove a portion of bone that will destroy areas crucial for osteological analysis. Sites that have antemortem or perimortem trauma or pathology formation must also be avoided. A typical sample size should be at least 5 grams, but consultation with the laboratory performing the DNA analysis is warranted, since protocols vary.

Teeth can be easier than bone to sample and are usually a good source of DNA, because the enamel covering protects the integrity of teeth. It is best to select teeth with closed, unbroken roots. Teeth should be intact without any caries or amalgamations. Molars and premolars are preferred, but all tooth types can provide suitable DNA. It is advisable to take at least two teeth for testing. Remains should be dried before they are packaged and placed into paper instead of plastic to inhibit the colonization of bacteria and fungi that may hinder DNA analysis.

DNA Extraction

The proper extraction of DNA from the biological matrix is critical to maximize a robust sample of DNA while excluding cellular materials known to inhibit downstream enzymatic reactions. Although there are many different laboratory-specific protocols and variations on extraction methodologies, standard procedures rely on one of three main methods of bone and tooth DNA isolation: (1) organic extraction, (2) Chelex, and (3) solid-phase methodologies.

Organic extraction is the original method used in forensic and ancient DNA analysis from bone and teeth and most effectively extracts high molecular weight DNA (Hagelberg and Clegg 1991; Stone and Stoneking 1993). In this procedure, sodium dodecylsufate (SDS) and proteinase K are incubated for several hours with ground bone or tooth powder to release DNA from the cell and to break down proteins. A phenol/chloroform solution is then added to separate the proteins from the DNA, followed by a series of alcohol precipitations to remove inhibitors. Some protocols have replaced the alcohol precipitations with a Centricon filter (Millipore, Billerica, MA) for a process called diafiltration (Comey et al. 1994). The drawback of the organic extraction method is that it involves the use of hazardous chemicals, requiring care to protect the user. In addition, small DNA fragments are not always extracted as efficiently with this method.

Chelex is a rapid DNA extraction procedure (Sivolap et al. 2001) that can be used for the extraction of DNA from bone; however, it does not eliminate organic inhibitors with the efficiency of phenol-chloroform extractions (Hoff-Olsen et al. 1999). The chelating-resin suspension Chelex 100® (Bio-Rad Laboratories, Hercules, CA) is an ion-exchange resin that is added as a suspension to the ground bone or tooth sample and boiled (Faerman et al. 1995; Walsh, Metzger, and Higuchi 1991). The sample is then washed and centrifuged to separate the Chelex resin and cellular debris from the DNA. The supernatant can be removed and used for polymerase chain reaction (PCR) amplifications.

Solid-phase methodologies, such as silica-based extractions, have also been employed. Silica extraction procedures have been proven effective for yielding DNA from ancient and degraded bone and tooth samples and purifying the DNA from inhibitors that are typically co-extracted (Baker, McCormick, and Matteson 2001; Götherström et al. 1986; Hoss and Pääbo 1993; Stone and Stoneking 1998). DNA is bound to silica particles in the presence of high concentrations of chaotropic salts (Boom et al. 1990). Because the DNA is bound to silica, the small fragments of degraded DNA are not lost during subsequent alcohol washes. This method is exceptionally sensitive and therefore extreme care must be taken to avoid contamination by extraneous DNA. There are several commercially available kits that have been developed that use silica-based DNA binding. QIAquick by QIAGEN, Inc. (Valencia, CA) and the DNA IQ System from Promega Corporation have both been effectively applied to bone DNA extraction (Yang et al. 1998; Ye et al. 2004).

Regardless of the extraction protocol used, proper cleaning techniques must be employed at all times. For example, only one sample should be cleaned and prepared for extraction at a time. Prepare for extraction by removing all traces of soft tissue and soil remnants using a sterile brush and detergent. The bone should be washed with bleach or soaked, sanded, washed again with bleach, and then rinsed with deionized water to remove traces of the bleach. The bone should be air dried in a sterile laminar flow hood in a DNA extraction clean room and then exposed to UV light irradiation on each side. Tooth samples should be soaked in bleach for 10 minutes, and a sterile brush should be used to remove any extraneous material. The tooth should be rinsed with deionized water, dried, and exposed to UV light on both sides to cross link any external contamination that may remain.

Modes of Analysis

Polymerase Chain Reaction (PCR)

Typing of bone DNA was extremely difficult prior to the invention of polymerase chain reaction (PCR), conceived by Kary Mullis in 1983. PCR makes copies of targeted regions of DNA at an exponential rate, ensuring that even a single copy of starting template can be examined. Prior to PCR, large amounts of DNA had to be extracted in order to be typed, or the DNA had to be cloned through painstaking processes. This restricted DNA analysis of bone in forensic investigations and relegated ancient DNA analysis to a novelty rather than a viable field of research. In addition, PCR analysis has been enhanced owing to the large number of commercially available high-fidelity polymerases and master mixes. The majority of forensic DNA testing now utilizes PCR technology.

Owing to the sensitivity of PCR, extreme caution must be taken to avoid contamination. Separate areas and equipment should be designated for pre- and post-amplified DNA. In addition, all lab personnel should have their DNA on file to facilitate the detection of contamination during laboratory processing. It is also advisable to analyze the DNA from anthropologists and archaeologist involved with excavating, collecting, and examining skeletal samples that are submitted to the laboratory for DNA testing.

The core PCR protocols are relatively straightforward. The components of the PCR reaction (target DNA, polyamerase, primers, dNTPs, buffer, MgCl2, and optional additives) are mixed and the reaction placed in a thermal cycler, an automated instrument that takes the reaction through a series of different temperatures for varying amounts of time. This series of temperature and time adjustments is referred to as one cycle of amplification. Each PCR cycle theoretically doubles the amount of targeted template sequence in the reaction production.

A PCR cycle consists of three important steps:

1. The template (original) DNA is first denatured or broken apart. The double stranded helix is separated into single strands. This is done by heating the DNA to 94°C.

2. The temperature is then reduced in order to allow the primer (synthesized piece of DNA) to bind to the single stranded original DNA.

3. Then the temperature is raised to allow the added bases to complete the remainder of the strand initiated by the primer.

Short Tandem Repeat (STR)

The most commonly used forensic DNA typing utilizes a core set of Short Tandem Repeat (STR) loci. STRs, or microsatellites, are DNA regions with repeated units 2–6 base pairs (bp) in length. The number of repeats for these highly polymorphic loci varies among individuals making them very effective for human identification purposes. Autosomal STRs are inherited biparentally and therefore are similar to each parent only by 50% and to each full sibling by 25%. As the number of STRs analyzed increases, the chance of two individuals having the same DNA profile is decreased. It has been determined statistically that a DNA profile of 13 loci gives a unique profile (Chakraborty et al. 1999). Lastly, STR alleles are small and therefore require only small target areas (~100–400bp) to be amplified. This makes STR markers useful in forensic applications where degraded DNA is common and potentially useful for the analysis of skeletal samples.

STR loci used in human identification are selected using the following criteria (Butler 2005; Carracedo and Lareu 1998; Gill et al. 1996): STR loci in human identification applications have a high discrimination power (>0.9, with observed heterozygosity >70%), are located on separate chromosomes, are robust when multiplexed with other markers, and have predicted allele lengths that fall into the range of 100–500 bp and therefore are suited for degraded DNA analysis. In fact, several ancient DNA studies have successfully used STR markers (Gill et al. 1994; Hummel et al. 1999; Ricaut et al. 2005; Zierdt, Hummel, and Herrmann 1996).

Standardization of STR loci used in forensic typing is important, because information is shared domestically between laboratories at the state and federal level as well as by the international community. A common nomenclature has been developed in the forensic DNA community to aid in comparisons of data and for database applications (Bar et al. 1994, 1997). The DNA Commission of the International Society of Forensic Haemogenetics (ISFH), now the International Society of Forensic Genetics (ISFG), issued guidelines for designating STR alleles in 1994 (Bar et al. 1994) and again in 1997 (Bar et al. 1997). The FBI Laboratory's Combined DNA Index System (CODIS) selected 13 genetic markers in 1997 that are used in the U.S. These 13 CODIS loci are CSF1PO, FGA, TH01, TPOX, VWA, D3S1358, D5S818, D7S820, S8S1179, D13S317, D16S539, D18S51, and D21S11 (Budowle et al. 1998; Butler et al. 2006). The International Crime Police Organization (Interpol) currently includes seven STR loci (THO1, VWA, FGA, D21S11, D35S1358, D8S1179, D18S51) used in all European laboratories (Martin et al. 2001; Schneider et al. 2001).

Commercially available kits have helped with standardization and quality control by providing high-quality products that contain core sets of loci. The largest commercially available STR multiplexes contain 15 STR loci and amelogenin. Applied Biosystems produces the Identifiler kit, which amplifies the 13 CODIS loci, amelogenin, and two tetranucleotide loci. Promega Corporation produces the PowerPlex 16 kit, which amplifies the 13 CODIS loci, amelogenin, and two pentanucleotide loci. The amount of time and effort needed to develop, validate, and reproduce multiplexes of this sort are beyond the ability of most laboratories, making commercially available multiplex kits essential to forensic DNA analysis. These commercial kits have become so important in forensic DNA analysis that in many ways they influence which loci will be used by the majority of laboratories.

There can be problems with the analysis of STRs. Bones that are exposed to high amounts of microbial organisms can be difficult or impossible to analyze (Calacal and De Ungria 2005). In addition, DNA used for STR typing must be quantified prior to amplification, because too little or too much DNA in an STR reaction will give poor or erroneous results (Andelinovic et al. 2005). Allele dropout or allele drop-in is increased when STR analysis of extremely low levels of DNA is attempted. The use of reduced-sized PCR products or miniSTRs has been examined to decrease this problem (Butler et al. 2003; Chung et al. 2004; Coble and Butler 2005; Opel et al. 2006; Parsons et al. 2007).

Mini-STRs

Although STR analysis works well on small quantities of DNA, there is still difficulty in the analysis of degraded samples. In particular, there are problems with alleles dropping out of the larger STRs. Hummel and colleagues (1999) demonstrated that the yield of products decreases with increasing product size. Large STR products fail to amplify with low quantities of degraded DNA. Analysis of forensic DNA typically includes a large number of samples that are degraded in nature, requiring the optimization of typing systems to maximize the amount of information that can be gathered from every sample.

There are several laboratories that have shown the utility of shorter STR amplicons for greater success in the amplification of forensic specimens containing low amounts of degraded DNA (Chung et al. 2004; Coble and Butler 2005). Research in ancient and forensic DNA has shown that DNA fragments as a function of time and environmental insults. By targeting smaller sections of DNA for amplification, one can increase the success rate of analysis.

Targeted STR loci have been reconfigured in multiple studies utilizing mini-STRs with increased success of degraded samples. Normal STRs range in size from 100–400 bp; mini-STR amplicon sets are smaller and range from 20–200 bp. Recently, the European Network of Forensic Science Institutes (ENFSI) and the European DNA Profiling Group (EDNAP) recommended the transition of existing STR multiplexes to mini-STR multiplexes and the addition of three new mini-STR loci (D10S1248, D14S1434, and D22S1045) (Gill et al. 2006).

The European Network of Forensic Science Institutes' (ENFSI) and the European DNA Profiling group's (EDNAP) recent recommendations were to add three new mini-STR loci, with alleles less than 130 bp (d10s1248, d14s1434, d22s1045), to the seven currently utilized in the International Criminal Police Organization (Interpol). They also recommended that the existing multiplexes be re-engineered to improve the success rate of analyzing degraded DNA. The enactment of these recommendations may be difficult for several reasons. Existing commercially available multiplex kits must be re-engineered to include any new loci, and each laboratory must undergo costly validation studies for these new loci. Additionally, databases have to be altered to incorporate the changes as well as maintain the ability to match future samples with previously analyzed DNA.

Analysis of DNA from skeletal remains utilizing mini-STR multiplexes will potentially help to produce more full profiles from difficult cases in the future. However, the reduced size of the amplicons has reduced the number of loci that can be analyzed per reaction. Multiplexes of mini-STRs will be able to contain only several loci at a time.

Mitochondrial DNA

The human mitochondrial genome is a maternally inherited small circular genome consisting of approximately 16,569 base pairs (Case and Wallace 1981; Giles et al. 1980; Hutchinson 1974) (see Figure 25.1). Hundreds to thousands of copies of the genome can be found per cell, making mitochondrial DNA (mtDNA) a very useful tool for genetic analysis of small amounts of degraded DNA such as that from skeletal remains.

The mitochondrial genome is divided into coding and noncoding regions. The mtDNA noncoding control region of the genome mutates 5–10 times faster than nuclear DNA and contains three hypervariable sections as well as two variable regions. The high rates of genetic polymorphisms in these areas decrease the likelihood that maternally unrelated individuals will share

the same sequence variation (Excoffier and Yang 1999; Greenberg, Newbold, and Sugino 1983, Meyer, Weiss, and von Haesler 1999; Stoneking 2000; Wakeley 1993). According to Budowle (2003), there is an average of eight nucleotide differences between any two Caucasian individuals and 15 differences between any two individuals of African descent. In addition to the coding region's utility in forensic examinations, this nucleotide segment has been targeted for population genetic studies. Its high mutation rate may provide insight into short- and long-term evolutionary events, as well as ancestry and population migrations (Krings et al. 1997; Relethford 2002).

Genetic analysis typically involves the sequencing of two of the hypervariable segments located in the control region; these two segments contain most of the genome variation between individuals. Hypervariable region 1 (HVI) spans nucleotide (nt) 16,024 to nt16,365 (342 bp in length) and hypervariable region II (HVII) spans nt73 to nt340 (268 bp in length). Ideally, each region can be amplified in one or two separate reactions and sequenced. Unfortunately, DNA degrades to fragments of 100–200 bp in length (Pääbo 1989; Pääbo, Gifford, and Wilson 1988), making the amplification of larger full-length fragments difficult or impossible. As a result of the typically degraded DNA obtained from forensic bone and tooth samples, laboratories are forced to amplify very small overlapping regions (~80bp) within the target sequence and reconstruct consensus sequences for HVI and HVII.

Sample sequence variation is determined by comparison with the published Cambridge Reference Sequence (CRS) (Anderson et al. 1981), which was slightly modified in 1999 (Andrews et al. 1999). The CRS assigns each nucleotide a specific number, and only the sites that differ from the CRS are reported by using the nucleotide number and the base that represents the change. For example, if position 16111 has a T instead of the C described in the CRS, it would be reported as 16111T. Any site not reported is assumed to have the same nucleotide base as the CRS.

MtDNA is inherited only from the mother and does not recombine. Therefore, direct comparison can be made between unidentified remains and any maternal relative, such as a mother, sibling, aunt, uncle, cousin, or grandmother, because they should have identical nucleotide sequences. The maternal mode of inheritance can be advantageous in cases involving missing persons, when often only extended relatives are available for comparison. Alternatively, a negative consequence of maternal inheritance of mtDNA is that many related family members share a common sequence, providing a circumstantial identification and not a positive identification. Although not as powerful as nuclear STR analysis, given the proper context, mtDNA provides a method for putative identification in many challenging cases.

There are several other limitations that should be noted with regard to mtDNA analysis. Most individuals are homoplasmic, having one detectable nucleotide at a given sequence position; however, heteroplasmy, indicated by two detectable nucleotides at a given sequence position, occurs on occasion and at different rates for different tissues (Bendall, Macaulay, and Sykes 1997; Carracedo et al. 2000; Comas, Pääbo, and Bertranpetit 1995; Gill et al. 1994; SWGDAM 2003; Wilson et al. 1997). In addition to heteroplasmy databases, reference population databases need to be maintained and increased for one to know the true frequency of sequence haplotypes (groups of samples with shared sequence variation). Paternal leakage and recombination have been claimed and disputed in the mitochondrial genome (Budowle et al. 2003). Lastly, inconsistent nomenclatures with regard to changes from the CRS and subjective interpretation of results have to be standardized among all those working in both forensic and anthropological genetics to ensure the most accurate assessments of population variation. Each of these issues should be monitored and evaluated in every laboratory; to ensure consistent results, general guidelines for mtDNA analysis have been addressed (Budowle et al. 1999, Carracedo et al. 2000, Holland and Parsons 1999, Tully 2001; SWGDAM 2003).

From a technical perspective, forensic mtDNA sequence analysis is a labor-intensive and time-consuming process. Sequence specific oligonucleotide probes (SSOP), as well as linear array analysis, have provided faster alternative methods to examine variation in the control region (Divine et al. 2005; Stoneking et al. 1991). Both systems target the most variable sites in the control region to screen for variants. This cuts down on the number of samples that have to be subsequently analyzed by sequencing. Linear array analysis is well suited for use in mass disasters and has been successfully utilized in the analysis of remains from mass graves (e.g., Gabriel et al. 2003).

Recently, single nucleotide polymorphisms (SNP) have been examined outside the control region and are found to further differentiate between individuals with similar mtDNA sequence haplotypes (Coble et al. 2004, 2006; Just et al. 2004; Kline et al. 2005; Niederstatter et al. 2006). The use of multiplex panels of SNPs to supplement control region sequencing has provided increased discrimination to mtDNA analysis.

Databases for missing persons often utilize mtDNA because of its unique characteristics. The FBI's National Missing Persons DNA Database in the United States currently holds DNA profiles on roughly 2,000 unidentified persons and family reference samples. In 2005, Mexico launched a new missing persons database that also has a DNA component named SIRLI, System for the Identification of Remains and Localization of Individuals (Baker 2006). The mtDNA analysis is performed at Baylor University and has focused on the identification of deceased, undocumented Mexico/U.S. border crossers. To date, the database has provided matches for over 25 skeletal cases from Arizona, California, and Texas. The Armed Forces DNA Identification Laboratory (AFDIL) is the most active lab for mtDNA analysis. AFDIL receives over 800 bone samples from unidentified bodies and between 1,500 and 2,000 family reference samples per year.

Y Chromosome

The Y chromosome has strictly paternal inheritance; therefore, paternal lineages can be traced through time like maternal lineages with mtDNA and are used frequently in anthropological studies. Unfortunately, it is present only in male individuals and, with only one copy per cell, is difficult to analyze in degraded samples. Y chromosome DNA can be useful in missing persons identifications but is much less variable than DNA found in the mitochondrial control region.

Increasingly, analysis of the Y chromosome is being utilized in forensic circumstances (de Knijff et al. 1997; Jobling, Pandya, and Tyler-Smith 1997; Kayser et al. 1997; Underhill et al. 2000). Although not useful for distinguishing between paternal relatives, it can be very useful in sexual assault cases where there is an overwhelming female component and a small male genetic component. The current recommendations of the Scientific Working Group on DNA Analysis Methods (SWGDAM) include 11 core Y loci for forensic analysis. These can be found in commercially available kits that also provide additional loci.

Sexing

Sexing skeletal remains is typically performed by forensic anthropologists or bioarchaeologists and can be a fairly straightforward task when a complete set of unfragmented adult remains is present (see Braz this volume). Unfortunately, postmortem taphonomic influences (see Chapter 22) can render remains difficult to sex, and the sexing of sub-adult remains is not currently possible with any reliability. Consequently, sexing through the use of genetic markers can provide information in certain circumstances that is impossible to obtain through other methods.

Human somatic cells contain two sets of each chromosome and therefore contain the sex chromosomes: an X and a Y chromosome in males and two X chromosomes in females. With the exception of extremely rare chromosomal abnormalities, the physical presence of a Y chromosome indicates male skeletal material. However, the failure of molecular techniques to detect Y-specific sequences is not sufficient evidence to classify samples as female. Errors in the PCR amplification process may provide alternative explanations for nondetection. For example, DNA may be too degraded for detection, or technical problems may inhibit the amplification process. As a result, it is imperative that genetic-based sex determination have an internal control.

The amelogenin gene is involved in the formation of tooth enamel and tooth development (Buel, Wang, and Schwartz 1995) and has copies on both the X and the Y chromosomes (Nakahori, Takenaka, and Nakagome 1991). The amelogenin gene on the X chromosome, however, contains a 6 base pair deletion of the first intron, creating a slightly smaller PCR product. Since the size differentiation is within the same PCR primer set, DNA from the X and the Y genes can be amplified simultaneously and distinguished from each other via a variety of methods, including gel and capillary electrophoresis. Because males and females carry at least one X chromosome, an error in amplification is indicated when the X copy is not detected. Genetic sexing using this methodology has been performed on numerous forensic and ancient skeletal remains (Mannucci et al. 1994; Matheson and Loy 2001; Palmirotta et al. 1997; Pascal et al. 1991; Santos, Pandya, and Tyler-Smith 1998; Stone et al. 1999). Typically, a small fragment is targeted for amplification (112 bp for the Y and 106 bp for the X because of the deletion), making amelogenin useful in the analysis of degraded DNA.

Several commercially available STR kits, such as AmpFLSTR® PCR amplification kits (Applied Biosysytems, Foster City, CA) and PowerPlex® System kits (Promega Corporation, Madison, WI) amplify as many as 15 STR loci as well as the amelogenin segment. Promega also offers the GenePrint® Sex Identification System in which amelogenin testing can be analyzed alone or added

to other reactions. Note that amplicons generated by these kits are 212 bp and 218 bp for the X and Y, respectively, rather than the more typical 106 bp and 112 bp. Amplification of these larger segments may not be possible from bone samples in which the DNA has degraded below the 200 bp threshold.

Although extremely useful, the amelogenin gene approach is not infallible (Michael and Brauner 2004). There have been reported cases in which the Y portion of the amelogenin gene used for sex identification has not amplified from known male samples owing to a deletion in the targeted area (Chang, Burgoyne, and Both 2003; Kashyap et al. 2006). The frequency of failure varies, depending on the population tested. Santos and associates (1998) reported a 0.6% frequency of failure from 350 specimens from around the world. Frequencies have been reported to be as high as 1.85% in Indian males (Chang, Burgoyne, and Both 2003; Thangaraj, Redyy, and Singh 2002) and as low as 0.018% in the Austrian National DNA database (Steinlechner et al. 2002). The addition of another Y locus can help to reduce mistyping of males in these situations. The sex-determining region Y (SRY) is important for testis formation and even most XX males who lack a Y chromosome still have a copy of SRY on their X chromosome. Therefore, the addition of this locus will confirm that the DNA is from a male individual (McKeown, Stickley, and Riordan 2000).

Advisory Boards

To ensure uniform quality between laboratories, one must standardize molecular techniques and nomenclature; there are several organizations around the world tasked with defining and reviewing standards and guidelines for forensic DNA analysis. The International Society of Forensic Genetics (ISFG) (www.isfg.org/) was founded in 1968 to promote scientific knowledge in the field of genetic markers analyzed for forensic purposes and now has members from over 50 countries. There are nine working groups recognized by the ISFG. These include the European DNA Profiling group (EDNAP), the DNA Commission, and seven language-specific working groups. EDNAP was established in 1988 by a group of European forensic scientists in order to ensure that each European country is represented, to facilitate the advancement of techniques and the exchange of data necessary when prosecuting cross-border crimes.

In the United States, the Scientific Working Group on DNA Analysis Methods (SWGDAM) meets twice a year to discuss possible alterations to the national DNA standards set forth by the DNA Advisory Board (DAB). The DAB was established by the Director of the Federal Bureau of Investigations (FBI) under the DNA Identification Act of 1994. It recommended standards for quality assurance guidelines for forensic analysts and laboratories performing DNA analysis. Consequently, these guidelines provide detailed information on how to arrange, organize, and establish standard operating procedures for laboratories performing forensic DNA analysis. The utilization of standard operating procedures, validation, accreditation, and quality assurance programs help to provide confidence in result reliability.

Conclusion

Forensic molecular analysis has become increasingly utilized as advances in technology have allowed for the DNA amplification from challenging sources such as bone, teeth, and hair samples. Forensic archaeologists are in many instances the first in the chain of protectors of genetic information and therefore are relied on to take necessary precautions to preserve a variety of potential data. Increasingly, archaeologists are working in genetic laboratories and learning first hand how current molecular applications may be employed in the context of the field of archaeology. With new advances in high-throughput genome sequencing technology, archaeologists and geneticists will continue to find a rich common ground for collaboration.

References

Alonso, A., Andelinovic, S., Martín, P., Sutlovic, D., Erceg, I., Huffine, E., Fernández de Simón, L., Albarrán, C., Definis-Gojanovic, M., Fernández-Rodriguez, A., García, P., Drmic, I., Rezic, B., Kuret, S., Sancho, M., and Primorac, D. 2001. DNA typing from skeletal remains: Evaluation of multiplex and megaplex STR systems on DNA isolated from bone and teeth samples. *Croatian Medical Journal* 42: 260–266.

Andelinovic, S., Sutlovic, D., Erceg Ivkosic, I., Skaro, V., Ivkosic, A., Paic, F., Rezic, B., Definis-Gojanovic, M., and Primorac, D. 2005. Twelve-year experience in identification of skeletal remains from mass graves. *Croatian Medical Journal* 46(4): 530–539.

Anderson, S., Bankier, A. T., Barrell, B. G., de Bruijn, M. H., Coulson, A. R., Drouin, J., Eperon, I. C., Nierlich, D. P., Roe, B. A., Sanger, F., Schreier, P., Smith, A., Staden, R., and Young, I. 1981. Sequence and organization of the human mitochondrial genome. *Nature* 290: 457–465.

Andrews, R. M., Kubacka, I., Chinnery, P. F., Lightowlers, R. N., Turnbull, D. M., and Howell, N. 1999. Reanalysis and revision of the Cambridge reference sequence for human mitochondrial DNA. *Nature Genetics* 23(2): 147.

Baker, L. E. 2002. *DNA analysis of the Holmes-Vardeman-Stephenson Cemetery.* Report to the Kentucky Transportation Cabinet.

———. 2006. SIRLI (Sistema de Identificación de Restos y Localización de Individuos): A Review of the First Year of Mexico's Database for Missing Persons. *Proceedings of the Journal of Forensic Sciences* 13.

Baker, L. E., McCormick, W. F., and Matteson, K. J. 2001. A silica-based mitochondrial DNA extraction method applied to forensic hair shafts and teeth. *Journal of Forensic Sciences* 46(1): 126–130.

Bar, W., Brinkmann, B., Budowle, B., Carracedo, A., Gill, B., Lincoln, P., Mayr, W., and Olaisen, B. 1997. DNA recommendations: Further report of the DNA Commission of the ISFH regarding the use of short tandem repeat systems. *International Journal of Legal Medicine* 110: 175–176.

Bar, W., Brinkmann, B., Lincoln, P., Mayr, W. R., and Rossi, U. 1994. DNA recommendations: 1994 report concerning further recommendations of the DNA commission of the ISFH PCR-based polymorphisms in STR (short tandem repeat) systems. *International Journal of Legal Medicine* 107: 159–160.

Bendall, K. E., Macaulay, W. A., and Sykes, B. C. 1997. Variable levels of heteroplasmic point mutation in individual hair roots. *American Journal of Human Genetics* 61: 1303–1308.

Boom, R., Sol, C., Salimans, M., Jansen, C., Wertheim-van Dillen, P., and van der Noordaa, J. 1990. Rapid and simple method for purification of nucleic acids. *Journal of Clinical Microbiology* 28: 495.

Budowle, B., Allard, M. W., Wilson, M. R., and Chakraborty, R. 2003. Forensics and mitochondrial DNA: Applications, debates, and foundations. *Annual Review of Genomics and Human Genetics* 4: 119–141.

Budowle, B., Moretti, T. R., Niezgoda, S. J., and Brown, B. L. 1998. CODIS and PCR-based short tandem repeat loci: Law enforcement tools. *Proceeding from the Second European Symposium on Human Identification*: 73–88.

Budowle, B., Wilson, M., DiZinno, J., Stauffer, C., Fasano, M., Holland, M., and Monson, K. 1999. Mitochondrial DNA regions HVI and HVII population data. *Forensic Science International* 103(1): 23–35.

Buel, E., Wang, G., and Schwartz, M. 1995. PCR amplification of animal DNA with human X-Y amelogenin primers used in gender determination. *Journal of Forensic Sciences* 40(4): 641–644.

Burger, J., Hummel, S., Herrmann, B., and Henke, W. 1999. DNA preservation: A microsatellite-DNA study on ancient skeletal remains. *Electrophoresis* 20: 1722–1728.

Butler, J. M. 2005. *Forensic DNA Typing: Biology, Technology and Genetics of STR Markers.* Amsterdam: Elsevier Academic Press.

———. 2006. Genetics and genomics of core short tandem repeat loci used in human identity testing. *Journal of Forensic Sciences* 51(2): 253–265.

Butler, J. M., Decker, A. E., Vallone, P. M., and Kline, M. C. 2006. Allele frequencies for 27 Y-STR loci with U.S. Caucasian, African American, and Hispanic samples. *Forensic Science International* 156: 250–260.

Butler, J. M., Shen, Y., and McCord, B. R. 2003. The development of reduced size STR amplicons as tools for analysis of degraded DNA. *Journal of Forensic Sciences* 48(5): 1054–1064.

Calacal, G. C., and De Ungria, M. C. A. 2005. Fungal DNA challenge in human STR typing of bone samples. *Journal of Forensic Sciences* 50(6): 1394–1401.

Case, J. T., and Wallace, D. C. 1981. Maternal inheritance of mitochondrial DNA polymorphisms in cultured human fibroblasts. *Somatic Cell Genetics* 7(1): 103–108.

Carracedo, A., Bar, W., Lincoln, P., Mayr, W., Morling, N., Olaisen, B., Schneider, P., Budowle, B., Brinkmann, B., Gill, P., Holland, M., Tully, G., and Wilson, M. 2000. DNA Commission of the International Society for Forensic Genetics: Guidelines for mitochondrial DNA typing. *Forensic Science International* 110: 79–85.

Carracedo, A., and Lareu, M. V. 1998. Development of new STRs for forensic casework: Criteria for selection, sequencing and population data and forensic validation. *Proceedings from the Ninth International Symposium on Human Identification*: 89–107.

Chakraborty, R., Stivers, D. N., Su, B., Zhong, Y., and Budowle, B. 1999. The utility of short tandem repeat loci beyond human identification: Implications for development of new DNA typing systems. *Electrophoresis* 20(8): 1682–1696.

Chang, Y. M., Burgoyne, L. A., and Both, K. 2003. Higher failures of the amelogenin sex test in an Indian population group. *Journal of Forensic Sciences* 48: 1309–1313.

Chung, D. T., Drabek, J., Opel, K., Butler, J., and McCord, B. 2004. A study on the effects of degradation and template concentration on the amplification efficiency of the STR miniplex primer sets. *Journal of Forensic Sciences* 49(4): 733–740.

Coble, M. D., and Butler, J. M. 2005. Characterization of new miniSTR loci to aid analysis of degraded DNA. *Journal of Forensic Sciences* 50(1): 43–53.

Coble, M. D., Just, R., O'Callaghan, J., Letmanyi, I., Peterson, C., Irwin, J., and Parsons, T. 2004. Single nucleotide polymorphisms over the entire mtDNA genome that increase the power of forensic testing in Caucasians. *International Journal of Legal Medicine* 118: 137–146.

Coble, M. D., Vallone, P., Just, R., Diegoli, T., Smith, B., and Parsons, T. 2006. Effective strategies for forensic analysis in the mitochondrial DNA coding region. *International Journal of Legal Medicine* 120: 27–32.

Colson, I., Bailey, J. F., Vercauteren, M., Sykes, B., and Hedges, R. E. M. 1997. The preservation of ancient DNA and bone digenesis. *Ancient Biomolecules* 1997(1): 109–118.

Comas, D., Pääbo, S., and Bertranpetit, J. 1995. Heteroplasmy in the control region of human mitochondrial DNA. *Genes Research* 5: 89–90.

Comey, C. T., Koons, B., Presley, K., Smerick, J., Sobieralski, C., Stanley, D., and Baechtel, F. 1994. DNA extraction strategies for amplified fragment length polymorphism analysis. *Journal of Forensic Sciences* 39: 1254–1269.

de Knijff, P., Kayser, M., Caglia, A., Corach, D., Fretwell, N., Gehrig, C., Graziosi, G., Heidorn, F., Herrmann, S., Herzog, B., Hidding, M., Honda, K., Jobling, M., Krawczak, M., Leim, K., Meuser, S., Meyer, E., Oesterreich, W., Pandya, A., Parson, W., Penacino, G., Perez-Lezaun, A., Piccinini, A., Prinz, M., Schmitt, C., Schneider, P. M., Szibor, R., Teifel-Greding, J., Weichhold, G., and Roewer, L. 1997. Chromosome Y microsatellites: Population genetic and evolutionary aspects. *International Journal of Legal Medicine* 110(3): 134–149.

Divine, A., Nilsson, M., Calloway, C., Reynolds, R., Erlich, H., and Allen, M. 2005. Forensic casework analysis using the HVI/HVII mtDNA linear array assay. *Journal of Forensic Sciences* 50(3): 548–554.

Excoffier, L., and Yang, Z. 1999. Substitution rate cariation among sites in mitochondrial hypervariable region I of humans and chimpanzees. *Molecular Biology and Evolution* 16(10): 1357–1368.

Faerman, M., Filon, D., Kahila, G., Greenblatt C.L., Smith, C. L., and Oppenheim, P. 1995. A sex identification of archeological human remains based on amplification of the X and Y amelogenin alleles. *Gene* 167: 327–332.

Gabriel, M. N., Calloway, C. D., Reynolds, R. L., and Primorac, D. 2003. Identification of human remains by immobilized sequence-specific oligonucleotide probe analysis of mtDNA hypervariable regions I and II. *Croatian Medical Journal* 44(3): 293–298.

Gabriel, M. N., Huffine, E. F., Ryan, J. H., Holland, M. M., and Parsons, T. J. 2001. Improved mtDNA sequence analysis of forensic remains using a "mini-primer set" amplification strategy. *Journal of Forensic Sciences* 46(2): 247–253.

Giles, R. E., Blanc, H., Cann, H. M., and Wallace, D. C. 1980. Maternal Inheritance of Human Mitochondrial DNA. *Proceedings of the National Academy of Sciences USA* 77(11): 6715–6719.

Gill, P., Fereday, L., Morling, N., and Schneider, P. M. 2006. The evolution of DNA databases: Recommendations for new European STR loci. *Forensic Science International* 156: 242–244.

Gill, P., Ivanov, P. L., Kimpton, C., Piercy, R., Benson, N., Tully, G., Evett, I., Hagelberg, E., and Sullivan, K. 1994. Identification of the remains of the Romanov family by DNA analysis. *Nature Genetics* 6: 130–135.

Gill, P., Urquhart, A., Millican, E., Oldroyd, N., Watson, S., Sparkes, R., and Kimpton, C. P. 1996. A new method of STR interpretation using inferential logic: Development of a criminal intelligence database. *International Journal of Legal Medicine* 109: 1.

Götherström, A., and Lidén, K. 1996. A modified extraction method for bones and teeth. *Laborativ Arkeologi* 9: 53–56.

Greenberg, B. D., Newbold, J. E., and Sugino, A. 1983. Intraspecific nucleotide sequence variability surrounding the origin of replication in human mitochondrial DNA. *Gene.* 21(1–2): 33–49.

Hagelberg E., and Clegg, J. B. 1991. Isolation and characterization of DNA from archaeological bone. *Proceedings of the Royal Society of London* 244(1309): 45–50.

Hoff-Olsen, P., Mevag, B. Staalstrøm, E., Hovde, B., Egeland, T., and Olaisen, B. 1999. Extraction of DNA from decomposed human tissue: An evaluation of five extracting methods for short tandem repeat typing. *Forensic Science International* 105: 171–183.

Holland, M., and Parsons, T. 1999. Mitochondrial DNA sequence analysis: Validation and use for forensic casework. *Forensic Science Review* 11: 21–50.

Hoss, M., Jaruga, P., Zastawny, T. H., Dizdaroglu, M., and Pääbo, S. 1996. DNA damage and DNA sequence retrieval from ancient tissues. *Nucleic Acids Research* 24(7): 1304–1307.

Hummel, S., Schultes, T., Bramanti, B., and Herrmann, B. 1999. Ancient DNA profiling by megaplex amplications. *Electrophoresis* 20: 1717–1721.

Hoss, M., and Pääbo, S. 1993. DNA extraction from Pleistocene bones by a silica-based purification method. *Nucleic Acids Research* 21: 3913.

Hutchinson, C. A., Newbold, J. E., Potter, S. S., and Edgell, M. H. 1974. Maternal inheritance of mammalian mitochondrial DNA. *Nature* 251: 536–538.

Iwamura, E. S. M., Soares-Vieira, J. A., and Muñoz, D. R. 2004. Human identification and analysis of DNA in bones. Revista do Hospital das Clínicas 59: 383–388.

Jobling, M. A., Pandya, A., and Tyler-Smith, C. 1997. The Y chromosome in forensic analysis and paternity testing. *International Journal of Legal Medicine*110(3): 118–124.

Just, R. S., Irwin, J., O'Callaghan, J., Saunier, J., Coble, M., Vallone, P., Butler, J., Barritt, S., and Parsons, T. 2004. Toward increased utility of mtDNA in forensic identifications. *Forensic Science International* 146S: S147–S149.

Kashyap, V. K., Sahoo, S., Sitaliaximi, T., and Trivedi, R. 2006. Deletions in the Y-derived amelogenin gene fragment in the Indian population. *BMC Medical Genetics* 7: 37.

Kayser, M., Caglia, A., Corach, D., Fretwell, N., Gehrig, C., Graziosi, G., Heidorn, F., Herrmann, S., Herzog, B., Hidding, M., Honda, K., Jobling M., Krawczak, M., K. Leim, K., Meuser, S., Meyer, S., Oesterreich, W., Pandya, A., Parson, W., Penacino, G., Perez-Lezaun, A., Piccinini, A., Prinz, M., Schmitt, C., Schneider, P. M., Szibor, R., Teifel-Greding, J., Weichhold, G., de Knijff, P., and Roewer, L. 1997. Evaluation of Y-chromosomal STRs: A multicenter study. *International Journal of Legal Medicine* 110(3): 125–133, 141–149.

Kline, M. C., Vallone, P. M., Redman, J. W., Duewer, D. L., Calloway, C. D., and Butler, J. M. 2005. Mitochondrial DNA typing screens with control region and coding region SNPs. *Journal of Forensic Sciences* 50(2): 377–385.

Krings, M., Stone, A., Schmitz, R. W., Krainitzki, H., Stoneking, M., and Pääbo, S. 1997. Neandertal DNA sequences and the origin of modern humans. *Cell* 90: 19–30.

Lowe, A., Murray, C., Whitaker, J., Tully, G., and Gill, P. 2002. The propensity of individuals to deposit DNA and secondary transfer of low level DNA from individuals to inert surfaces. *Forensic Science International* 129: 25–34.

Mannucci, A., Sullivan, K. M., Ivanov, P. L., and Gill, P. 1994. Forensic application of a rapid and quantitative DNA sex test by amplification of the X-Y homologous gene amelogenin. *International Journal of Legal Medicine* 106(4): 190–193.

Matheson, C. D., and Loy, T. H. 2001. Genetic sex identification of 9400-year-old human skull samples from Cayonu Tepesi, Turkey *Journal of Archaeological Science* 28: 569–575.

McKeown, B., Stickley, J., and Riordan, A. 2000. Gender assignment by PCR of the SRY gene: An improvement on amelogenin. *Progress in Forensic Genetics* 8: 433–435.

Meyer, S., Weiss, G., and von Haeseler, A. 1999. Pattern of nucleotide substitution and rate heterogeneity in the hypervariable regions I and II of human mtDNA. *Genetics* 152(3): 1103–1110.

Michael, A., and Brauner, P. 2004. Erroneous gender identification by the amelogenin sex test. *Journal of Forensic Sciences* 49(2): 1–2.

Nakahori, Y., Takenaka, O., and Nakagome, Y. 1991. A human X-Y homologous region encodes "amelogenin." *Genomics* 9: 264–269.

Niederstatter, H., Coble, M., Grubwieser, P., Parsons, T., and Parson, W. 2006. Characterization of mtDNA SNP typing and mixture ratio assessment with simultaneous real-time PCR quantification of both allelic states. *International Journal of Legal Medicine* 120(1): 18–23.

Opel, K. L., Chung, D. T., Drabek, J., Tatarek, N. E., Jantz, L. M., and McCord, B. R. 2006. The application of miniplex primer sets in the analysis of degraded DNA from human skeletal remains. *Journal of Forensic Sciences* 51(2): 351–356.

Pääbo, S. 1989. Ancient DNA: Extraction, characterization, molecular cloning, and enzymatic amplification. *Proceedings of the National Academy of Sciences USA* 86(6): 1939–1943.

Pääbo, S., Gifford, J. A., and Wilson, A. C. 1988 Mitochondrial DNA sequences from a 7000-year-old brain. *Nucleic Acids Research* 16(20): 9775–9787.

Palmirotta, R., Verginelli, F., Di Tota, G., Battista, P., Cama, A., Caramiello, S., Capasso, L., and R. Mariani-Costantini, L. 1997. Use of a multiplex polymerase chain reaction assay in the sex typing of DNA extracted from archaeological bone. *International Journal of Osteoarchaeology* 7(6): 605–609.

Parsons, T. J., Huel, R., Davoren, J., Katzmarzyk, C., Milos, A., Selmanovic, A., Smajlovic, L., Coble, M. D., and Rizvic, A. 2007. Application of novel "mini-amplicon" Str multiplexes to high-volume casework on degraded skeletal remains. *Forensic Science International: Genetics* 1(2): 175–179.

Pascal, O., Aubert, D., Gilbert, E., and Moisan, J.P. 1991. Sexing of forensic samples using PCR. *International Journal of Legal Medicine* 104(4): 205–207.

Poinar, H. N., Hoss, M., Bada, J. L., and Pääbo, S. 1996. Amino acid racemization and the preservation of ancient DNA. *Science* 272: 864–866.

Relethford, J. H. 2002. *Genetics and the Search for Modern Human Origins*. New York: John Wiley and Sons, Inc.

Ricaut, F., Keyser-Tracqui, C., Crubezy, E., and Ludes, B. 2005. STR-genotyping from human medieval tooth and bone samples. *Forensic Science International* 151(1): 31–35.

Roffey, P. E., Eckhoff, C. I., and Kuhl, J. L. 2000. A rare mutation in the amelogenin gene and its potential investigative ramifications. *Journal of Forensic Sciences* 45: 1016–1019.

Santos, F. R., Pandya, A., and Tyler-Smith, C. 1998. Reliability of DNA-based sex tests. *Nature Genetics* 18: 103.

Schmerer, W. M., Hummel, S., and Herrmann, B. 1999. Optimized DNA extraction to improve reproducibility of short tandem repeat genotyping with highly degraded DNA as target. *Electrophoresis* 20: 1712–1716.

Scientific Working Group on DNA Analysis Methods (SWGDAM). 2003. Guidelines for mitochondrial DNA (mtDNA) nucleotide sequence interpretation. *Forensic Science Communication* 5(2), www.fbi.gov/hq/lab/fsc/backissu/april2003/index.htm.

Sivolap, Y., Krivda, G., Kozhuhovan, N., Chebotar, S., and Benecke, M. 2001. A homicide in the Ukraine: DNA-based identification of a boiled, skeletonized, and varnished human skull, and of bone fragments found in a fireplace. *American Journal of Forensic Medicine and Pathology* 22(4): 412–414.

Steinlechner, M., Berger, B., Niederstatter, H., and Parson, W. 2002. Rare failures in the amelogenin sex test. *International Journal of Legal Medicine* 116(2): 117–120.

Stone, A., Milner, G. R., Pääbo, S., and Stoneking, M. 1999. Sex determination of ancient human skeletons using DNA. *American Journal of Physical Anthropology* 99(2): 231–238.

Stone, A., and Stoneking, M. 1993. Ancient DNA from a pre-Columbian Amerindian population. *American Journal of Physical Anthropology* 92: 463–471.

———. 1998. mtDNA analysis of a prehistoric Oneota population: Implications for the peopling of the New World. *American Journal of Human Genetics* 62: 1153–1170.

Stoneking, M. 2000. Hypervariable sites in the mtDNA control region are mutational hotspots. *American Journal of Human Genetics* 67(4): 1029–1032.

Stoneking, M., Hedgecock, D., Higuchi, R. G., Vigilant, L., and Erilich, H. A. 1991. Population variation of the human mtDNA control region sequences detected by enzymatic amplification and sequence-specific oligonucleotide probes. *American Journal of Human Genetics* 48: 370–382.

Sullivan, K. M., Mannucci, A., Kimpton, C. P., and Gill, P. 1993. A rapid and quantitative DNA sex test: Fluorescence-based PCR analysis of X-Y homologous gene amelogenin. *BioTechniques* 15: 636–639.

Thangaraj, K., Reddy, A., and Singh, L. 2002. Is the amelogenin gene reliable for gender identification in forensic casework and prenatal diagnosis? *International Journal of Legal Medicine* 116(2): 121–123.

Tully, G., Bar, W., Brinkmann, B., Carracedo, A., Gill, P., Morling, N., Parson, W., and Schneider, P. 2001. Considerations by the European DNA profiling (EDNAP) group on the working practices, nomenclature and interpretation of mitochondrial DNA profiles. *Forensic Science International* 124(1): 83–91.

Underhill P. A., Shen, P., Lin, A., Jin, L., Passarino, G., Yang, W., Kauffman, E., Bonne-Tamir, B., Bertranpetit, J., Francalacci, P., and Ibrahim, M. 2000. Y chromosome sequence variation and the history of human populations. *Nature Genetics* 26(3): 358–361.

van Oorschot, R. A. H., and Jones, M. K. 1997. DNA fingerprints from fingerprints. *Nature* 387: 767.

Wakeley, J. 1983. Substitution rate variation among sites in hypervariable region 1 of human mitochondrial DNA. *Journal of Molecular Evolution* 37(6): 613–623.

Walsh, P. S., Metzger, D. A., and Higuchi, R. 1991. Chelex 100 as a medium for simple extraction of DNA for PCR-based typing from forensic material *BioTechniques* 10: 506–513.

Wilson, M. R., Polanskey, D., Replogle, J., DiZinno, J. A., and Budowle, B. 1997. A family exhibiting heteroplasmy in the human mitochondrial DNA control region reveals both somatic mosaicism and pronounced segregation of mitotypes. *Nature Genetics* 100: 167–171.

Yang, D. Y., Eng, B., Wave, J. S., Dudar, J. C., and Saunders. S. R. 1998. Technical note: Improved DNA extraction from ancient bones using silica-based spin columns. *American Journal of Physical Anthropology* 105(4): 539–543.

Ye, J., Ji, A., Parra, E., Zheng, X., Jiang, C., Zhao, X., Hu. L., and Tu, Z. 2004. A simple and efficient method for extracting DNA from old and burned bone. *Journal of Forensic Sciences* 49(4): 754–759.

Zierdt, H., Hummel, S., and Herrmann, B. 1996. Amplification of human short tandem repeats from medieval teeth and bone samples. *Human Biology* 68(2): 185–199.

27

FORENSIC ODONTOLOGY

John Gerald Clement

This chapter presents a broad overview of forensic odontology. Beginning with defining the discipline of odontology, it then discusses the role that forensic dentists play in identifying deceased individuals. A brief overview of dental structures is provided, followed by a discussion of the types of dental records that may be used by the forensic dentist. The odontologist's contribution to dental ageing and superimposition are also discussed. Current research being undertaken to improve ageing adults is outlined. The chapter concludes with a discussion of forensic odontology's shared responsibilities in advocacy for human rights.

Definition of the Discipline

Within the panoply of dentistry *odontology* is taken to mean "forensic odontology." It is currently one of the fastest emerging subspecialties within the practice of dentistry and in the context of the broader subject of dental science. In the past, it has been known as "forensic dentistry" and in Scandinavia as "forensic odontostomatology," but neither of these alternate names really encompasses the scope of the discipline. As implied by its modern generic title, the legal process requires dental experts to observe, gather, record, and interpret meaningfully dental evidence in all its manifestations for the benefit of courts of law and the justice system. In essence, the forensic odontologist has to be an experienced practitioner of clinical dentistry and is, as such, usually required to be currently registered with the local professional licensing authority. However, many of the leaders and pioneers in the field often have academic appointments and higher degrees in dentistry or expertise in a relevant related discipline, such as anatomy (comparative and human) and biological anthropology. These additional skills obviously broaden the skill base of the forensic odontologist to the point where his or her expertise may overlap the margins of closely related disciplines such as archaeology and mainstream physical anthropology.

In the last two decades, opportunities—although rare—have arisen for postgraduate training specifically in forensic odontology. Hence, in the past, dentists have largely had to be self-taught, and it took many years to amass sufficient experience to become truly expert in all aspects of the discipline. When a practitioner does have the benefit of specifically targeted training, one can safely assume that he or she is not only expert in his or her own right but has a broad familiarity with the fields of expertise of all the other experts with whom he or she may have to work in a professional capacity. Although these experts obviously include pathologists, anthropologists, and archaeologists, they also include cultural heritage officers, the police, and other officers of the legal system in the prevailing jurisdiction.

Although forensic odontologists may have an increasingly important role to play in the investigation of circumstances and situations that have led to claims of negligence and malpractice against other dentists and paradental professionals, their main focus in day-to-day casework still remains primarily the corroboration of identity of deceased persons from a comparison of antemortem records and postmortem findings. Visual identification from the face or body is vulnerable to genuine mistakes and fraud or other attempts to pervert the course of justice and should not be used without corroborating evidence. The role of forensic odontology extends beyond contemporary events to the interpretation of ancient remains and therefore clearly has significance to archeological and cultural investigations as well.

Even before contemporary scientific investigative methods were conceived, let alone applied, there were numerous historical accounts of famous persons being identified accurately postmortem by the recognition of certain peculiarities within their dentitions. Keiser-Neilsen (1984) collated many of these cases. Over the last decade, and growing out of both historic and contemporary areas of activity, there has been an increasing emphasis on the ethical context of the application of forensic dental expertise. In dental practice this may relate to such issues as fitness for intellectually impaired persons to consent to treatment or an examination for the purposes of a criminal investigation. At the other end of the scale, it may relate to the position of the dental profession at large with respect to issues related to its complicity in torture (International Dental Ethics and Law Society 2006).

Forensic odontology has a vital role to play in identification for three main reasons. First, the teeth are durable in life and postmortem, often in extremely adverse conditions that have destroyed many other parts of the body. Second, the teeth are the only skeletal elements to have been visible and hence recorded in life by means of photographs or dental records in their various forms. Finally, there is a wide range of variability in the form of the teeth and the dental arches and paradental anatomy.

Success in using odontology for identification has recently been emphasized by the outcome of the Disaster Victim Identification (DVI) process in Phuket, Thailand, following the Boxing Day 2004 tsunami in which thousands of people perished. The widespread assumption of investigators at the outset of the investigation (including the

odontologists involved) was understandably that DNA would provide the major means of identification, particularly because Phuket is a region where many foreign tourists died and where it would be possible to obtain well provenanced antemortem biological samples for comparison. Unfortunately, and surprisingly, this proved not to be the case. Although it remains difficult to get reliable figures for the success rates of the various methods used to identify the victims, the disparity between the success of forensic odontological methods and DNA was huge, with dental methods contributing to the identification of approximately 70% of the victims identified, whereas DNA identified approximately only 1% in its own right. The problems with DNA analysis in very large-scale investigations are numerous: these range from an inability to obtain antemortem samples for comparison when the victims' homes have disappeared, the problems of locating close relatives (many of whom may also have perished), to problems of an inability to maintain continuity of evidence for samples, laboratory overload, multiple centers using different analytical protocols, and technical problems related to sample degradation caused by postmortem putrefaction (see Baker this volume).

Durability and Uniqueness of Dental Structures

The teeth are the most durable organs in the bodies of vertebrates, and thus interpretations of our past and evolution rely heavily on remnant dental evidence found as fossils (Tobias 1990). Teeth can persist long after other skeletal structures have succumbed to organic decay or destruction by some other agency, such as fire. Teeth and bone can be heated to temperatures approaching the melting point of skeletal mineral (>1,600°C) without appreciable loss of microstructure or tertiary architecture (Clement, Olsson, and Phakey 1992; Holden, Clement, and Phakey 1995a, 1995b, 1995c) (Figure 27.1). This seems paradoxical for the ashing of tissues implies that all which remains is powder. Anyone who has seen the remains of a modern human cremation knows this is not the case. It may be argued that dental enamel, the hardest skeletal tissue, is not a tissue at all in the strictest sense but virtually a fossilized secretion from the time of tooth formation within the bony crypts of the alveolar processes of the jaws and hence prior to tooth emergence into the mouth. The amount of organic matrix remaining in mature enamel is minimal (<2% w/w), but the inorganic fraction is 96% w/w, comprising submicroscopic crystals of an impure form of hydroxyapatite (HA)

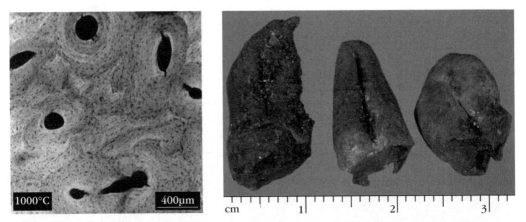

Figure 27.1 (*Left*) Transverse section of mid-shaft of human femoral cortex incinerated for 2 hours at 1,000°C. Haversian systems and osteocyte lacunae can still be clearly recognized despite some cracking and shrinkage of the original tissue. No organic matrix remains, and yet the structure appears almost intact. This mineral skeleton is very friable, and such evidence needs to be identified, stabilized, and collected by an expert. (*Right*) Three human teeth recovered from a fatal fire. Much of the bone of the craniofacial and appendicular skeleton was destroyed, but the teeth are remarkably intact. Dark colour would indicate incomplete combustion of the organize matrix owing to brevity of the fire or temperatures lower than 800°C (or a combination of both factors).

that are very long compared to their width (so long to have eluded measurement by any method applied to date). Nevertheless, the crystals' aspect ratio can definitely be expressed in many orders of magnitude, with the "c" axis of the crystals being very long compared to either the "a" and "b" axes, which are similar to each other. Following combustion of the residual organic matrix and the purging of any moisture in the enamel, it could be argued that the complex tertiary structure of enamel (in which long crystals are woven into complex prismatic patterns during tissue formation) holds the tissue together. Although this may have a role to play, other factors are at work.

When bone is heated similarly, it, too, retains its structure, albeit in a friable state; yet it is known that bone mineral is deposited as much smaller, shorter crystals lacking the filamentous nature of those found in enamel (see also Thompson this volume). Why then does burnt bone not disintegrate? As the collagenous and mucopolysaccharide components of bone burn and the accompanying water is driven off, the remaining inorganic components (also an impure form of HA) retain structure so well that osteons and even bone cell spaces are preserved. This occurs because, on heating and cooling, the original, impure apatite recrystallizes with its smallest crystals becoming sintered to their larger neighbors. It is this sintering that holds the remnants of the tissue together and enables it to be collected and examined histologically or in a scanning electron microscope. The recrystalized

mineral results in a more purer apatite than the original together with small quantities of a minor, secondary phase, beta-tricalcium-phosphate. From the relative proportions of major and minor phases, the lack of stoichiometry (the calculation of measurable relationships of the reactants and products in chemical equations) of the original mineral can be calculated, and from this inferences can be made about taxonomic origins of the tissue. The combination of histology and knowledge of crystal chemistry can reveal genus differences, and in the case of morphologically unidentifiable fragments of skeleton comprising any of the collagen-based hard tissues (bone, dentine, and cementum), this may be important for the correct interpretation of both crime scenes and archaeological sites (Miles 1963).

Dental Treatment, Dental Records, Nomenclature, and Notation

Much of the utility of dental findings for identification purposes derives from the almost universal need for people in economically developed countries to attend a dentist for an examination of their oral health status. The inevitable by-products of such visits are the dental records of the person in life. Such records comprise much more than just written clinical notes; plaster casts of the patient's mouth, clinical photographs, and, in particular, radiographs (dental "X rays") are invaluable for the forensic odontologist's comparison of antemortem status and postmortem findings (Figure 27.2). However,

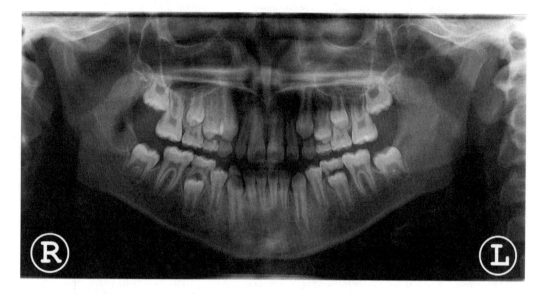

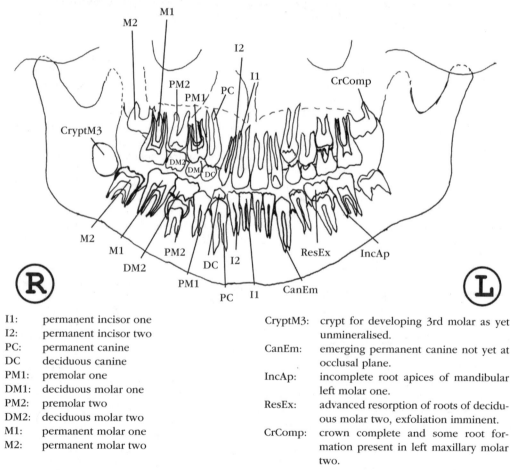

I1:	permanent incisor one	CryptM3:	crypt for developing 3rd molar as yet
I2:	permanent incisor two		unmineralised.
PC:	permanent canine	CanEm:	emerging permanent canine not yet at
DC	deciduous canine		occlusal plane.
PM1:	premolar one	IncAp:	incomplete root apices of mandibular
DM1:	deciduous molar one		left molar one.
PM2:	premolar two	ResEx:	advanced resorption of roots of decidu-
DM2:	deciduous molar two		ous molar two, exfoliation imminent.
M1:	permanent molar one	CrComp:	crown complete and some root for-
M2:	permanent molar two		mation present in left maxillary molar
			two.

Figure 27.2   Clinical radiograph of a 10-year-old Caucasian girl.

in the past it is was commonly (and erroneously) assumed that if no treatment has been provided, then dental records would be of little or no use for identification. This was a serious misconception.

With the optimization of the fluoride content of the drinking water supply (to maximize its anti-caries effects), combined with educational efforts to improve diet and oral hygiene, many young people in economically developed countries no longer have any dental decay. Although such people obviously do not have any dental restorations, which themselves are made of durable materials and that might have been used for identification purposes, most still have radiographic examinations of their teeth done routinely to check for early signs of dental decay beginning at the regions of contact between adjacent teeth in the dental arches. In older people, similar radiographs are taken to monitor periodontal health.

Furthermore, a decline in dental decay in modern, prosperous populations is invariably accompanied by an increasing societal emphasis on aspects of oral health status that were once generally considered less important, or a luxury. The growth in orthodontic practice in Western societies is a good example of this change in attitude and sophistication (Kingman 1997). Typically, full, lateral cranial radiographs are taken as part of the orthodontic examination. Plaster casts of the patients' mouths are always made for assessment, diagnosis, and treatment planning. These casts record tooth number, size, crown form, and tooth position very accurately. Occlusal relationships are also recorded and can also be important for identification purposes, particularly if reconstruction of facial features on remnant skull evidence or the use of superimposition techniques is required. Given the combination of the durability of the dental structures, the likelihood that the dental status of many people is recorded in detail by professionals known to be hoarders and who retain records for as long as is practicable, often far in excess of that mandated by law, there obviously exists a very powerful resource for the identification of remains. However, using this resource is not without its difficulties.

One problem frequently encountered in international situations relates to the fact there are several different conventions currently in use for the dental nomenclature used by dentists in their records. In part these can be divided crudely across geopolitical boundaries. The United States and smaller countries within its direct sphere of influence use a system of dental nomenclature known as The Universal System. The rest of the world tends to employ a system agreed on by the Federation Dentaire International (FDI).

Some older United Kingdom/European systems, such as Palmer/Zigmondy and the Scandinavian Haderup system, still have some exponents; however, these tend to be older dental practitioners. But we remember that not all bodies are examined promptly after death, and not all dental treatment was carried out in the last six months. The remains of many people are discovered only many years after they have died and in a skeletonized state. In such circumstances, the only antemortem records that may exist could well be recorded in archaic form. Applying the analogy of languages to this situation, we should also remember that dialects and even individual variations exist to the main charting conventions. For this reason, it is very unwise for anyone without dental training to attempt to decipher clinical dental notes. Experience has shown that when such an attempt is made, not only are mistakes made with respect to the interpretation of the records to hand but, worse still, the existence of other records, made by specialists elsewhere, often goes unnoticed.

Another reason why the expertise of a forensic odontologist needs to be drawn on relates to the fact that the dental and radiographic examination of a corpse or skeletonized remains is quite different from the more common dental examination of a living person, irrespective of whether he/she is awake and cooperative or anaesthetized and unresponsive. These skills in postmortem radiography are not taught as part of any undergraduate dental curriculum.

Another difficulty relates to the fact that some practitioners chart only work to be done and not work done previously, perhaps by a previous dentist. Modern codes of practice deem this to be unethical, yet many incomplete records still exist and are still useful. When combined with other partial records, they can build up a complete composite antemortem record that can then be compared with the postmortem findings.

It has been estimated that with 160 tooth surfaces existing in a full adult human dentition, the combination of sites of dental decay and the fillings placed in teeth to restore them and other features of the mouth could provide "an astronomical" number of unique combinations that may be depicted in a single dental chart, and when radiographic evidence is added, then the number of possibilities "approaches infinity" and "no two sets of teeth are identical" (Mertz 1977: 47). Although this set of circumstances may exist theoretically, such statements can also be highly misleading. Dentists are aware that certain tooth surfaces are more likely to decay before others and are therefore more likely to have been restored in a similar way (Clement 1998). Comparisons between ante-mortem and postmortem dental charts alone can erroneously create the incorrect impression that a "match" exists when an examination of the body or the inclusion of radiographic comparisons would show that it does not. For this reason, it is important to note that although modern, purpose-built software for the handling of large quantities of dental data, such as might constitute a missing persons' database or be used in DVI situations and can suggest "candidate matches," the final arbiter has to be a clinician capable of appreciating all the subtleties between records. Detailed morpho-logical characteristics of teeth and individual res-torations need to be sought and compared before the expert can determine a match and make the appropriate recommendation to the investigating authorities for their final arbitration on the identity of the deceased.

Less Commonly Used Features for Comparison

Antemortem X-ray images of the head and oro-dental region are excellent evidence for identification pur-pose. The size, shape, and dimensions of many structures are very stable in the skeleton of the head after early childhood, particularly those relating to the cranial base in the region of the anterior cra-nial fossa. The paranasal sinuses are small early in life, but the pneumatization of the bones of the face and base of skull with growth to adulthood gives rise to a series of large air-filled cavities that are complex in form and unique in outline. The frontal sinuses housed in the ridge of bone just above the eye sockets have numerous chambers with lobes separated by walls or septae. These sinuses are ideal for comparison between antemortem records and corresponding postmortem views. The com-parison can be made by overlaying the antemortem and postmortem films either directly, if to the same scale and taken with the same geometry, or in an electronic environment where some adjustments can be made (Andersen and Wenzel 1995; Clement, Officer, and Sutherland 1995; Ranta and Kerusuo 1995), provided an audit trail of image manipula-tions is recorded. The biggest impediment to the more widespread use of this technique is attribut-able to the relative rarity of antemortem postero-anterior (PA) radiographs of the skull. This situation applies to many types of medical treatment, and when the medical and/or dental records exist they are excellent. Unfortunately, from an identification requirement, they are rare; far more people still have their teeth checked, compared to, for example, having their hips replaced.

The maxillary sinuses are similarly both com-plex and stable in form in adulthood. Their images are frequently recorded on dental radiographs. It is only in panoramic views such as an orthopanto-mograph (OPG) that they are seen in their entirety. Their images are often poorly recorded, because the bones surrounding them are very thin. The films taken to record the health status of the teeth and their associated alveolar processes (both of which are much more radiopaque than the some-times eggshell thin bones of the face) overexpose air-filled sinuses in antemortem dental films (see Figure 27.2). However, when their shape and form are clearly depicted, they are excellent for com-parison purposes, and postmortem many different exposures can be taken in the same projection so that if one combines all the information, both teeth and bones can be imaged clearly and their ana-tomical relationships visualized.

In addition to skeletally based methods for cor-roborating identification, the characteristics of the oral soft tissues and lips have occasionally been used (Kasprzak 1990). The less deformable and the better protected such structures are, the more potential value they possess. Therefore, whereas lip prints on rigid objects can be compared with impressions or photographs of the lips of living subjects, postmortem changes or other destructive processes such as burning quickly destroy any indi-vidualizing characteristics. Conversely, structures such as palatal rugae, protected within the mouth from fire and predation, survive for comparison (Thomas and Kotze 1983). Mirror-image impres-sions of these features, which are stable in life and durable postmortem, are commonly recorded on the fitting surface of dentures.

What Can Be Achieved in the Absence of Antemortem Records?

In some cases when skeletal remains are found, it is not immediately obvious whether the remains are human or not. Fortunately, the teeth and facial skeleton of humans are highly characteristic, dif-fering significantly even from anthropoid apes, our nearest evolutionary relatives. Nevertheless, a good knowledge of comparative dental anatomy finds application from time to time. This may be for the identification of certain genera from skel-etal and dental remains *per se* in archaeological finds through to the identification of a particular species of shark and calculating the size of an indi-vidual fish from fragments of teeth and wound patterns found in victims of shark attack. Other bitemarks, such as those inflicted by dogs, large cats, and crocodiles, can be interpreted fully only if the dental anatomy of the animal implicated is understood.

Once remains have been determined to be human (see Mulhern this volume), then one must consider the possibility of commingling of multiple remains (see Adams and Byrd this volume). This requires the expertise of the anthropologist, but the forensic odontologist can assist by inferring age from patterns of calcification and emergence of teeth in subadults and commenting on the age-related changes to erupted teeth in the adult. Most of the postemergence features, such as tooth wear, are highly dependent on culture, diet, and lifestyle of the deceased. For this reason, it is hazardous to allow oneself to be pressed to give opinions in cases involving living persons, because the precision demanded of the courts just cannot be provided, and the consequences of error can be catastrophic for the individual.

A common situation encountered today is that involving recent immigrants or refugees charged with a serious offence. If deemed a minor (say, <16 years of age in some jurisdictions), then the person will be subjected to a more lenient and supportive experience within the legal system. Problems arise when the alleged offender is suspected of having lied about his or her age previously in order to gain residency within a particular country—there can then exist an incompatible discrepancy between the previously declared age and the current claim to still be a minor. Unfortunately, the precision of age estimation from dental maturity, although better than any other physical indicator in early life, is just not good enough to definitely determine whether a person is 15 or 17 years old, and yet that may be what the law seeks to discover. Notwithstanding this problem, during the 19th century in Britain, children were precluded from working in factories until their second permanent molars had erupted (Saunders 1837), which occurs approximately around 12 years of age.

Combining age estimates based on dental maturity with other anthropological age indicators may add to precision and accuracy, but it is highly unsafe to be too didactic when ancestral variation, past nutritional status, and population statistics reflecting secular trends are unavailable. Unfortunately, much of the original data on which widely accessible tables of tooth emergence (often misleadingly described as "eruption") were based were gleaned from small samples of dubious validity. Logan and Kronfeld's studies (for example, 1933) that were brought to a much wider readership by Schour and Massler's later publication (1941) were based on the chronology of dental development in a small group of terminally ill children. Even in dental schools, this fact is not widely known, and for convenience Schour and Massler's charts of tooth development are still very widely used for reference. Add to this fundamental problem the general trend toward earlier attainment of physical maturity in recent times, and it becomes apparent that the old data should not be regarded as directly applicable today. Lastly, it is important to draw a distinction between dates of tooth emergence into the oral cavity, in which there is considerable individual variation, and the chronology of tooth development. Although the two processes are linked, there are important opportunities for discrepancies to arise. A more reliable indicator of age would appear to be radiographic assessment of the level of the chronology of the whole process of tooth development for every individual tooth within the dentition, but ethical constraints should limit this application in living subjects unless they give informed consent.

A representative reassessment of tooth development and emergence patterns for all contemporary populations is urgently required. Because of differences in genetic background and general environmental conditions in the world, it is extremely inappropriate to use what may be excellent data gathered in one place long ago (Moorrees, Fanning, and Hunt 1963) and apply them to an entirely different population without first establishing their validity in the new context. In each case, published standards need to be validated for the population to which they are going to be applied (Liversidge 2003).

The excellent system of "scoring" tooth development devised by Demirjian and Goldstein (1976) has recently been refined by Willems (2000). It would be particularly valuable if other researchers could use this methodology, which, requiring only quite low technology and often simply access to patients' notes, would enable data from various sources to be compared. Meanwhile, the courts rely on experts who, through years of experience, have acquired sufficient experience to make the necessary local adjustments to the standard data tables, often without realising it.

Age Estimation in Adulthood

Although there remains room for improvement for studies of chronology of dental development, age estimation in adulthood is even more problematic (see Rogers this volume). In Sweden, a system for ageing extracted or lost, previously fully erupted teeth was developed by Gustafson

(1966). Essentially, Gustafson made longitudinal ground sections of teeth and then scored features known to change over time. These changes included progressive wear on the biting surfaces of the teeth; the reduction in the volume of the pulp chamber by continued slow, hard tissue formation on its walls (secondary dentine accretion); the continued deposition of cementum, a bone-like tissue, on the external root surface; and the increase of translucency in the dentine due to continued mineralization together with changes that may take place as the soft tissues of the periodontal tissues recede over time. By examining many teeth taken from individuals of known age and combining scores of the status of the age-related changes, Gustafson was able to construct a regression curve. Thereafter, when unknown teeth were found, they would be sectioned, the various features scored, and then, by reference to the regression curve, the age of the person from whom they came was derived.

Although this method worked well in Sweden at the time, it very likely would be much less applicable, even in Sweden, 40 years later. At the time that Gustafson's method was developed, Sweden was a remarkably stable society. Not having experienced much recent migration and virtually none from outside Scandinavia and Northern Europe, the gene pool was settled, and the prevailing political system effectively meant most people experienced a similar level of prosperity, education, living conditions, and diet.

By contrast, in other countries, or even Sweden in the 21st century, Gustafson's method, or its derivatives, is unlikely to be very useful. In many parts of the world, political instability and poverty have forced people to move from countries each with their own idiosyncratic customs, lifestyles and diets to other countries where these conditions may be very different. This can, and often does, have a profoundly confusing effect on age-related changes to the dentition; although some, such as the slow increase in root translucency with increased deposition of intratubular dentine (commonly misnamed "peritubular dentine") over time may be largely physiological, others such as occlusal wear and the pulpal reactions to it may be dictated much more by the abrasiveness of the diet than increasing age *per se*.

Ancestral Traits in the Teeth and Dentition

Dental anatomists and anthropologists study the human dentition in two ways: metrically and nonmetrically. There have been a multitude of studies in which the sizes of tooth crowns have been measured. Foremost among the exponents of this "metric" methodology are Garn, Lewis, and Kerewsky (1965, 1968); Goose (1963, 1971); Kieser (1990); Moorrees (1957); Moorrees and associates (1957); Moorrees and Chandha (1962); Moorrees and Reed (1964); Townsend (1980); and Townsend and Brown (1978). The populations studied usually represent geographically or culturally separate populations who are therefore assumed to share some common genetic features or exhibit the effects of some important environmental effects. The resulting measurements are therefore taken to be descriptive of, and may be unique to, that particular group. Large numbers of measurements are made on large numbers of teeth from large numbers of individuals. For living subjects, plaster casts are frequently used as an intermediate step, whereas with skeletal remains of past populations measurements can frequently be made directly from the remains. Obviously, care has to be exercised. It is possible for a particularly important reference set of remains to have been examined so frequently that they become abraded by frequent measuring and then become less useful. Although such studies are very useful for identifying evolutionary change within the dentition or investigating general patterns of inheritance of tooth size and form or the shape of the dental arches on a population basis, they can be used with much less certainty in the forensic situation that often requires the examination of the dentition of a specific individual.

Another way in which tooth form has been studied has been to recognize the presence, absence, or degree of expression of features that vary in their prevalence among individuals. These "nonmetric" studies have been made semiquantitative to bring some consistency to the interpretations made by widely separated investigators. To this end, identical sets of dental casts have been manufactured from type specimens and distributed in an attempt to standardize scoring of any particular feature that is being described (Buikstra and Ubelaker 1994; Dahlberg 1945, 1949, 1963; Turner, Nichol, and Scott 1991). It is more common for nonmetric variations of tooth form to find application in forensic cases, because the local forensic odontologist is very well aware of the prevalence of certain characteristics, for example, the prevalence of Carabelli's trait, in the teeth of some of the people making up their own local populations. Again, it must be emphasized that experience has shown that there is no dental trait that is proof-positive of any ethnic group under all circumstances.

Predictable Future Scientific Advances

The determination of age at death of unidentified remains is still problematic, particularly when the remains of adults are involved and when the effects of environmental factors known to modify the dentition during life are unknown. One method that has had some sporadic exploration of its usefulness but that is certainly worthy of further research is the slow but irreversible conversion of left-handed (levo) amino acids into their right-handed (dextro) enantiomers in proteins following the time of their deposition (Arany et. al. 2004; Davies 1975; Kvenvolden and Peterson 1973; Ogino and Ogino 1985, 1988; Ohtani and Yamamoto 1990a, 1990b, 1992).

Aspartic acid has, to date, been shown to be the amino acid with a suitably rapid conversion rate that also correlates better with period-since-deposition than either glutamic acid or alanine (Ohtani and Yamamoto 1991). At some time, all the hard tissues of the body have been investigated as source material for such determinations, but bone is problematic, because it is in a constant state of turnover, so an elderly person may have bone tissue within the bone organs that may be only very recently deposited. Cementum is very sparse and exhibits continued deposition throughout life, with the later deposited material possibly swamping any determinations derived from the scant veneer of first-deposited material closest to the tooth root surface. Dental enamel has been explored (Ohtani and Yamamoto 1992), but because it is 96% mineral by weight, again there is very little organic material to be collected and sampled.

Because collagen is the major proteinaceous component of dentine and dentine constitutes the bulk of all teeth, there is a strong possibility that time-related chemical transformations shown to occur in collagen will be useful for ageing of dentine. This situation is made more favourable since in most adult teeth the period of deposition in any single tooth would rarely exceed nine years, and any secondary dentine laid down during later life always resides on the pulpal surface from which it can be removed if required.

Furthermore, if from its morphology the particular tooth can be identified, then the time window during which it was formed can be estimated. If this information can be combined with an estimation of the degree of aspartic acid racemization that has taken place, then using regression equations, one can determine age at death. One recent study concluded that age determination using this technique with fresh cadavers predicted age to

within two to four years of the true age (Ohtani 1995). Unfortunately, other laboratories have not always been so successful, with Mornstad, Pfeiffer, and Teivens (1994) predicting age with a confidence interval of 95% of about +/-12 years, which would be much less useful. The anatomical position of the teeth sampled has been shown to have an effect, and it has been postulated that teeth (and tooth surfaces) deepest from the body surface and farthest from the opening of the mouth undergo a more rapid conversion of aspartic acid, because they are held at a higher temperature than are their more superficial counterparts (Ohtani 1997; Ohtani, Ito, and Yamamoto 2003).

Postmortem conditions are also an important consideration in evaluating the usefulness of aspartic acid racemisation. Fixation of tissues in formalin stops the racemization of aspartic acid (Ohtani et al. 1997), as does desiccation. Conversely, the conversion rate may be accelerated in alkaline environments, becoming progressively slower through water, acid, and dry conditions (Ohtani 1995). Reviews by Waite and associates (1999) and Yekkala and colleagues (2006) suggest that the general method is rather technique sensitive, and there are other factors to be taken into account before too much reliance can be placed solely on the results of a biochemical assay. For example, the dentine from deciduous teeth has been shown to exhibit double the conversion rate of dentine from permanent teeth (Ohtani, Kato, and Sugeno 1996). There are problems with the interpretation of very old skeletal material (Kvenvolden and Peterson 1973), and the consequences of sampling slabs of material cut transversely from various parts of the tooth, compared with longitudinal sections, does not always seem to have been understood. A midline longitudinal section collects material from the whole period of the tooth's formation, which is a longer time window than any horizontal section through crown or root would provide.

Nevertheless, given all of the above-mentioned shortcomings, aspartic acid racemization would still offer the possibility of providing objective estimates of time since death. It also offers opportunities for ageing living persons if biopsy techniques can be developed and ethical issues addressed (Helfman and Bada 1975; Ritz et al. 1995).

Another area of forensic odontological practice that is still problematic, yet highly likely to benefit from further scientific study, is the inference of facial appearance from the skeletal remains of the cranium, mandible, and associated dentitions. This process of reconstructive anatomy has been called "facial reconstruction" or rather more pedantically "facial approximation" (see Stephan this volume).

The techniques for achieving results are many and varied yet all rely on an assumption that the external form of the face can be inferred from the form of the underlying skeleton. This has never been proven. Moreover, in all attempts to visualise, or harder still quantify, the range of variation obtained when multiple operators using a range of methods—but all working from identical replicas of the same skull and given the same details about body mass index (BMI) and sex—have been so widely divergent that the value of attempting facial approximation has to be questioned (Stephan and Henneberg 2001). This observation is countered by practitioners who claim high success rates over chance with reconstructions (approximations) obtained in their laboratories. Such claims are rarely verifiable. (A good review of the history of facial reconstruction is provided by Wilkinson (2004).

Nevertheless, the scepticism of investigators often finally succumbs to the fact that facial reconstruction is a technique of last resort, and nothing is to be lost by attempting it. Haglund (1998) argues that the success of forensic art has as much to do with the timing and style of publicity afforded to any reconstruction of facial likeness as it has to do with the fidelity of the reconstruction itself. At the time that Haglund wrote this, it was highly likely to be the case, but more recently facial reconstruction is moving from empirical artistic roots to a science much more rooted in engineering and computer modelling and 3D visualization, which are innately more amenable to quantitative methods.

One very exciting possibility that will add greatly to knowledge in this area is the capacity to utilize data arising from the routine CT scanning of cadavers as part of the forensic autopsy to study interrelationships among skull, dentition, and face for the first time in a truly holistic manner. Modern mathematical methods of analysis free the investigator from historical reliance on hard-to-locate landmarks, and the access to modern contemporary data from relevant populations gives the results immediate applicability.

Forensic Odontology's Shared Responsibilities in Advocacy for Human Rights

In common with other colleagues in the forensic disciplines, the forensic odontologist has a responsibility to ameliorate any potential harm to those incarcerated and/or subjected to torture. The forensic odontologist is expert in the examination, documentation, and, when early treatment can be instigated, the healing of those with oro-facial injuries. These injuries can take several forms and collectively may clearly represent a systematic pattern of abuse over time. Prisoners may be beaten and suffer fractures of oro-facial structures. Alternatively, they may have been forced to consume corrosive liquids or have been burned, both of which may leave characteristic patterns of scarring. Careful documentation including the use of photographs and radiographs can provide compelling evidence for courts at a later date. In the case of examination of skeletal remains of past populations, the prevalence of oro-facial trauma in the skeletons of children can be used to estimate whether domestic violence was more or less common in societies that no longer exist. This can then be compared with the circumstances under which those people are thought to have lived (Walker, Collins-Cook, and Lambert 1997).

At the other extreme, the humanitarian responsibilities of the odontologist extend to a role in the prevention of massacres and other atrocities. In concrete, practical terms, perhaps the most important role for the forensic odontologist and others such as the pathologist and anthropologist is to gather evidence that mass murder has been committed. Again, the role of all forensic professions is to document the evidence from mass gravesites in such a meticulous and comprehensive manner that it can withstand the closest scrutiny by the courts, international tribunals, and the most critical historians of future generations. This type of evidence has been used in The Hague for the prosecution of those charged with crimes against humanity, including mass murder. A clear understanding from the outset on the part of potential perpetrators that crimes committed against humanity will be investigated and the perpetrators will be brought to trial may deter some who may be contemplating genocidal acts. However, we should not be naïve about such hopes; monsters go, or are deposed, often only to be replaced by others of the same ilk, the situation in Iraq in 2006 being a ghastly example in recent times. However, in a civilised society all of us have a duty to hope and, if nothing else by our actions as expert witness forensic odontologists with our peers in other related disciplines carry the responsibility to bear witness and document the facts for future generations to hear and judge. For this reason, reputation and a capacity to demonstrate independence from those with vested interests are vital.

People missing as a result of armed conflict, internal violence, or civil unrest are currently a harsh reality for many families around the world. This is not only very distressing for those directly concerned, but it may also hamper reconciliation and peace efforts by contributing to further out-breaks of violence. Of course, it is impossible to document every atrocity. To give some perspective to recent events, Human Rights Watch gives an estimate for the numbers of victims who "disappeared," many presumed murdered, during Saddam Hussein's reign in Iraq at almost 300,000 (Human Rights Watch). In addition and more controversially, Burnham and associates (2006) have estimated that following the invasion by America and its allies a further 655,000 extra deaths have occurred, many of these as a result of sectarian violence. For the remains of a significant number of these people to be exhumed and identified and have the manner of their death recorded are beyond the capacity of the world's forensic community at this time, and so new strategies have to be formed to bring finality to the next of kin and allow the affected communities to rebuild themselves. The International Committee of the Red Cross has begun work on "The Missing," a project that aims to shift the emphasis of investigations into the fate of persons who disappear during civil conflict from a prosecution focus to one with broader humanitarian objectives (The Missing Project 2003).

In the past, when mass murderers were caught or handed over to the authorities, it was necessary only to prosecute them for the deaths of a few identified persons rather than identify all the victims. This situation left the traumatized communities with no definite end-point to their wish to know for certain the fate of their friends, neighbours, and kith and kin. "The Missing" project has been exploring the feasibility of identifying all the deceased as far as is practicable and developing strategies to do so. The expert forensic odontologist will certainly have an important role to play in the education and training of local workers, who will inevitably have to shoulder the bulk of the burden for the identification of victims of atrocities to the satisfaction of their surviving relatives. The aim of "The Missing" project is to heighten awareness among governments, the military, international and national organizations—including the worldwide Red Cross and Red Crescent networks—and the general public about the tragedy of people unaccounted for as a result of armed conflict or internal violence and about the anguish of their families.

Conclusion

The identification of persons from the unique peculiarities of their teeth and oral structures has been practiced since antiquity. In the last century,

this practice became a scientific discipline within dentistry but with close links to related disciplines, particularly anthropology. In common with other forensic sciences, forensic odontology is practiced on behalf of the family and friends of the deceased. For people to know for certain of the death of a loved one can be a comfort from the anguish of continuous uncertainty. In this way, individuals may find it easier to rebuild shattered lives and, in the aftermath of atrocities that have resulted in mass murder, it may form a basis for a gradual reconciliation between past adversaries.

References

Andersen, L., and Wenzel, A. 1995. Digital subtraction radiography applied to bitewing radiographs, in B. Jacob and W. Bonte (eds.), *Advances in Forensic Sciences*, Vol. 7, *Forensic Odontology and Anthropology*, pp. 193–195. Berlin: Verlag Dr. Köster.

Arany, S., Ohtani, S., Yoshioka, N., and Gonmori, K. 2004. Age estimation from aspartic acid racemization of root dentin by internal standard method. *Forensic Science International* 141(2–3): 127–130.

Buikstra, J. E., and Ubelaker, D. H. (eds.). 1994. *Standards for Data Collection from Human Skeletal Remains*. Arkansas Archeological Survey Research Series no. 44 Fayetteville: Arkansas Archeological Survey.

Burnham, G., Lafta, R., Doocy, S., and Roberts, L. 2006. Mortality after the 2003 invasion of Iraq: A cross-sectional cluster study. *The Lancet* 368: 1421–1428.

Clement, J. G. 1998. Dental Identification, in J. G. Clement and D. L. Ranson (eds.), *Craniofacial Identification in Forensic Medicine*, pp. 63–81. London: Arnold.

Clement, J. G., Officer, R. A., and Sutherland, R. D. 1995. The use of digital image processing in forensic odontology: When does "image enhancement" become "tampering with evidence?" in B. Jacob and W. Bonte (eds.), *Advances in Forensic Sciences*, Vol. 7. *Forensic Odontology and Anthropology*, pp. 149–153. Berlin: Verlag Dr. Köster.

Clement, J. G., Olsson, C., and Phakey, P. P. 1992. Heat-induced changes in human skeletal tissues, in L. K. York and J. W. Hicks (eds.), *Proceedings of an International Symposium on the Forensic Aspects of Mass Disasters and Crime Scene Reconstruction*, FBI Academy Quantico 1990. Laboratory division of the FBI, Washington, D.C., U.S. Government Printing Office.

Dahlberg, A. A. 1945. Paramolar tubercle (Bolk), *American Journal of Physical Anthropology* 3: 97–103.

———. 1949. The dentition of the American Indian, in W. S. Laughlin (ed.), *The Physical Anthropology of the American Indian*, pp. 138–176. New York: Viking Fund.

Dahlberg, A. A. 1963. Analysis of the American Indian dentition, in D. R. Brothwell (ed.), *Dental Anthropology*, pp. 149–178. London: Pergamon Press.

———. 1975. Aspartic acid racemization of dentine as a measure of ageing. *Nature* 262: 279–281.

Demirjian, A., and Goldstein, H. 1976. New systems for dental maturity based on seven and four teeth. *Annals of Human Biology* 3: 411–421.

Garn, S. M., Lewis, A. B., and Kerewsky, R. S. 1965. Size interrelationships of the mesial and distal teeth, *Journal of Dental Research* 44: 350–354.

———. 1968. Relationship between buccolingual and mesiodistal crown diameters. *Journal of Dental Research* 47: 495.

Goose, D. H. 1963. Dental measurement: An assessment of its value in anthropological studies, in D. R. Brothwell (ed.), *Dental Anthropology*, pp. 125–148. London: Pergamon Press.

———. 1971. The inheritance of tooth size in British families, in A. A. Dahlberg (ed.), *Dental Morphology and Evolution*, pp. 263–270. Chicago: University of Chicago Press.

Gustafson, G. 1966. *Forensic Odontology*. London: Staples Press.

Haglund, W. 1998. Forensic "art" in human identification, in J. G. Clement and D. L. Ranson (eds.), *Craniofacial Identification in Forensic Medicine*, pp. 235–242. London: Arnold.

Helfman, P. M., and Bada, J. L. 1975. Aspartic acid racemization in tooth enamel from living humans. *Proceedings of the National Academy of Science, USA* 72(8): 2891–2894. Alan Clift Associates.

Holden, J. L., Clement, J. G., and Phakey, P. P. 1995a. Age and temperature related changes to the structure and chemistry of human bone mineral. *Journal of Bone Mineral Research* 10(9): 1400–1409.

———. 1995b. Scanning electron microscope observations of incinerated human femoral bone: A case study. *Forensic Science International* 74: 17–28.

———. 1995c. Scanning electron microscope observations of heat-treated human bone. *Forensic Science International* 74: 29–45.

Human Rights Watch December. 2002. Justice for Iraq. *A Human Rights Watch Policy Paper*. Washington, D.C., www.hrw.org/mideast/iraq.php

International Dental Ethics and Law Society (IDEALS). 2006. www.ideals.ac.

Kasprzak, J. 1990. Possibilities of cheiloscopy. *Forensic Science International* 46: 145–151.

Keiser, J. A. 1990. Human adult odontometrics. *Cambridge Studies in Biological Anthropology* 4. Cambridge: Cambridge University Press.

Keiser-Neilsen, S. 1984. Historical cases, in I. R. Hill, S. Keiser-Neilsen, Y. Vermylen, E. Free, E. de Valck, E. and Tormans (eds.), *Forensic Odontology: Its*

Scope and History, pp. 35–100. IOFOS Solihull: Alan Clift Associates.

Kingman, A. 1997. Statistics in community oral health, in C. M. Pine (ed.), *Community Oral Health*, pp. 147–161. Oxford: Wright.

Kvenvolden, K. A., and Peterson, E. 1973. Racemization of amino acids in bones. *Nature* 245: 308–310.

Liversidge, H. M. 2003. Worldwide variation in human dental development, in J. L. Thompson, A., Nelson, and G. Krovitz (eds.), *Growth and Development in the Genus Homo*, pp. 73–113. Cambridge: Cambridge University Press.

Logan, W. H. G., and Kronfeld., R. 1933. Development of the human jaws and surrounding structures from birth until the age of fifteen years. *Journal of the American Dental Association* 20: 379–427.

Mertz, C. A. 1977. Dental identification. *Dental Clinics of North America* 21(1): 47–67.

Miles, A. E. W. 1963. Dentition in the assessment of individual age in skeletal material, in D. R. Brothwell (ed.), *Dental Anthropology*, pp. 191–209. London: Pergamon Press.

Moorrees, C. F. A. 1957. *The Aleut Dentition*. Cambridge, MA: Harvard University Press.

Moorrees, C. F. A., and Chandha, J. M. 1962. Crown diameters, of corresponding tooth groups in the deciduous and permanent dentition. *Journal of Dental Research* 41: 466–470.

Moorrees, C. F. A., Fanning, E. A., and Hunt, E. E. 1963. Age variation of formation stages for ten permanent teeth. *Journal of Dental Research* 42: 1490–1502.

Moorrees, C. F. A., and Reed, R. B. 1964. Correlations among crown diameters of human teeth. *Archives of Oral Biology* 9: 685–697.

Moorrees, C. F. A., Thomsen, S. O., Jensen, E., and Yen, P. K. J. 1957. Mesiodistal crown diameters of deciduous and permanent teeth. *Journal of Dental Research* 36: 39–47.

Mornstad, H., Pfeiffer, H., and Teivens, A. 1994. Estimation of dental age using HPLC-technique to determine the degree of aspartic acid racemization. *Journal of Forensic Sciences* 39(6): 1425–1431.

Ogino, T., and Ogino, H. 1985. Applications of aspartic acid racemization to forensic odontology: Postmortem designation of age at death. *Forensic Science International* 29: 259–267.

———. 1988. Applications to forensic odontology of aspartic acid racemization in unerupted and supernumary teeth. *Journal of Dental Research* 67: 1319–1322.

Ohtani, S. 1995a. Estimation of age from the teeth of unidentified corpses using amino acid racemization method with reference to actual cases. *American Journal of Forensic Medicine and Pathology* 16(3): 238–242.

Ohtani, S. 1995b. Estimation of age from dentin by utilizing the racemization of aspartic acid: influence of pH. *Forensic Science International* 75 (2–3): 181–187.

———. 1997. Different racemization ratios in dentin from different locations within a tooth. *Growth, Development and Ageing* 61(2): 93–99.

Ohtani, S., Ito, R., and Yamamoto, T. 2003. Differences in the D/L aspartic acid ratios in dentin among different types of teeth from the same individual and estimated age. *International Journal of Legal Medicine* 117(3): 149–152.

Ohtani, S., Kato, S., and Sugeno, H. 1996. Changes in D-aspartic acid in human deciduous teeth with age from 1–20 years. *Growth, Development and Ageing* 60(1): 1–6.

Ohtani, S., Ohhira, H., Watanabe, A., Ogasawara, A., and Sugimoto, H. 1997. Estimation of age from teeth by amino acid racemization: influence of fixative. *Journal of Forensic Science* 42(1): 137–139.

Ohtani, S., Susumu Yamada, Y., and Yamamoto, I. 1998. Improvement in age estimation using amino acid racemisation in a case of pink teeth. *American Journal of Forensic Medicine and Pathology* 19(1): 77–79.

Ohtani, S., and Yamamoto, K. 1990a. Racemization velocity of aspartic acid in dentine. *Japanese Journal of Legal Medicine* 44(4): 346–351.

———. 1990b. Estimating age through the amino acid racemization of acid-soluble dentinal peptides. *Japanese Journal of Legal Medicine* 44(4): 342–345.

———. 1991. Age estimation by amino acid racemization in teeth: A comparison of aspartic acid with glutamic acid and alanine as indicators. *Japanese Journal of Legal Medicine* 45(2): 119–123.

———. 1992. Estimation of age from a tooth by means of racemization of an amino acid, especially aspartic acid—comparison of enamel and dentin. *Journal of Forensic Sciences* 37(4): 1061–1067.

Ranta, H., and Kerosuo, E. 1995. Computerized image analysis of panoramic tomograms, in B. Jacob and W. Bonte (eds.), *Advances in Forensic Sciences*, Vol. 7. *Forensic Odontology and Anthropology*, pp. 178–180. Berlin: Verlag Dr. Köster.

Ritz, S., Stock, R., Schutz, H. W., and Klaatsch, H. J. 1995. Age estimation in biopsy specimens in dentine. *International Journal of Legal Medicine* 108(3): 135–139.

Saunders, E. 1837. The teeth as a test of age, considered with reference to the factory children:

Addressed to the members of both Houses of Parliament. London: H. Renshaw.

Schour, I., and Massler, M. 1941. The development of the human dentition. *Journal of the American Dental Association* 28: 1153–1160.

Stephan, C. N., and Henneberg, M. 2001. Building faces from dry skulls: Are they recognized above chance rates? *Journal of Forensic Science* 46(3): 432–440.

The Missing Project. 2003. ICRC (International Committee of the Red Cross), www.icrc.org/web/eng/siteeng0.nsf/iwpList509/.

Thomas, C. J., and Kotze, T. J. V. W. 1983. The palatal rugae in forensic odontostomatology. *Journal of Forensic Odontostomatology* 1(1): 11–20.

Tobias, P. V. 1990. *Olduvai Gorge Vol: The Skulls, Endocasts and Teeth of Homo habilis*. New York: Cambridge University Press.

Townsend, G. C. 1980. Heritability of deciduous tooth size in Australian aboriginals. *American Journal of Physical Anthropology* 53: 297–300.

Townsend, G. C., and Brown, T. 1978. Heritability of permanent tooth size. *American Journal of Physical Anthropology* 49: 497–505.

Turner, C. G., Nichol, C. R., and Scott, G. R. 1991. Scoring procedures for key morphological traits of the permanent dentition: The Arizona State University Dental Anthropology System, in M. A. Kelly and C. S. Larsen (eds.), *Advances in Dental Anthropology*, pp. 13–31. New York: Wiley-Liss.

Waite, E. R., Collins, M. J., Ritz-Timme, S., Schutz, H.-W., Catteano, C., and Borrman, H. I. M. 1999. A review of the methodological aspects of aspartic acid racemization analysis for use in forensic science. *Forensic Science International* 103: 113–124.

Walker, P., Collins-Cook, D., and Lambert, P. M. 1997. Skeletal evidence for child abuse, American Physical Anthropology Perspective, in *Journal of Forensic Sciences* 1997 42(2): 196–207.

Wilkinson, C. 2004. *Forensic Facial Reconstruction*. Cambridge: Cambridge University Press.

Willems, G. 2000. Dental age estimation and computers, in G. Willems (ed.), *Forensic Odontology*: Proceedings of the European IOFOS Millennium Meeting, Leuven (Belgium), p. 199 (Abstract). Belgium: Leuven University Press.

Yekkala, R., Meers, C., Van Schepadael, A., Hoogmartens, J., Lambrichts, I., and Willems, G. 2006. Racemization of aspartic acid from human dentin in the estimation of chronological age. *Forensic Science International* 159 Suppl 1: S89–94.

PART

FOUR

THE CRIME AND DISASTER
SCENE: CASE STUDIES IN
FORENSIC ARCHAEOLOGY
AND ANTHROPOLOGY

28

DOMESTIC HOMICIDE INVESTIGATIONS: AN EXAMPLE FROM THE UNITED STATES

Dawnie Wolfe Steadman, William Basler, Michael J. Hochrein, Dennis F. Klein, and Julia C. Goodin

The role of forensic anthropology in domestic cases in the United States has expanded tremendously in the last two decades. In addition to working on traditional cases of personal identification of skeletal remains, forensic anthropologists routinely assist in missing person searches, apply forensic archaeological techniques at recovery scenes, estimate postmortem intervals, explain burning patterns of bone, and interpret trauma. Forensic pathologists also increasingly consult with forensic anthropologists in cases for which identity is known. For instance, forensic anthropologists assist in interpreting the direction of impact in car-pedestrian accidents and detecting suites of healed and acute injuries in child abuse cases. Forensic anthropologists also must ensure that the methods they employ satisfy the current criteria for evidence admissibility in court.

This chapter provides a detailed report of a complex federal case illustrating the multidisciplinary nature of domestic homicide investigations that highlights the role of forensic anthropology. This case demonstrates the various forms of physical evidence that can be recovered from mass graves when standard archaeological procedures are correctly applied and underscores the critical need for cooperation between forensic pathologists and anthropologists in trauma analysis. Like many anthropological cases, the lengthy period between disappearance and recovery necessitated consistent investigative attention until critical information came to light.

In July of 1993, Lori Duncan,[1] her two little girls, Kandace and Amber, and her friend, Greg Nicholson, disappeared from Lori's home in Mason City, Iowa. Four months later, another man, Terry DeGeus, disappeared as well. The sole known connection between the cases was that both men had been involved in a drug distribution ring headed by Dustin Honken. Nicholson had recently agreed to cooperate with federal prosecutors and testify against Honken in an upcoming federal trial. Months and then years passed without any trace of the five missing persons. Although it became increasingly apparent to the federal authorities that the missing people were victims of foul play, it took over a decade for a team of investigators, prosecutors, and forensic scientists from a variety of federal, state, and local agencies to locate and recover the victims' bodies and bring to justice their murderers, Dustin Honken and his girlfriend and accomplice, Angela Johnson.

The Investigation

Dustin Honken was born and raised in northern Iowa. Though intellectually gifted, he was an academic underachiever. Upon graduation from high school, he attended a local community college and excelled in chemistry but eventually dropped out of school and moved to Arizona to live with his older brother. While in Arizona, Honken perfected a methamphetamine production method and began distributing this drug to two individuals in north Iowa, Greg Nicholson and Terry DeGeus, who, in turn, sold the methamphetamine to street level dealers. When one of Nicholson's customers was arrested, he agreed to cooperate with the police, and Nicholson was arrested. Nicholson was also given the opportunity to cooperate with the police, which led to Honken's arrest during March of 1993.

Honken was charged in federal court for distribution of methamphetamine and, during the pretrial proceedings, learned that Nicholson had been responsible for his arrest. On July 8, 1993, Honken negotiated a plea agreement and was scheduled to plead guilty on July 30. He was released from jail in the interim. Before his arrest, Honken had become romantically involved with Angela Johnson, the exgirlfriend of Terry DeGeus. Johnson was a high school dropout with a history of drug abuse and an assortment of occupations. Near the time of Honken's release, Angela Johnson purchased a Tec-9, a semiautomatic 9-mm handgun, from an area pawnshop. Investigators would later locate witnesses who described efforts by Honken and Johnson to learn the whereabouts of Greg Nicholson. A few days before Nicholson's disappearance, Honken was directed to the home of Lori Duncan.

Following his release, Greg Nicholson had lived at a variety of locations around Mason City, Iowa. In early July, a friend had introduced him to one of her coworkers, Lori Duncan. Lori was a divorced mother who worked at a factory to support herself and her two daughters, Kandace, age 10, and Amber, who was 6 years old. Nicholson moved into the Duncan home in mid-July. All four members of the household were last observed by relatives, friends, and neighbors on Sunday, July 25, 1993.

On Monday morning, July 26, Lori Duncan uncharacteristically failed to report to work. Later that day a welfare check at Lori's home turned up only a note indicating that Lori had to leave on short notice but would be in contact soon. Nicholson, Lori, Kandi, and Amber were never seen alive again. Just four days later, at his scheduled court appearance on July 30, 1993, Honken informed the federal prosecutor that he no longer intended to plead guilty and told the prosecutor that the case against him was "not as good as you think it is."

With Nicholson unavailable and his whereabouts unknown, the case against Honken was in jeopardy. The government attempted to resurrect its case by pursuing information regarding Terry DeGeus, Honken's other drug distributor. On October 27, 1993, Angela Johnson was subpoenaed to testify before the grand jury and was questioned about DeGeus's drug business and his involvement with Honken. A few days later, on November 5, Johnson left a telephone message for Terry DeGeus telling him to meet her that evening in Mason City. After leaving for that meeting, DeGeus was never seen alive again.

Because Nicholson and DeGeus could not be located, all charges against Honken were dismissed in September of 1995. However, Honken was arrested again during the early spring of 1996 for assembling a methamphetamine laboratory in Mason City. Honken was released from jail pending trial, this time wearing an ankle bracelet that allowed authorities to monitor his whereabouts. Honken's best friend was also arrested and investigators pressured him to tell them about Honken's drug activities. He cooperated with the authorities in a plea arrangement. Honken's friend told the police that Honken was trying to learn how to electronically defeat the ankle device and that his intentions were to kill the current witnesses against him, including police, informants, and laboratory personnel. He also stated that, although Honken never told him so directly, Honken had hinted that he had killed the people who were missing since 1993. Finally, Honken's friend told investigators that he had helped Honken cut up, melt, and discard the remnants of a gun during the winter of 1993–1994. Although the friend was unfamiliar with firearms, he drew a sketch that closely resembled the profile of a Tec-9, the model that had been purchased by Angela Johnson.

Honken's pretrial bond was revoked in light of this new information, and he was incarcerated until his trial. However, Honken apparently believed he could continue to escape justice by killing witnesses. While awaiting trial in jail in 1996, Honken unsuccessfully solicited the murder of his best friend, who had betrayed him. Years later, this conspiracy would be added to the murder charges arising from the 1993 disappearances.

Although the investigation into the disappearances in 1993 had continued, it was re-energized in 1996 with the new information supplied by Honken's best friend. The investigation now focused on both Honken and Johnson as the persons responsible. Finding the bodies became even more crucial, yet there were few reliable leads, and investigators hit several dead ends. For instance, one investigative theory was that DeGeus, who had worked at his father's excavation/demolition business at the time of his disappearance, may have participated in the killings of Nicholson, Duncan, and her two daughters and that the bodies may have been buried at the site where DeGeus was working at the time. It was further theorized that DeGeus may have later been killed to ensure his silence. Following this theory, the investigators found the site where DeGeus was working on July 26, 1993, a farm field where buildings had been knocked down and buried. Investigators examined the site utilizing ground-penetrating radar and cadaver-trained search dogs, but no human remains were found.

The investigation continued without significant progress until 1999. Honken had finally pled guilty to the 1996 federal drug charges and was serving a 20-year sentence in a Colorado prison. In the summer of 1999, the first of several prisoners contacted federal authorities in Iowa to provide information that Honken was bragging to fellow inmates that he had "killed his rats." Honken shared details of the killings to at least one inmate that would ultimately be corroborated by forensic scientists.

In November 1999, prosecutors began presenting evidence to the grand jury in pursuit of murder indictments against Honken and Johnson. One of the persons subpoenaed was Angela Johnson's best friend during 1993. Though this woman had been interviewed and summoned to the grand jury several times, she always claimed that she had no information about the disappearances. During the summer of 2000, she was interviewed yet again and finally admitted that Angela Johnson had confessed to assisting Honken with the kidnapping and eventual murders of Nicholson, Duncan, and the two young girls. Specifically, Johnson had obtained entry to the Duncan home by posing as a lost saleslady and then used a handgun to control the victims until Honken arrived. They bound the adults then transported all four victims to a wooded area in the country. Johnson related to her friend that Honken took Greg Nicholson and Lori Duncan a distance from the car before shooting and killing them both. He then returned to the car, where Johnson was holding the two frightened girls. Honken executed each with a bullet to the head. All four were buried in a grave. Johnson further told her friend that Nicholson was killed so that he could not testify against Honken, and the others had been murdered because they were potential witnesses to Nicholson's abduction. Johnson's friend further disclosed that, on a separate occasion, Johnson had confessed that she and Honken had murdered Terry DeGeus. On the

day DeGeus disappeared, Johnson told her that she had called DeGeus and asked him to meet her in Mason City, which he did. Johnson then took DeGeus to a remote location where Honken was waiting. Honken killed DeGeus with a gun and an aluminum baseball bat and buried him in a hand-dug grave.

Unfortunately, Johnson did not disclose the location of either grave to her friend. Nevertheless, with this information the case against Johnson was now stronger than the case against Honken, since rules of evidence based on the 6th Amendment Right to Confrontation would prevent using Johnson's confession against Honken. Thus, changing the focus of the investigation, and despite the fact that the bodies of the five murder victims had still not been recovered, authorities sought and obtained an indictment of Angela Johnson on five counts of murder. On the seventh anniversary of the Nicholson-Duncan disappearances, Angela Johnson was arrested and transported to the Benton County jail to await trial.

The Benton County jail is a relatively small facility, housing both male and female prisoners in separate cells on the same floor. Prisoners are able to communicate with one another by talking through the walls and passing notes, often using books on the jail's book cart. Using these methods, Johnson was befriended by a male inmate who, though currently serving a life sentence in another state for conspiring to import heroin into the United States, was temporarily in Iowa to testify in another case. He told Johnson that he knew a prisoner at the federal prison in Leavenworth, Kansas, who was serving a life sentence and had no hope of ever being released. He told her that he thought he could convince this federal prisoner to admit to committing the five murders, which would set Johnson free and she could then sue the federal government for false arrest. The only problem with this plan, he explained, is that the prisoner would need something to prove his credibility to the authorities, such as maps of where the bodies had been buried. Johnson eventually provided two maps to her jailhouse friend, detailing where the bodies could be found and information about the bodies themselves. In hopes of exchanging this information for potential leniency in his own case, the inmate turned the maps over to federal authorities.

Recovery of a Mass Grave

Johnson's two hand-drawn maps identified street names and other landmarks. Iowa detectives quickly located two areas near Mason City, which, according to the maps, should contain the clandestine graves. Iowa authorities then contacted the St. Louis, Missouri, FBI Evidence Response Team (ERT) for forensic assistance. Additional assistance was requested of Omaha Division's FBI ERT and the ERT Unit (ERTU) based out of the FBI Laboratory in Quantico, Virginia. After securing federal search warrants that authorized examination of two possible burial sites, the ERT began its site investigations on October 11, 2000. The first scene was an abandoned farmstead and adjacent corn field along Killdeer Avenue in Cerro Gordo County. Soil coring and probing limited further subsurface searching to an area approximately 10 m x 50 m along the actively cultivated corn field. A cadaver dog and handler were unable to locate buried or surface-scattered remains. However, geophysical prospecting in the form of ground-penetrating radar identified so many subterranean anomalies as to make the technique ineffective (see Holland and Connell this volume for further discussion on the search and detection of human remains). The ERT selected what appeared to be the most promising area among the numerous anomalies and dug a 1 x 1 m test pit. However, the excavation revealed only the approximately 30-year-old burial of a calf, a large segment of metal rail, and other debris buried 63 cm (24.8 in) below the surface. Following a day of test excavations and sampling, the ERT decided to complete a site map of the farmstead and preliminary surveys for future searches that would entail removal of the upper levels of the cornfield plow zone using heavy equipment. This work proved crucial: investigators would return to this site a month later and find the remains of Terry DeGeus.

The following morning the ERT continued mapping the Killdeer Avenue site while other investigators began to search the second potential site, located on Lark Avenue. Here, certain landmarks were found that appeared consistent with one of Angela Johnson's jail house maps. Searchers were drawn to two vehicle tires beneath a bush in the area of Lark Avenue and a railroad right of way. They understood from Johnson's description that tires were placed over or near the grave. Again, a cadaver dog failed to alert to the area. Ground-penetrating radar indicated the existence of an anomaly below ground surface. Confirmation of possible buried remains was first received when a small piece of bone was found in the upper 20 cm of a soil core sample. This sample prompted more intrusive testing of the spot.

The excavation began by digging a small, controlled test pit, or "window," in what was thought to be the center of the anomaly as delineated by ground-penetrating radar. That small (40 cm x 35 cm x 30 cm) (16 x 14 x 12 in), rectangular pit revealed commingled animal and human bones. Above and among the clavicles of an adult human were what would later be identified as the bones of an opossum (*Didelphis virginiana*) and short-tailed shrew (*Blarina brevicauda*). If this was a mass grave of murder victims, the commingling of nonhuman remains at the top of the grave was initially puzzling. However, subsequent excavation revealed an infilled burrow, or "krotovina," which extended from the area of the opossum and shrew bones toward and through the eastern edge of the grave. What originally appeared as the intentional burial of road-kill, or a family pet, on top of human victims was demonstrated through archaeological excavation, geological characteristics, and zoological consultation to be the natural wintering and death of an opossum inside another rodent's abandoned chamber. A less controlled excavation and documentation of the remains and associated geotaphonomic evidence of bioturbation could have resulted in an incorrect or inconclusive explanation for the coexistence of the nonhuman and human occupants of the grave (see also Nawrocki this volume).

The creation of the initial excavation window, beyond offering the first confirmation of buried human remains, established a starting point for full excavation. It also offered an idea of how to orient the mapping system that would be used to record those excavations and their finds in three dimensions. A grid system of 1 x 1 m stringed units was established at ground surface over the interpreted size and orientation of the grave. After the existing surface was defoliated and its contours and cultural debris were mapped in relation to the three-dimensional grid system, excavation proceeded by expanding the initial excavation window across the exposed human remains toward the original edges of the grave feature. This expansion involved carefully slicing, in effect thin-sectioning, the fill from above the remains, keeping a vertical wall or profile of fill in front of the excavator throughout the process. As a result, evidence encountered in the excavated vertical profiles could be photographed and mapped *in situ* preserving their contexts in relation to the human remains and other features of the general scene. To preserve potential geotaphonomic tool marks, and to better clean the excavation, a vacuum was carefully used to clean loosened fill. All excavated fill was screened through a minimum ¼-in hardware cloth to recover smaller evidence possibly overlooked in the excavation. Screening was critical in that a decision was made to collect the skeletal remains

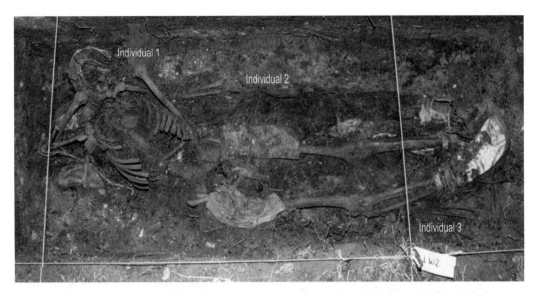

Figure 28.1   Full excavation to the top of Individual 1 resulting in the partial exposure of Individuals 2 and 3 (photograph Lavone Tienken, used with permission of M. Hochrein).

of each victim's hands and unclothed feet en masse rather than detail each phalange or carpal/tarsal. Although this technique did reduce excavation time in a situation in which multiple victims were interred, its downside was that some hand bones became commingled between victims, and a small number were not recovered.

After 24 hours of continuous excavation Individual 1, the uppermost skeleton in the grave, was completely exposed. Individual 1 was lying supine and slightly curved at the waist on top of Individual 2 (Figures 28.1 and 28.2). The wrists were bound by a clothesline-type ligature. Duct tape was wrapped around the eyes and nasal regions of the individual. A green synthetic fabric sock protruded from the mouth. Stitching around the torso indicated this individual was interred while wearing a natural fiber shirt or undershirt. Remnants of jeans or denim type pants included only the pocket linings, stitching, zipper, and some rivets. Behind the right hip was a billfold found to contain a driver's license bearing information for Gregory Nicholson. The right foot of the individual bore a white athletic sock and athletic shoe, and the left foot was covered only by a white athletic sock (Hochrein 2000: 57–58).

A large root that had grown over the femora of Individual 1 was later examined by a University of Missouri botanist. The dendrochronological conclusions were that a minimum of four growing seasons had passed in order for the root to grow to its collected size from the bush located on the south side of the grave. This did not contradict the purported timing of the victims' disappearances and supposed deaths approximately 7 years before. Bioturbation and root activity effectively sewed the remains of Individual 1 to the fill and to portions of Individual 2, extending the excavation time. Below the plow, or root, zone, subsequent victims were less affected and more easily extracted from the grave.

Individual 2 was found immediately below Individual 1 at depths between 40 cm (15.7 in) and 65 cm (25.6 in), and there was no stratigraphic evidence of fill or detritus between the skeletal remains. The skeleton was face down with clothesline-type ligatures around the left wrist and both ankles. As with Individual 1, duct tape was wrapped around the head, and a green synthetic fiber sock protruded from the mouth. Deteriorated segments of cloth and stitching indicated a shirt-type garment was worn at the time of disposal. Beneath the remnants of that garment was an intact brassiere. Additionally, this victim appeared to wear dark-colored sweat pants and white athletic socks. One athletic shoe was found between the feet (Hochrein 2000: 58).

As with Individuals 1 and 2, the lack of stratigraphy between Individuals 2, 3, and 4 indicated all were buried contemporaneously. Individual 3 was found immediately below Individual 2 at depths between 40 and 70 cm (15.7 and 27.6 in). The articulated remains were situated face down. Clothing associated with Individual Number 3 included a dresslike garment and apparent underpants, or panties. At depths between 50 and 77 cm

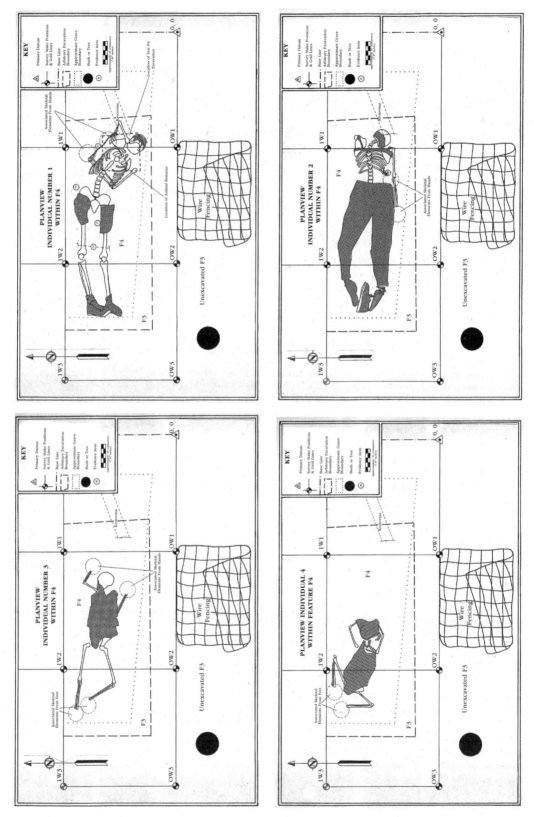

Figure 28.2 Plan views of Individuals 1–4 recovered from the mass grave (map by M. Hochrein).

(19.7 and 30.3 in), the remains of the smaller of the two juvenile victims were encountered directly beneath those of Individual Number 3. The articulated remains of the fourth victim lay supine. Most of the torso lay under and between the legs of Individual Number 3, and the legs were flexed into a frog or squatlike position. A shirt-type garment was pulled up and over the head, thus trapping the hands in the garment sleeves above the head. Other clothing associated with Individual Number 4 included a single piece, multicolored synthetic fiber swimsuit covering the torso.

Following 36 hours of excavation, mapping, and photography, all the human remains were removed from their secret interment. Documentation of the geotaphonomic record continued, however; as the grave was measured, a metal detector was used to search for additional evidence, and the grave walls were examined for evidence of possible tool marks. No additional ballistic evidence was recovered from the grave fill or beyond the grave walls. Although no tool marks were identified, clues of the grave's construction were reflected in its dimensions and microstratigraphy above the remains of Individual 1. The horizontal dimensions of the grave seemed just large enough to accommodate Individual 1, the tallest of the victims. All four victims were deposited in a grave that had a maximum depth of 77 cm (2.5 feet). The stratigraphy above Individual 1 consisted of individual lenses of soil consistent with the amounts of soil held in each shovel-full of backfill. Given these geotaphonomic characteristics, the conclusion was reached that this grave was excavated and filled using one or more hand shovels rather than heavy equipment.

Anthropological Analysis

Methodology

The autopsies of the first four victims were conducted jointly by the forensic pathologist and anthropologist. Each set of remains was placed on a gurney to be unwrapped, washed, and analyzed separately. The protocol was the same for all individuals and included an inventory of the bones and teeth present, a description of all clothing, ligatures, and personal effects, radiography, development of a biological profile, description and interpretation of perimortem and postmortem trauma, and photographic documentation. Soil from the clothing and pelvic and cranial cavities were carefully screened for additional physical evidence, such as projectiles. There was commingling of bones, principally of the subadults, at the bottom of the grave.

These were reassociated with the youngest two victims based on size and development. The biological profiles were consistent with the missing individuals, and the identifications of the adults were ultimately confirmed by dental analysis (see Clement this volume) and that of the subadults by mitochondrial DNA (mtDNA) (see Baker this volume). Thus, the importance of the anthropological analysis rested on the interpretation of perimortem trauma (see Loe this volume).

It was quickly evident that all four individuals suffered gunshot trauma. Typically, when a bullet penetrates a bone at or about a 90° angle it produces a beveled, circular defect that is widest away from the weapon. In other words, beveling occurs on the internal surface of a bone in an entrance wound and on the external surface for an exit wound (DiMaio 1999; Smith, Berryman, and Lahren 1987). These physical characteristics allow reconstruction of the trajectory of the bullet as it passed through the bone. If a projectile strikes the bone tangentially, then the bullet may graze the bone and produce a keyhole-shaped defect. The circular, internally beveled portion represents the entrance wound, whereas the adjacent triangular portion, surrounded by external beveling, is created when all or part of the bullet exits (Dixon 1982). Thus, the triangular portion points to the direction of fire.

In any case of violent death, blunt trauma to the skeleton must also be a concern for the anthropologist. However, since the bodies were buried for over 7 years, it is possible that fractures occurred after death and decomposition via bioturbation, surface pressures, and excavation. Thus, it is necessary to distinguish perimortem and postmortem fracture patterns. In general, perimortem fracture margins will be the same color as the surrounding bone because they have gone through the same postmortem processes. In this case, the bones were dark brown, the color of the soil, and so recent fresh postmortem fractures were easy to discern because the margins were much lighter in color than the surrounding bone. In addition, perimortem long-bone fractures may splinter and have adherent fragments with jagged edges, whereas dry bone is more brittle and will shatter into fragments of similar size (Maples 1986; Sauer 1998).

Analysis of the Victims

The skeleton of Individual 1, found at the top of the grave, was nearly complete and well preserved. Bindings of the face and appendages were observed as described above (Figure 28.3). The individual was estimated to be a 30–40 year-old

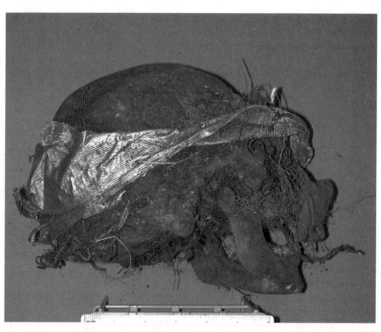

Figure 28.3   Skull of Individual 1, Greg Nicholson, with duct tape and a child's sock over the face (photograph permission of D. W. Steadman).

male of European descent who stood between 67 and 73 inches (175–183 cm). Antemortem pathology included spinal arthritis, a healed fracture of the right second metatarsal, and antemortem tooth loss. Dental records confirmed these were the remains of Greg Nicholson, who was 34 years old at the time of his disappearance.

A circular defect was located on the left occipital, immediately behind the left mastoid process. The internal beveling indicated this defect was a gunshot entrance wound and was accompanied by fractures that radiated through the basicranium, face, and left side of the skull. A bullet was located in the posterior nasal aperture, and there was no exit wound. The trajectory of the gunshot was therefore back to front and slightly left to right. Another gunshot wound was observed on the right 5th rib near the vertebral end. Beveling characteristics indicated a back to front trajectory. Finally, multiple perimortem fractures of the neural arch of the 4th cervical vertebra suggested direct trauma and/or severe rotation of the neck.

Individual 2 was buried immediately below Individual 1 in the mass grave and was similarly bound. The remains were of a 30–40 year-old female of European descent with a stature of 61–67 inches (159–167 cm). The spine and left shoulder exhibited osteoarthritis, and there were multiple dental restorations and some antemortem tooth loss. The remains were identified via dental

records as those of Lori Duncan, who was 31 years old when she disappeared.

Of all of the victims in the grave, Lori suffered the greatest amount of perimortem skeletal trauma. A large defect above the left orbit had extensive external beveling, indicating a gunshot exit wound. The shape was irregular, since it abutted a preexisting fracture radiating from the other side of the skull (Figure 28.4), but appeared to be an example of an exit keyhole wound (Dixon 1984). Both the circular and triangular portions exhibited external beveling and there was little internal beveling. A semicircular defect in the fractured greater wing of the right sphenoid was suspected to be the entrance wound, although this area of bone is too thin to demonstrate beveling (Quatrehomme and İşcan 1999). If this was the entrance wound, then the trajectory of the bullet was right to left and slightly upward. The facial skeleton was extremely fragmented and detached, as was the right side of the skull. There was also gunshot trauma of the proximal left ulna and at least two ribs. Though the trajectory of the bullet could not be determined for the ulna, one of the ribs demonstrated clear beveling that indicates a back to front bullet path. The findings suggested that there was a minimum of two gunshots, one to the head and one to the thorax. This is a conservative estimate, since it cannot be ruled out that the two rib wounds resulted from the same projectile and that the ulna could

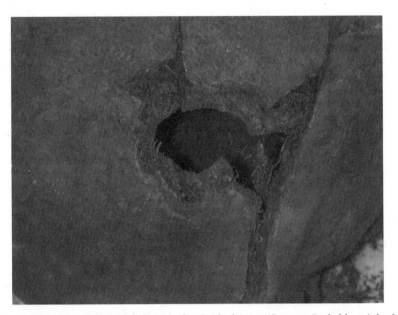

Figure 28.4   Gunshot wound of the left frontal of Individual 2, Lori Duncan. Probable exit keyhole wound (photograph permission of D. W. Steadman).

have been wounded by the same bullet that hit either the thorax or skull. Finally, the left 4th metacarpal and right ilium exhibit perimortem fractures due to blunt trauma.

Individual 3 was buried just below the adults and is the older of the two subadults. Sex cannot be estimated reliably for subadults because the pelvic and cranial characteristics do not diverge until after puberty (see Braz this volume). Based on the dental and long-bone development, age was estimated to be between 8 and 11 years. The skeleton did not exhibit antemortem pathology.

A gunshot entrance wound was present on the right superior occipital bone immediately below the Lambdoid suture and approximately 1.7 cm to the right of midline (Figure 28.5). Fractures radiated from the defect onto the right frontal, basicranium and left and right parietals. No distinct exit wound was identified, but the bullet likely exited through the upper facial region near the midline as evidenced by the jagged margins around areas of missing bone in the superior nasal aperture and left maxillo-orbital region. The facial bones were traumatically separated. The findings were consistent with a gunshot wound to the back of the head.

The last victim, Individual 4, was placed in the grave first and was the youngest. Based on dental and epiphyseal development, the age was estimated to be between 5 and 7 years. Sex was not estimated, and there were no skeletal pathologies.

A gunshot entrance wound was on the superior occipital bone just right of Lambda, very similar in location to that of Individual 3. Fractures radiated from the defect onto the right side of the skull and the basicranium. Part of the right temporal and sphenoid was detached from the skull, and the facial bones were too fragmentary to reconstruct.

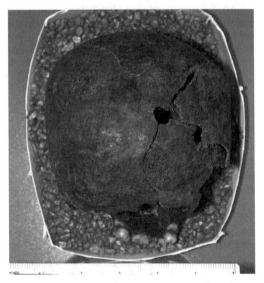

Figure 28.5   Gunshot entrance wound on the occipital of Individual 3, Kandace Duncan (photograph permission of D. W. Steadman).

The bullet likely exited the face near the midline, as evidenced by the jagged margins of the fractured superior nasal aperture. As with Individual 3, the trajectory of the gunshot was back to front.

Lori Duncan's children lacked dental records, so mitochondrial DNA (mtDNA) was sampled from the bones of Individuals 3 and 4 and compared to mtDNA of Lori Duncan's mother, who was still living. Unlike nuclear DNA, which is contributed by both parents, mtDNA is inherited only from the mother. In addition, mtDNA has a much lower statistical specificity than does nuclear DNA, since all maternally related individuals have identical mtDNA. Thus, confirming identifications in this case relied on multiple modalities. The mtDNA of both subadults were identical to each other and to Lori's mother, and the biological profiles were consistent with the missing girls. In addition, the clothing was identified by Lori's mother, and Lori's children were known to disappear at the same time as Lori. Through these means, 10-year-old Kandace and 6-year-old Amber Duncan were positively identified.

Although it is not possible for the anthropologist or pathologist to reconstruct which victim was killed first, it is clear that the Amber and Kandi were each shot in the back of the head, and the adults suffered multiple gunshot wounds as well as blunt trauma. The two children were placed in the grave first, followed by the two adults. The bullet recovered from Nicholson's skull, the only projectile recovered from the grave site, was too badly damaged to yield significant class information.

The Search for Terry DeGeus

Following the identification of the first four victims, investigators turned their attention to finding the body of Terry DeGeus. By November of 2000, the Killdeer Avenue site that had previously been searched by the ERT without success was now more accessible because the corn had been harvested. Using heavy equipment, investigators gradually removed thin layers of topsoil until they observed an area of soil that differed in color. When a boot was brought to the surface by heavy machinery, hand excavation of the grave began. The grave revealed the skeletonized remains of an adult buried face down with the legs bent such that the feet were above the buttocks. This matched the description on Johnson's map on which she had written: "The 1 is buried on his knees like he would make me be when I would beg for my life (face down)." The skeleton was clad in a hooded sweatshirt that covered the head, a jean jacket, metal accoutrements of pants, underwear with a handwritten name of "DeGeus, Terry"

on the band, a leather belt with a Harley Davidson buckle, socks and leather work boots. Several personal effects were also recovered from the grave, including a pack of cigarettes, money, a cigarette lighter, nail clippers, and a watch.

The anthropologist employed the same protocol as before to derive the biological profile and to interpret perimortem injuries. The remains were those of a 30–40-year-old male of European descent who stood between 65 and 71 in (170 and 178 cm) tall. Antemortem pathologies included osteoarthritis of the spine, a healed fracture of the left acromion process, and a well-healed fracture of the left fibula. The remains were positively identified as those of Terry DeGeus, aged 34 years, by comparison of antemortem and postmortem dental X rays.

The skeleton exhibited extensive perimortem trauma. The skull was highly fragmentary, and much of the anterior frontal bone and right inferolateral vault were missing, each area exhibiting multiple radiating fractures. Green staining, consistent with oxidizing copper, was noted on the internal aspect of the right temporal fragments. The location and distribution of the stains suggested perimortem fragmentation of the temporal bone, after which some bone fragments were in contact with metal during decomposition. A copper jacket was found inside the sweatshirt hood that covered the skull. A semicircular defect was present on the greater wing of the right sphenoid. As this is a naturally thin area of bone, beveling characteristics were not present. The bullet likely entered the right side of the skull and exited the left frontal.

A gunshot wound of the third thoracic vertebra was evidenced by bone loss of the anterior centrum and copper staining. Further, radiographs revealed metallic fragments embedded in the margins of the wound. The left proximal humerus also exhibited gunshot trauma and fragments of bone and metal remained embedded in the medullary cavity. The trajectory of these wounds could not be determined. There was also a gunshot wound on the iliac crest of the left ilium. Beveling indicated a back to front and slightly right to left trajectory. A minimum of three bullets penetrated this individual—the skull, thorax, and pelvis. The gunshot to the humerus could have been coincident with the skull or thorax trauma. Perimortem fractures of the dentition indicated Terry DeGeus also suffered blunt trauma.

The Prosecutions of Honken and Johnson

With the discovery and successful identification and analysis of perimortem trauma of all five missing persons, criminal proceedings could move forward against Dustin Honken and Angela Johnson. The investigation of the murders was over 10 years old, and hundreds of witnesses and informants had been interviewed. Prosecutors waded through scores of boxes of evidence and records to decide who to subpoena to testify in court. The prosecution sought to demonstrate that Dustin Honken masterminded the efforts to eliminate DeGeus and Nicholson so they could not testify against him on the earlier drug charges. The Duncan family was simply collateral damage.

On August 30, 2001, Dustin Honken, now 33 years old, was charged with five counts of federal witness tampering murder, five counts of drug conspiracy murder, five counts of continuing criminal enterprise murder, one count of soliciting murder of a witness, and one count of conspiracy to tamper with and solicit the murder of a witness. Honken was tried in the United States District Court for the Northern District of Iowa. In addition to informants, several forensic expert witnesses testified. The maps drawn by Angela Johnson that led investigators to the graves were introduced into evidence, and an FBI ERT specialist testified as to the location and recovery of the remains. Two forensic pathologists from the Office of the Iowa State Medical Examiner testified that the cause of death was gunshot trauma and the manner of death was homicide for each individual. In the United States, only forensic pathologists are legally empowered to determine manner of death (homicide, suicide, accidental, natural, or undetermined). Next, the forensic anthropologist provided lengthy testimony on the perimortem trauma suffered by each individual. Finally, a firearms expert testified that spent bullets recovered from DeGeus had class characteristics consistent with having been fired from a Tec-9.

Following a lengthy defense, the jury received the case. After deliberating for 17 hours over three days, the jury returned guilty verdicts on all counts. After a penalty proceeding that lasted several days, the same jury sentenced Dustin Honken to life in prison for the counts relating to the murders of the three adults and sentenced him to death for the murders of Kandi and Amber Duncan. The trial, including the penalty phase and deliberations, lasted 11 weeks.

The trial of Angela Johnson began in the same courtroom approximately five months later. She faced five counts of drug conspiracy murder and five counts of continuing criminal enterprise murder. The forensic experts again presented their evidence. A different jury found Angela Johnson guilty as charged on all counts. After a short penalty phase proceeding, the jury sentenced Johnson to life in prison for the two counts relating to the murder of Greg Nicholson and imposed a penalty of death in connection with the counts relating to each of the other four murder victims. Johnson's trial took 10 weeks.

These cases were remarkable in several respects, not the least of which was the application of the death penalty in the state of Iowa. Though Iowa does not have the death penalty, the death penalty could be applied because these proceedings were in federal court. Although prosecution of a federal death penalty case in a non-death-penalty state is not unprecedented, it is rare. Some local controversy was generated by the fact that for the first (and second) time in more than 40 years a jury of Iowans was called on to deliberate in a death penalty case. In addition, Angela Johnson achieved the dubious distinction of being the first woman in America to receive a federal death sentence since the early 1950s, when Ethel Rosenberg resided on death row.

Conclusion

This case exemplifies the multidisciplinary cooperation required for murder investigations. Dogged perseverance on the part of the investigators kept this from becoming another missing persons "cold case." It must be noted that our discussion has focused on only a small portion of the total forensic effort; there are many other important facets of the investigation not described here, including firearms, document, DNA, and fingerprint analyses.

This case also demonstrates how archaeology, properly applied in concert with other forensic specialties, can be used as a tool for reconstructing the events of a crime rather than merely collecting evidence from a scene. The archaeological excavation of the Lark Avenue grave site demonstrated the amount of contextual information that can be gleaned beyond the victims' skeletons. In this case, plant activity offered chronological information about the victims' interments. The recorded remnants of each victim's clothing, such as a bathing suit, suggested the time of year the murders took place. Geological evidence explained the presence of nonhuman animal activity within the grave. Zoology helped to distinguish the natural versus intentional placement of nonhuman animal remains. Finally, stratigraphic evidence and three-dimensional mapping of each victim's position within the grave helped to clarify and confirm perimortem activity and to compare that with witness and subject statements.

Perhaps the most salient effect of applying archaeology at this crime scene was the manner in which it allowed for the recreation of the scene for juries in Dustin Honken's and Angela Johnson's federal trials. They could better imagine the horrors of that night in 1993 in seeing how the children were thrown into the grave, their hands so close to their mother's. The jury could reflect on the last moments of Greg Nicholson and Lori Duncan lives—each bound with duct tape around their faces and the children's socks in their mouths. Similarly, the detailed anthropological description of the perimortem injuries, especially of the little girls, created a great deal of tension and sympathy in the courtroom. Although juries have come to expect much forensic fanfare (the so-called CSI effect), careful investigation and analysis allow investigators to accurately and respectfully tell the story of each victim without sensationalism.

Note

1. The authors received permission to use real names of the defendants and victims by the U.S. Attorney General's office, since the trials of those charged for the murders detailed in this case study are complete. All information provided at the trial by the authors is in the public record via trial transcripts. The authors chose not to use the names of various informants.

References

DiMaio, V. 1999. *Gunshot Wounds: Practical Aspects of Firearms, Ballistics and Forensic Techniques* (2nd ed.). Boca Raton, FL: CRC Press.

Dixon, D. 1982. Keyhole lesions in gunshot wounds of the skull and direction of fire. *Journal of Forensic Sciences* 27(3): 555–566.

———. 1984. Exit keyhole lesion and direction of fire in a gunshot wound of the skull. *Journal of Forensic Sciences* 29(1): 336–339.

Hochrein, M. J. 2000. Federal Bureau of Investigation Evidence Response Team Crime Scene Investigation, Killdeer Avenue and Lark Avenue Sites, Cerro Gordo County, Iowa, October 11–13, 2000. Unpublished manuscript.

Maples, W. R. 1986. Trauma analysis by the forensic anthropologist, in K. J. Reichs (ed.), *Forensic Osteology: Advances in the Identification of Human Remains*, pp. 218–228. Springfield, IL: Charles C. Thomas.

Quatrehomme, G., and İşcan, M. Y. 1999. Characteristics of gunshot wounds in the skull. *Journal of Forensic Sciences* 44(3): 568–576.

Sauer, N. 1998. The timing of injuries and manner of death: Distinguishing among antemortem, perimortem and postmortem trauma, in K. J. Reichs (ed.), *Forensic Osteology: Advances in the Identification of Human Remains* (2nd ed.), pp. 321–332. Springfield, IL: Charles C. Thomas.

Smith, O. C., Berryman, H., and Lahren, C. 1987. Cranial fracture patterns and estimate of direction from low velocity gunshot wounds. *Journal of Forensic Sciences* 32(5): 1416–1421.

Domestic Homicide Investigations in the United Kingdom

John Hunter

Forensic archaeology is now a relatively well-accepted discipline among police forces in the United Kingdom (U.K.). Operational work stems from the late 1980s, and the development of the discipline is well recorded together with summary case studies (Hunter and Cox 2005). The work has to be understood within the context of U.K. policing and law enforcement structure; there is no national police force as such, but instead there are over 40 individual regional forces, each of which is largely autonomous and responsible to its own public Police Authority (44 forces in England, Wales, and Northern Ireland; eight in Scotland). The government department known as the Home Office coordinates certain activities, notably training, specialist types of operational support from the National Crime and Operations Faculty (NCOF), and central intelligence databases, but police forces otherwise operate independently. There are no full-time professional forensic archaeologists in the U.K. Individuals tend to be invited to incidents either because they are known to, or have worked for, the police force on the case or because a police force has requested specialist assistance from the NCOF, which keeps a central register of experts.

It is now also likely that a force may consult the register of the Council for the Registration of Forensic Practitioners (CRFP) for suitable personnel. The register was established in 2000 at the behest of the Home Office in order to ensure that forensic personnel working in laboratories or at crime scenes were competent to do so and that the courts could be satisfied that evidence given was of appropriate weight and value (www.crfp.org). The long-term intention of the CRFP is to provide a future environment in which all forensic practitioners working in the U.K. are registered and revalidated on a regular basis. Identified sectors of expertise (including archaeology and anthropology) were encouraged to identify criteria by which individuals could be deemed "competent" by their peers. In the U.K., *archaeology* is concerned with the recovery and recording of buried remains whereas *anthropology* is more strictly concerned with the study of (human) skeletal remains, buried or otherwise. At the time of writing, registered numbers are high in certain disciplines (for example, scene investigation and fingerprints) but relatively small in others, such as forensic archaeology, where the professional community is also small. Inevitably, U.K. courts now place emphasis on querying why some expert witnesses are *not* registered in their particular field, and therefore may query their level of competence.

The Investigation of a Scene of Crime

As elsewhere, the investigation of a homicide scene in the U.K. can involve many individuals under the overall management of a senior detective, in the U.K. known as a Senior Investigating Officer (SIO). The scene itself will be coordinated by a Crime Scene Manager (CSM) and draw on Scene of Crime Officers (SOCOs), sometimes known as Crime Scene Investigators (CSI) or Forensic Scene Investigators (FSI), for much of the basic recording, sampling, and recovery of evidence. There will also be a Scientific Support Manager (SSM) in each force whose responsibility it is to advise the SIO on techniques, specialist equipment, and skill areas that individual incidents might require. There is no state-funded forensic science service in the U.K., and the deployment of specialists must be within budget. Nor is there any obligation for the SIO to take advice or to utilise any forensic specialist (including an archaeologist). However, the growing number of court cases in which defence counsel is requesting independent archaeological comment is making this situation less likely.

Other experts drawn in might typically include forensic scientists (including specialists in entomology, palynology, fingerprints, and fibres) with whom the archaeologist may need to work closely. It is not a matter of imposing rigid archaeological methodology but ensuring that there is mutual understanding of each person's evidential requirements. Given the diverse nature of skill backgrounds among the personnel involved in the U.K., there can be a strong element of "mission" in the archaeologist's work, as well as the need to understand the theory and processes of others. Nowhere is this more important than in the relationship with the forensic pathologist, who plays a pivotal role in any incident in which human remains are involved. Unlike in the United States (U.S.), where the equivalent individual (the Medical Examiner) will be largely familiar with the work of anthropologists, in the U.K., the evolution of both anthropology and archaeology is distinctive.

Here, archaeology has a very specific field-based origin, whereas in the U.S. it has a more specific historical association with human remains under the umbrella of anthropology. Because of these differences, the need to build operational relationships with the forensic pathologists in the U.K. has been more complex (see also Cox this volume for discussions about anthropology) but also more rewarding in its success. At the end of the day, it is the forensic pathologist who probably carries the greatest weight in court in providing evidence for cause and manner of death, and as a result his or her wishes at a scene will almost certainly be given priority by the SIO. As in all cases, the best results derive from considered planning and briefings between those in the front line, typically the pathologist, the archaeologist and the scene of crime officer; this is illustrated in some of the cases discussed below.

The U.K. criminal justice system also presents some idiosyncratic features that may affect the manner in which an investigation occurs and with which the forensic archaeologist will certainly need to be familiar. There are three pieces of legislation of particular importance to the forensic archaeologist: the Prosecution of Offences Act 1985 (POA 1986); the Criminal Procedure and Investigations Act (CPIA 1996), and the Police and Criminal Evidence Act 1984 (PACE 1984).[1]

In the U.K., the police no longer prosecute offences themselves; this process is undertaken by a body known as the Crown Prosecution Service (CPS) under the terms of the Prosecution of Offences Act 1985 (POA 1986). The CPS is an independent authority that undertakes prosecutions in court; it advises police whether sufficient evidence has been gathered to enable the likelihood of a successful prosecution, or indeed whether it is even in the public interest to prosecute at all. Although archaeologists may be brought into an enquiry and remunerated by the police, they are, like any other forensic expert, expected to provide objective scientific evidence. They will be independent witnesses of the court, whether they have been called by either the CPS or the defence. The process is aimed at ensuring that the criminal justice process is played fairly, and this intent now also extends to the sharing of evidence, a process known as "disclosure," by both adversarial parties under the terms of the Criminal Procedure and Investigations Act (CPIA 1996). Put simply, they require that all records made by investigating personnel in whatever form—written, tape-recorded, photographed, planned, or sketched—are disclosable. All this information is collected, collated, and logged, is made available to the court to both prosecution and defence counsels, and can be used as evidence. In archaeological terms, this information includes plans, section drawings, record sheets, notes, and, on longer-term projects, day-books or similar. These will be open to scrutiny; hence any altered plans, changed interpretations, illegible sketches, lack of completed fields on record sheets, and such can be used to criticise professional integrity. Equally, verbose reports will provide greater opportunity for questioning under cross-examination. There is a fine balance to be made.

The final piece of legislation is particularly relevant in those operations that take place while a suspect is being detained in custody in England and Wales. According to the terms of the Police and Criminal Evidence Act 1984 (PACE 1984), detention in custody is strictly time-limited (see Dilley 2005: Figure 7.3). Initially set at 24 hours, this period of detention can be extended to 96 hours via a series of legal stages after which the suspect must be formally charged with an offence or released; in Scotland, the period is much less. The operational effect of this is that the recovery of appropriate or necessary evidence (for example, locating and excavating of human remains) may have clearly defined time limits imposed. Failure to respond successfully during this period of detention may result in the suspect tampering with or moving buried evidence on release. To counter this, the precise archaeological parameters, as well as the logistics in terms of equipment, mechanical excavators, personnel, and other resources, need to be determined well in advance. Knowledge of site history will need to be commensurate with working within the timeframe available.

These general points provide the context for a range of domestic case studies in the U.K. that have had an archaeological involvement. All scenarios are different, and it is difficult to divide the various criminal investigations in which archaeology contributes into "types." Nevertheless, general case experience suggests that archaeological input falls broadly under the four main headings: (1) disappearances of named individuals; (2) search and recovery of nonhuman buried items; (3) allegations of anonymous human remains buried in specific locations; (4) accidental discovery of human remains. These are by no means exclusive, but they embrace a typical range of scenes.

Disappearances of Named Individuals

This type of input probably constitutes only a minor part of the forensic archaeological case load but is given preference in this chapter, because it tends to illustrate the full nature of the archaeologist's role and contribution. It is always a reminder that forensic searching for buried human remains is as much about elimination as it is about finding and recovering. Search methodologies tend to target specific locations as being significant, or as priority, according to suspect movement, psychological profiling, witness account, or other methodologies. Each target area needs to given defined boundaries, searched thoroughly, and if unproductive, eliminated.

Many investigators of disappearances now tend to utilise archaeologists very early in the process, especially if there is a high probability of burial. A case in point was that of a young male, believed murdered during a drugs dispute. His disappearance was reported to the police by family members, but it was unclear where he may have been deposited. The police had very few starting points but had identified through intelligence a number of locations around the country that were known to have been used by the drugs gang. Each of these became the target of a specific search, and an archaeologist was invited to each briefing to give advice and help devise an appropriate strategy.

The availability of aerial photographs was essential to each site, particularly for those sites that might be sensitive to a police presence. Some of the target areas (building sites or wasteland) could be visited safely before devising a strategy. Others relied only on covert helicopter photography, one in particular being a large country house with outbuildings. Nevertheless, this photograph could be used to identify possible foci of interest such as disturbed ground; it could determine which types of geophysical survey (if any) might be effective according to landscape and, by comparison with earlier photographs, show if any outbuildings or terraces had been built since the victim disappeared. On the basis of this, a search plan for the land and the buildings was devised between the investigation team and the police force in whose area the building was located. It involved using the local Police Search Advisors (POLSAs), who worked closely with the archaeologists to establish an optimum strategy. After careful preparation, this strategy was implemented early one morning after the issuing of a search warrant. Specialist search teams scoured the house and outbuildings, the geophysicists undertook survey work on new terraces and outbuildings, the archaeologists tested potential disturbances identified from the air, and a cadaver dog was used to test any anomalies. The process took less than one working day but was sufficiently thorough to ensure that the whole complex could be eliminated with a high degree of confidence.

Attention then moved to other sites, one in particular lying in the north of England in an open rural area. This site had also been photographed, and a possible disturbed target excavated and eliminated. However, intelligence had also pointed to a corner of a water-logged field nearby that merited attention; it measured some 70 x 50 m and was used as a storage area for horse manure. The practicalities of the exercise were such that machine stripping was seen as the best way forward, given that the topsoil/manure layers were relatively shallow and that any disturbance into the yellow clay substrate would be readily visible once the topsoil had been removed. The machine used a wide toothless ditching bucket and was supported by a cadaver dog to test any anomalies found; it stripped the higher part of the area, but water-logging made it impossible to machine on the lower part. No large intrusions were found, but the machining did expose a narrow linear feature cut into the clay, presumably a field drain that allowed water to flow down into the water-logged area. Because of its indistinct nature when first exposed, it was vented for the cadaver dog (that is, probed carefully to allow any gasses to be emitted). The dog responded in a half-hearted way, but despite further venting in the immediate area it was not possible to focus the dog's response. It was assumed that any source might be higher up the pipeline, but the machine stripping had identified no intrusion.

A few months later, when the water-logging was less inhibiting, the lower part of the field was stripped and revealed a grave-shaped disturbance. This feature was cleaned and defined using trowels and partially excavated by careful sectioning at one end. Evidence of human remains were found, the area was immediately designated a crime scene, and a forensic pathologist was called. Reference to the previous search plans showed that the grave was located along the line of the field drain and only a few metres from the point where the dog had previously responded, but downstream. The sensitivity of the dog appears to have been such that it had picked up the scent of the cadaver *upstream*, rather than downstream from the source as had been assumed.

The discovery was made at approximately 11.00 A.M., but the casework of the pathologist was such that his arrival was not until about 5.00 P.M. During this time the area was made secure, the scene was tented and additional uniformed officers drafted in from the local police force. The pathologist had already worked with archaeologists on previous occasions, which led to a mutually comfortable operational arrangement. After discussion, it was agreed that the two archaeologists would each work in a different half of the grave, leaving a narrow baulk between the two in order to record the nature of the burial infill. This allowed the process to proceed more quickly, given that it was winter, the temperature was around zero, and there were strong winds and heavy rain. The method of excavation was to remove the infill in each half in arbitrary spits of about 10 cm each and record them on context sheets. Each spit was numbered, and any exhibit seized was numbered

in a different sequence but cross-referenced to the spit number. This approach allowed a coarse but effective method of relocating exhibits in three dimensions at either end of the grave. Electronic recording systems would have been less effective, given the small nature of the area being excavated and the prevailing weather. The deposits of each spit were retained in sealed, numbered plastic dustbins for later attention if required. As the body became more exposed, the pathologist became progressively more involved, checking for trauma, and advising on how the individual might have been deposited, in order to facilitate the excavation and lifting. Water-logging became a major problem: even in the early stages of excavation the grave would fill up, and the excavation of a drainage channel running downhill out of the grave appeared to make little impression. However, it soon became clear that when the grave was originally dug, the field drain had been severed, allowing water to flow continuously into the grave (Figure 29.1).

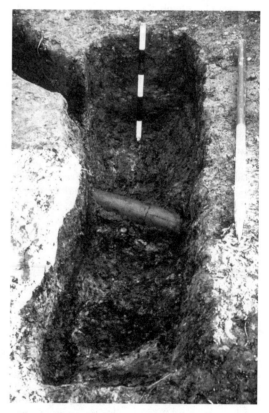

Figure 29.1 Photograph showing the excavated grave. The fractured field drain served to provide both positive and negative aspects to the excavation. The channel to the left was the result of an attempt to drain the grave during excavation.

This problem was eventually resolved by using the machine excavator to remove a large sump through the field drain upstream of the grave allowing the water to be channelled away from the scene.

The victim had become substantially skeletonised as a result of the bacteria present in the horse manure, and very little soft tissue had survived. This situation made the collection of the smaller skeletal elements difficult in the muddy infill, but it also had the advantage of exposing the bone surface and with it evidence of any hard-tissue trauma. For example, the body was face down and exhibited a projectile entry wound in the back of the head. Until this point, the archaeologists had been concerned with maintaining the physical integrity of the remains prior to lifting and postmortem examination, identifying correctly the grave edges, recording accurately, and checking for foreign materials in the fill. The bullet wound required a new interrogation of the data. Had the victim been shot in the grave, or had he been shot elsewhere and transported to the disposal site? And would it be possible to determine this archaeologically? Would there be projectiles still lodged in the body, or would they have penetrated the grave bottom? With all this in mind, the body was then fully exposed, the baulk recorded and removed, and the body then lifted into a body bag and taken away for postmortem examination. This recovery exercise lasted some 8 hours, and the archaeologists returned the following morning to remove the lowest deposits in the grave (that is, those under the body), record the grave profile, and check the grave bottom and walls for projectiles with a metal detector.

A statement was subsequently prepared by each archaeologist detailing the process and the findings, supported by all disclosable material such as plans, record cards, and photographs. Under the terms of the CPIA, the statements were made available to the defence. When the case came to trial many months later, the archaeological evidence was used as part of the CPS argument but was not cross-examined. The defendant was found guilty and was sentenced to life imprisonment.

Another case involved the disappearance of a young woman and her 3-year-old son in 1976. It represents a "cold-case" review, and the case remains an issue of local intrigue in the Inverness area of Scotland.

Cold-case reviews of major unsolved crimes occur at regular intervals. Different officers are used, partly to review what has already been undertaken and to consider new options and developed technologies but equally to provide a fresh set of ideas and attitudes. In several long-standing cases,

DNA techniques that were unavailable at the time a crime was committed have enabled well-publicised convictions to be made. Similar developments have been made in search techniques, and there is now increased awareness of the availability of geophysics, the relevance of offender profiling, and of search strategies and recording. Officers faced with a search review may well draft in areas of expertise that were not available or utilised in the original enquiry. Being a relatively recent part of the forensic scenario, archaeology often falls within this category.

The woman had been having an affair; she had separated amicably from her husband and had settled in a different area. Months later her burned-out car was discovered on the main A9 road in Scotland, and subsequent large-scale searches failed to find either her or her young son. A disused sand/gravel quarry nearby was infilled a matter of only days afterward and appears not to have been searched by police until the following year, when excavation work commenced. Part of the infill was removed, but the investigation was halted two weeks later through lack of resources. By then, the open quarry had been landscaped, filled with debris and building materials from the road workings, and covered in top soil. The police excavations of 1977 were unproductive, but in the years that followed, local interest and curiosity developed, culminating in a television programme broadcast in 2003 that pointed to the disused quarry as needing renewed investigation.

To their credit, the local police force, Northern Constabulary, reviewed the situation and agreed to have the quarry excavated archaeologically in order either to find the remains of the two victims or to have it eliminated from the enquiry and from local folklore. Various briefings took place with archaeologists, anthropologists, and others through the Centre for International Forensic Assistance, and a strategy was devised for its excavation. By then, the former quarry was barely identifiable: the edges were unrecognisable, and planted pines had grown to a height of over 12 m. Earlier aerial photographs had enabled the quarry perimeter to be defined, and arrangements were made to remove the trees across an area of over 100 m in diameter. The depth to the quarry floor was unrecorded, and it was difficult to ascertain exactly how long the project would take. The area was fenced off, temporary office facilities brought in, and the site was manned and made secure for a period predicted to be between four to six weeks. Geophysics was not feasible owing to the potential depth and size of the targets, but ground-penetrating radar (GPR) was considered as a possible method of identifying the sand and gravel quarry base and walls. However, because much of the infill was also of sand and gravel, this was rejected as a useful way forward. Before excavation work commenced, a company specialising in 3D-recording using an automated reflectorless system surveyed the area.

A machine trench was used to ascertain the depth of the quarry. Trial work showed that at least 3–5 m of deposits needed to be removed before the original quarry bottom and terraces could be exposed. Any human remains were considered to lie within the scree on the quarry terraces rather than in the infill. Nevertheless, when excavation took place archaeologists and anthropologists were assigned to each of the two 360° excavators and 20-ton dumper trucks on a watching brief basis. The quarry was effectively half-sectioned, excavated stratigraphically like a large archaeological pit, and recorded contextually: the latest infills were removed first; the trench dug by the police in 1977 was identified and excavated; the quarry landscaping was reversed, and the terraces and floors were returned to their original state of 1976 (Figure 29.2).

Throughout the operation, spatial records were made using a total station electronic measurement system (EDM) supplied and operated by the police Accident Investigation Unit. The entire process took over four weeks and required the excavation of an estimated 37,000 tons of material. The result was the return of the quarry to its original state allowing the terraces and floors to be examined in order to locate any victims. These surfaces were searched thoroughly, including the use of cadaver dogs, but no human remains were found. The ledges were then overcut by machine with a watching brief in order to confirm absence of any further anthropogenic activity. The exercise initially involved two anthropologists and two archaeologists, but as the extent and nature of the exercise became clearer this was changed to three archaeologists and one anthropologist with another anthropologist on stand-by. There were daily briefings with the police, but the strategy decisions were largely made by the archaeologists. At the end of the excavation, it was possible to assert that no remains had been deposited there, as opposed to the fact that no remains had been found. The distinction is significant. The search was also concentrated in the area immediately adjacent to the quarry with detailed records maintained. These will be of value if the area is again subjected to enquiry.

Search and Recovery of Nonhuman Buried Items

The scale of the operation can be contrasted with the search of a small garden of an urban terraced house measuring c. 10 x 5 m. Neither case had used archaeology previously. However, the focus of the search here was a possible buried firearm, which may (or may not) have been concealed during a particular period of tenancy that lasted only a few years. The investigation was planned very carefully and involved numerous briefings for all concerned. It also necessitated compiling a history

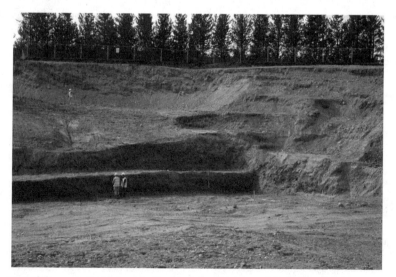

Figure 29.2   Part of the excavated quarry in Scotland showing the original shape of the quarry ledges before infilling and landscaping in 1976.

of the garden in order to ascertain which elements of the garden (for example, layers of terrace, flower borders, pathways) were created or were used by particular tenants during the occupancy of the house throughout its 40-year life. Operational police personnel had been trained by the archaeologists, and a simulated site had been prepared for trial purposes in advance of the actual operation. On site, before excavation took place, both GPR and magnetometry were used, but only after substantial ferrous features, including doors, were physically removed from the surrounding environment to minimise background "noise."

Each geophysical method produced its own set of responses and anomalies, some in common; these were investigated by hand and a small number of ferrous objects recovered. However, the nature of the enquiry necessitated more sensitive evidence, including DNA from appropriate relevant stratigraphic contexts. In view of this, all the personnel (which consisted of two archaeologists, one of whom was a specialist in conservation, and a small number of archaeologically trained police search officers) were suitably clothed to prevent DNA contamination, and all equipment used was new and additionally cleaned with anticontaminant gel. The garden was excavated stratigraphically, and all soil layers (a total of only some 6 tons, compared to the 37,000 tons in Scotland) were hermetically sealed in polythene bags before removal from the scene. On the basis of the background history of the garden, it was possible to identify particular layers or contexts as being of priority value for further attention by sieving. The net result was that the rear garden of the property was "deconstructed" down to the natural bedrock by appropriate stratigraphic means. This gave the police and forensic teams the opportunity to examine individual archaeological contexts of proven chronological association in order to further their enquiry. This was very much a team effort; the operation lasted two days, but the sieving and further scrutiny of the layers continued for several weeks thereafter. The results of the sieving are not known.

On another occasion, a kidnapper had successfully eluded a police trap and had escaped with a substantial sum of money packed into a holdall. When eventually apprehended, he was charged with both kidnapping and with the murder of a previous victim. However, the ransom was nowhere to be found, and the incident enquiry team set up an investigation for its location. Evidence was drawn in from a number of sources, including eyewitness accounts, criminal profilers, and military fieldcraft experts and others, and a focal area

of interest was eventually identified. This centred on a bridge adjacent to a main railway line with cultivated fields either side of the railway cutting. An archaeologist was brought in to support the enquiry, essentially to determine whether any disturbances were visible in the railway cutting and to add comment on the overall search focus. It was initially clear that the railway had been cut through bedrock and that burial of even a holdall would have been impossible. However, at the top of one side of the cutting, fenced from a cultivated field, was a strip of scrub woodland running parallel with the railway. It was agreed that this should be searched using geophysical survey techniques. In this case, GPR was the most feasible method. The target area was some 50 m in length and some 3 m wide. It contained some fly tipping and a few areas of loose rubble. Later it was found that one of these rubble patches was acting as a marker for the buried holdall. The GPR survey identified a large number of anomalies, each of which was investigated by hand until the holdall was found. This investigation was seen as a major achievement for teamwork and led to the successful conviction of the offender.

Allegations of Anonymous Human Remains Buried in Specific Locations

There are a substantial number of instances in which members of the public feel obliged, after years of soul searching, to confess to having witnessed serious crimes in the distant past. Typically, a person will admit to having seen a victim being buried in a particular location, but invariably there is never a missing person or a named offender to place in context. However, the location is always specific, such as in the corner of a garden, or by a certain tree in woodland. There is rarely any corroborating evidence, but the police have an obligation to take the information seriously. From an archaeological point of view, the situation is relatively straightforward and involves simple testing or ground-truthing of the location in question. One such case involved the edge of a golf course in a woodland clearing. The informant took officers to a small hollow at the edge of the course and pointed to a low-lying area of vegetation in the middle. The officers and the archaeologist agreed that any investigation should be bounded within an area measuring some 3 × 2 m centred on this location. Systematic probing demonstrated consistent hard-compacted substrates across the whole area but indicated softer ground in the lowest-lying parts at the centre. This was subsequently sectioned and shown to be an area of softer earth presumably resulting from water-logging. There was no evidence of any previous anthropogenic activity, and the file was closed.

Incidents such as this can usually be resolved directly by careful invasive means. Other methods, such as geophysical survey, are rarely necessary, especially if the location can be pinpointed and will need to be excavated anyway. In one case, the release of a notorious paedophile from gaol, marked by intense media interest, caused one elderly lady apparently to recognise him from the newspaper photograph. She had seen him, she claimed, years earlier trampling down loose earth at the edge of woodland. She was adamant that he was the man in question, but she was unable to define the location other than the general area of a field corner. Fieldcraft showed no suspicious vegetational or topographic features. Geophysics was commissioned in order to narrow down the area in question, and a cadaver dog was introduced in order to check any resulting anomalies. Again, boundaries were defined, and the geophysical (resistivity) survey identified two anomalies, neither of which was of appropriate size. Each was tested by the dog, which responded to neither. One was in very open landscape, but the other was more secluded, and this was sectioned by the archaeologists before being fully eliminated (Figure 29.3).

Geophysics was also used to eliminate the garden of a property in which a woman claimed her father had murdered and buried a prostitute. The alleged incident had occurred almost two decades earlier and the woman had a history of drug abuse.

Nevertheless, it was felt that the allegation could not be ignored, and archaeologists were brought in to devise a search strategy. The house in question was a council property with a relatively secluded rear garden measuring some 20 x 10 m and a very small front garden that was open to the road and in full view of other houses. Both were flat and grass covered. It would have been possible to excavate both parts of the garden fully using Operational Support Unit (OSU) officers, but this approach would have been both obtrusive and costly and unlikely to have been justified on the strength of the information received. It was also in a city area that was not particularly police-friendly. Instead, both parts of the garden were gridded out for a resistivity survey, and the work was carried out in a few hours. After data processing, it was seen that there were no significant anomalies in the rear garden but that there was an oblong lower resistance anomaly in the front garden. This was subsequently sectioned by the archaeologists (dressed in the guise of workmen) and found to be a former flowerbed. The file was then closed. In this case, as in all others, investigation progressed from the non-invasive to the invasive in order to minimise any potential loss of evidence.

However, a greater problem arises when one is dealing with alleged infanticide or neonatal disposals, which, given the victims' size, are probably the hardest to search for. Adult victims are rarely physically transported very far because of the weight factor, but newborn or premature individuals can be more easily carried and disposed of. Nevertheless, if they are buried, the minimum size

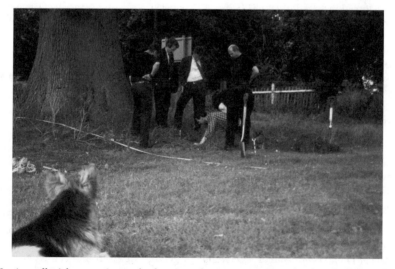

Figure 29.3 A small trial excavation took place in order to test an anomaly identified through geophysical survey. A cadaver dog was also used.

is likely to be that of a spade width, perhaps some 30 × 30 cm, and likely to be detectable in otherwise undisturbed ground by a careful geophysics or clearance strategy.

In one instance, the allegation was that the individual was located in an unused grassy part of a graveyard measuring about 4 × 4 m. This area was surveyed using resistivity at 25-cm intervals, and a small number of anomalies were found, all of appropriate size. The turf was carefully removed in a square around each and the topsoil trowelled back to undisturbed natural deposits. In each case, the anomaly had been created by tree or plant roots. After this, the SIO asked for the whole area of 4 × 4 m to be cleared; turf was removed and the topsoil trowelled down to undisturbed substrates. No further disturbances were identified and the file was closed.

A similar allegation involved the rear garden of a terraced house, but here, in order to avoid suspicion, access could not be made until the morning of the search. However, a covert aerial photograph had identified that the garden was predominantly of grass, and as a result a resistivity survey was planned. However, it was discovered that the grass and topsoil had been superimposed over concrete, effectively making the technique unviable. Fortunately, a GPR system was also available. GPR is unique in being able to penetrate dense materials, and this case identified a number of anomalies. The entire concrete was lifted and disposed of into a pre-arranged skip, and the underlying deposits investigated by hand. None of the anomalies or any of the other features contained human remains.

Accidental Discovery of Human Remains

All the preceding examples were investigated as a result of careful planning and briefing, but there are many cases that occur at short notice, usually because human remains have been discovered during building operations or by people enjoying leisure activities. One such instance occurred when articulated skeletal remains were discovered by children playing in woodland. The remains lay on the side of a steep bank and were partially covered in soil and obscured by vegetation. The area was immediately taped off, and the SIO kept the site secure until an archaeologist and an anthropologist could be brought in at short notice. The archaeologist was able to determine that the remains had not been intentionally buried but had become covered (buried) through a process of hillwash and natural accumulation of deposits. This was an important distinction, because it demonstrated that a third party had not been involved. Had the remains been moved before this examination, this distinction would have been lost. The anthropologist was able to provide preliminary information regarding age, stature, and sex in order that the enquiry could move forward before the postmortem the following day. It transpired that the individual was

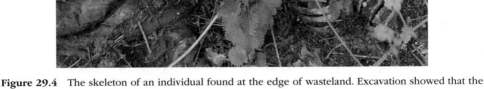

Figure 29.4 The skeleton of an individual found at the edge of wasteland. Excavation showed that the lower half of the body had been removed by an earth-moving machine.

likely to have been a young male adult who had discharged himself from a local hospital, had wandered off, and who had died from natural causes. His identity was later confirmed by DNA.

In a similar scenario, building workers came across part of a human skeleton on wasteland that was being redeveloped. The skull and upper torso were visible against a wall behind some low bushes, but the rest appeared to be buried (Figure 29.4). The area was sealed off until archaeologists could attend. Preliminary examination of the remains and the soil layers showed that the body lay on the surface and that its lower part, far from being buried, had been severed above the pelvis, probably by the earth moving machine that had been clearing the site and landscaping the site perimeter with low banking. A few skeletal elements were observed in the immediate vicinity, notably a foot, but otherwise the skeleton was incomplete.

Fortunately, the upper torso retained a heart pacemaker with a reference number that could be associated with a specific individual. He was an elderly man and a known alcoholic who lived in a local hostel and who was known to wander off. Reference to the manner of landscaping and machine activity suggested that the missing remains could lie anywhere within a large area. It would have been impractical to excavate and sieve the entire disturbed area of some 80 x 50 m, and the collected remains were returned to the family for burial. Cause of death was never established but was assumed to be from natural causes.

The final case concerns skeletal remains found by a member of the public while walking along a beach. The bones were taken to the local police station and were identified by the police surgeon as being human. The general area of the discovery was secured until an archaeologist was called in to examine the location. His first question was to ascertain whether they belonged to a burial or whether they had been introduced as disarticulated remains in a redeposition of material. His findings demonstrated that the former was the case: they were part of a complete buried skeleton that had been partly exposed by marine erosion at the shore edge (Figure 29.5).

The task then was to ascertain the age of the burial. In similar instances where there had been no associated material such as clothing, jewellery or modern dental treatment radiometric dating was able to offer some solution, but here there was good stratigraphic evidence to indicate an "archaeological" timescale of deposition. Once cleaned up, the exposed grave section was shown

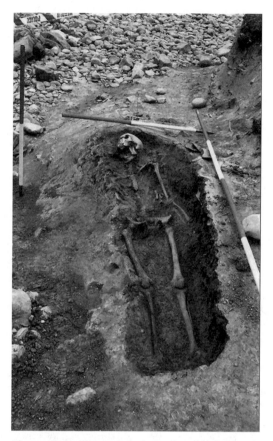

Figure 29.5 The excavated remains of an "archaeological" burial. The right arm of the individual had been eroded out of the shoreline and caused the enquiry to take place.

to underlie anthropogenic deposits, including the unbroken surface of a footpath that had been in use for over a century. Moreover, reference to local museum collections revealed that the area was part of a known prehistoric burial ground. The remains were formally excavated and dispatched to the museum for further attention.

Conclusion

The case studies under these four broad themes provide a reasonable insight into the types of work in which a forensic archaeologist might expect to feature. Much of the work will be routine and most will be concerned with elimination or with giving advice. Ten years ago, involvement at this level would have been relatively rare: input would have been restricted to a few individual cases involving a known missing person or occasionally to situations where skeletal remains had been found.

Awareness of the discipline has developed significantly since then, partly through teaching and research in the subject and partly through the effectiveness of operational involvement and the provision of training programmes. These have been delivered not only to law enforcement groups but also to other archaeologists in a two-way process of awareness. There is, nevertheless, still some misunderstanding as to what archaeology and anthropology actually are as disciplines, and how they differ. Unlike in the United States, where archaeology tends to be subsumed and practised under the discipline of anthropology, in the United Kingdom, the roles are very clearly defined—the archaeologist deals with buried material of whatever type and the anthropologist with human skeletal materials, buried or not (see Cox this volume). Of course, some individuals are skilled in both areas. Nevertheless, the misunderstanding is more than compensated for by an increasing use of archaeological evidence in court and through recognition by the Council for the Registration of Forensic Practitioners (CRFP). Archaeologists still wince at certain crime reports in the media, in which it is clear that archaeological involvement should have been used but was not, but such reports are becoming fewer. However, the fact that any exist at all is still a cause for concern.

Acknowledgment

I am grateful for the advice of Mr. Barrie Simpson in the preparation of this chapter.

Note

1. See Dilley (2005) for a detailed discussion of other legal matters relating to forensic archaeology.

References

CPIA 1996. *Criminal Procedure and Investigations Act 1996.* C.25. London: HMSO.

Dilley, R. 2005. Legal matters, in J. R. Hunter and M. Cox (eds.), *Forensic Archaeology: Advances in Theory and Practice*, pp. 177–203. London: Routledge.

Hunter, J. R., and Cox, M. (eds.). 2005. *Forensic Archaeology: Advances in Theory and Practice.* London: Routledge.

PACE 1984. *Police and Criminal Evidence Act 1984.* Public General Acts and Measures of 1984. London: HMSO.

POA 1986. *Prosecution of Offences Act 1985.* Public General Acts and Measures of 1985. London: HMSO.

30

FORENSIC ANTHROPOLOGY IN DISASTER RESPONSE

Paul S. Sledzik

When struck by disaster, humans attempt to control the associated effects on their lives. The first response to controlling the immediate chaos gives way to the recovery process: rebuilding infrastructure, homes and businesses, and support services. If the disaster kills large numbers of people, the recovery process becomes more complex. The affected community must deal with the retrieval of the dead, the identification of the remains, and personal and social grief processes made more intense by the sudden death of the victims.

Although not typically considered first responders, forensic scientists are invaluable to mass-fatality response. They are the specialists in the arena of disaster victim identification, an arena often overlooked by first responders who are trained to rescue survivors, treat the injured, and provide for the living. As part of the medico-legal systems required to conduct fatality identification, forensic scientists bring both technical capabilities to identify the dead and a unique understanding of the complexities of managing large numbers of deceased individuals. Mass-fatality forensic teams are multidisciplinary and usually include forensic pathologists, forensic anthropologists, forensic dentists, fingerprint specialists, DNA analysts, medico-legal investigators, funeral directors, and forensic managers.

The involvement of forensic anthropology in mass-fatality response encompasses traditional roles and newly established contributions (Table 30.1). The traditional approaches are extensions of those applied in skeletal casework: the application of archaeological methods in the search for, and recovery of, human remains from disaster sites and the examination of human remains to determine biological characteristics useful for identification. In recent years, anthropologists have moved into managing overall victim identification efforts, examining the importance of antemortem data in the identification process (with particular attention on the cultural factors that affect the process) and working with family members of the deceased to help answer their questions and address their concerns. With broad training in biological interpretations of human identification, anatomy, taphonomy, and human biology, and supported by knowledge of the cultural considerations of religion, death, and mourning, anthropologists are uniquely suited to make important contributions to the field of disaster victim identification.

Although large-scale disasters may overwhelm local medico-legal agencies, the agencies are still legally responsible for victim identification and determination of cause and manner of death. Soon after the disaster, a tension develops between individual and societal needs for remains (for funerals and other grief rites) and medico-legal requirements for proper identification. Family members of the victims and civic leaders often begin to

Table 30.1 Forensic anthropological skills in mass-fatality incidents.

Disaster Scene	Devise appropriate system for search for and recovery of remains based on size and scope of event. Locate, recognize, and recover human remains, especially burned and fragmented. Train search personnel to recognize human remains (based on taphonomic factors). Provide field assessment of condition of remains.
Incident Morgue	Assist in triage of remains. Separate commingled remains. Describe incomplete/fragmentary remains and condition of remains. Determine sex, age, race, stature, and distinguishing characteristics. Interpret radiographs for age estimation and unique skeletal features. Determine minimum number of individuals based on remains recovered. Assist in identifications using anthropological features. Assist in sex and age assessment of remains. Analyze trauma evidence and incident related injuries. Conduct quality assurance of remains before release from morgue. Serve as morgue manager.
Disaster Management	Examine processes used to document remains to ensure all appropriate biological data is collected. Speak with family members concerning methods of identification. Assess and solve problems in management of antemortem and postmortem data. Examine antemortem data collection issues, including availability and accuracy. Serve as manager of overall victim identification efforts.

question the forensic response, particularly the length of time needed for the identification process. When informed about the details of the identification process and the need for medico-legal investigation, family members and the public begin to understand the issues involved. Cultural and religious beliefs also affect methods of identification, and whether attempts at identification are undertaken at all. Because societal expectations for the level of identification vary across the globe, the use of scientific methods to identify disaster victims is not universal.

Overview of Mass-Fatality Response Operations

The response to a mass-fatality event usually sees three distinct areas of work develop: the disaster site, the disaster morgue, and the family assistance center, where families of the deceased gather to receive and provide information.

At the disaster site, forensic personnel work with first responders to document the remains before they are recovered. The tenet used by site personnel is to treat the scene as a crime scene and document it accordingly using photographs, diagrams, and mapping, using total station or global positioning hardware and software. Remains are numbered on scene and removed to a temporary storage location to await their transfer to the disaster morgue.

In the flow of events following a disaster, the search for and recovery of human remains comes after life-saving efforts, fire suppression, and other first-responder requirements are completed. The size of the affected area, the number of fatalities, the condition of remains, time of day/night, and the location and weather during the efforts influence the methods and time required for search and recovery. The methods used to process a crime scene are logically applicable to the disaster scene, and some disaster scenes are crime scenes. When remains are distributed across a disaster site, appropriate search procedures document the scene, ensure that all areas are searched, and make certain that human remains are recognized and recovered properly. Standard collection processes also permits sharing of information between response and recovery agencies.

Forensic anthropologists trained in forensic archaeological methods easily adapt those methods to disaster scenes (Dirkmaat, Hefner, and Hochrein 2001). Because of the large amount of physical evidence requiring documentation at terrestrial disaster scenes, Dirkmaat and colleagues stress a more rigorous approach to the location, documentation and recovery protocols, and the routine use of sophisticated, electronic surveying instrumentation. Archaeological training helps in determining the size and scope of the search. Using their knowledge of taphonomy, anthropologists can train search and recovery personnel about the unique aspects of scenes where fragmentation, burning, and decomposition of remains are a concern. The ability to recognize otherwise unrecognizable remains (to the non-anthropologist) allow for the recovery of remains that might otherwise be overlooked. An on-scene assessment of material can often reveal if the items are human, non-human, or nonbiological.

The disaster morgue resembles an assembly line where human remains are systematically documented and analyzed (Sledzik and Kauffman 2007; Wagner and Froede 1993). Figure 30.1 portrays a typical disaster morgue operation process and indicates some of the considerations that affect how remains are processed. Selecting the site of the disaster morgue requires considerations regarding proximity to the disaster site, the size of the facility needed to document the remains, and logistics concerns, such as heating, air conditioning, lighting, security, water, restrooms, and office space. Once selected, portable morgue equipment and supplies are brought in to outfit the facility.

Remains are taken from the site and placed in storage, to await processing in the morgue. Storing remains in refrigerator trucks or holding morgues allows forensic analysts to control the flow of remains into the examination portion of the morgue. Once admitted into the morgue, the remains are radiographed in the container they are stored in, usually a body bag or pouch. This radiograph allows personnel to look for items in the remains that may be a safety concern (such as sharp metal items or unexploded ordinance) and helps in assessing the remains for processing. In the case of fragmented or dismembered remains, the radiographs also aid in the triage process. In the morgue, the anthropologist's knowledge of skeletal biology and anatomy is critical in analyzing and interpreting remains that are fragmented, burned, and decomposed, typical of many types of mass disasters.

Triage allows sorting of remains from other materials (for example, personal effects, wreckage, nonbiological material), and the assessment of remains using a probative index to systematically classify human remains according to their identification potential or investigative value (Kontanis and Sledzik 2008; Mundorff 2008). This categorization system relates the number of positive and presumptive identifying features to the potential for a DNA, dental, fingerprint, or medical identification. Those remains with the greatest potential for identification (for example, jaw fragments with teeth, hands with ridge skin for fingerprints, bones with prosthetic devices) are placed into the morgue stream for further analysis. Small pieces of soft tissue and organs are not typically placed into the stream, because their likelihood for identification is small. These remains are placed in a separate container and may be analyzed further if all victims are not identified. Most often, these remains will become common tissue, remains that cannot be identified. As the only morgue section staffed by a multidisciplinary team, triage can reveal patterns in the types of remains as they relate to search areas. When recognized, the presence of these patterns may require changes in the recovery process and help guide search and recovery efforts.

Remains that are placed into the morgue flow for analysis are then photographed, radiographed (as an individual specimen) a second time, and numbered sequentially. The various forensic specialties then analyze the remains. In the case of complete or nearly complete remains, each discipline participates in the analysis. For fragmentary remains, the most appropriate disciplines will examine the specimen (for example, a hand would be examined by the pathology, anthropology, and fingerprint sections). Data from the examinations are then entered into a database that allows comparison with antemortem data.

While the postmortem data are being collected at the morgue, antemortem information is being obtained from family members and friends of the deceased. This process typically happens at a family assistance center. Using standard interview forms, specialists in funeral service and forensic identification interview the family members, obtaining contact information for dentists and doctors (for obtaining antemortem records and radiographs), data on the unique biological aspects of the deceased, DNA samples, and information related to personal effects with the deceased.

In most disaster situations involving recently deceased, the methods used for positive identification are unique, biologically based attributes. These methods include prints (for instance, fingerprints, handprints, toe prints, and footprints), odontology, radiology, DNA analysis, and permanently installed medical devices with recorded serial numbers. Distinctive physical characteristics (for example, ears, scars, moles, tattoos) with appropriate antemortem photographic documentations may be used to for a positive identification in a closed population

Mass Fatality Morgue Operational Plan

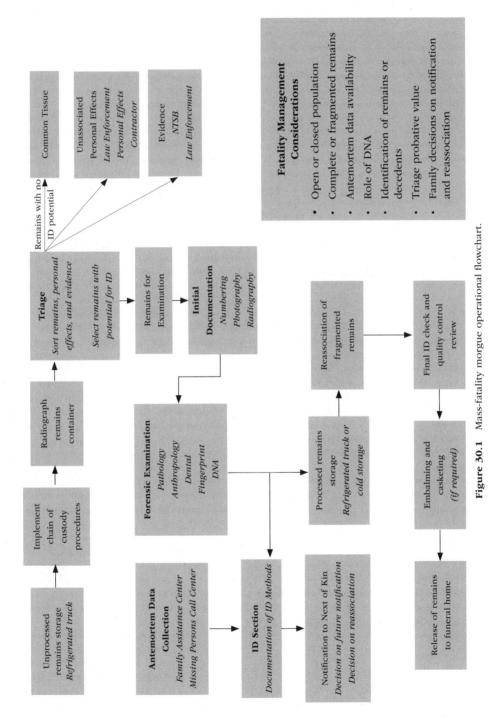
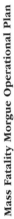

Figure 30.1 Mass-fatality morgue operational flowchart.

(such as an aircraft accident). Using such characteristics for positive identification in an open population should be done with caution. Presumptive identification using personal effects, clothing, and the like is a preliminary step toward confirmatory identification using some or all of the procedures listed above. Regularly scheduled identification meetings are held between the medico-legal authority and the identification scientists to examine, critique, and decide on identifications. The forensic specialist from the appropriate discipline documents the details of the identification in a report, and the identification is presented to the medical examiner or coroner for agreement and authorization.

Once remains are identified, the next of kin are notified of the identification and arrangements for the release of the remains are made. Following a final check of the remains for quality assurance, the remains are released to the funeral home or other designated party.

Fatality Management Considerations

Each disaster poses unique challenges for fatality management, a term defining forensic-based decisions influencing how the victims, their families, and the identification efforts are managed. Fatality management encompasses the focus of the overall identification efforts and the influence of taphonomic factors on the process, and it also addresses the expectations of both the family members of the dead and society about the identification process. Before victim identification begins, the medico-legal authority and the primary forensic responders must answer several important questions:

- What is the number of fatalities?

- What are the challenges in searching for and recovering the victims?

- Is the victim population open or closed (that is, unknown or known number of fatalities)?

- What is the condition of the remains (for example, complete, fragmented, burned, dismembered)?

- What are the types, availability, and accuracy, of antemortem information?

- Will forensic efforts focus on identifying all victims or all remains?

- What is the role (and the limitations) of DNA in the identification efforts?

- What are the concerns and expectations of society and the next of kin for the identification efforts?

Answers to these questions focus the work of the forensic teams, determine the length of the identification process, expose potential limits to identifications, and determine the role of forensic science in the response (Tun et al. 2005; United States Department of Justice 2005, 2006).

Commonly, it is thought that the greater the number of fatalities, the more complex the identification process. Although the number of fatalities is important (particularly when the figure rises into the thousands), the associated factors of taphonomy and antemortem data availability have a more profound effect on the ability of the jurisdiction to conduct identifications.

As an example, consider two hypothetical disasters, each resulting in 100 fatalities. The first disaster has left the remains complete, with little taphonomic change, and antemortem records are available. The second disaster caused fragmentation of remains (with nearly 8,000 fragments representing the 100 victims), and little is known about the victims and their available antemortem information. If the same amount of forensic resources is applied to each case, the second disaster will take longer, cost more, and require more complex fatality management decisions than the first.

Characterizing the group of victims highlights one important fatality management concern. Victim populations are categorized as open or closed, based on the information known about them at the time of the disaster. In a closed population, some basic data about the number and identity of the victims (usually a name) are easily obtainable. With a victim's name or other type of contact information, authorities can reach next of kin to obtain antemortem information. The most common example is an aircraft accident wherein a flight manifest (supported by positive identification checks, ticket purchasing procedures, and airport security) becomes the initial source of antemortem information. Under United States law, for example, passenger names and contact information are provided to the authorities within a matter of hours following an accident, and the collection of antemortem information can begin shortly thereafter.

Conversely, an open population defines a victim group in which neither the number of victims nor their names are known. To create an accurate list of victims, response personnel sort those who are reported missing from those who are actually missing. Ideally, a designated missing persons or casualty call center receives all missing-persons calls and develops a comprehensive list of those persons reported as missing. From this list, investigators establish a list of those actually missing through winnowing duplicate reportings, clarifying misspellings, and verifying the status of a missing person. A single central call center for reporting disaster missing is essential for effective victim identification. Once a victim is known to be missing, the process of obtaining and examining antemortem data begins.

Often the initial reports of the number of fatalities in an open population disaster differ significantly from the final figures. For example, in the September 11, 2001, World Trade Center disaster, initial media reports indicated as many as 10,000 dead or missing. In subsequent days, the number of reported missing ranged between 3,958 and 6,453 (Simpson and Stehr 2003). As of November 2005, the total number of missing from the disaster was 2,749, of which 1,594 had been identified (Biesecker et al. 2005). In the Asian tsunami of 2004, the World Health Organization reported 10,000 dead, and within ten days the number expanded to 153,000 (Fleck 2005). The final death toll was nearly 250,000, with an understanding that the final number will never be known (Morgan et al. 2006; Thieren 2005). Following the bombing of several trains and buses in London on July 7, 2005, a centralized casualty call center was established (per previous planning efforts) to handle missing persons calls (Great Britain, Greater London Authority 2006). The center received 42,000 calls within the first hour of operation. The number of missing-persons calls, for an event that killed 38 and injured over 700, underscores the intense public response following a disaster and the need for authorities to implement a coordinated missing-persons system.

The process of positive identification requires comparing the postmortem data with antemortem information, with a focus on unique biological genetic characteristics. Thus, two areas of forensic work develop: the morgue and the collection of antemortem information. Analyzing remains for postmortem information occurs relatively quickly and simply as forensic scientists analyze remains in the morgue. However, locating, obtaining, and evaluating antemortem data are often more time consuming and complex (Blau et al. 2006; Brannon and Kessler 1999; De Valck 2006).

Antemortem records in the form of dental and medical documents, radiographs, fingerprints, and DNA reference samples are the most frequently used and reliable methods for identification. However, to be used for identification, these records must be available, obtainable, and accurate. For example, some disasters may destroy potential antemortem records. If records do exist, they are usually obtainable only if family members can report the victim's dentist and doctor contact information. Similarly, some victims may have never visited a doctor or dentist, or are transient. Many people have never been fingerprinted or were printed as part of a process not allowing for locating and retrieval of the record. Other factors such as age, socioeconomic status, cultural practices, and religious beliefs of the victims and their next of kin may limit antemortem record availability. For example, religious beliefs about death may cause family members to refuse to provide DNA reference samples. Some victims' socioeconomic status may have prevented them from visiting a dentist.

The accuracy and applicability of antemortem records also limits their usefulness. Reports from the forensic dental literature routinely point out the issues of accuracy, completeness, and legibility of dental records, in addition to the inability of next of kin to locate dentist contact information for the deceased (Brannon and Kessler 1999).

When antemortem data are unavailable, authorities often turn to identifications based on visual means or personal effects, both methods known to be inaccurate, particularly when remains are not well preserved or when next of kin are under stress (Fierro, 1993; Lain, Griffiths, and Hilton 2003; Weedn 1998).

Efforts required to locate and analyze antemortem data have received little attention from forensic scientists, despite the nature of this essential requirement for victim identification. Anthropologists have begun to apply their research skills to this important area, which has the potential to enhance disaster-fatality identification practices (Simmons and Skinner 2006; Tyrrell et al. 2006).

Taphonomy (see Nawrocki this volume) also affects fatality management. The taphonomic spectrum of a disaster ranges from complete bodies to small, fragmentary remains. Along this spectrum, fire, chemicals, decomposition, and water cause additional damage to remains (Sledzik and Rodriguez 2002).

In the case of fragmentary remains, one critical decision concerning the examination of remains is whether to identify all remains or all victims—a decision tempered by the type of disaster (open or closed) and the social/cultural beliefs of the population affected by the disaster. In the case of an unknown number of victims, the decision should focus on the identification of all remains, with DNA analysis used to reveal the profiles of all remains and, consequently, of all victims (if results are interpretable). In a closed-population disaster resulting in fragmentary remains, such as an aircraft accident, identifying as many remains from each victim as possible is often the focus.

The limitations of forensic identification methods, especially DNA, and the availability of antemortem data may prevent all remains from being identified, yet all victims have been identified. Because certain fragmented remains possess the individualizing anatomical structures needed to conduct identification (for example, dental structures or hands with ridge skin), when the fragment is identified, there is both proof of death and identification of the victim. However, many fragments have no unique physical identifier, and DNA becomes the sole method for identification.

Despite the application of all human identification techniques, some fragmentary remains will not be identified. These unidentifiable remains are often referred to as "common tissue." The concept of unidentified remains and the actual remains themselves must be managed carefully, and families are informed of their existence and involved with their final disposition.

History of Forensic Anthropology in Mass Disasters in the United States

Over the past several decades, forensic anthropologists have played an increasingly important role when disaster strikes. Complex human identification efforts, such as those seen in wars, human rights abuses, and disasters, require the broad training and specific skills of forensic anthropologists. The experience of forensic anthropologists in disasters is visible in the scientific literature, viewed largely through the reporting of activities at specific events. A synthesis of these reports underscores the range of involvement of the science in disaster response (see Black; see Briggs and Buck this volume).

Forensic anthropology's exposure to mass-fatality work is rooted largely in its support of the U.S. military war dead identification efforts during World War II, the Korean War, and the Vietnam War. Although anthropologists focused on identifying individual service members killed in battle, their skills were also useful when accidents killed large numbers of troops (Sledge 2005). Starting with the work of Shapiro, Trotter, Snow, and Stewart during World War II (Ubelaker 2000; Wood and Stanley 1989) and continuing to the efforts of Warren, Kerley (Hinkes 2001), and McKern during the Korean and Vietnam Wars, anthropologists assisted in disaster situations when they arose. In fact, the Vietnam War era job descriptions of anthropologists employed by the military specifically mentioned examining remains from disasters and resolving commingling issues (Warren 1981).

The culmination of this military support work was Stewart's (1970) edited volume *Personal Identification in Mass Disasters*. The volume, comprising papers from a 1968 seminar sponsored by the Support Services of the U.S. Army and the Smithsonian Institution, reflected the military's desire to apply new scientific methods to war dead identification efforts. The volume dealt little with management issues of disaster victim identification but did present new anthropological methods useful in identification. Stewart was initially approached by the military to organize a seminar dealing with war dead identification. However, after discussing the proposal with several forensic colleagues, he decided to expand the scope of the seminar to address both mass-disaster and war dead identification, thus tying the techniques presented in the volume to both applications.

In the 1960s and 1970s, the Federal Aviation Administration's Civil Aeromedical Institute (CAMI) employed anthropologists Richard Snyder and Clyde Snow. Although their research focused mainly on biomechanics and anthropometry, they also responded to aviation accidents to examine survivability and interpret traumatic injuries of victims. Their reports for CAMI reveal unique applications of anthropology to aviation accident survivability, including issues such as seat and lap belt injuries and trauma resulting from impact with water (Collins and Wayda 2003). Anthropologists have not continued their work, remarkable for its focus outside victim identification and morgue operations, in any significant way.

In 1976, Charney responded to the Big Thompson River flood in Colorado. Because of fragmentation and decomposition, Charney's team of anthropologists assisted in identifying the 139 victims. Based on his experiences, Charney, who served as codirector of the disaster morgue, called for a centralized national system to identify disaster fatalities (Charney and Wilbur 1984).

Using the 1986 U.S. military aircraft accident in Gander, Newfoundland, as a starting point, Hinkes (1989) examined the role of forensic anthropology in resolving the problems of disaster victim identification. In highlighting the field's technical capabilities, she argued for the inclusion of anthropologists in all stages of the response (from recovery through final evaluation). Overall victim identification efforts would benefit, Hinkes claimed, because anthropologists produce biological profiles on remains previously considered unidentifiable.

The conditions encountered after the burning of the Branch Davidian compound in Waco, Texas, in 1993, allowed anthropologists to conduct scene documentation, search and recovery, trauma analysis, and victim identification (Houck et al. 1996; Owsley et al. 1995; Ubelaker et al. 1995). The burned remains required careful excavation of the scene to protect evidence and document the sequence of events. The methods used by the anthropological team underscore the comprehensive technical approach anthropologists bring to disaster response. For example, the team applied demographic analyses to examine the victim population, which ranged greatly in age. Research comparing actual victim age with anthropological age assessments revealed that the methods applied were accurate (Houck et al. 1996).

That same year, Sledzik and colleagues became involved in the identification efforts following the flooding of a rural Midwestern cemetery (Sledzik and Hunt 1997; Sledzik and Willcox 2003). Floodwaters from the Missouri River carved away several hundred burials from the town cemetery in Hardin, Missouri. Thousands of skeletal elements and hundreds of complete embalmed bodies in various states of preservation required anthropological analysis. The team documented the remains, determined the minimum number of individuals represented by the individual bones, and identified several individuals despite limited antemortem information.

The fragmentation of remains following the 1996 crash of Valujet 592 required radiographic age assessment of the wrist and hands to determine the ages of the juvenile victims (Warren et al. 2000). The radiographic interpretations helped isolate and seriate the hands of these victims, a majority of whom were identified based on their age. Radiographic identification based on unique skeletal features seen in postmortem radiographs has been applied by anthropologists in other disasters and is a common technique for positive identification (Kahana et al. 1997; Lichtenstein, Fitzpatrick, and Madewell 1988; Saul and Saul 2003).

With the creation in the United States of the Disaster Mortuary Operational Response Team (DMORT) in the 1990s, anthropologists became key personnel in forensic disaster response (Sledzik and Willcox 2003). DMORT is a federal volunteer team of forensic scientist and mortuary personnel who are trained in disaster-victim identification and mass-fatality management. Similarly, the Interpol Disaster Victim Identification teams (DVI) are composed of forensic specialists. Interpol DVI responds to fatality events in most countries around the world, whereas DMORT responds only within the United States.

In 2002, the operator of a crematorium in northwest Georgia chose to bury and dispose of remains sent to his business rather than cremate the remains. Hundreds of bodies, in various states of preservation, were located in burial pits, buildings, and vehicles. This scene posed anthropologists with several challenges (Steadman et al. 2008). The complex nature of the site and the condition of the remains required varied approaches to search and recovery. Anthropologists analyzed most of the remains because of advanced decomposition and partial mummification. When family members began to question the authenticity of the cremated remains in their possession, anthropologists again became involved in the analysis.

The events of September 11, 2001, posed an unprecedented challenge for forensic scientists. Taphonomically, fragmentation and commingling posed anthropological challenges in recovery and analysis. The 9/11 events also marked an important change in the anthropological role in disaster response. Anthropologists emerged to serve as directors of victim identification teams, quality control managers, morgue managers, and coordinators of long-term identification efforts (London et al. 2003; Mundorff 2003; Rodriguez 2003; Sledzik et al. 2003; Warren et al. 2003), and their efforts highlight the capabilities of forensic anthropologists as broadly trained experts in human identification who can manage complex human identification events.

Two unique applications of the anthropological involvement in mass-fatality identification took place at the World Trade Center disaster (Budimlija et al. 2003; Mundorff et al. 2005; Wiersema et al. 2003). The immense administrative effort of managing the data related to thousands of fragments resulted in procedural errors, such as misnumbering, incorrect data, and siding errors. DNA cross-contamination caused by the forces of the building collapse (for example, two right feet producing identical DNA profiles) also became evident. To resolve these problems, a quality control project referred to as "anthropological verification" was created. The project required the reexamination of over 16,000 specimens and their associated case file information and DNA results. After examining 16,915 of a total of 19,963 cases, the anthropology team's work revealed both new identifications and associations between previously unassociated remains.

The second process requiring anthropological involvement was the "final anthropological review," a quality assurance procedure created to ensure the certainty of the identification and reduce the possibility of misidentification. Once identification was made, usually by DNA, the anthropologist examined the identified remains to ensure the biological attributes of the remains were congruent with the file and identification information. The remains were then compared to other remains identified from the same individual to look for duplication or other inconsistencies in the set of remains belonging to that individual. Problems were resolved by using document reviews, additional anthropological analysis, and reanalysis of DNA. MacKinnon and Mundorff (2007: 495) indicate that the review was important to "resolve any final and outstanding issues of commingling and contamination, and ultimately provided the opportunity to reconfirm the correlation between the case files, the identification modality/ies, and the physical remains, before final repatriation of the victim occurred."

Anthropologists from the U.S. Army Joint POW/MIA Accounting Command and a private disaster-consulting firm responded to the Asian tsunami of December 2004. The dual role of the anthropologist was again implemented: as technical experts to assess biological features useful for identification and as coordinators in the identification efforts (Martrille et al. 2006; Tyrrell et al. 2006). Following Hurricane Katrina in 2005, anthropologists with DMORT served again in these dual roles (Fulginiti et al. 2006).

Recent guides and documents related to mass-fatality management have included anthropological understandings, both forensic and cultural. The 2005 National Institute of Justice publication *Mass Fatality Incidents: A Guide for Human Identification* was produced by the National Center for Forensic Science with the assistance of a group of experienced mass-fatality forensic responders, including several anthropologists. The guide also contains a section on the work that anthropologists conduct at disaster sites. The 2004 publication by the Pan-American Health Organization, *Management of Dead Bodies in Disaster Situations*, discusses a variety of mass-fatality issues, including preparedness for mass-death response, medico-legal work, health considerations in mass fatalities, sociocultural issues, psychological aspects, legal concepts, and several case studies from recent South and Central American disasters. The principles outlined in this document are being implemented and promoted by a variety of organizations, including the Pan American Health Organization, the World Health Organization, the International Committee of the Red Cross, and the International Federation of Red Cross and Red Crescent Societies.

Providing information to family members of disaster victims has also developed as a relatively new area for anthropologists in North America (Mundorff and Steadman 2003; Sledzik et al. 2006),

although forensic anthropology practitioners in South America have a long history of interaction with family members (see Fondebrider this volume). Family members often express concerns about the condition of remains and the process of identification (Blakeney 2002; Levin 2004). Forensic anthropologists doing this work must be able to provide factual information about taphonomic and identification concerns in a compassionate manner.

Managing Concerns of Family Members

Disaster victim identification takes place for two reasons: legal and humanitarian. Remains need to be identified because of legal requirements such as issuance of death certificates, settlement of wills and insurance claims, and remarriage. The legal reasons underlie the humanitarian reasons: the empathy and compassion that compel us to aid those affected by a disaster.

The term *family assistance* defines a set of standard practices supporting the unique needs of family members of those killed or injured in disasters. Family assistance differs from traditional disaster services (which encompasses the delivery of food, water, shelter, medical care, and similar needs). Although family members of the deceased and injured may need this support, they also seek information about the victim or injured person. Family members of deceased victims often have questions about the search, recovery, and identification of remains, the cause of the disaster, and the return of personal effects (Eyre 2002). Family assistance support models create a structure whereby family members can receive accurate and timely answers to their questions.

In the United States, a primary focus of family assistance was the passage of the United States law entitled the Aviation Disaster Family Assistance Act of 1996. The law requires the National Transportation Safety Board to coordinate the resources of the federal government, the airline, the local authorities, and identified organizations to meet the needs of aviation disaster victims and their families (United States National Transportation Safety Board 2000). The support families receive often encompasses travel to and from the accident site, lodging, informational briefings (including information on victim recovery and identification), mental health counseling, site visits, memorial services, and long-term information sharing (Slater and Hall 1997). This model of family assistance has been applied to other transportation accident modes and terrorism bombings in the United States and the United Kingdom.

To address family members about the topics of search and recovery of remains and the process of victim identification, the medical examiner or coroner (or their representative) is often involved. Family members of the disaster dead deserve frank and compassionate discourse from forensic responders. Although families are involved in the identification process by providing antemortem information, they must also make decisions about death notification, final disposition, and other concerns related to the remains of the deceased. For example, in cases where multiple fragments from one individual may be identified over a lengthy period, families choose how often they wish to be notified of identifications (initially or each time an identification of the victim is made) and when the remains will be provided to them for final disposition. The sometimes-lengthy process of DNA identification is also explained, and families may be asked to provide DNA reference samples.

In nearly all disasters causing fragmentary remains, not all fragmented remains are identified. To manage these unidentified remains (also known as common tissue), the medical examiner or coroner must be informed of the presence of these unidentified remains and their disposition. Preferably, family members will work as a group to decide the final disposition of the remains. If families cannot decide, the medico-legal authority takes action under the jurisdiction's laws to dispose of the remains.

Anthropologists are well suited to analyze the complex issues related to the condition of remains, the desire of family members, and the technical limitations of the identification sciences. The cultural, social, and scientific implications of this work are reflected in a series of questions often asked early in a disaster response. The questions are asked of, and by, forensic scientists, family members, and society and examine how remains are identified, the extent to which science should go to identify them, and expectations about what is provided the family for final disposition. Although these questions are not unique to disaster work (Williams and Crews 2003) they do require careful consideration and public and professional discourse. Among these questions:

- Should the limited resources available to conduct identification be used to identify all fragmentary remains or all victims?
- How large does a specimen need to be for testing?
- Should every specimen be analyzed and tested for DNA?

- What if a specimen is identified by DNA, yet is consumed entirely in testing?
- At what point does the identification process end?
- Should remains recovered years after a disaster be processed for identification?
- What should be done with unidentifiable remains?

Forensic scientists endeavor to apply all applicable technology to identify the disaster dead. Often, in the first days following a disaster, families expect that identifications will happen quickly and that whole bodies will be returned. The process of making their expectations more consistent with the taphonomic reality of the disaster is difficult but necessary if families are to truly understand the reasons behind the answers to these questions. Answers to these questions are dependent on the particulars of the disaster, desires of the family members (individually and as a disaster-specific group), cultural beliefs about death and final disposition of remains, societal expectations about what science can provide, and the availability of appropriate forensic identification tools and techniques (Pan American Health Organization 2004).

Impact of Disaster Work on Anthropologists

Forensic disaster responders work in a highly stressful, challenging, chaotic environment. The disaster environment poses challenges to all responders, and the stress of handling the dead is unique (Ursano and McCarroll 1990). Although disaster forensic work is physically and psychologically demanding, forensic scientists often overlook the effect of these stressors. Early studies by disaster mental health researchers focused on the psychological impact of body recovery and morgue work on inexperienced, nonforensic personnel. Recently, this research has expanded to examine experienced forensic responders, with a particular focus on forensic dentists (McCarroll et al. 1996; Webb, Sweet, and Pretty 2002).

Research examining the physical and psychological impact of mass-fatality work on experienced forensic personnel reveals several interesting points. In general, experienced forensic responders managed the physical and psychological stresses of mortuary work more effectively than did inexperienced responders (e.g., Wright 2006). The anticipation of mass-fatality work leads to psychological and physiological stress, although experience reduces the amount of anticipatory stress. Mortuary workers reported an increase in somatic symptoms (such as nausea, chest pains, fainting, and weakness) during and after working in the disaster morgue (McCarroll et al. 2002). The condition of the victim's remains, particularly aspects of visual grotesqueness, odor, and tactile features, is considered a stressor. Working with the remains of children has a significant impact on stress. Identifying or personalizing with the victims increases emotional attachment to the remains, may reduce objectivity, and may increase vulnerability to psychological distress. Handling personal effects has also been shown to be difficult for mortuary workers (Ursano and McCarroll 1990).

In a study of the psychological stress encountered by experienced and inexperienced forensic dentists who identified victims following the Branch Davidian event, McCarroll and associates (1996) found that about half reported psychological reactions that included anxiety prior to the work beginning, difficulty working with the remains of children, and the stress dealing with the chaos of the identification process. The stress was significantly related to the amount of exposure to the remains, previous experience in mass-fatality events, age, and the level of coworker and spouse support.

The most effective coping strategies are the use of humor and the opportunity to talk with colleagues involved the disaster response. Indeed, the on-site and postdisaster camaraderie was an important source of positive feelings about a disaster response (Webb, Sweet, and Pretty 2002). Forensic responders also reported that, despite the stress, assisting in the response was a valuable experience, provided a sense of accomplishment, and increased their appreciation of life.

Conclusion

Although cultural anthropologists have examined the behavioral, organizational, economic, and other cultural responses of humans to disasters (Hoffman and Oliver-Smith 2002), they do not often delve into the treatment of deceased resulting from a disaster. The complex cultural questions arising from dealing with the realities of victims of disasters are often overlooked: search, recovery, identification, management, familial grief, societal grief, memorialization, and recovery. Forensic anthropologists, with their broad training in many of these areas, are ideally suited to take on the study and management of these complex topics.

This new application of the field has begun. Forensic anthropologists employed in medical examiner offices and law enforcement laboratories in the United States are taking on the responsibilities of mass-fatality planner as an additional responsibility beyond their casework. This is a logical extension of the daily casework and a trend underscoring the important application of broad anthropological training in human identification. Anthropologists in other parts of the world, such as those working for the Pan American Health Organization, the International Committee for the Red Cross, and the World Health Organization, are making significant contributions to the publications focusing on managing victims of disasters.

Similar forensic and management concerns affect forensic anthropologists involved in disaster work and human rights responses. The methods used to solve the problems encountered by each group would benefit from a shared approach. As large-scale, complex human identification efforts, both require broad knowledge of forensic science, an ability to work within an existing cultural framework, and balancing family member/societal and scientific concerns about the identification efforts (Williams and Crews 2003). Oddly, these two groups of practitioners have not interacted in a comprehensive way that would share lessons learned and advance methods for large-scale human identification efforts.

More broadly, however, these new applications of the field highlight the need for the discipline of forensic anthropology to be redefined. A new definition should encompass forensic anthropology as a science that deals with a range of anthropological issues, as well as medico-legal questions. Such a definition would include applications of other fields of anthropology and would allow for a broader understanding of human interaction with the environment (physical, social, cultural, and linguistic) and resulting medico-legal interpretations. From the perspective of disaster response, forensic anthropologists will continue to take on responsibilities that go beyond the technical requirements of remains identification and delve into the management of the scientific response, interactions with family members, and the needs of society to understand the complex issues of disaster victim identification.

References

Biesecker, L. G., Bailey-Wilson, J. E., Ballantyne, J., Baum, H., Bieber, F. R., Brenner, C., Budowle, B., Bulter, J. M., Carmody, G., Conneally, P. M., Duceman, B., Eisenberg, A., Forman, L., Kidd, K. K., Leclair, B., Niezgoda, S., Parsons, T. J., Pugh, E., Shaler, R., Sherry, S. T., Sozer, A., and Walsh, A. 2005.

DNA identifications after the 9/11 World Trade Center attack. *Science* 310(5751): 1122–1123.

Blakeney, R. L. 2002. *Providing Relief to Families after a Mass Fatality: Roles of the Medical Examiner's Office and the Family Assistance Center.* Washington, D.C.: Department of Justice, Office for Victims of Crime Bulletin, November.

Blau, S. Hill, A., Briggs, C. A., and Cordner, S. A. 2006. Missing persons–missing data: The need to collect antemortem dental records of missing persons. *Journal of Forensic Sciences* 51: 386–389.

Brannon, R. B., and Kessler, H. P. 1999. Problems in mass disaster dental identification: A retrospective review. *Journal of Forensic Sciences* 44: 123–127.

Budimlija, Z. M., Prinz, M. K., Zelson-Mundorff, A., Wiersema, J., Bartelink, E., MacKinnon, G. Nazzaruolo, B. L., Estacio, S. M., Hennessey, M. J., and Shaler, R. C. 2003. World Trade Center Human Identification Project: Experiences with individual body identification cases. *Croatian Medical Journal* 44: 259–263.

Charney, M., and Wilbur, C. G.. 1984. The Big Thompson flood, in T. A. Rathbun and J. E. Buikstra (eds.), *Human Identification: Case Studies in Forensic Anthropology*, pp. 107, 112. Springfield, IL: Charles C. Thomas.

Collins, W. E., and Wayda, M. E. 2003. *Index to FAA Office of Aerospace Medicine reports: 1961 through 2002.* Oklahoma City, OK: Civil Aerospace Medical Institute, Federal Aviation Administration, DOT/FAA/AM-03/1.

De Valck, E. 2006. Major incident response: Collecting antemortem data. *Forensic Science International* 159: S15–S19.

Dirkmaat, D. C, Hefner, J. T., and Hochrein, M. J. 2001. Forensic processing of the terrestrial mass fatality scene: Testing new search, documentation and recovery methodologies. *Proceedings of the American Academy of Forensic Sciences* 7: 241.

Eyre, A. 2002. Improving procedures and minimizing stress: Issues in the identification of victims following disasters. *Australian Journal of Emergency Management* 17: 9–14.

Fierro, M. F. 1993. Identification of human remains, in W.U. Spitz (ed.), *Spitz and Fisher's Medico-Legal Investigation of Death: Guidelines for the Application of Pathology to Crime Investigation*, pp. 71–117. Springfield, IL: Charles C. Thomas.

Fleck, F. 2005. Tsunami body count is not a ghoulish numbers game. *Bulletin of the World Health Organization* 83: 88–89.

Fulginiti, L. C., Warren, M. W., Hefner, J. T., Bedore, L. R., Byrd, J. H., Stefan, V., and Dirkmaat, D. C. 2006. Anthropology responds to Hurricane Katrina. *Proceedings of the American Academy of Forensic Sciences* 12: 305.

Greater London Authority. 2006. *Report of the 7 July Review Committee.*

Hinkes, M. J. 1989. The role of forensic anthropology in mass disaster resolution, *Aviation, Space, and Environmental Medicine* 60: A18–A25.

———. 2001. Ellis Kerley's service to the military. *Journal of Forensic Sciences* 46: 782–783.

Hoffman, S. M., and Oliver-Smith, A. 2002. *Catastrophe and Culture: The Anthropology of Disaster.* Santa Fe, NM: School of American Research Press.

Houck, M. A., Ubelaker, D., Owsley, D., Craig, E., Grant, W., Fram, R., Woltanski, T., and Sandness, K. 1996. The role of forensic anthropology in the recovery and analysis of Branch Davidian Compound victims: Assessing the accuracy of age estimations. *Journal of Forensic Sciences* 41: 796–801.

Jones, D. J. 1985. Secondary disaster victims: The emotional effects of recovering and identifying human remains. *American Journal of Psychiatry* 142: 303–307.

Kahana, T., Ravioli, J. A., Urroz, C. L., and Hiss, J. 1997. Radiographic identification of fragmentary human remains from a mass disaster, *American Journal of Forensic Medicine and Pathology* 18: 40–44.

Kontanis, E. J., and Sledzik, P. S. 2008. Resolving commingling issues during the medicolegal investigation of mass fatality incidents, in B. J. Adams and J. E. Byrd (eds.), *Recovery, Analysis, and Identification of Commingled Human Remain*, pp. 317–336. Totowa, NJ: Humana Press.

Lain, R., Griffiths, C., and Hilton, J. M. N. 2003. Forensic dental and medical response to the Bali bombing: A personal perspective. *Medical Journal of Australia* 179: 362–365.

Levin, B. G. L. 2004. Coping with traumatic loss: An interview with the parents of TWA 800 crash victims and implications for disaster mental health professionals. *International Journal of Emergency Mental Health* 6: 25–31.

Lichtenstein, J. E., Fitzpatrick, J. J., and Madewell, J. E. 1988. The role of radiology in fatality investigations. *American Journal of Radiology* 150: 751–755.

London, M. R., Mulhern, D. M., Barbian, L. T., Sledzik, P. S., Dirkmaat, D. C., Fulginiti, L. C., Hefner, J. T., and Sauer, N. J. 2003. Roles of the biological anthropologist in the response to the crash of United Airlines Flight 93. *Proceedings of the American Academy of Forensic Sciences* 9: 279.

MacKinnon, G., and Mundorff, A. Z. 2007. The World Trade Center—September 11th, 2001, in T. J. U. Thompson and S. M. Black (eds.), *An Introduction to Biological Human Identification*, pp. 485–499. Boca Raton, FL: CRC Press.

Martrille, L., Cattaneo, C., Schuliar, Y., and Baccino, E. 2006. Anthropological aspect of mass disasters. *Proceedings of the American Academy of Forensic Sciences* 12: 304.

McCarroll, J. E., Fullerton, C. S., Ursano, R. J., and Hermsen, J. M. 1996. Posttraumatic stress symptoms following forensic dental identifications: Mt. Carmel, Waco, Texas. *American Journal of Psychiatry* 153: 778–782.

McCarroll, J. E., Ursano, R. J., Fullerton, C. S., Liu, X., and Lundy, A. 2002. Somatic symptoms in Gulf War mortuary workers. *Psychosomatic Medicine* 64: 29–33.

Morgan, O. W., Sribanditmongkol. P., Perera. C., Sulasmi. Y., Alphen. D. V., and Sondorp, E. 2006. Mass fatality management following the South Asian tsunami disaster: Case studies in Thailand, Indonesia, and Sri Lanka. *PloS [Public Library of Science] Medicine* 3: e195.

Mundorff, A. Z. 2003. The role of anthropology during the identification of victims from the World Trade Center disaster, *Proceedings of the American Academy of Forensic Sciences* 9: 277.

———. 2008. Anthropologist directed triage: Three distinct mass fatality events involving fragmentation of human remains, in B. J. Adams, and J. E. Byrd (eds.), *Recovery, Analysis, and Identification of Commingled Human Remains*, pp. 123–144. Totowa, NJ: Humana Press.

Mundorff, A. Z., Shaler, R., Bieschke, E. T., and Mar, E. 2005. Marrying of anthropology and DNA: Essential for solving complex commingling problems in cases of extreme fragmentation. *Proceedings of the American Academy of Forensic Sciences* 11: 315–316.

Mundorff, A. Z., and Steadman, D. W. 2003. Anthropological perspectives on the forensic response at the World Trade Center Disaster, *General Anthropology* 10: 2–5.

Owsley, D. W., Ubelaker, D. H., Houck, M. M., Sandness, K. L., Grant, W. E., Craig, E. A., Woltanski, T. J., and Peerwani, N. 1995. The role of forensic anthropology in the recovery and analysis of Branch Davidian Compound victims: Techniques of analysis. *Journal of Forensic Sciences* 40: 341–348.

Rodriguez, W. C. 2003. Attack on the Pentagon: The role of forensic anthropology in the examination and identification of victims and remains of the 9/11 terrorist attack. *Proceedings of the American Academy of Forensic Sciences* 9: 280.

Saul, F. P., and Saul, J. M. 2003. Planes, trains, and fireworks: The evolving role of the forensic anthropologist in mass fatality incidents, in D. W. Steadman (ed.), *Hard Evidence: Case Studies in Forensic Anthropology*, pp. 266–277. Upper Saddle River, NJ: Prentice Hall.

Simmons, T., and Skinner, M. 2006. The accuracy of ante-mortem data and presumptive identification: Appropriate procedures, applications and ethics. *Proceedings American Academy Forensic Sciences* 12: 303–304.

Simpson, D. M., and Stehr, S. 2003. Victim management and identification after the World Trade Center collapse, in *Beyond September 11th: An Account of Post-Disaster Research*, pp. 109–120. Program on Environment and Behavior Special Publication #39, Institute of Behavioral Science, Natural Hazards Research and Applications Information Center, Boulder, CO: University of Colorado.

Slater, R. E., and Hall, J. E. 1997. *Final Report: Task Force on Assistance to Families of Aviation Disasters*. Washington, D.C.: U.S. Department of Transportation and National Transportation Safety Board.

Sledge, M. 2005. *Solider Dead: How We Recover, Identify, Bury, and Honor our Military Fallen*. New York: Columbia University Press.

Sledzik, P. S., and Hunt, D. R. 1997. Disaster and relief efforts at the Hardin cemetery, in D. A. Poirier and N. B. Bellantoni (eds.), *In Remembrance: Archaeology and Death*, pp. 185–198. Westport, CN: Bergin and Garvey.

Sledzik, P. S., Jantz, L. M., Mundorff, A. Z., Vidoli, G. M., Holland, T. D., Mileusnic-Polchan, D. X., Doretti, M., and Frodebrider, L. 2006. Working with Family Members of Decedents: A Discussion of Techniques for Forensic Scientists. *Proceedings of the American Academy of Forensic Sciences*, 12: 301–302.

Sledzik, P. S., and Kauffman, P. J. 2007. The mass fatality incident morgue: A laboratory for disaster victim identification, in M. W. Warren, H. A. Walsh-Haney, and L. E. Freas. (eds.), *The Forensic Anthropology Laboratory*. Boca Raton, FL: Taylor and Francis/CRC Press.

Sledzik, P. S., and Kontanis, E. J. 2005. Resolving commingling issues, in P. S. Sledzik and E. J. Kontanis. 2005. Resolving commingling issues in mass fatality incidents. *Proceedings of the American Academy of Forensic Sciences* 11: 311.

Sledzik, P. S., Miller, W., Dirkmaat, D. C., de Jong, D. L., Kauffman, P. J., Boyer, D. A., and Hellman, F. P. 2003. Victim identification following the crash of United Airlines flight 93. *Proceedings of the American Academy of Forensic Sciences* 9: 195–196.

Sledzik, P. S., and Rodriguez, W. C. 2002. Damnum fatale: The taphonomic fate of human remains in mass disasters, in W. D. Haglund and M. H. Sorg (eds.), *Advances in Forensic Taphonomy: Methods, Theories and Archaeological Perspectives*, pp. 321–330. Boca Raton, FL: CRC Press.

Sledzik, P. S., and Willcox, W. A. 2003. Corpi Aquaticus: The Hardin cemetery flood of 1993, in D. W. Steadman (ed.), *Hard Evidence: Case Studies in Forensic Anthropology*, pp. 256–265. Upper Saddle River, NJ: Prentice Hall.

Steadman, D. W., Sperry, K., Snow, F., Fulginiti, L., and Craig, E. 2008. Anthropological investigations of the Tri-State Crematorium incident, in B. J. Adams and J. E. Byrd (eds.), *Recovery, Analysis, and*

Identification of Commingled Human Remains, pp. 81–96. Totowa, NJ: Humana Press.

Stewart, T. D. (ed.). 1970. *Personal Identification in Mass Disasters*. Washington, D.C.: Smithsonian Institution.

Thieren, M. 2005. Asian tsunami: Death-toll addiction and its downside. *Bulletin of the World Health Organization* 83(2): 82.

Tun, K., Butcher. B., Sribanditmongkol, P., Brondolo, T., Caragine, T., Perera, C, and Kent, K. 2005. Forensic aspects of disaster fatality management. *Prehospital and Disaster Medicine* 20: 455–458.

Tyrrell, A. J., Kontanis, E. J., Simmons, T. L. V., and Sledzik, P. S. 2006. Restructuring data collection strategies in investigation priorities in the resolution of mass fatality incidents. *Proceedings American Academy Forensic Sciences* 12: 165.

Ubelaker, D. H. 2000. The forensic anthropology legacy of T. Dale Stewart (1901–1997). *Journal of Forensic Sciences* 45: 245–252.

Ubelaker, D. H., Owsley, D. W., Houck, M. M., Craig, E., Grant, W., Woltanski, T., Fram, R., Sandness, K., and Peerwani, N. 1995. The role of forensic anthropology in the recovery and analysis of Branch Davidian Compound victims: Recovery procedures and characteristics of victims. *Journal of Forensic Sciences* 40: 335–340.

United States Department of Justice, Office of Justice Programs. 2005. *Mass Fatality Incidents: A Guide for Human Forensic Identification*. Washington, D.C.

———. 2006. *Lessons learned from 9/11: DNA Identifications in Mass Fatality Incidents*. Washington, D.C.

United States National Transportation Safety Board. 2000. *Federal Family Assistance Plan for Aviation Disasters,* Washington, D.C.

Ursano, R. J., and McCarroll, J. E. 1990. The nature of the traumatic stressor: Handling dead bodies. *Journal of Nervous and Mental Disease* 178: 396–398.

———. 1994. Exposure to traumatic death: The nature of the stressor, in R. J. Ursano, B. G. McCaughey, and C. S. Fullerton (eds.), *Individual and Community Responses to Trauma and Disaster: The Structure of Human Chaos*, pp. 46–71. New York: Cambridge University Press.

Wagner, G. N., and Froede, R. C. 1993. Medico-legal investigation of mass disasters, in W. U. Spitz (ed.), *Spitz and Fisher's Medico-Legal Investigation of Death: Guidelines for the Application of Pathology to Crime Investigation*, pp. 567–584. Springfield, IL: Charles C. Thomas.

Warren, C. P. 1981. Forensic anthropology in a military setting. *Human Organization* 40: 172–180.

Warren, M. W., Eisenberg, L. E., Walsh-Haney, H., and Saul, J. M. 2003. Anthropology at Fresh Kills: Recovery and identification of the World Trade Center victims. *Proceedings of the American Academy of Forensic Sciences* 55: 278.

Warren, M. W., Smith, K. R., Stubblefield, P. R., Martin, S. S., and Walsh-Haney, H. A. 2000. Use of radiographic atlases in a mass fatality. *Journal of Forensic Sciences* 45: 467–470.

Webb, D. A., Sweet, D., and Pretty, I. A. 2002. The emotional and psychological impacts of mass casualty incidents on forensic odontologists. *Journal of Forensic Sciences* 47: 539–541.

Weedn, V. W. 1998. Postmortem identification of remains. *Clinics in Laboratory Medicine* 18: 115–137.

Wiersema, J. M., Bartelink, E., Budimlija, Z., Prinz, M., Shaler, R., Mundorff, A. Z., and MacKinnon, G. 2003. The importance of an interdisciplinary review process in the World Trade Center mass disaster investigation. *Proceedings of the American Academy of Forensic Sciences* 55: 194.

Williams E. D., and Crews, J. D. 2003. From dust to dust: Ethical and practical issues involved in the location, exhumation, and identification of bodies from mass graves. *Croatian Medical Journal* 44: 251–258.

Wood, W. R., and Stanley, L. A. 1989. Recovery and identification of World War II dead: American Graves Registration activities in Europe. *Journal of Forensic Sciences* 34: 1365–1373.

Wright, R. 2006. Tales of atrocity from the grave. *The Australian* 17th May, www.theaustralian.news.com.au/story/0,20867,19158508-12332,00.html.

31

MEDICO-LEGAL INVESTIGATIONS OF ATROCITIES COMMITTED DURING THE SOLOMON ISLANDS "ETHNIC TENSIONS"

Melanie Archer and Malcolm J. Dodd

Fifty exhumations and autopsies were conducted in the Solomon Islands between 2003 and 2006 as part of the medico-legal investigation into the "Ethnic Tensions" murders. This investigation was unusual for two main reasons. First, all autopsies were carried out by one Australian forensic pathologist (Dodd) over the course of several visits to the country. Second, most gravesites were accessible to exhumation teams only by air or sea, and this created significant logistical challenges. Difficulties were exacerbated by a need for rapid results to charge alleged perpetrators. This was partly because some former militants were a flight risk while at liberty, but also because swift criminal indictment demonstrated to the traumatised community that positive results could be achieved. The operations were ultimately successful, with over 50 former militants having been arrested by April 2004 (Wainright 2004).

The 1998 to 2003 Ethnic Tensions was a brutal conflict that received scant media attention. This civil war centred on Guadalcanal Island (Figure 31.1), and was predominantly between the people of Guadalcanal (Guales) and the neighbouring Island of Malaita. Fractiousness between these people has been recorded since colonial times (Fraenkel 2004), but the recent Ethnic Tensions caused economic and political chaos for the Solomon Islands, because its capital city, Honiara, was engulfed in the turmoil.

The influx of Malaitans onto Guadalcanal following World War II was a major step in the evolution of the recent troubles. A large United States military base was established in Guadalcanal during the South Pacific campaign, and Honiara became the capital. Malaitan settlers were among those exploiting its postwar economic and employment opportunities and many acquired land, which often contravened Guale customs of matrilineal land inheritance and tribal land ownership. Additionally, many Guales felt that their power base was eroded by Malaitan domination of various institutions. For example, by 1998, Malaitans accounted for approximately 75% of the Royal Solomon Islands Police Force (RSIP). Immigrants also held many jobs in Honiara and occupied many surrounding residences (Dinnen 2002; Fraenkel 2004).

In 1998, tensions between Guales and settlers escalated, and a clandestine Guale militia organisation, the Guadalcanal Revolutionary Army, began evicting migrants (mainly rural Malaitans). The pro-indigenous movement later split into factions, the most notorious of which was Harold Keke's Guadalcanal Liberation Front (GLF). A Malaitan opposition group, the Malaita Eagle Force (MEF), eventually formed under the leadership of Jimmy

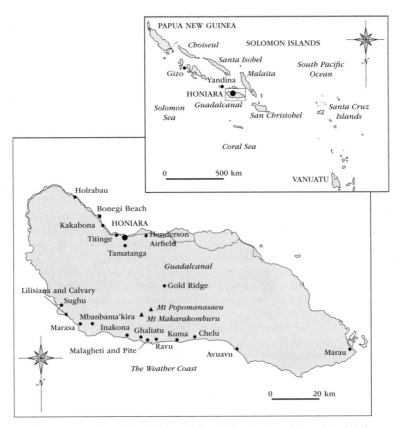

Figure 31.1 Map of the Solomon Islands showing Guadalcanal in detail.

"Rasta" Lusibaea. Honiara became the MEF's stronghold, whereas pro-indigenous groups held rural areas such as the remote Weather Coast. The Tensions culminated in the MEF-led coup on June 5, 2003, and international intervention was requested by the Solomon Islands Parliament following the Prime Minister's forced resignation (Fraenkel 2004).

It is estimated that around 100 fatalities resulted from the Tensions (Anonymous 2003; Fraenkel 2004), and thousands were internally displaced and terrorised before the first contingent of the Regional Assistance Mission to the Solomon Islands (RAMSI) arrived on 24 July 2003 (Fraenkel 2004). Member countries comprised Australia, New Zealand, Papua New Guinea, Samoa, Fiji, Vanuatu, Kiribati, Cook Islands, Nauru, Tuvalu, and Tonga; these countries initially provided among them 2,225 police, military, and other personnel (Anonymous 2003). The end of the Tensions was swift and bloodless following RAMSI's commencement, but the Operation is still active and now mainly concerned with capacity building and tackling official corruption.

Another of RAMSI's main aims is to prosecute perpetrators of crimes committed during the lawless Tensions period. A proportion of the offences were murders for which RAMSI investigations have yielded detailed witness statements and victim grave locations. Therefore, exhumations and autopsies of 50 victims were undertaken to verify witness statements, provide victim identifications, and determine cause and manner of death. This process began two months after RAMSI arrived, and the initial murder trials in the Honiara High Court (Guadalcanal) have already resulted in life imprisonment for several key militants.

Exhumation Protocol

The remoteness of most exhumation sites necessitated air or sea travel, and few exhumations were conducted close enough to Honiara to utilise road travel. There are no vehicular tracks to the Weather Coast, so a combination of helicopters and Short Take Off and Landing aircraft (Caribous and Twin Otters) was used to transport equipment, personnel, and human remains. A naval ship was also once used to travel from Honiara to the Weather Coast, with helicopter transfer to land. These specialised transport needs presented a challenge, because exhumation teams were competing for air support with personnel from other RAMSI sections. Tight drop-off and pick-up schedules were therefore necessary, and teams often had to extract bodies within six hours. An additional requirement for speed was the risk of unpredictable tropical downpours flooding exhumation sites.

There was a high degree of consultation with the local people prior to each exhumation, although they were not directly involved with body extraction. Local ministers of religion were also invited to conduct ceremonies at several graves prior to exhumation. Villagers were predominantly relied on to locate remains, because graves were usually dug by them after militants abandoned the bodies of their victims. Even when murderers buried their victims, this was often done within several hundred meters of villages and in full view of witnesses.

Most exhumations were led by an Australian and New Zealand Police Disaster Victim Identification (DVI) team, and the remainder were led by police investigative and crime scene personnel. An experienced anthropologist/archaeologist was not included with the team for unknown reasons, perhaps partly because of the relative novelty of the discipline in Australasia and a corresponding unawareness of the valuable contribution that anthropologists can make to body recovery. The forensic pathologist fulfilled one major role of the archaeologist by attending gravesites where extensive commingling of remains was expected. Most remains were relatively easy to extract from the surrounding soil without archaeological expertise, which was especially true of those enclosed within wrappings. However, an archaeologist prepared to work under the necessary time constraints could possibly have further increased the pace of some exhumations and probably would have been able to prevent the single case of exhumation fracture that damaged one victim's skull. This unfortunate accident was due to the inexperience of a DVI team member in distinguishing skeletal elements from the surrounding soil and detritus.

Autopsy Protocol

The first three Ethnic Tensions autopsies were performed at Weather Coast gravesites using trestle tables and tents as a makeshift mortuary. Despite the rudimentary nature of the setup, basic autopsy technique was applied, including detailed photography. Remaining cases were examined at the Honiara National Referral Hospital mortuary (Guadalcanal).

Remains were classified as "decomposing" if ≥60% of soft tissues was present and "skeletonised" if <60% of soft tissue was present. All cases had focal areas of skeletonisation and varying degrees of disarticulation; several also had focal areas of mummification or adipocere (the insoluble fatty acids remaining as a residue from pre-existing fats following decomposition). Autopsy technique was therefore somewhat flexible to accommodate these differences. There was no radiographic equipment available, so extra time and care were necessary to locate metallic ballistic evidence.

Bones were placed in buckets of water and cleaned if they were relatively devoid of soft tissues. When skulls were washed, care was taken to avoid loss of teeth and cranial fragments. Bones were then dried, reassembled to anatomical position, and photographed. Traumatised skeletal elements were placed on white paper and injuries clearly annotated with marker pens prior to photography.

Victim Identification

DNA samples were taken from the femoral head and teeth, and these were processed at the Australian Federal Police laboratories. Skeletal indicators of identity were of limited value in distinguishing individuals: all victims except one were male, all were Melanesian, and most were between 20 and 30 years old and of a similar stature. In addition, healed fractures were found in only two cases, and no medical prostheses were recovered. Odontological methods were similarly unhelpful in most cases, since only two victims had evidence of dental treatment. There were no distinctive dental features, such as diastemas, although four cases of periodontal disease were seen that could potentially have caused enough pain that associates of the victim may have been aware of their condition.

No identifying documents or cards were located, which is unsurprising given that the majority of people are rural subsistence farmers. But hairstyles are distinctive in the living population, and, in particular, there are many combinations of dreadlock configuration and length. Dreadlocks were commonly preserved intact on decomposed bodies and were therefore an excellent feature on which to base putative identifications.

Clothing was usually light because of the tropical climate and was often remarkably well preserved. T-shirts usually bore distinctive logos and designs that sometimes allowed establishment of a putative identity. Some groups of victims also wore similar clothing, which grouped them as casualties of particular incidents. For example, seven priests from the Melanesian Brotherhood were murdered (six in one incident), and these men wore a distinctive uniform supplied by a single clothing company. Jewellery and property were also helpful putative identifiers, and either or both were present in 56% of cases.

Decomposition and Burials

All 50 individuals had been buried. The majority (52%) were in beach graves <50 m from the beach front. Beach sand at most grave locations is coarse and wet, with a layer of pebbles beginning at approximately 50–100 cm deep. Graves were seldom dug below this level, which is probably because pebbles are difficult to dig through, and grave edges collapse beneath this depth. Thirty-six percent of cases were jungle burials ≥50 m from the beach front. Jungle soil is humic, and extensive networks of tree roots hinder digging. There was also heavy bone erosion in the jungle environment, especially in thin areas such as scapulae; this was sometimes hard to differentiate from trauma. Only 12% of cases were buried in village cemeteries; one in a coffin and the remainder with

or without fabric wrappings. Cemetery graves were sometimes marked by planting coconut trees at the head and foot of the body. Tree roots grew throughout several skeletons, even penetrating the cortex of some bones and holding others in anatomical position.

There was more than one victim in 57% of "killing incidents," defined here as a militia killing (or killings) in the same village or municipal location on the same day. However, 61% of graves were single, which probably arises from the high number of graves reportedly dug by people not involved with the killings and who knew the victims. But the high number of single graves may also be due partly to the comparative ease of digging single graves (especially in loose beach sand), as opposed to pits large enough to accommodate multiple bodies. Most remaining graves were double and triple burials, although there was one mass grave containing eight of ten mercenaries who journeyed to the Weather Coast to capture certain GLF commanders. Commingling of skeletal elements between bodies was seen in 42% of cases, which is the majority of bodies buried in multiple graves.

Many variables are likely to have affected decomposition rate: postmortem interval; antemortem trauma; initial body mass; rainfall, clothing; wrappings/coverings; grave depth; soil type;

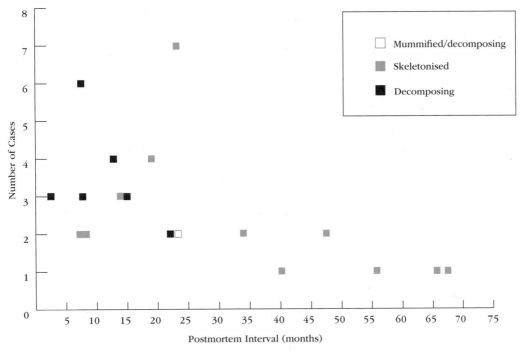

Figure 31.2 Number of cases in each decomposition category for Ethnic Tensions victims medico-legally examined by RAMSI ($n = 50$).

soil moisture; number of bodies in the grave; degree of decomposition prior to burial and type of overlying vegetation. Evidence of scavenging was seen in 30% of cases; this may also have affected decomposition rates (local scavengers include pigs, dogs, birds, cats, and rodents). The combined effect of variables that affect decomposition produced amazing differences in the state of remains of the same age, burial type, and even within mass graves (Figure 31.2). Therefore, postmortem interval was a poor predictor between about six months and two years of whether a body would be decomposing or skeletonised (see Figure 31.2). Indeed, graves dug within the same month, and within meters of one another, could contain a mixture of decomposing and skeletonised bodies.

Potential ligatures were associated with 44% of remains and were predominantly around the wrists and arms; no potential blindfolds were located. In one case, a loop of material encircled the left lower thigh in the region of skeletal gunshot damage and may have been a tourniquet rather than a ligature. Several individuals had multiple unconnected ligatures encircling areas such as the wrists and waist, and two victims were bound together at the ankles. The material from which ligatures were fashioned was variable: rope, vine, cloth, wire, and fishing line were all used.

Injury Patterns

Most victims sustained blunt-force trauma combined with gunshot trauma; however, exclusive blunt or gunshot trauma was also common (Table 31.1). Sharp-force trauma was rarely seen, which may have been because soft-tissue defects had decomposed. But our figures (Table 31.1) may be accurate, because there were correspondingly few witness reports of sharp-force trauma being inflicted.

Gunshot Trauma

Thirty-five victims sustained at least one gunshot injury, although, because of decomposition, only the minimum number of gunshot wounds could be determined. In all gunshot cases, ballistic trauma would have been sufficient to cause death, and police information indicates that modern military-style weapons were generally used (for example, "SLR" and "SR88 A" semi-automatic assault rifles).

Gunshot trauma to the thoracic and abdominal skeleton was usually differentiated with ease by morphology and extent from other forms of trauma. Rib fractures caused by gunshot injury were often of the shatter type, rather than linear, vertical, or oblique. Incomplete circular defects on rib margins caused by projectile transit were additionally present in three cases. Similarly, pelvic gunshot trauma was of the extensive shatter type, rather than the relatively clean curvilinear fractures seen in low-grade blunt-force trauma.

Projectile entry points were concentrated around the head and torso, and few cases of gunshot injury to the limbs were seen. In 46% of gunshot cases, the presence of coexistent blunt trauma strongly suggested that beating accompanied the shooting. Witness statements support the proposition that many of these fracture patterns represent a form of menacing or torture prior to execution by gunshot.

Cranial gunshot cases incurred massive fracture with the shatter patterns typically caused by the passage of high-velocity projectiles. Clear internal and external bevelling was seen in some skulls, and most displayed fracture and dissociation of the cranial plates with the characteristic pattern of symmetrical facial skeletal separation. This is the hallmark of rapidly expanding cranial contents.

The trajectory of fire could be reconstructed in some cases and was most striking for a group of mercenaries allegedly killed by the GLF. Witnesses claim that the men were lined up on the beach with their backs to the ocean and that their executioners stood facing the victims, elevated above them on a sandy shelf. Bullets had passed from the frontal chest to the dorsal lumbar structures in several bodies examined, which could occur only if the shooter was elevated above the standing victim or if the victim was hunched or leaning forward before a standing shooter.

Table 31.1 Patterns of injury sustained by victims of Ethnic Tensions murders medico-legally examined by RAMSI. Numbers of individuals ($n = 50$) sustaining each type or combination of trauma are given, along with percentage of cases in each category.

Gunshot Trauma Only	Blunt Trauma Only	Combined Gunshot and Blunt Trauma	Combined Gunshot, Blunt and Sharp Trauma	Combined Blunt and Sharp Trauma
12 (24%)	13 (26%)	22 (44%)	1 (2%)	2 (4%)

Most high-velocity jacketed military-style projectiles should exit the body, leaving only shattered skeletal elements. But in 15 gunshot cases, ballistic evidence was recovered. In 5 cases, deposits of friable blue-green material that represented oxidised bullet jacketing were present. These were carefully differentiated from brass studs and degraded green clothing, which can appear similar. Surprisingly, 10 cases also yielded large uncorroded bullet jacket and core fragments, and 3 cases retained largely intact projectiles. Projectile remnants were sometimes deeply embedded in bone but were also located in decomposed soft tissues or soil contained within body bags. A further 2 cases had NATO 7.62 short-cartridge cases contained within debris in the body bag, which highlights the need for meticulous examination of detritus accompanying remains.

There are possible explanations for the high percentage of cases that retained ballistic evidence. First, much of the high-velocity ammunition used by the GLF and IFM was obtained from World War II underground stock piles. Police investigators reported to us that this ammunition was unreliable, with misfires being common: not only can the casing of ammunition corrode as it ages, but the propellant can degrade. Some militants also used weapons of World War II vintage that are likely to have become unreliable, and some may also have used homemade weapons (Fraenkel 2004). This combination of factors can reduce muzzle velocity of projectiles and cause instability in trajectory, which would result in a high retention rate within bodies.

Blunt Trauma

Blunt-force trauma was most commonly inflicted in the thoracic region (58%), followed by the head and neck (32%). Definitively lethal blunt-force trauma to the head was identified in only two victims who had both sustained massive occipital fractures. In the 14 cases where blunt force was thought to be the leading cause of death, analysis of injury patterns strongly suggests a bias toward repeated and aggressive thoracic trauma.

Thoracic trauma involved predominantly the ribs, although complex and often depressed fractures of the manubrium and/or sternum were documented in 14 cases. Sternal fractures are frequently present in victims of high-velocity motor vehicle accidents but rarely result from beatings. At least one rib fracture was present in 70% of remains, probably due mainly to blunt trauma. Two victims suffered clavicular fractures (one bilateral), and six victims suffered scapular fractures (two bilateral).

These again probably represent blows with sticks and gun butts, as was frequently recorded in witness statements.

Most blunt-force trauma deaths were probably caused by extreme compressive forces applied to the anterior chest, with or without intercurrent blows to the lateral rib cage. In these cases, extensive bilateral rib fractures (often resulting in flail segments) were identified. The most common fracture plane was lateral, followed by posterior and anterior, and this pattern is typical of forceful front to back compressive force. Two potential mechanisms derived from witness reports could be stomping and dropping rocks onto the chests of victims. Death would be caused by a combination of lung collapse following puncture by broken ribs, haemopneumothorax formation (air and blood in the chest cavity), and cardiac contusion and/or laceration.

Analysis of fracture frequency for individual ribs shows virtual sparing of the well-protected 1st and 2nd ribs, and complete sparing of the small and flexible 12th rib (Figure 31.3). Maximal trauma involved ribs 4–9, often in multiple planes, and a bilaterally symmetrical pattern was frequently seen. In some cases, focal aggregates of fracture were also seen on the lateral rib cage, often involving three to four sequential ribs, indicating areas of kicking or striking.

Blunt trauma involving the middle one-third of the face (four cases) and mandible (seven cases) further indicated that blows to the face may often have been delivered prior to killing by crushing the chest. In one case, few injuries were identified apart from two rib fractures overlying the spleen. Witnesses report that the victim became very thirsty before he collapsed and died, indicating that death was probably due to splenic rupture and internal blood loss. This is a particular risk in malaria-ridden countries, where splenomegaly is common, and Dodd autopsied a recently deceased murder victim in the Solomon Islands (unrelated to the Ethnic Tensions) who had similar injuries. She was kicked in the ribs, resulting in rupture of her grossly enlarged spleen and internal loss of approximately 2 L of blood.

Pelvic fractures were seen in only two cases, probably because the pelvis is largely protected by overlying fatty tissue and deep musculature. One victim had an uncomplicated pelvic fracture, perhaps from a kick or gun butt blow, and this injury was coupled with repeated chest trauma. The second case (see Case Studies: Honiara Murder at the end of the chapter) was attributed to motor vehicle impact.

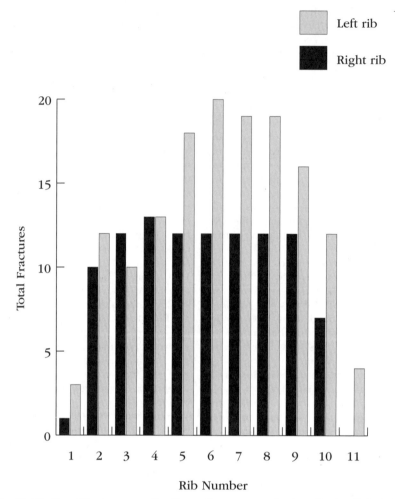

Figure 31.3   Distribution of fractures over the ribcage for cases examined medico-legally by RAMSI. Values are numbers for each rib of victims who sustained at least one fracture to that rib.

Blunt trauma to vertebrae, often with bone loss, was frequently seen in combination with repeated thoracic trauma. Seven victims demonstrated spinal trauma involving 13 separate vertebrae between them. Maximal trauma extended from T5–T10, again in keeping with kicking or blows from a gun butt. It is impossible to determine exactly how these injuries were caused, but it is worth noting that this segment of the spine is prominent if a defensive foetal posture is adopted.

Blunt trauma to the extremities was seen in four cases and was restricted to the upper arm, forearm, and hand. In each case, these injuries were combined with blunt-force trauma to the chest. A higher incidence of defence-type injury to the upper limbs may be expected in cases of repeated blunt-force assault, but the paucity

of injuries to the extremities may be explained in two ways. First, there was a high incidence of ligature binding (either of the limbs themselves or the binding of the victim to an object, such as a tree). Second, many victims may quickly have been immobilised through loss of consciousness.

Sharp-Force Trauma

Sharp-force trauma was identified in three victims only. This is in stark contrast to atrocities in East Timor, where blows by jungle knives and machetes were recorded in 43% of deaths investigated (Pollanen 2003). One victim was allegedly struck with a machete across the upper right back/shoulder area (see Case Studies: Marasa Village Incident at the end of the chapter). This wound involved soft tissue only, and according to witnesses constituted part of the torture phase prior to death. Another victim, who was reportedly stabbed, had a solitary shaved and incised defect to a single rib. Examination of his T-shirt showed three independent incised defects to the lower anterior chest/upper abdominal area. Two of these defects did not correspond with skeletal trauma, so were deemed to overlie soft-tissue trauma obscured by decomposition.

Case Studies

In these two case studies, victims' names are coded for privacy. These are not the most horrific incidents investigated but demonstrate some typical pathology and illustrate aspects of investigative methods.

Marasa Village Incident

A Joint Operations Group (JOG) of collaborating militants and police operated on the Weather Coast in 2003 attempting to capture GLF leaders. On June 15, 2003, two boats were sent to Marasa village by the RSIP to reprovision JOG members further inland. Their radio communications were allegedly intercepted by the GLF, who gained information about the landing of the resupply party and ambushed them while they were unloading their boats. An RSIP Special Constable (victim F3) was allegedly shot dead while attempting to start the boat's outboard motor. The remaining JOG forces and resupply party fled, and the body of F3 was taken to Sughu village and buried by locals. The body was wrapped in a tent and buried in a beach grave approximately 175 cm deep.

Two local villagers (F1 and F2) were captured on June 16, 2003, by the GLF. Victim F2 was a former RSIP Special Constable, and F1 was a teenager who had been accused by the GLF of being a government spy. The two victims were allegedly tortured, humiliated, and beaten until their deaths some hours later. Money delivered by the resupply boat to pay JOG members was seized, and some was allegedly torn up and rammed down the throats of F1 and F2 with a stick. Surprisingly, RAMSI forensic officers found numerous fragments of material that appeared to be Solomon Islands bank notes under the stones on Marasa Beach in September 2003.

Over 400 villagers were abducted along with F1 and F2 and forced to watch the entire incident, but they were instructed to refrain from showing emotion under threat of death. Most of their village was burned down the day after F1 and F2 died.

The hostage villagers were also used to attempt to lure RSIP boat patrols into the area, but the militants did not succeed and eventually abandoned the area. The bodies of F1 and F2 were buried by villagers in a jungle grave approximately 75 cm deep.

The three heavily decomposed victims were autopsied at the exhumation sites approximately three months after death. There were ligatures associated with the wrists of F1 and F2, and both had several nonlethal injuries that corroborated witness statements of prolonged torture. For example, each sustained blunt-force mandibular fractures, and F2 additionally had a blunt-force nasal bridge fracture and a superficial incised injury to the upper right back, supporting a witness report that he was struck across the shoulder with a machete. F2's oral cavity also had an area of focal swelling and haemorrhage in keeping with the allegation of forceful cramming of paper money fragments into the back of his throat with a stick.

The possibility of mechanical asphyxia following this treatment cannot be excluded, although the cause of death for both victims F1 and F2 was ultimately designated as blunt-force trauma to the chest. Examination of the thoraces of both victims disclosed multiple bilateral fractures, and F2 additionally sustained a sternal fracture. There was accompanying haemorrhage into the upper right anterior, lateral and posterior intercostal muscles of F1. Death would have resulted from a combination of lung collapse following puncture by broken ribs, haemopneumothorax formation (air and blood in the chest cavity), and cardiac contusion and/or laceration.

Victim F3 was allegedly shot while trying to start the boat's motor, and witnesses reported seeing a plume of blood discharged from the head or neck at the moment of projectile impact. Autopsy revealed a "through and through" defect through his laryngeal cartilage, and the right lateral surface showed a degree of external bevelling. There was also a shatter-like fracture to the medial one-third of the left and right clavicles, and the right 1st rib showed a central shatter-like fracture with complete separation of the lateral and medial halves. A vertically oriented fracture was identified through the manubrium, and there was also bullet jacketing and core associated with the remains.

All injuries to F3 were deemed to have been caused by the path of a single high-velocity projectile through the neck and upper right chest. The projectile is likely to have severed major blood vessels and caused aspiration of blood, asphyxia, and significant internal blood loss. Its trajectory would be in keeping with the stooped and partially rotated position that may be adopted while trying to start an outboard motor.

Honiara Murder

Three RSIP Special Constables were allegedly conveyed to Jimmy Lusibaea's compound on 26 January 2002, because they were believed to have been involved in the killing of several MEF members. Victim W1 escaped but was reportedly rammed by a four-wheel-drive vehicle, after which he continued into long grass, where he was recaptured and shot dead. His body was later recovered from the Lunga River (Honiara), and he was buried within a body bag and a wooden coffin at Titinge cemetery (Honiara City Outskirts). One of the other captive Special Constables was also reportedly killed during this incident, but his body was never found.

W1's remains were exhumed two years after death. The soft tissues had been liquefied by their enclosed environment, and approximately 40 L were retained within the body bag with minimal flesh adherent to the skeleton. Copious ammonia had formed from the liquefied flesh, and fumes were sufficiently strong to require mortuary personnel to take frequent breaks outside.

The liquid flesh was sieved, and fragments of bullet jacketing were found. There was also a 6-mm diameter defect through the iliac fossa of the left hemipelvis and a small contralateral conical and ovoid defect representing the point of projectile impact. This indicated that a bullet passed into the pelvis from right to left, impacting and rebounding.

There was evidence of extensive blunt-force trauma as seen after impact with the bumper of an oncoming vehicle. A comminuted fracture accompanied extensive chipping-type bone loss through the body of the left ischium, and this extended over the posterior half of the left acetabulum. There was also a transverse oriented fracture with anterior bone loss of the promontory of the sacrum and a comminuted fracture with extensive bone loss of the left neck of femur.

The cause of death was intra-abdominal/flank high-velocity gunshot wounding in tandem with extreme blunt-force trauma to the left hip (in keeping with motor vehicle impact), and the mechanism of death would have been extensive internal haemorrhage.

Conclusion

The number of Ethnic Tensions victims was relatively small compared with large-scale fatalities in Kosovo, Iraq, and East Timor. Witness statements were detailed in most cases and were often given by relatives or associates of the deceased. This meant that corroboration of witness statements linked to individual victims assumed greater judicial importance than in many large-scale or clandestine killings where such statements are frequently unavailable (e.g., Cordner 2005; Pollanen 2003).

There has been considerable success in bringing to justice those responsible for the crimes described here. Many people endured campaigns of terror and intimidation mounted by criminals, and the prosecution of prominent militants has made a significant difference to the community rebuilding process.

Acknowledgments

We thank John McIntyre (AFP/Operation RAMSI), who corrected many of the facts about the circumstances surrounding cases. Brian Dobrich, Neville Spradau, Harry Hains, Penny Spies, and Andy Thorpe (AFP/Operation RAMSI) also checked our facts on the investigations with which they were involved. Steve Williamson (Operation RAMSI) very kindly gave us permission to access the Panatina Investigation findings, and Dale Potter (Operation RAMSI) made us feel at home when we read through these files at Rove Police Station. Finally, thanks to VIFM's Director, Professor Stephen Cordner. He not only put up with our absences but also has been supportive of our desire to document our experiences.

References

Anonymous. 2003. Peacekeeping: The changing face of the Solomons. *Platypus* 80: 9–13.

Cordner, S. M. 2005. The missing: Action to resolve the problem of those unaccounted for as a result of armed conflict or internal violence, and to assist their families. *VIFM Review* 3: 2–6.

Dinnen, S. 2002. Winners and losers: Politics and disorder in the Solomon Islands 2000–2002. *The Journal of Pacific History* 37: 285–298.

Fraenkel, J. 2004. *The Manipulation of Custom: From Uprising to Intervention in the Solomon Islands.* Wellington: Victoria University Press.

Pollanen, M. S. 2003. *Forensic Investigation of Mass Killing in East Timor*, 1999. East Timor: Report prepared for the Office of the Prosecutor General.

Wainright, E. 2003. Responding to state failure: The case of Australia and the Solomon Islands. *Australian Journal of International Affairs* 57: 485–498.

———. 2004. Solomon Islands, Papua New Guinea and Australia's policy shift. *The Sydney Papers*, Autumn edition: 123–132.

32

DISASTER ANTHROPOLOGY: THE 2004 ASIAN TSUNAMI

Sue Black

Until relatively recently, forensic anthropology was not routinely employed in mass-fatality investigations. Opinion began to change when anthropological expertise came to the fore in the identification of the victims of war crimes and violations of human rights in South America and then in Rwanda (Ferllini 1999), followed in rapid succession by the atrocities witnessed in East Timor, Sierra Leone, and the former Yugoslavia, (Baraybar and Gasior 2004; Glenny 2000; Komar 2003; Steadman and Haglund 2005). Now, as a result of terrorist-related incidents (for example, Bali bombing [see Briggs and Buck this volume], 9/11, London bombings, and Sharm el Sheikh, to name a few) and natural disasters (for example, Asian Tsunami, hurricane Katrina), the position of forensic anthropology has been more firmly secured within war crimes investigations and global Disaster Victim Identification (DVI) response requirements (Lain, Griffiths, and Hilton 2003; MacKinnon and Mundorff 2007). Indeed forensic anthropology is a major component of the national DVI training programme for the U.K. (Black et al. 2008).

Anthropology has a significant role to play at both a national and an international level in assisting the judicial investigation of homicide, mass disaster incidents, crimes against humanity, war crimes, and genocide (Steadman and Haglund 2005). The context under which many

anthropological cases are undertaken has changed during the last decade owing to a number of factors that have affected not only how forensic anthropologists perform their job but also the types of jobs they are now requested to undertake, and the 21st century has seen an increasing likelihood of practitioners involved with mass-fatality incidents. Thus, it may be argued that viewing the forensic anthropologist as someone who "*deals with the analysis of human skeletal remains resulting from unexplained deaths*" (as defined by Byers 2004; italics added) is unrealistically restrictive, given the multidisciplinary nature of the demands of human identification in the 21st century.

This chapter briefly discusses the background of the Asian Tsunami of 2004 and the international disaster victim identification (DVI) response that arose. The role that different forensic disciplines, including forensic anthropology, played in the disaster scenario is addressed.

Background

Tsunami is Japanese for "harbour wave." Japanese fishermen would return to port to find utter devastation in the settlements surrounding their harbour (*tsu*) although they had been oblivious to any impending wave-(*nami*)-related disaster while they had been at sea.

A tsunami can be defined as a series of waves that are generated by an impulsive disturbance (normally an earthquake, although not exclusively) that displaces a large volume of water. These waves form as a result of the water mass attempting to regain its equilibrium, and because water cannot be compressed, the energy is dissipated in an outward direction as "shallow-water" waves. The term is somewhat confusing but in fact refers to the ratio between water depth and wavelength. Unlike normal waves, which might have a wavelength of about 91 m (300 ft) a tsunami wave may have a length in excess of 483 k (300 miles). Waves move at a speed that is equal to the square root of the product of the acceleration of gravity (9.8 m/s²) and water depth. Because the ratio between water depth and wavelength is very small for a tsunami, it can move at a speed in excess of 805 k (500 miles) per hour, and because of a shoaling effect when the wave reaches the coastline, it can grow to over 30 m (100 ft) in height before it breaks land, although the popular concept of a "wall of water" is not always realised. A wave loses energy at a rate inversely proportional to its wavelength, and therefore a tsunami wave can travel at high speeds over prolonged distances for an extended period of time and lose very little of its initial energy before it hits land (Bryant 2001; Lautrup 2005; Tibballs 2005).

Environmental and human devastation occur when the wall of water pushes and floods inland, destroying all in its path through the energy and volume of the water, with most of the damage caused by the large mass of water behind the initial wave front. The sheer weight of the water is sufficient to pulverise objects in its path, often reducing buildings to their foundations and scouring exposed ground to the bedrock; large objects such as ships can be carried several kilometres inland before the tsunami subsides. The destruction continues as the wave then retreats, sucking debris and people back out to sea in the trough in front of the succeeding wave.

Normal waves have a regular periodicity of approximately 10 seconds (that is, distance between successive crests), but a tsunami wave may have a periodicity of up to an hour. Therefore, there can be a considerable time delay between successive waves of destruction, which can lead to increased fatalities when survivors feel it is safe to go back to their homes to look for other survivors or collect possessions. However, the first wave is not always the most powerful or destructive, and many more lives can then be lost in subsequent waves.

Most tsunamis occur in the Pacific Ocean as a result of the large number of active volcanic island

arcs, mountain ranges, and subduction zones (Dudley and Lee 1998). Although the last pan-Pacific tsunami occurred in 1964, over 146 warnings have been issued in the past six years for the Pacific Rim (PTWC). This high propensity for tsunamis has led to the development of an elaborate system of early-warning devices by the 26 member states that border the Pacific Rim. However, tsunamis in the Indian Ocean are rare, with the penultimate major event occurring in 1883 as a result of the Krakatoa volcanic eruption. Because of the infrequency of their occurrence there, the Indian Ocean had no early warning capabilities before 2005.

The 2004 Tsunami

At 00:58:53 UTC or Zulu time (07:58:53 local time) on 26 December 2004, an undersea earthquake measuring 9.3 on the Richter scale was recorded with a hypocentre just north of Simeulue Island off the west coast of northern Sumatra (3.316°N, 95.854°E). This has been labelled the "Indian Ocean earthquake" or the "Sumatra-Andaman earthquake," and it occurred some 30 k (19 miles) below sea level. Approximately 1,207 k (750 miles) of a north-south oriented faultline slipped 15 m (50 ft) along the subduction zone where the India plate passes under the Burma tectonic plate. The rupture proceeded at a speed of over 10,137 kmph (6,300 mph) and lasted over 200 seconds— the longest duration of faulting ever recorded. It took place in two phases, with the first occurring off the coast of Aceh and the second toward the Nicobar and Andaman islands. Approximately 11 cubic kilometres (7 cubic miles) of water was displaced as the seabed rose by several metres, and a series of tsunami waves radiated out from the entire length of the rupture line. Technically, this was therefore a *teletsunami,* because it resulted from a vertical rather than a horizontal displacement of the seabed. The seismic energy release was calculated to be equivalent to 0.25 gigatons of TNT and was sufficient to slightly alter the Earth's rotation—mathematicians have calculated that it may result in a shortening of the day by approximately 2.68 microseconds (Cook-Anderson and Beasley 2005). It was reported that the Andaman and Nicobar islands were displaced to the south west by around 1.2 m (4 ft) and sunk by around 1 m (3 ft) (*Science Now* 2005).

The North/South orientation of the fault ensured that some landmasses to the north (for example, Bangladesh) remained relatively unaffected as the full brunt of the force was meted out on coastlines to the east and west of the hypocentre as the waves emanated along the full length of the fault-line. Even many of the landmasses that were technically in the shadow of the waves (for instance, the west coast of Sri Lanka) did not remain unaffected, because a tsunami can diffract, producing a "wrap-around" effect.

Variously referred to as the "Asian tsunami" or the "Boxing Day tsunami," it resulted from the second largest ever-recorded seismic event in history, with a periodicity of over 30 minutes between each crest—and the third wave proved to be the most powerful and fatal, arriving a full hour after the first devastation. Eighteen countries were affected around the boundaries of the Indian Ocean—Indonesia, Thailand, India, Sri-Lanka, Malaysia, Myanmar, Bangladesh, Maldives, Reunion Island, Seychelles, Madagascar, Mauritius, Somalia, Tanzania, Kenya, Oman, South Africa, and Australia. Some of the tsunami's energy escaped into the Pacific Ocean and produced small but measurable tsunamis along the coasts of North and South America, and a wave was even registered at Japan's Syowa Base in Antarctica (Japan Coast Guard 2004).

Of the fatalities, almost half were in Indonesia, with the highest proportion of European tourists being killed in Thailand. The disaster occurred at the height of the Christmas/winter tourist season, and holidaymakers from over 40 countries were involved. Sweden was most heavily affected with 428 dead and 116 missing. This was the most devastating tsunami in history, claiming the lives of over 200,000 individuals with a further 40,000 reported missing and millions rendered homeless and displaced. The United Nations Secretary-General at the time, Kofi Annan, stated that this was probably the most expensive natural disaster in history and could take anything up to 10 years to see full reconstruction achieved.

Disaster Victim Identification (DVI) Responses

With regard to the death toll, Indonesia (approx. 220,000), Sri Lanka (approx. 31,000), and India (approx. 16,000) suffered the largest number of fatalities, and over half of the Thailand fatalities (5,395) were foreign tourists (Tun et al. 2005; UNOSETR 2006). Note that most international DVI teams were not mobilised under the direction of providing humanitarian assistance but were more commonly under home political direction to facilitate matters of national repatriation. Therefore, over 30 DVI teams from around the world descended on Thailand within days of the event, while the other countries with significantly larger death tolls

(Indonesia, India, and Sri Lanka) were largely left to deal with their own dead with little or no international assistance. There was a small but temporary international presence in Sri Lanka, but each international team pulled out once all its nationals had been identified. This situation frequently led to dissatisfaction expressed by the international team members and left indigenous workers no alternative but to opt for a mass-burial solution with limited attention to identification issues (Perera 2005). In the early days, many Interpol DVI teams remained fiercely parochial, focusing their efforts on "finding their own" deceased, which led to some animosity. This approach served to hinder the larger operation, but common sense prevailed largely through good communication and sound diplomacy (Tun et al. 2005).

Not surprisingly, the response to this enormous natural disaster was managed in very different ways in different countries (Morgan et al. 2006a), and for the most part there was little prior local planning that would assist with the enormity of the operation. This chapter is restricted to the international DVI situation in Thailand, where multinational disaster victim identification teams operated for a complete calendar year.

The Response in Thailand

International teams began to arrive in Thailand around 27 December, and an agreement was reached with the Thai authorities that the international teams would work in collaboration with the Royal Thai police and the Thai forensic experts. On 12 January, the Thai Tsunami Victim Identification (TTVI) centre was established in Phuket. Over 30 international DVI teams would work for nearly a full calendar year to establish the identity of the deceased in Thailand. The teams variably comprised police officers, forensic biologists, fingerprint experts, pathologists, odontologists, anthropologists, radiographers, and mortuary technicians. The British team in the early stages comprised police officers and fingerprint experts and in time would be supplemented with CIFA odontologists who would assume the principal identification conduit for the operation.

It was agreed that Interpol protocols and procedures would be adopted utilising the relevant yellow antemortem and pink postmortem forms (Interpol 2002). Antemortem data from families was directed through Consular or Embassy interactions with the Royal Thai Police, and antemortem/postmortem comparisons were undertaken at the Information Management Centre

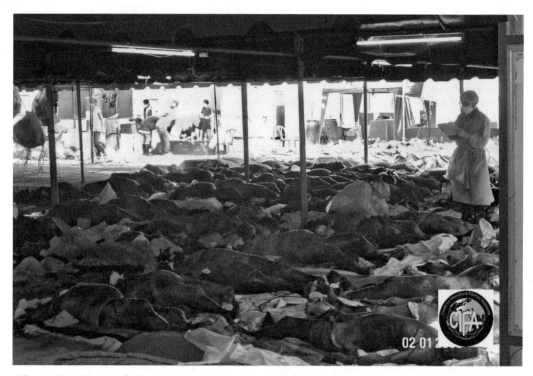

Figure 32.1 Remains laid out in lines prior to arrival of refrigerated containers. Bloating and discoloration of the corpses is evident (photograph courtesy of the author; used with permission of CIFA).

(IMC) in Phuket utilising the Danish *Plass Data* computer software.

Initial body recover in Thailand was a largely uncoordinated event with the deceased transported to temples on the back of trucks by survivors, local volunteers, NGO personnel, military, reservists, and police. No records were kept of which bodies had been found together or the location from where the bodies had been recovered. At the temples, the bodies were laid out in rows (several hundred at a time), and some temporary shade from the sun was achieved by the erection of makeshift awnings (Figure 32.1). The lack of refrigerated containers in the early stages resulted in a decision being taken by many local authorities to bury the bodies in mass graves in an attempt to lower the temperature and slow decomposition. This action led to inflammatory accusations of attempts to bury bodies without addressing identification issues. An attempt was, however, made to surround many of the bodies with dry ice to halt escalating decomposition. This proved largely unsuccessful, although a modicum of result was achieved when the bodies were placed in surrounding cells of ice and then the entire area was covered with a tarpaulin (Figure 32.2). However, a considerable number of health and

safety casualties resulted from the dry-ice packing process: workers received burns from touching and moving the corpses. Largely to prevent such injuries, workers tried to achieve the same goal using water-based ice, but this led to unacceptable groundwater contamination issues and unsanitary working conditions.

Temporary mortuary sites were initiated in the early days at temples in Khao-Lak, Phuket, and Krabi. Each body was photographed as it arrived at the temple, and the images were made available on computer for families to attempt visual identification. However, the heat, humidity, and lack of refrigeration meant that most bodies had passed beyond facial recognition within 48 hours of death. In this regard, children were particularly difficult to identify, because the decomposition process rendered facial identification virtually impossible from the outset. The resulting images became too distressing for families to view, and so this practice was halted. When postmortem images were misleading and inappropriate for public view, forensic artists were employed to recreate facial appearance from the soft-tissue remains. The images were cleaned to remove debris, and any clothing was highlighted. The effects of decomposition, bloating, deformation, and discolouration were

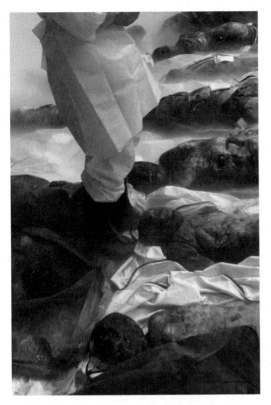

Figure 32.2 Remains waiting for analysis were packed with dry ice in an attempt to slow decomposition (photograph David I. Gross; used with permission of David I. Gross).

eliminated, and characteristic facial details were emphasised in an attempt to stimulate recognition (Figure 32.3).

Although some remains were allegedly identified through either visual means or personal effects, mistakes were inevitably made, and several cases of incorrect identification were picked up later in the process as more refined and reliable methods of identification were employed. It was established in the investigation of the Bali bombing in 2002 (see Briggs and Buck this volume) that visual identification of the deceased proved to be incorrect in approximately one-third of cases (Lain, Griffiths, and Hilton 2003). Consequently, as Interpol advises, visual identification should not be encouraged. Within the first week, Thai authorities had released over 1,000 bodies to families, and approximately 500 bodies were released by local physicians and police without recourse to forensic assistance (Morgan et al. 2006). Misidentification inevitably leads to an incorrect outcome for two individuals and their families.

Many of the early problems in the tsunami identification programme arose through the inability to separate Indigenous from Western deceased with any degree of reliability. The heat, humidity, and effect of water resulted in rapid decomposition that primarily affected the external appearance of the body—where the most immediate indicators of ancestry are located, for example, skin colour, hair type, epicanthic folds). This led to quite considerable international animosity that was sufficiently vociferous at one stage to actually threaten the continuation of the entire international programme. A unilateral decision was taken by the local authorities to bury all Indigenous personnel and concentrate on repatriation of the Western nationals. Such a sorting process is problematic, particularly considering the demographics of a country such as Australia, where many citizens are of Asian descent. In the tsunami event in Thailand, although many individuals may well have been of Thai descent, victims could not automatically be assigned Thai national status—in some cases, they were more appropriately classified as "foreigners." This led to accusations that the primary sorting process based on biological identity was fundamentally flawed and not sufficiently robust, and it was suspected that Western nationals were inadvertently being included in the mass graves. Ultimately, this concern led to all mass graves being exhumed at a later date to allow one additional recording of information before the deceased were re-interred.

Clearly, the lack of scientific anthropological input pertaining to indicators of ancestry was contributing to a volatile situation that required resolution, but anthropological advice was never sought and when given was generally not welcome, because it would have required a realignment of adopted procedures. Misidentification was addressed in some cases at a later date, when DNA analysis would indicate the identity of an interred individual—resulting in that individual being exhumed for a third time. This situation could largely have been prevented if anthropological expertise had been introduced at an early stage in the preliminary deployments.

When the steady flow of corpses arriving at the mortuaries showed no sign of abating, health and safety practical issues had to be addressed. Although there is some acceptance of the fact that an accumulation of a large number of corpses does not necessarily escalate into pandemic high-risk infections (Morgan, Tidball-Binz, and Van Alphen 2006; PAHO 2004), issues relating to personal protective equipment, disposal of waste, and long-term storage and processing issues all had to be addressed. Late in March it was decided to consolidate mortuary efforts by building new facilities at the site of the largest temporary mortuary in Wat

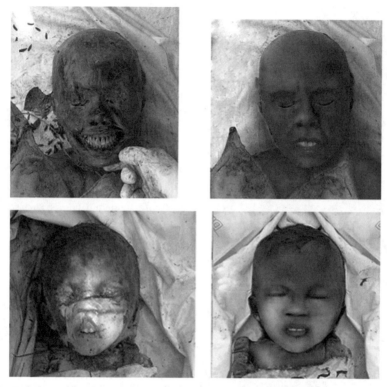

Figure 32.3 Early loss of facial recognition led to attempts to assist via reconstructive art (photograph Dr. C. Wilkinson; used with permission of Dr. C. Wilkinson).

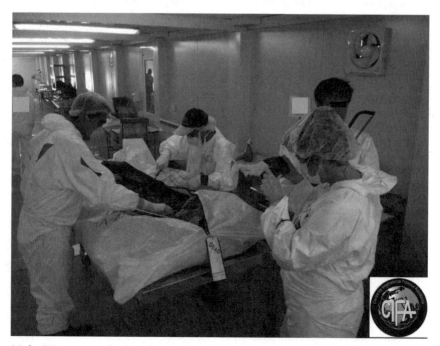

Figure 32.4 DVI mortuary facilities (photograph courtesy of the author; used with permission of CIFA).

Yan Yao in the northern Thai Province of Phang Na (Figure 32.4). This was the largest of the temporary mortuary sites and had handled over 3,000 corpses during the first three months of the operation while housing over 300 people in a working day.

Sources of Identification

Each mass-fatality scenario dictates its own requirements and solutions, and the Asian tsunami was largely an issue of identification of the deceased rather than a collection of evidence for prosecutorial purposes (for example, Kosovo war crimes investigations) or for establishing cause of death (for instance, domestic homicides). The main characterising issues for the Asian tsunami were the condition of the remains, the mode of recovery, and the number of victims. By the time international teams were involved, the issue of body recovery was largely moot. It was decided at an early stage of the proceedings that there would be three primary identifiers: fingerprints, dentition, and DNA. Each of these processes was not without problems, laying down challenges and lessons to be learned for future responses (Alonso et al. 2005; Kieser, Ling, and Herbison 2006). The role of identification is clearly portrayed in the TTVI mission statement—to identify victims of the Thai tsunami and release them for repatriation to their families in accordance with the Thai law, Interpol DVI guidelines, and TTVI protocols.

The comparison of antemortem and postmortem fingerprints has a relatively short utilisation period, because skin slippage resulting from advanced decomposition renders the contact ridge pattern too damaged or faint for recording. Therefore, in Thailand the antemortem recovery of fingerprints was likely to be an identification option for a restricted time period owing to the rapid rate of decomposition in the early stages. Because there is no genetic basis to fingerprints, recovery for comparison with relatives was not an option but relied on circumstantial recovery. The initial prospect for fingerprint identifications was not promising, but surprisingly over 24% of the identifications between January and March 2005 were achieved by this method. This was largely due to fingerprint records being kept by countries that issued identification cards where this was a recorded biometric.

Comparison of antemortem and postmortem dental information was chosen wisely as the principal means for speedy identifications of the deceased Western tourists. Dental records were sourced from family dentists and the information converted into the antemortem Interpol format. This was then transferred to the IMC in Phuket, where comparisons were made with postmortem forms. Although the *Plass data* system worked quite well in this regard, the final confirmation of identity often required the experience of forensic odontologists to refine the detailed aspects (Figure 32.5). Between January and March 2005, approximately 73% of

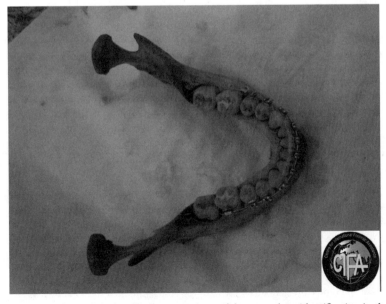

Figure 32.5 Dental analysis proved to be the most successful approach to identification in the early stages (photograph Dr. J. Robson; used with permission of CIFA).

identifications were achieved through dental comparisons, highlighting the importance of accurate dental recording and record keeping (see Clement this volume).

A variety of national and international laboratories were initially contracted to undertake the DNA analysis. Collection of antemortem DNA generally relied on buccal swab samples from surviving relatives and the generated profiles being compared with profiles retrieved from bone or tooth samples of the deceased. This process, of course, did not achieve separation of siblings or close family relations. Owing to the extensive and increasing levels of decomposition, many laboratories found it difficult to extract a full DNA profile to a level that was acceptable by many Western countries. Eventually the Royal Thai Police entered into an agreement that the DNA profiling would be undertaken by the International Commission on Missing Persons (ICMP), which has an international reputation for extraction of DNA from degraded samples. In the early stages, few identifications were made through DNA analysis (less than 3%), but this number will inevitably rise as the final analysis approaches.

Between January and March 2005, over 4,000 postmortem examinations were undertaken, and over 2,000 antemortem files had been listed. Within 8 months, nearly 70% of identifications had been achieved. For comparison, after the World Trade Center terrorist attack on September 11, 2001, identification of 50% of the 3,025 took 18 months (Schwartz et al. 2002), and the 202 deceased of the Bali bombing in the same year took approximately 6 months (Lain, Griffiths, and Hilton 2003).

The Role of the Forensic Anthropologist in Mass Disasters

Where was the forensic anthropology in this largest mass disaster of modern times? Unfortunately, the discipline remained largely marginalised throughout the entire proceedings. Although issues pertaining to ancestry could have been addressed, they were not, and a great opportunity was missed. Most anthropologists served to assist pathologists and odontologists in the general recording of data, and they played virtually no part in the reconciliation of antemortem with postmortem data. Was this a reasonable approach, or are the anthropologists aggrieved at their lack of involvement?

A mass-fatality situation requires that the most appropriate disciplines be involved to meet the needs of the situation in hand (see Sledzik this volume). In the war crimes investigations of the former Yugoslavia (see Sterenberg this volume) and Rwanda, the bodies were generally severely decomposed, and the anthropologist's role was in reconstructing biological identity from the remains and assisting the pathologist in the reconstruction of trauma injuries to establish a cause of death or the trajectory of a missile. Comparison of antemortem and postmortem data was the primary remit of the tsunami scientific effort in an attempt to identify the deceased and to assign a name to the individual. This identification can best be achieved through markers that can be established via other professional disciplines (for example, fingerprints, dental information, and DNA). Each scientific discipline takes on a level of responsibility that is appropriate to the questions being asked about the remains and the purposes of the deployment. Anthropology could have assisted greatly in the determination of ancestry, which could have prevented unnecessary hostilities, but this problem was largely overcome through diplomatic means. However, anthropology is likely to play a continuing role in Thailand and other countries where there will be a continuous uncovering of human remains over time as redevelopment continues. Many countries do not have forensic anthropological training (for instance, Sri Lanka and Thailand), and so there will be a need to equip and assist these countries to adapt to changing identification issues in the ongoing humanitarian response to the aftermath of the largest natural disaster in recent history.

In the United Kingdom, the Asian tsunami heralded the development of an organised DVI response capability. This was launched in 2006, and anthropology is involved in both the training and deployment capabilities of the team. The Centre for International Forensic Assistance (CIFA) has been tasked with coordination of the medical, scientific, and technical component of the team and has identified the British Association for Human Identification (BAHID) as the nominated repository for contact with forensic anthropologists in the United Kingdom. Due credit will be given to those forensic anthropologists who have evidenced their professionalism through accreditation with the Council for the Registration of Forensic Practitioners (CRFP 2006), which is rapidly becoming a recognised source for professional registration within the forensic disciplines.

Conclusion

The people who survive such mass disasters as the tsunami are also victims, and although Laurence Binyon's poem "The Fallen" serves to commemorate those whose lives were lost in the First World War, it applies equally to those who were lost in

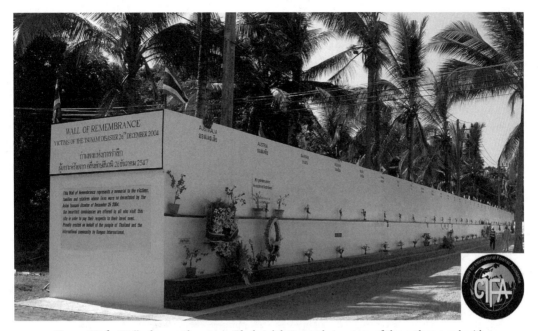

Figure 32.6   Wall of remembrance in Phuket (photograph courtesy of the author; used with permission of CIFA).

the most recent worldwide disaster and serves as a comfort to those who have survived: "They shall not grow old as we who are left grow old. Age shall not weary them, nor the years condemn. At the going down of the sun and in the morning, we will remember them."

Remembrance is a vitally important part of the healing process, and the chosen focus for that act is intimately personal. The Asian Tsunami Wall of Remembrance commemorates the disaster and ensures that the world will not forget those who died on 26 December 2004 (Figure 32.6); it also offers a focus for annual pilgrimage. We can never forget that the results of our labours in forensic identification primarily aid the living.

About the Figures: The Tamaki Makau-rau Accord on the Display of Human Remains and Sacred Objects

I recognise that the display of human remains is a sensitive issue for a variety of reasons. The disaster of the south Asian tsunami affected hundreds of thousands of individuals and represented a mass disaster on a scale that has never been encountered before. The use of these images attempts to inform not only with regard to the enormity of the mass scale of events that but also to the dedication and care of attention given to each and every

case. At the time of writing, none of the individuals depicted had been positively identified, and no cultural or community appropriateness could be observed other than the international standards of decency, dignity, and respect. The right of the individual to the retention of his or her identity is recognised. Permissions have been given by the Thai authorities, the DVI teams, and NGO organisations involved for images to be made available for publication—lest we forget the scale of devastation. The survivors, families, and friends could not be consulted for permission, because they were not known at the time of writing. These images are a powerful record of an unprecedented humanitarian disaster and serve to facilitate scientific and humanitarian learning.

References

Alonso, A., Martin, P., Albarran, C., Garcia, P., Fernandez de Simon, L., Jesus Iturralde, M., Fernandez-Rodriguez, A., Atienza, I., Capilla, J., Garcia-Hirschfeld, J., Martinez, P., Vallejo, G., Garcia, O., Garcia, E., Real, P., Alvarez, D., Leon, A., and Sancho, M. 2005. Challenges of DNA profiling in mass disaster investigations. *Croatian Medical Journal* 46(4): 540–548.

Baraybar, J. P., and Gasior, M. 2004. Forensic anthropology and the most probable cause of death in cases of violations against International Humanitarian

Law: An example from Bosnia and Herzegovina. *Journal of the Royal Society for the Promotion of Health* 124(6): 271–275.

Black, S., Walker, G., Hackman, L., and Brooks, C. 2008. *Disaster Victim Identification: The Practitioner's Guide.* Dundee: Dundee University Press.

British Association for Human Identification (BAHID). www.bahid.org (accessed 26/08/06).

Bryant, E. 2001. *Tsunami: The Underrated Hazard.* Cambridge: Cambridge University Press.

Byers, S. N. 2004. *Introduction to Forensic Anthropology.* Upper Saddle River, NJ: Prentice Hall.

Centre for International Forensic Assistance (CIFA). www.cifa.ac (accessed 24/08/06).

Cook-Anderson, G., and Beasley, D. 2005. NASA details earthquake effects on the earth. *National Aeronautics and Space Administration* (press release), 10 January 2005.

Council for the Registration of Forensic Practitioners (CRFP). www.crfp.org.uk (accessed 24/ 08/06).

Dudley, W. C., and Lee, M. 1998. *Tsunami!* Honolulu: University of Honolulu Press.

Ferllini, R. 1999. The role of forensic anthropology in human rights issues, in K. Reichs (ed.), *Forensic Osteology: Advances in the Identification of Human Remains*, pp. 287–301. Springfield, IL: Charles C. Thomas.

Glenny, M. 2000. *The Balkans 1804–1999 Nationalism, War and the Great Powers.* London: Granta Books.

International Commission on Missing Persons (ICMP). www.ic-mp.org/downloads/press/Tsunami_TChart.pdf (accessed 24/08/06).

Interpol 2002. Interpol Disaster Victim Identification Guide. www.interpol.int/Public/DisasterVictim/guide/chapitre3.asp (accessed 24/08/06).

Japan Coast Guard. 2004. Indian Ocean tsunami at Syowa Station, Antarctica. www1.kaiho.mlit.go.jp/KANKYO/KAIYO/KOUHOU/iotunami/iotunami_eng.html, Hydrographic and Oceanographic Department, Japan Coast Guard (accessed 24/08/06).

Kieser, J. A., Laing, W., and Herbison, P. 2006. Lessons learned from large-scale comparative dental analysis following the South Asian tsunami of 2004. *Journal of Forensic Sciences* 51(1): 109–112.

Komar, D. 2003. Lessons from Srebrenica: The contributions and limitations of physical anthropology in identifying victims of war crimes. *Journal of Forensic Sciences* 48: 713–716.

Lain, R., Griffiths, C., and Hilton, J. M. 2003. Forensic dental and medical response to the Bali bombing:

A personal perspective. *Medical Journal of Australia* 179: 362–365.

Lautrup, B. 2005a. Tsunami physics. www.nbi.dk/~lautrup/continuum/tidbits/tsunami.english.pdf#search=%22tsunami%20physics%22 (accessed 24/08/06).

———. 2005b. Tsunamiens fysik. *Kvant: Tidsskrift for Fysik og Astronomi* 1: 22–25.

MacKinnon, G., and Mundorff, A. Z. 2007. The World Trade Centre: September 11, 2001, in T. Thompson and S. Black (eds.), *Forensic Human Identification: An Introduction*, pp. 485–501. Boca Raton, FL: CRC Press.

Morgan, O., Sribanditmongkol, P., Perera, C., Sulasmi, Y. Van Alphen, D., and Sondorp, E. 2006. Mass fatality management following the south Asian tsunami disaster: Case studies in Thailand, Indonesia and Sri Lanka. *Plosmedicine* 3(6): e195.

Morgan, O., Tidball-Binz, M., and Van Alphen, D. 2006. *Management of Dead Bodies after Disasters: A Field Manual for First Responders.* PAHO/WHO/ICRC.

Pan American Health Organization (PAHO). 2004. *Management of Dead Bodies in Disaster Situations.* Washington, D.C.: PAHO.

Perera, C. 2005. After the tsunami: Legal implications of mass burials of unidentified victims in Sri Lanka. *Plosmedicine* 2(6): e185.

PTWC (Pacific Tsunami Warning Centre). www.prh.noaa.gov/ptwc/bulletins/pacific/ (accessed 24/08/06).

Schwartz, S. P., Li, W., Berenson, L., and Williams, R. D. 2002. Deaths in World Trade Center terrorist attacks: New York City, 2001. *Morbidity and Mortality Weekly Report* 51: 16–18.

Science Now. 2005. *After the earth moved.* http://sciencenow.sciencemag.org/, January 28.

Steadman, D. W., and Haglund, W. D. 2005. The scope of anthropological contributions to human rights investigations. *Journal of Forensic Sciences* 50: 23–30.

Tibballs, G. 2005. *Tsunami: The World's Most Terrifying Natural Disaster.* London: Carlton Books ltd.

Tun, K., Burcher, B., Sribanditmongkol, P., Brondolo, T., Caragine, T., Perera, C., and Kent, K. 2005. Panel 2.16: Forensic aspects of disaster fatality management. *Prehospital and Disaster Medicine* 20(6): 455–458.

United Nations Office of the Special Envoy for Tsunami Recovery (UNOSETR). www.tsunamispecialenvoy.org/country/humantoll.asp (accessed 24/08/06).

33

THE ROLE OF THE ANTHROPOLOGIST IN DISASTER VICTIM IDENTIFICATION: THE BALI INCIDENTS OF 2002 AND 2004

Christopher A. Briggs and Alanah M. Buck

Disaster Victim Identification (DVI) is the term given to the procedures used to positively identify deceased victims of a multiple-casualty event (*Victorian Disaster Victim Identification Manual* 2005). In all mass fatalities, the deceased need to be identified to the satisfaction of the local jurisdictional authorities, such as the Coroner (in Australia and Great Britain) or the Chief Medical Examiner (in the United States of America). In a domestic context, forensic experts usually work as an extension of the local legal process, and individual identification goes hand in hand with determination of cause of death. However, in mass disasters the cause of death may already be known or strongly suspected (for example, shrapnel type injury, inhalation of fire fumes), and identification therefore becomes the most difficult and resource-intensive task. Identification is, however, not just a legal requirement but has moral, ethical, and financial ramifications. For both legal and compassionate reasons, forensic specialists need to ascertain how many individuals are represented and, as far as possible, match the remains against available records of known persons involved in the disaster.

According to international standards as outlined by the International Criminal Police Organisation (INTERPOL), the DVI process is carried out in five separate phases (Figure 33. 1). Traditionally, the examination of human remains in the DVI process has been carried out by the pathologist and the dentist. However, with advances in identification technology, such as DNA profiling, the procedures for individual identification have expanded to include a number of specialist areas, including anthropology, medical science, and archaeology. The role of the anthropologist is to support the identification and investigation process by supplying information that would not easily be determined from a routine examination (see Sledzik this volume).

The Nature of Mass Fatalities

Mass fatalities can occur in a variety of ways but commonly involve extreme forces affecting the body (Figure 33.2). Natural disasters are often large in scale and "open" in nature, that is, they involve large numbers of bodies where there are no clues as to identity. In contrast, a "closed" human-made disaster, such as a plane crash, may result in a large number of bodies; however, the identities of the victims are generally known. Recent examples of open human-made disasters include the terrorist train bombings in Madrid in 2004, the bombings of London's public transport system in 2005, and terrorist attacks in Dahab in Egypt in 2006. These disasters all highlight the problems associated with human identification when the victims' ages and ethnic backgrounds are widely varied.

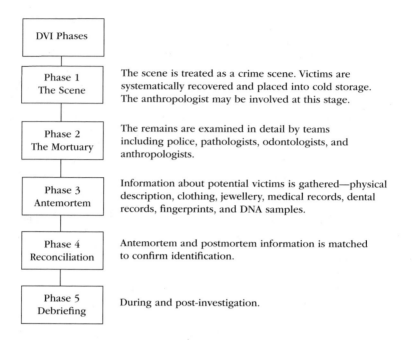

Figure 33.1   Interpol phases of disaster victim identification.

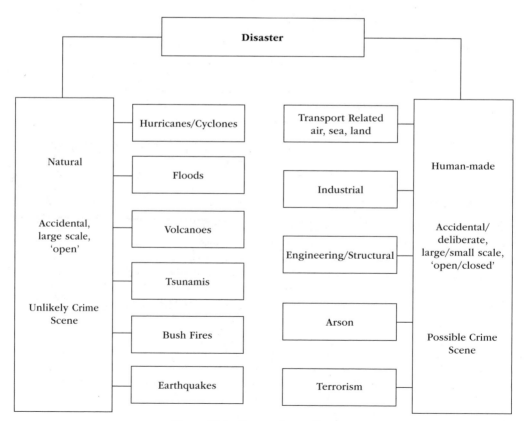

Figure 33.2   Nature of mass disasters.

The extreme forces associated with mass disasters that affect the body result in a variety of differentially preserved human remains. Natural disasters generally result in complete bodies, which may exhibit incineration and/or decomposition. Human remains following human-made disasters are often more disrupted, with varying degrees of incineration, fragmentation, and/or decomposition. Such conditions have a significant effect on identification processes.

Other factors that influence the nature of the DVI process include these:

- *record keeping*: Most Western nations have detailed and relatively easy-to-access antemortem (AM) records. In contrast, AM records are absent or at best often difficult to locate in most developing nations.

- *criminal activity*: When a criminal act has taken place before or during a mass disaster, further forensic investigation is required.

- *multinational involvement*: Incidents that involve individuals in locations other than their country of origin or in transport-related accidents (for example, ferry or plane).

The Role of the Anthropologist in DVI

By definition, a forensic anthropologist should have a background in physical anthropology. The discipline relies on a sound knowledge of human anatomy and in particular, osteology. As the pathologist and odontologist, the anthropologist should be experienced in coronial mortuary work and have the appropriate academic qualifications. Following are recommendations for the selection of anthropologists required for DVI deployment:

- appropriate tertiary qualifications;
- experienced forensic practitioners with recent casework history;
- affiliation with recognised forensic institution;
- experience with mortuary material (for example, badly disrupted, burnt, and/or decomposed human remains).

Required Skills

A forensic anthropologist's role at a DVI scene will be determined by the nature of the event.

However, certain skills will be required in most circumstances. The forensic anthropologist must be able to:

- identify small fragments of bone from any region in the body;
- identify left and right elements (often from small fragments);
- identify cross-sections of bone in soft tissue masses;
- assess incinerated (no soft tissue) remains;
- where possible, assess age, sex, and ancestry in heat-damaged and/or disrupted remains.

Depending on the type of incident, the role of the anthropologist may change over the time of the investigation. In a natural disaster, the anthropologist might be introduced at a later stage of examination, as the bodies become more decomposed and are unable to be identified by other methods. In a human-made disaster, where bodies are disrupted and scattered, the anthropologist can be involved during Phase 1, in the recovery of bodies from the scene.

Medical Advisory Team (MAT) Member

At a mass disaster, the anthropologist will usually work in conjunction with a pathologist and an odontologist. Combined, these three professionals form a strong team, covering all areas of assessment of human remains (Buck 2004). The DNA specialist is also involved in the assessment of remains for sample suitability. Examination by the anthropologist and assessment of whole bodies that are partially disrupted or incinerated can provide information useful for identification relating to:

- personal age estimation;
- sex;
- ancestry;
- stature;
- trauma or individualising bony anomalies.

The assessment of body parts is ideally undertaken with a pathologist, who evaluates soft-tissue structures. Protocols for the sampling of body parts for DNA profiling should be established before the sampling begins (that is, standard size of sample, policy for exclusion of unsuitable material). These protocols are best determined by a team of anthropologist, pathologist, and DNA expert.

The 2002 Bali Bombings

On Saturday, 12 October 2002, just after 11:00 P.M., at a time when foreign tourists as well as locals were out enjoying the night life in Bali's Kuta district, an explosion ripped through Paddy's Irish Bar, a popular destination with holidaymakers, causing massive damage to the building and to the surrounding tourist strip (Figure 33.3). This explosion was followed 10 to 15 seconds later when a second bomb, concealed in a white Mitsubishi van, was detonated outside the Sari Club (just across the road from Paddy's Bar), another nightspot frequented by Western tourists. Less than a minute later a third bomb was detonated in the suburb of Renon, just 100 m from the United States Consulate.

Indonesian authorities immediately started the task of removing the deceased from the wreckage of the two buildings and commenced disaster victim identification procedures. It was thought the death toll might be in the vicinity of 180–200 individuals, and was likely to include people of many nationalities. It was anticipated that up to 50% of the casualties were Australian, with the majority being young people in their 20s and 30s. The Australian government response was immediate and, in consultation with the Indonesian government, formed a multi-agency support team, incorporating expertise from state police services, the Australian Security Intelligence Organization (ASIO), and the Department of Foreign Affairs and Trade (DFAT), as well as contributions from the various Australian state forensic institutions, which sent pathologists, odontologists, technical support staff, and other specialists (e.g., Lain, Griffiths, and Hilton 2003). They were soon joined by forensic experts from Holland, Hong Kong, Japan, Sweden, Taiwan, the United Kingdom, and the United States. Teams were initially rostered on 14-day rotations, although this was modified as the work proceeded. The work undertaken in Bali was not the first time that Australian forensic specialists had been involved in the investigation and identification of large numbers of deceased in overseas jurisdictions; however, it was the first time that the Australian Federal Police (AFP) and forensic experts from across the continent had been asked by a foreign sovereign government (Indonesia) to assist in the determination of identity of Australians abroad.

Phase 1: The Scene

The scene was treated as a crime scene. Victims were systematically recovered and, when possible, placed into cold storage. The scene was photographed and videotaped and the position of human remains recorded. Although this phase of such operations is usually delayed until all survivors are removed, in Bali it was instituted as quickly as possible to negate the rapid rate of decomposition in the hot and humid conditions. Twelve hours after the blasts, both Sari Club and Paddy's Bar were still ablaze; however, recovery personnel had to begin the task of extricating bodies from the ruins. Body parts were not only in the buildings but also widely dispersed within and around the two major bomb

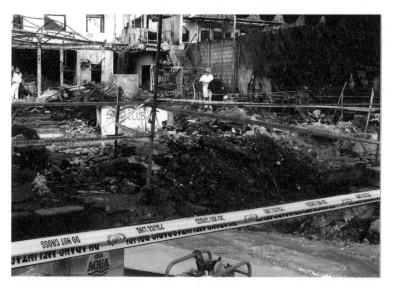

Figure 33.3 Image of nightclub explosion (photograph courtesy of the author).

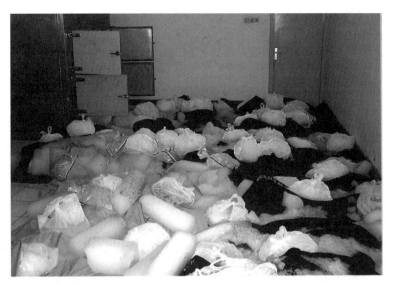

Figure 33.4 Body parts in cold storage, Sanglah Hospital (photograph courtesy of the author).

sites (for example, on nearby roofs) and scattered over a wide area. Many body parts were not easily recognisable. All immediately accessible bodies and body parts were labelled with a unique identification tag, bagged, and delivered by Indonesian authorities, including local volunteers, to Denpasar's Sanglah Hospital mortuary (Figure 33.4). Property located at the scene was collected, labelled, and its location recorded.

Phase 2: The Mortuary

Owing to a lack of portable refrigeration units, the deceased victims were placed under awnings in the space connecting the mortuary to the hospital administration wing and covered with ice. On arrival in the mortuary, the remains were logged and placed into storage until space and personnel were available to begin examination. Bodies were examined in detail, initially by teams of pathologists, odontologists, and anthropologists.

Unlike in a normal autopsy examination of a deceased person, in Bali the emphasis was on clues that might reveal identity rather than on determination of cause of death (which in most cases was already established). The face and the entire body of victims were photographed (clothed and unclothed). Jewellery, personal effects, and clothing were photographed in situ, examined, cleaned, rephotographed, then secured. When appropriate, the external examination took note of the individual's skin and hair colour, sex, likely age, height, weight, and body build. The unclothed body was examined for distinctive features such as tattoos,

birthmarks, scars (for example, of previous surgical procedures), nicotine staining of fingers, and obvious deformities and malformations. Visual identification is, however, known to carry a significant risk of misidentification (e.g., Watts 2002). Of the 16 bodies that had been visually identified by families immediately following the incident, nine had been incorrectly identified, reinforcing the need for consistent and reproducible procedures (Lain, Griffiths, and Hilton 2003).

Police conducted fingerprint analysis, and molecular biologists waited for DNA samples to be taken. When possible, at least three DNA samples were removed from different body sites. This was not always possible, owing to the calcined or decomposed nature of many of the bodies. A bone sample, preferably the proximal femur, muscle tissue from unburned regions of the body, and hair and blood were taken, stored in dry ice, and immediately shipped back to the Australian Federal Police DNA laboratory in mainland Australia. Following examination, the remains were returned to storage to await further examination in light of accumulating antemortem information. Anthropological examinations were conducted to answer the following questions:

- Do the remains represent more than one individual? When there are multiple fragments from different individuals (as was the case in Bali), efforts are made to apportion these to one person, through identification of left and right elements and specific anatomical location.

- Is it possible to deduce from the skeletal remains clues as to the deceased's sex, age, stature, ancestry, and physique?

- Are there any skeletal traits or anomalies present to positively identify the individual, or other personal characteristics that might aid the process of identification?

After the initial examination of whole bodies, attention turned to the significantly disrupted, fragmentary, and incinerated remains, and efforts were then made to attribute these separate parts to the appropriate individual. The experiences gained from investigations of the New York Twin Towers terrorist attacks (e.g., Budimlija et al. 2003), as well as examinations of skeletonised victims of genocide in the former Yugoslavia (e.g., Rainio et al. 2001), in Latin America (e.g., Steadman and Haglund 2005), and in Rwanda (e.g., Kirschner and Hannibal 1994) indicate that skilled forensic anthropologists can play an important role in the identification process. The nature of the Bali incident, with multiple fatalities involving incineration and fragmentation of remains, particularly among those close to the center of the explosion, indicate a need for expertise in the analysis of bone fragments.

The body parts were recovered from a wide area and over a protracted period of time. Remains were still being recovered up to two weeks after the event, and, as a result, many of the body parts were in an advanced state of decomposition. A procedure for assessment and sampling was determined by the pathologist, anthropologist, and DNA specialists before commencing the examination, and this procedure was maintained throughout the entire process. Every body part was sampled (soft tissue and bone when possible), except when decomposition or incineration was considered too severe. A basic description of the body part was required, which included anatomical location (for example, left mid-shaft of femur). It was at this stage that the anthropologist was able to contribute valuable information.

General observations of the body parts from the Bali incident included these:

- A high degree of fragmentation of individuals close to the blast site was found in both locations.

- The distal limb segments (in particular the legs) were severely incinerated.

- Mid-shafts of most long bones exhibited breakages.

- A high percentage of major joint complexes (knee, shoulder, hip) was often intact.

These types of findings are consistent with exposure to a high explosive with associated pressure wave and incendiary effects.

Phase 3: Antemortem Data

The antemortem phase of the Bali bombing commenced on Thursday, 17 October, with the release of a list of missing persons, five days after the incident. Although previous experience has shown that the number of persons reported as missing inevitably exceeds the number actually involved, one of the immediate tasks faced by authorities in the event of a disaster on this scale is the collection of antemortem data. In all Australian states, police teams accompanied by counsellors were organised to visit families of those suspected of being among the victims. In Bali, police forensic teams visited hotel rooms. Authorities began interviewing friends and relatives, collecting photographs, details of clothing and jewellery commonly worn by the deceased, and other items such as hair combs and toothbrushes that might be useful in the event of DNA analysis. Surfaces were sampled for finger and even footprints. Names of family doctors and dentists were assembled so that medical and dental histories could be obtained from the victims' places of residence. All individuals potentially involved were initially listed, and then those known to have survived were subtracted, resulting in the final estimate of 200 victims. Not all of these were immediate victims of the bomb attack. Some, especially those with severe burns who were airlifted to Australia, died of their injuries in the following days and weeks.

Phase 4: Reconciliation

In the reconciliation phase, antemortem information and postmortem information are matched to confirm identification. Leaders of specialist sections—fingerprint, dental, medical, anthropological, DNA, and physical (property and photography)—are coordinated to confirm the identity of the deceased. In Bali, reconciliation commenced on Friday, 25 October, with representatives of the Indonesian military, the AFP, foreign DVI teams, a dentist, a pathologist, and a medical scientist in attendance. Results of the various sections were compared, if inconsistencies were found, and, when possible these were reconciled and a formal report prepared. In Bali, anthropologists were involved in only the reconciliation phase, as observers; the stand-alone identifiers were a pathologist, a forensic odontologist, and a DNA expert.

The Bali DVI closed on Friday, 15 February, 2003—one year, four months, and three days after the explosions. There were in total 202 fatalities from 21 countries of which 199 were positively identified, including 88 Australians (several body parts remained unidentified). Thirty-nine body parts have been linked to one unidentified body, which may be that of the bomber, and three body parts produced DNA profiles that have not been identified to date.

The 2004 Australian Embassy Bombing

On September 9, 2004, a bomb exploded outside the Australian Embassy in Jakarta killing 12 people (Figure 33.5). Many of the individuals involved were Embassy security personnel, along with civilians and a suspected ordinance carrier. A medical advisory team from Australia, including a forensic pathologist, a mortuary manager, and a forensic anthropologist, was deployed to assist the Indonesian authorities with the DVI process and subsequent criminal investigation. A good working relationship had been developed between Australian DVI experts and their Indonesian counterparts during the Bali disaster incident of 2002.

The main tasks of the medical advisory team were to assess and record all body parts, to identify two civilian bodies, and to identify any possible bomb carriers. The anthropologist, in conjunction with the pathologist, identified and recorded all the body parts recovered from the scene. Each body part had been allocated a locational number. Once the identification of the body part had been determined, it could then be related to the scene, and distribution patterns could be assessed. Over 90 body parts were identified, and an inventory was constructed (Figure 33.6). Body parts were examined and allocated to one of the following categories: bone only, soft tissue, or a combination of both. Specific anatomical location was also recorded. This type of inventory is useful for later consultation for estimates of the amount of soft and hard tissue available for sampling. It is also a useful indicator of the degree of fragmentation involved in the incident.

Most of the bodies were identifiable by routine methods; however, two civilians were close to the blast when it detonated. These bodies were badly disrupted (distal limb segments missing and heads extensively damaged) and displayed a high degree of incineration. Visual identification was not possible, and antemortem records (dental and medical) were not available. Two suggestions were put forward as possible identities for the individuals; however, the age, sex, and ancestry were very similar. Because a preliminary identification was required (identity was subsequently confirmed by DNA), it was necessary to find a biological parameter that would distinguish the individuals. It was decided that the height of the individuals (antemortem estimates obtained by Indonesian authorities)

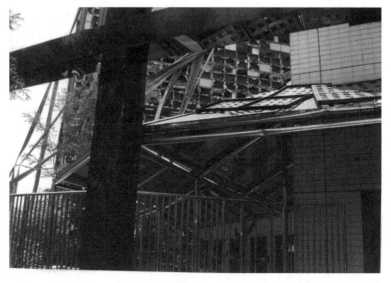

Figure 33.5 Damage to the Australian embassy and surrounding buildings (photograph courtesy of the author).

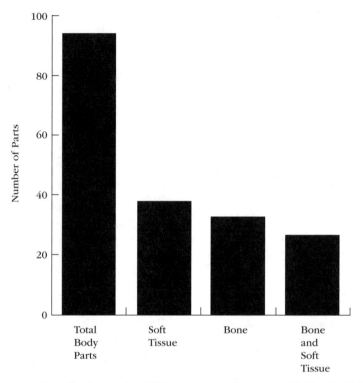

Figure 33.6 Total number of body parts (*n* = 98) by anatomical location and further breakdown into broad categories; Australian Embassy Bombing, Jakarta 2004.

was sufficiently disparate that it could be used to establish a preliminary identification. A stature estimate was calculated by the anthropologist together with Indonesian pathologists from the remaining intact femora. The regression equation was calculated from Southern Chinese male data (Krogman and İşcan 1986), the closest available to an Indonesian sample. The stature estimate identification was later confirmed by DNA testing, thereby highlighting the usefulness of anthropological parameters when antemortem records are difficult or impossible to obtain.

The final task for the medical advisory team was the tentative identification of a possible bomb carrier. This was carried out by the anthropologist and the pathologist, who, based on experience and observations of postblast injuries from previous cases, systematically examined each body part looking for postblast injuries that were consistent with proximity to the blast site. A process of elimination was used to identify body parts that may have originated from a possible bomb carrier. For example, a superior articular facet of the atlas was identified that could not have belonged to any of the other victims,

because all other neck regions were intact. The size and condition of the atlas fragment was also consistent with it being in close proximity to the explosion. Subsequent DNA tests confirmed the bone belonged to a person of interest to the authorities.

Lessons Learned from the Bali Bombing Incidents

The Bali incidents had serious implications for regional governments, forcing both Indonesia and Australia to take the threat of terrorism more seriously (Dupont 2003). At the time, Bali and Indonesia were placed at the top of Australia's restricted countries list. Australia also started to take the threat of terrorist attack on home soil seriously and to plan for the possibility of future attacks closer to home. DVI units were established in most Australian States and Territories and comprise teams fully trained to respond to disaster and terrorist situations including chemical, biological, and radiological events, with the capacity to call in additional expertise if and when required. The value of having a forensic anthropologist on the DVI teams is now widely recognised in Australia. This person, rotating on a state basis, is available for an immediate response, with responsibility to liaise with other members of the DVI team.

Conclusion

Mass disasters, in particular, incidents with a criminal element, have become increasingly prominent in recent times. Forensic services have been called on to attend these types of incidents, and a wide range of forensic specialists have been involved in both the human identification process and the criminal investigations. Along with the more traditional practitioners, namely, the pathologist and the odontologist, the forensic anthropologist has also come to play an increasing role in incidents involving mass fatalities.

Although the anthropologist's role may change during an investigation and vary in conjunction with the type of incident, as part of the medical advisory team the anthropologist can contribute to both the recovery and the analysis aspects of DVI. The anthropologist is able to offer expertise in the assessment of highly fragmented and incinerated human remains, determine the minimum number of individuals, differentiate human from nonhuman remains, and elicit biological profiles (age, sex, ancestry) from otherwise unidentifiable remains.

With the increased awareness of the usefulness of forensic anthropologists at mass-fatality incidents comes the necessity that the experience and academic background of the practitioner be able to satisfy international requirements. Given the importance of the DVI process and possible associated criminal investigations, the discipline of forensic anthropology in Australia will need to consider the establishment of a register of practitioners accredited to recognised standards for the future. With these standards in place, forensic anthropology can continue to bring valuable skills to the DVI process.

References

Buck, A. 2004. DVI Forensic Anthropology Procedures. Appendix K. *Australasian DVI Standards Manual*: 127–130.

Budimlija, Z. M., Prinz, M. K., Zelson-Mundorff, A., Wiersema, J., Bartelink, E., MacKinnon, G., Nazzaruolo, B. L., Estacio, S. M., Hennessey, M. J., and Shaler, R. C. 2003. World Trade Center human identification project: Experiences with individual body identification cases. *Croatian Medical Journal* 44 (3): 259–263.

Dupont, A. 2003. Transformation or stagnation? Rethinking Australia's defence. *Australian Journal of International Affairs* 57(1): 55–76.

INTERPOL. Disaster Victim Identification. www.interpol.int/Public/Search.asp?ct=Data&q1=DVI&cboNbHitsPerPage=20 (accessed 12/07/06).

Kirschner, R. H., and Hannibal, K. E. 1994. The application of the forensic sciences to human rights investigations. *Medicine and Law* 13(5–6): 451–460.

Krogman, W. M., and İşcan, M. Y. 1986. *The Human Skeleton in Forensic Medicine*. Springfield, IL: Charles C. Thomas.

Lain, R., Griffiths, C., and Hilton, J. M. N. 2003. Forensic dental and medical response to the Bali bombing: A personal perspective. *The Medical Journal of Australia* 179(7): 362–365, www.mja.com.au/public/issues/179_07_061003/lai10499_fm.html (accessed 06/07/04).

Rainio, J., Hedman, M., Karkola, K., Lalu, K., Peltola, P., Ranta, H., Sajantila, A., Soderholm, N., and Penttila, A. 2001. Forensic osteological investigations in Kosovo. *Forensic Science International* 121(3): 166–173.

Steadman, D. W., and Haglund, W. D. 2005. The scope of anthropological contributions to human rights investigations. *Journal of Forensic Sciences* 50(1): 23–30.

Victorian Disaster Victim Identification Manual. 2005. Publication of Victoria Police and Victorian Institute of Forensic Medicine. Victoria, Australia.

Watts, J. 2002. Kuta Bali bombing offers lessons for disaster relief. *The Lancet* Nov 2; 360 (9343): 1401.

34

DEALING WITH THE REMAINS OF CONFLICT: AN INTERNATIONAL RESPONSE TO CRIMES AGAINST HUMANITY, FORENSIC RECOVERY, IDENTIFICATION, AND REPATRIATION IN THE FORMER YUGOSLAVIA

Jon Sterenberg

This chapter is not intended to be an exact history of the atrocities and crimes committed during the conflicts that resulted from the break up of the former Yugoslavia between 1991 and 2002. Nor is it an exact account of the international response to the recovery, identification, and final repatriation of the remains of victims from the various conflicts of the former Yugoslavia. Rather, the chapter acquaints the reader with some of the problems and issues that I observed over nine years of work within the region.

Because of the sheer numbers of cases involved, I have concentrated on the effort within Bosnia and Herzegovina (BiH) and some of the complexities of working as an international within a national framework, and I briefly outline the process of assistance in other regions of the former Yugoslavia. As with any recovery and identification program of this magnitude, the process within BiH would not be where it is today without the dedication and incredible hard work of many hundreds of international and national experts working together toward a common goal: to resolve the fate of the missing.

Background

The exact number of persons missing and killed as a result of the conflict in BiH will possibly never be known. Estimates range anywhere from 200,000 overall (Nation 2003) to 96,000 individuals (RDC 2006). In any postconflict situation, numbers can vary greatly even between organizations and governments. For example, whereas the International Committee of the Red Cross (ICRC) states that it has approximately 20,286 records for whom family members have opened a tracing request, another international organisation, the International Commission on Missing Persons (ICMP), has as of August 2006 information on 22,129 missing individuals represented by blood samples from surviving family members in BiH (ICMP 2006).

It is also estimated through research that between 97,000 (RDC 2006) and 102,000 (Tabeau ICTY 2004) civilian and military casualties are thought to be dead or missing out of a total of approximately 350,000 war victims (RDC 2006). These records take into account all of the break-away regions, including Croatia, Serbia, Montenegro, Kosovo, and Macedonia, throughout this period.

Witness accounts of mass killings and the subsequent discovery of hundreds of graves (many of them large, complicated secondary mass graves) together with accounts of an untold number of skeletal remains observed scattered across fields and hillsides or located within caverns confirmed fears regarding the fate of most of the missing and forced the international community to take action.

Yet it was not until the signing of the Dayton Peace Accord in 1995, which effectively split the country into two regions, the Federation of Bosnia and Herzegovina (FBiH) and the Republika Srpska (RS), that a process could be established to assist the scientific recovery and identification of the missing in BiH.

During the war, many bodies and remains were simply traded across inter-entity borders. This continued until the development of the Joint Exhumation Process (JEP) in 1996, which, together with an Expert Group on Exhumations and Missing Persons established by the Office of the High Representative (OHR), took on the main responsibility for resolving the fates of missing persons. The JEP, once established, undertook investigations within the legal jurisdiction of the local authorities. To facilitate this work, three commissions were established: the State Commission of Bosnia and Herzegovina for the Tracing of Missing Persons; the Office for the Exchange of Prisoners and Missing Persons of the Croatian Side of the Federation of Bosnia and Herzegovina; and the State Commission of the Republika Srpska for the Exchange of Prisoners of War and Missing Persons. At the time, these commissions had a legal obligation to cooperate with other entity authorities, that is, the opposing side, as well as with any international organization involved (such as ICRC, Physicians for Human Rights—PHR, ICMP, and Stabilization Force—SFOR)[1] to conduct "humanitarian" recovery and repatriation operations.

To keep this process politically neutral, OHR requested guidance and assistance from international organizations such as Physicians for Human Rights (PHR) and the recently created International Commission on Missing Persons (ICMP), established in 1997. Much needed support from the international community, both financial and in the form of expertise and equipment, gave recovery teams of all three commissions the practical ability to begin the daunting task of exhuming and identifying the thousands of mortal remains buried in the region. Very slowly, the commissions began to push forward with the object of addressing the issue of the missing.

The operations of JEP, initiated in 1996 under the Banja Luka Agreement, began in earnest in 1997. This was seen as a truly progressive approach to promoting cooperation between former warring parties and, more important, a means of bringing closure to grieving families of the missing. All recoveries were undertaken by local teams who had a variety of skilled staff at hand, including forensic pathologists who acted as court representatives at sites. Formal training in either anthropology or archaeology was virtually non-existent in BiH, and certainly no training in the forensic application of these skills existed at this time. This meant that authorities in BiH lacked the capacity to deal with the complicated problems of scientific recovery and forensic examination, and it was quickly realized that international assistance was required.

A pilot project was undertaken, funded by various governments, which enabled a scientific process of identification to begin. Initial operations supported by the Governments of Finland (Rainio 2002) and the Netherlands in 1996 were continued in 1997 through the intervention of Physicians for Human Rights (PHR), who provided training and advice to local forensic teams. Based in the Bosnian town of Tuzla, PHR also established the first antemortem database and DNA analysis of recovered remains. Tuzla was identified as the major area where survivors from Srebrenica had established themselves and the area to which the majority of remains were known to relate. Even with these key developments, it was clear to the international organizations involved in the process that BiH, owing to the lack of nationally trained or identified experts, would continue to require the largest support from international experts.

The International Criminal Tribunal for the Former Yugoslavia (ICTY)

In 1997, small-scale recovery operations were being undertaken by the local Bosnian commissions on missing persons with limited assistance from international anthropologists. At the same time, large-scale forensic archaeological recoveries of remains, mainly concentrating on the fall of Srebrenica in July 1995, were being conducted by forensic teams of international experts employed by the International Tribunal for the Prosecution of Persons Responsible for Serious Violations of International Humanitarian Law Committed in the Territory of the Former Yugoslavia since 1991, more commonly known as the United Nations International Criminal Tribunal for the Former Yugoslavia (ICTY). Under the ever-present eye of national and international media, these excavations, and subsequent anthropological and pathological examinations, focused on the "forensic" recovery of information in order to recover evidence that could be used in the trials of those indicted criminals alleged to be responsible for the large-scale killings of up to 8,000 Muslim men and boys. A large number of these victims were believed to be buried in large "primary" mass graves located in the area of control of the then Bosnian Serbian

Army (BSA) Drina Corps. The aim of the investigations was also to ensure that exhumations were conducted in a dignified manner and according to international standards.

These excavations were the largest ongoing forensic investigation operations in the world at the time, employing a full forensic team with personnel from virtually every continent, including members of already established forensic teams such as the Argentine Forensic Anthropology Team (EAAF) and the Fundación/Equipo de Antropología Forense de Guatemala (F/EAFG). Experienced archaeologists, anthropologists, crime scene personnel, pathologists, mortuary technicians, and radiographers worked together with additional support from administrative staff to fulfil the investigative tasks assigned from The Hague-based court. The majority of the excavations were undertaken under the direction of a highly experienced forensic archaeologist who was previously employed to investigate mass graves in the Ukraine as part of an Australian investigation of war criminals (Wright 1995). A full mortuary facility, under the direction of an experienced international forensic pathologist (Clark 2000, 2001; Hunt 1998; Lawrence 1998), was also in place to undertake the postmortem examination and anthropological analysis of remains recovered by the ICTY field team. Owing to commitments in their home countries mortuary staff, specialized technical staff and field staff rotated throughout the season.

An ICTY excavation team could typically comprise 13–20 archaeological, anthropological, crime scene, and logistics staff with either United Nations or International military security. The examination team could consist of 20–30 staff, including forensic pathologists, anthropologists, radiographers, crime scene personnel, data-management personnel, and photographers. National staff were employed by ICTY mainly to act in a support role at mortuary facilities. Owing to climatic constraints, the excavation of sites by ICTY was usually undertaken between the months of March and November. During the season, excavation teams worked on 3–4 large mass graves and also undertook smaller invasive "probes" of suspected sites in order to confirm or eliminate sites for future investigation. Autopsies and consequent analysis was also undertaken throughout the excavation season at ICTY facilities located in areas of the country where security was deemed satisfactory to allow operations to occur. Ethnic tensions were still fairly active during these early investigations (1997–1998), and so facilities were usually housed within "safe" Muslim Federation areas with logistical support located on existing military

bases where security was already in place. These large-scale forensic investigations, excavations, and examinations continued until the end of 2001. A small-scale ICTY forensic monitoring operation working with local commissions continued between 2001 and 2003.

ICTY, PHR, and ICMP were always conscious of the large number of graves that would need to be exhumed; however, one major problem that was still to be resolved related directly to the identification of remains recovered from secondary mass graves. The majority of these secondary sites was created over a short time period, often months after the original burial of the victims in primary graves, which were then deliberately concealed. The catalyst for the destruction of these primary sites was the release of U2 spy plane images in August 1995 by the United States Government showing suspected mass gravesites. The publication of these images by the international media forced an immediate reaction: the ethnic Bosnian Serb forces returned to the original primary locations, crudely excavated the bodies using heavy machinery, and transported them in trucks to other (secondary) sites.

This action had two effects: First, all this new activity was monitored by the intelligence community, who continued to image the country using spy planes, giving detailed information to ICTY investigators that allowed the location of secondary sites to be presumptively linked to primary sites. Second, and more difficult to predict, disturbing the primary sites meant that heavy commingled and fragmented remains were further scattered across the region. Often one or two deposits of remains from different primary sites were located at a single secondary site. Conversely, deposits from one single primary site were identified in several separate secondary sites. Scientific excavation of these sites also indicates that the process of disarticulation and fragmentation continued as wheeled heavy machinery was employed to further compact remains within the secondary sites.

Whatever the rationale behind the construction of secondary gravesites, the investigation of these sites has proved to be the most problematic exercise. ICTY's solution was to use experienced "rescue" or "classically" trained archaeologists who could identify differences in the graves deposits, undertake detailed recording of the grave itself and the interred remains, and also identify and recover forensic information from the graves' context and surrounding areas. Physical anthropologists were given the often daunting task of trying to examine traditional markers of skeletal anatomy for sex, age, and stature while at the same time identifying post- and perimortem trauma. Forensic pathologists experienced in dealing with largely fleshed remains now had the assistance of both archaeology and anthropology expertise to assist in determining cause and manner of death from these often largely skeletonized remains.

Because of the requirement to produce evidence that could quickly be integrated into ongoing trial proceedings, the main responsibility for recovery and examination remained with the international experts, who were already using "best practise" and standards within ICTY (Sterenberg 2002). Following the end of full ICTY operations in 2001, a shift in the approach of recovery and examination of remains was made. With the establishment and expansion of ICMP operations, the emphasis was based on recovery and identification, that is, humanitarian forensic archaeology and less full forensic information recovery (for the court). International practitioners, experienced in applying best practice at ICTY sites, were now faced with working within what was essentially a legal process in which the focus was on humanitarian recovery. To compound this, the issue of national prosecutions of war crimes cases within BiH itself had not been fully addressed; thus ICTY was seen as the final solution to prosecution of such trials.

The use of international forensic archaeologists in ICTY operations was designed to maximize the collection of critical forensic evidence along with the accurate mapping and recovery of remains that would then assist anthropologists and pathologists involved in the examination process. Thus, the use of archaeology within the process played a crucial role in the task of ensuring that absolutely everything was recorded in detail and that the mass grave site was completely investigated to the highest international standard. All the data were then compiled into a report that could then aid the court in its proceedings (ICTY United Nations 2001). Archaeological and anthropological evidence had previously been presented in court proceedings. This information had been used to disprove claims by military and political leaders that certain graves contained the remains of military and not civilian casualties (for example, in Argentina's cases of the "Disappeared" from the 1976–1983 military regime (Fondebrider et al. 2000) and Srebrenica-related cases (Clark 2003; Wright 1999, 2000, 2001).

Realising this fact, ICMP, the organization, which is now advocating the continuation of best practice and standards in BiH, was and is faced with how to assist the prosecution of war crimes while acting in a neutral humanitarian role. ICTY staff had the legal authority and support to affect judgments on what and how evidence and remains should be recovered. ICMP, which has a less powerful legal position within the current legislation of BiH, is therefore seen as only "assisting" in the process of recovery, placing ICMP excavation staff, predominantly international, in a less than ideal situation on site. This problem will continue to exist unless a change in the legal system of BiH places these experts on a par with BiH state-authorized forensic pathologists, who are recognized by the courts as being in charge of any recovery.

Present Level of Support within BiH

Although other organizations exist within BiH, support for recoveries, examinations, and identifications within the region reside mainly with the ICMP. Of the various departments within ICMP, the forensic science department (FSD) is the largest. Similar to ICTY, FSD has an excavation division that combines archaeologists and anthropologists, plus logistical support staff, who work on a wide variety of site types and locations. These can include primary and secondary mass graves where the full weight of ICMP archaeological input is employed in order to maintain the highest level of recovery of both human remains and associated evidence from any site. Other site types include underground caves, wells, burned and damaged buildings, and surface-scattered mortal remains. On average, the excavation of a complex mass gravesite can take between one month and six weeks to complete, whereas a standard "exhumation" would usually last for one day. Work is dependent on the complexities that are associated with the site—for example, unexploded ordnance (UXO) and other possible health and safety issues.

ICMP undertake many of the "inter-entity" recoveries; local commissions also undertake recoveries within their own theatre of operation, that is, "intra-entity" and often without support from internationals. This situation has led to many problems in the later stages of identification, when frequently the emphasis is on DNA identification and traditional methods of presumptive identification.

When requested, ICMP forensic anthropologists, experienced in the analysis of human skeletal remains, are also employed at commission recoveries, undertaking the field examination of skeletal elements and bone fragments to determine whether the remains are human or nonhuman. If the remains are human, advice is given on how to properly recover them to prevent commingling of bones from different individuals. In cases of a single exhumation, the anthropologist can further define whether the correct set of remains are being recovered; for example, the missing person may have been an older male but the skeletal elements in the grave were those of a young woman. The ICMP archaeologist often works in extremely tense political situations and has to deal, on a daily basis, with interpersonal conflicts and differing attitudes among national staff of particular pathologists, national court representatives, and local commissions (Skinner and Sterenberg 2005).

ICTY's specific mandate did not include the final identification of recovered remains. Examined remains were simply signed over to the relevant legally recognized commission, where they were then stored while pathologists pondered how to identify an ever-increasing number of recovered and very often highly fragmented remains. ICMP staff frequently use autopsy and anthropological data released by ICTY in order to identify and bring closure to cases that are still classed as open. To maintain a virtually seamless transition between ICTY and ICMP, ICMP excavation teams have adopted and adapted many of the original forms developed for use in ICTY operations (Wright 1997–2000), including the use of a sequential case number system that also acts as the main evidence log for each site.

ICMP anthropologists undertake and continue to apply internationally recognized standards and procedures when examining remains. This is undertaken at facilities large enough to allow appropriate storage of remains, physical analysis, and DNA sampling. In response to the realities of the postconflict situation, and more specifically the nature of the disposal of victims, ICMP has three fully staffed facilities currently in operation within BiH. Each facility works on and deals with slightly differing caseloads, ranging from the examination of largely intact (75% or more) remains related to Srebrenica 1995 to the examination of NN (No Name) cases specific to one region of BiH dating from 1992 and also to the examination and re-association of remains from all 1995-dated secondary mass gravesites. Integral to the process of identification is a fully functional database that combines all possible available data so that they can be cross-referenced or queried for many thousands of cases. Experienced anthropologists undertake a full electronic inventory of remains while focusing on identifying trauma, pathology, and skeletal markers of sex and age and determining which particular element should be sampled for DNA profiling. The experts work in pairs following DNA profiling to ensure quality control and quality assurance and also to employ their skills

to re-associate fragmented remains using DNA-matched profiles.

PHR, ICTY, and ICMP acknowledged, very early, that the state of the remains, combined with the lack of detailed medical and dental information, dramatically reduced the effectiveness of traditional forensic methods of identification. The development of high-throughput DNA profiling (the ability to screen large numbers of samples in order to obtain large numbers of DNA profiles in a short amount of time) has provided a tool that, when combined with anthropology and pathology, can give positive identifications to recovered remains even in the cases of extremely fragmented skeletal elements. Without the development of DNA analysis, the process of positive identification would have been horrendous; few if any remains could have been identified through traditional "presumptive" techniques. It was estimated that even a full autopsy by a pathologist combined with solid antemortem data (such as physical dimensions, clothing, and jewellery) would permit, at most, accurate identifications in only 5–8% of cases related to the fall of Srebrenica in July 1995.

Analysis of thousands of bone samples (to date 19,102 bone samples have produced unique DNA profiles for 14,290 individuals [ICMP 2006]), has allowed ICMP scientists to analyse that not every sample taken for DNA can or will yield a profile. Ongoing analysis has identified which skeletal element provides the best DNA profile and has given the anthropologist additional information on what samples should be taken and from where. Where DNA samples have failed to provide a profile, the pathologist in charge of closing the case has to turn to other more traditional methods of identification. This may mean gathering additional antemortem data from families or examining artefacts found in association with the remains during the excavation, or even other possible linkages—for example, clothing, injuries, skeletal trauma, and archaeological evidence—in order to affect closure.

The Future of Recovery within BiH

Unfortunately, funding the process of recovery and examination cannot continue for an indefinite period, and it is now time for the government of BiH to address and resolve the issue. The Special Rapporteur for the United Nations recommended in 1997 "that the relevant authorities in both entities adopt an approach to the issue of missing persons based on cooperation with authorities of the other entity or other national backgrounds" (Rehn 1997). To achieve this, talks finally commenced in 2001 on the creation of a new state led institute for the missing. The Agreement on Assuming the Role of Co-Founders of the Missing Persons Institute (MPI) of Bosnia and Herzegovina was signed by ICMP and the Council of Ministers on 30 August 2005. The Agreement entails the merger of the respective entity bodies, such as the Federation Commission on Missing Persons and the Republika Srpska Office on Missing and Detained Persons, into MPI, along with affiliated funding from the entity-level governments. Supported by the BiH government and ICMP, the MPI will have legislation, a mandate, and the ability, once formalized, to depoliticize the process of recovery and identification across the country and unite the entity groups into one single response to addressing the issue of the missing. Key to the success of MPI and its standing within the international arena will be its ability to place acceptable levels of work practice within the current BiH legal framework. Local standards or codes of criminal procedure are presently too vague regarding exhumations and examinations, and these difficulties are further exacerbated by the small number of state pathologists involved in the process.

For ICMP, the issue now is how to continue to support and assist the process in a way that ensures the correct scientific control of site work while helping to build on the limited capacity of forensic training and to place more responsibility for recovery and repatriation back into the hands of the BiH government and its legal structure. To date, this process of excavation and examination has been used as a "political tool" since the end of the conflict. One has only to read the daily papers in BiH, or to monitor international press, to realize that the political power of the missing is still huge. Recent articles have brought this issue back into the public arena (Haxhaj 2006; Rakic 2006; Sarac 2006).

Documenting the truth is an important part of any reconciliation process within a postconflict society. Central to any operation is the ability to provide good scientific data and information that explain in detail the historical record of events. MPI has a huge responsibility to provide answers regarding actual numbers of killed and missing on all sides. A decade after the end of the 1992–1995 conflict, BiH is still struggling to develop a central electronic database that will combine all known data on the missing gathered from all inter-entity government offices, ICMP, ICTY, and the International Committee of the Red Cross (ICRC). This electronic database will also have to be capable of expansion in order to facilitate the input of further information relating to unrecovered remains currently interred within suspected mass graves across the country.

First and foremost, recovery teams must locate the sites. At present, the most successful way to find clandestine or hidden burials is through reliable witness testimony. The local commissions have had considerable success in finding these burial grounds during the first few years following the conflict, largely thanks to sympathetic and highly motivated witnesses who reported the graves' whereabouts to local authorities. However, after a decade of investigation and recovery, the precise details of many of these sites are rapidly being lost, quickly fading in the memories of witnesses and informers. Thus as witnesses' memories fade and landscapes are transformed, the roles of archaeologists and anthropologists take on ever-increasing importance.

Developments in the field of satellite and non-invasive geophysical analysis of sites may aid MPI to locate these remaining mass graves. Based on an expansion of ideas developed in Iraq (Sterenberg 2004; Wessling 2003), combinations of various non-invasive techniques of location have already been tested in BiH (Scott and Hunter 2004; Watters 2003; Watters and Hunter 2004). A series of previously identified mass gravesites "probed" by ICTY forensic teams in 1998 were chosen as test cases by which to ascertain whether a specific set of geophysical parameters could be identified and then be used in the wider context of BiH in general.

In 2005, ICTY and ICMP forensic archaeologists working with other specialists trained in analyzing botanical evidence and geological analysis of suspected burial grounds made some progress toward identifying indicators to locate mass gravesites in BiH. These techniques have been further refined through the application of various remote non-invasive methods of investigation, including satellite and spectral analysis, electrical imaging, and ground-penetrating radar (Hunter et al. 2005; Karaska 2005; Watters and Hunter 2004). The results of the exercise (undertaken over a one-week period) indicated that satellite and spectral imagery could influence the selection of an area for investigation of suspected sites and that non-invasive electrical imaging could be used to identify and locate discrete anomalies and potentially indicate separate body masses within known mass graves. Further enhancement through the use of Geographical Information Systems (GIS) (Reddick 2005) allowed a series of predictive models to be developed that may assist in identifying potential locations of mass gravesites in a given region by excluding those already investigated or deemed inappropriate for the type of disturbance.

Assistance in Other Regions of the Former Yugoslavia

Although BiH has borne the major burden of identifying and recovering the missing from a decade of conflict and war, other regions within former Yugoslavia were affected and are also actively addressing the issue of the missing. Croatia has been undertaking exhumations through The Government Commission for Detained and Missing Persons and Yugoslavia's Commission for Humanitarian Issues and Imprisoned Persons, who met in March 1997 to accelerate the resolution of cases of those who are missing, abducted, or detained, and with the assistance of the Croatian military, exhumed the remains of some 3,000 missing, primarily from operations "Flash" and "Storm" in 1991 and the conflict in the Krijina areas during 1992. As a result of these exhumations, a total of 1,075 individuals have been identified.

Serbia and Montenegro have also recovered the remains of approximately 700 individuals from a variety of sites. As in Croatia, little international assistance has been sought other than the use of DNA profiling and match reports provided by ICMP. Macedonia and Slovenia are also completing their own recovery of remains.

Kosovo is a slightly different situation, because the interim civilian administration is currently led by a United Nations mission (UNMIK) and as such has its own forensic capability coordinated through the Office of Missing Persons and Forensics (OMPF). OMPF has the capacity to employ various forensic skills to its ongoing investigations. Unlike the victims in the mass graves of Bosnia, a large proportion of the victims of the 1999 war with Serbian Para-Military forces in Kosovo were buried in single graves. Although the bodies of approximately 2,500 individuals have been recovered and undergone anthropological and pathological examination, the fate and the location of some 2,000 more individuals from the conflict are still under debate.

Serbia, to some extent, escaped the large-scale killings seen within the other regions of former Yugoslavia, apart from civilian and military casualties as a result of air strikes on various military targets during the push to remove then Serbian President Slobodan Milosevic in 1999. Reports of bodies being moved from Kosovo to Serbia were confirmed in 2001 and 2002, when excavations on several large mass graves were undertaken through the District Court of Belgrade (Ciric 2002). The excavation was undertaken in combination with the Institute of Forensic Medicine, Belgrade, who provided forensic pathologists and forensic anthropologists and ICMP archaeologists and anthropologists (Sterenberg et al. 2002). DNA analysis of the remains was undertaken by ICMP, resulting in a large number of identified individuals being returned to families for reburial.

Training and Capacity Building

Unlike ICTY, whose investigative mandate meant that nationals could not be included in the recovery operations, PHR and ICMP realised that in order for the standard of operations to continue once ICTY had ceased operations in the former Yugoslavia, the regional national capacity for forensically trained anthropologists and archaeologists had to be addressed. Unfortunately, the lack of nationally trained experts is still a stumbling block to the continuation of the process within BiH. Training of national staff within PHR and ICMP has resulted in only a small degree of trained DNA staff and an even smaller number of trained forensic archaeologists and anthropologists. Finding suitable candidates to train in archaeology and anthropology was a problem of job security. Unlike in Western Europe or the United States, where a postgraduate archaeologist or anthropologist with a degree can apply for many positions in a variety of employment over many years, the situation in the Balkans means that many young people tend to take up careers that provide job security for the long term. So although DNA scientists will continue to be required within BiH, making a long-term career possible, archaeology and anthropology are not considered to be a good career for long-term employment.

Conclusion

International experts (including ICTY, PHR, ICMP, and Kenyon International Emergency Services [subcontracted through ICMP]) have spent over ten years working together with national governments, institutes, commissions, pathologists, and families in an attempt to address the issue of the missing. Despite many problems in the process, there have also been many positive advances in several fields of forensic science. Many of the world's best practitioners have at one time or another worked in BiH and honed their skills poring over thousands of cases, enabling them to transfer those skills to other countries of the world.

There is still some debate as to why international standards are needed in the current process. Often the cause of arguments is the pace of recovery. If full forensic recovery is not required, then why place so much emphasis on scientific recovery (excavation) that includes total electronic mapping of remains and artefacts and the full recording of remains, when simple nonscientific recovery (exhumation) with total dependency on the results of DNA analysis—for example, positive identification—is acceptable to the courts and families of BiH? Good scientific excavation can save money and resources during the analysis phase of the operation. Put simply, recovering as much of one individual as possible at site means that fewer DNA samples have to be taken, thus reducing costs and shortening the time that the repatriation process takes as a whole (Tuller and Đurić 2006).

The use of high throughput DNA analysis in the current identification process has enabled ICMP to process to date between 12,000 to 13,000 body bags of mortal remains recovered between 1996 and 2006. Work is continuing on at least 5,000 cases that are still to be identified, and the ongoing investigation of potential gravesites is constantly adding to the numbers. Working with recovered remains raises ethical, medical, and moral questions all of which have an impact on what can be realistically achieved. It is the physical anthropologist who has to undertake analysis of remains and make a judgment on how much of an individual can be re-associated. Ossuary remains will continue to expand owing to the nature of the recovered remains and the constant pressure to identify and repatriate remains before the death of surviving family members. Knowing that the identified individual may be returned in one of several states, (complete, partial, or as a single skeletal element) is something that has to be addressed early in the process. Civil society initiatives (CSI) programs can educate the populace about why it is important to give a blood sample and can explain why certain parts of the process fail; for example, if original DNA samples have not been dried or stored correctly then they will fail to produce a DNA profile. This situation, when it occurs, often necessitates the re-exhumation of buried remains, putting relatives through the ordeal of having to re-experience the horrors of the conflict. Families will often ask why this is necessary—why was there a mistake, and who is going to pay for this to be done? Certainly it has been an issue in BiH, Kosovo, and other regions of the Former Yugoslavia. Fortunately for BiH, it has been agreed through formal channels that, if necessary, the re-exhumations will be paid for by the government.

In addition to the impediments to postconflict institution-building, peace initiatives, and reconciliation that unresolved missing-persons issues create, families of the missing are often poorly informed about existing and possible mechanisms to seek the truth about the fate of their missing loved ones. CSI programs have assisted through empowering surviving families, allowing them to be independent and fully engaged in clarifying the fate of their missing relatives, through networking and communication with other family associations.

The stage on which organizations undertake humanitarian forensic archaeology is typically crowded and difficult. Unfortunately, the issue of what is considered as morally the correct thing to do regarding identifications is rapidly losing out to other factors, the main being budgetary. International organizations and international and local governments in this situation are faced with not only having to deal with hard-pressed civilian populations desperate to find the remains of their loved ones but also working under pressure from local, political, religious, and legal systems—often resulting in a complex and infuriating environment.

It is estimated that over 15,000 persons are still unaccounted for from the recent BiH conflicts, of which the remains of 10,000–12,000 individuals are believed to be located in grave sites. The remains of 4,000 alone are known to relate to the fall of Srebrenica. Given the current rate of recovery, even with all the resources and international expertise being provided to MPI, the process of recovery and final identification may take an additional 8 to 10 years to complete. From a humanitarian point of view, the identification of those missing allows families and relatives to finally be able to carry out customary funeral rights, provide a proper burial, and mourn their dead, and in some cases to facilitate probate. The rate of exhumations and collection of blood from family donors will continue to be the main factors in determining how fast the DNA-led identification process can proceed within the former Yugoslavia as a whole.

Finally, in the world context, the need to "marry" the immediate needs of the postconflict political situation with the bigger picture of long-term truth and reconciliation means that everything from databases to the final handover of remains should ideally be in place before any operation begins. I hope that the experiences of forensic experts in the region of the former Yugoslavia, and other postconflict situations, will mean that, should a similar situation occur in the future, every lesson learned (such as the benefits of a consistent, controlled, and impartial approach) will provide a quick, effective, and nontraumatizing solution to the process of recovery of human remains.

Just as pertinent today as it was during the early postwar recoveries is the fact that questions are constantly being asked by a population scarred by the effects of conflict and war. Resolving the fate of missing persons is of paramount importance for the process of reconciliation. Internationals are struggling to assist and build capacity that hopefully will make full use of modern, classical, and future technologies in order to answer the basic question "what happened to my loved one." In the words of Carl Bildt, former High Representative for Bosnia and Herzegovina: "For postconflict societies, moving forward depends on overcoming the fears of the past. The recent conflicts in former Yugoslavia vividly illustrate the perils that result from failure to address the past, in particular as regards the existence of mass graves" (1997).

Note

1. SFOR was a NATO-led multinational force based in Bosnia and Herzegovina tasked with upholding the Dayton Agreement and capturing those responsible for alleged Bosnian Serb war crimes, including Radovan Karadžić and Ratko Mladić, deemed responsible for the Srebrenica massacre. SFOR was divided into three zones of operation with forces based in Mostar, Banja Luka, and Tuzla. It operated between 1996 and 2004. SFOR took over from a previous multinational force, IFOR (Implementation Force), which operated between 1995 and 1996, having taken over from a United Nations Protection Force (UNPROFOR). In 2004, SFOR was replaced by the European Union's EUFOR (European Union Force), which is still in operation.

References

Bildt, C. 1997. Press conference with Carl Bildt, former High Representative for Bosnia and Herzegovina.

Ciric, A. 2002. Second season of "freezer truck" excavations, Batajnica Archaeology, *Vreme Weekly*, November 7.

Clark, J. 2000. *ICTY Operations in Bosnia-Herzegovina 1999 Season*. Report of the Chief Pathologist, Srebrenica Related Grave Sites. ICTY Evidence Report (unpublished document in possession of the author).

———. 2001. *ICTY Operations in Bosnia-Herzegovina 2000 Season*. Report of the Chief Pathologist, Srebrenica Related Grave Sites. ICTY Evidence Report (unpublished document in possession of the author).

———. 2003. *ICTY Operations in Bosnia-Herzegovina 2001 Season*. Report of the Chief Pathologist,

Srebrenica Related Grave Sites (with incorporation of findings from 1999 and 2000). ICTY Evidence Report (unpublished document in possession of the author).

Fondebrider, L., Turner, S., Ginarte, A., Brenardi, P., Olmo, D., Sominliana, C., Burrell, J., LeBaron, R., Rousch, L., and Doretti, M. (eds.). 2000. *Argentine Forensic Anthropology Team [EEAF]. Annual Report*. New York.

Haxhaj. S. 2006. Failure of international and local institutions to address the issue of missing persons criticized. *Zeri* August.

Hunt, A.C. 1998. *Report on Autopsies of Human Remains from Brcko, September to October 1997*. ICTY Evidence Report (unpublished document in possession of the author).

Hunter, J., Karaska, M., Scott, J., Tetlow, E., and Reddick, A. 2005. *Location of Mass Graves Using Non-Invasive Remote Sensing Equipment, Geophysics, and Satellite Imagery* (unpublished internal report in possession of the author). Sarajevo, Bosnia-Herzegovina: International Commission on Missing Persons (ICMP).

ICMP 2006. *System Wide Tracking Chart: Tracking Chart by Conflict and Area of Disappearance* (unpublished document in possession of the author).

ICTY United Nations 2001. *Prosecutor V. Radislav Krstic—Judgement ICTY, 2001*. ICTY United Nations, www.worldlii.org/int/cases/ICTY/2001/8.html, accessed 10/02/05.

Karaska, M. 2005. *The Potential of Using Satellite Imagery to Locate Mass Graves in Bosnia*. Power point presented to the International Commission on Missing Persons (ICMP). Sarajevo Bosnia-Herzegovina: Applied Analysis Inc.

Lawrence, C. H. 1998a. *Report on Autopsies of Human Remains from Cancari Road Site 3*. August–September. ICTY Evidence Report (unpublished document in possession of the author).

———. 1998b. *Report on Autopsies of Human Remains from Cancari Road Site 12*. August. ICTY Evidence Report (unpublished document in possession of the author).

———. 1998c. *Report on Autopsies of Human Remains from Liplje Site 2*. October. ICTY Evidence Report (unpublished document in possession of the author).

———. 1998d. *Report on Autopsies of Human Remains from Hodzici Road Site 5*. October. ICTY Evidence Report (unpublished document in possession of the author).

———. 1998e. *Report on Autopsies of Human Remains from Hodzici Road Site 4*. October. ICTY Evidence Report (unpublished document in possession of the author).

———. 1998f. Report *on Autopsies of Human Remains from Hodzici Road Site 3*. October. ICTY

Evidence Report (unpublished document in possession of the author).

Lawrence, C. H. 1998g. *Report on Autopsies of Human Remains from Zeleni Jadar Site 5.* October. ICTY Evidence Report (unpublished document in possession of the author).

Nation, C. R. 2003. *War in the Balkans, 1991–2002.* Carlisle, PA: Strategic Studies Institute, U.S. Army War College.

Rainio, J. 2002. Independent Forensic Examination of Victims of Armed Conflict: Investigations of Finnish Forensic Experts in the Balkans Area. Ph.D. dissertation. Department of Forensic Medicine University of Helsinki, Finland.

Rakic, R. 2006. Representatives of all family associations from BiH unsatisfied with the treatment of authorities: Families request full implementation of law. *Oslobodjenje,* August 29.

Reddick, A. J. 2005. The Use of Spatial Techniques in the Location and Excavation of Contemporary Mass Graves. M.Phil. dissertation Institute of Archaeology and Antiquity School of Historical Studies, The University of Birmingham (U.K.).

Rehn, E. 1997. *Situation of Human Rights in the Former Yugoslavia,* Note by the Secretary-General. Human Rights Questions: Human Rights Situations and reports of Special Rapporteurs and Representatives. General assembly, fifty-second session, Agenda item 112 (c).

Research and Documentation Center. 2006. Casualty figures according to RDC (as reported in March).

Sarac, E. 2006. The problem of the missing is often used for political purposes. Letter to BiH and international representatives, *Dnevni Avaz,* August 29.

Scott, J., and Hunter, J. 2004. Environmental influences on resistivity mapping for the location of clandestine graves, in K. Pye and D. J. Croft (eds.), *Forensic Geoscience: Principals, Techniques and Applications,* pp. 33–38. London: The Geological Society (GLS).

Skinner, M., and Sterenberg, J. 2005. Turf wars: Authority and responsibility for the investigation of mass graves. *Forensic Science International* 151(2–3): 221–232.

Sterenberg, J. 2002. Archaeological Techniques and Methods for the Excavation and Recording of Contemporary Primary and Secondary Mass Graves. Thesis (M.Sc.) Forensic Archaeology, School of Conservation Sciences, Bournemouth, U.K.

———. 2004. *Assessment on the Use of Ground Probing Radar by the Finish Forensic Assessment Team at a Suspected Area Located to the South of Baghdad. Baghdad, Iraq:* Coalition Provisional Authority Forensic Team (unpublished document in possession of the author).

Sterenberg, J. with contributions from H. Tuller, A. Starovic, and S. Daley. 2002. *Exhumation and Examination Division; A Report on the Archaeological Findings Relating to the Excavation and Recovery of Human Remains from a Series of Related Features Located at Batajnica, Yugoslavia (Serbia), August to December 2002* (unpublished ICMP document in possession of the author).

Tabeau, E. 2004. Casualty figures according to the Demographic Unit at the ICTY.

Tuller, H., and Đurić, M. 2006. Keeping the pieces together: Comparison of mass grave excavation methodology. *Forensic Science International* 156(2–3): 192–200.

Watters, M. 2003. *Results of Ground Probing Radar Survey on Several Suspected Mass Gravesites in Bosnia* (unpublished PowerPoint presentation in possession of the author).

Watters, M., and Hunter, J. R. 2004. Geophysics and burials: Field experience and software development, in K. Pye and D. J. Croft (eds.), *Forensic Geoscience: Principals, Techniques and Applications,* pp. 21–31. London: The Geological Society (GLS).

Wessling, R. 2003. Various geological survey results, in *Inforce Foundation Site Assessment Summaries* (unpublished document in possession of the author).

Wright, R. 1995. War crimes: The archaeological evidence. *International Network on Holocaust and Genocide* 11(3): 8–11.

———. 1997–2000. *Protocols and Procedures for the Excavation of ICTY Gravesites* (unpublished document in possession of the author).

———. 1999. *Exhumations in Eastern Bosnia in 1998.* ICTY Evidence Report (unpublished document in possession of the author).

———. 2000. *Report on Excavations at Kozluk in 1999.* ICTY Evidence Report (unpublished document in possession of the author).

———. 2001. *Report on excavations and exhumations at the Glogova 1 Mass Grave in 2000:* p. 9. ICTY Evidence Report (unpublished document in possession of the author).

Wright, R., Hanson, I., and Sterenberg, J. 2005. The archaeology of mass graves, in J. Hunter and Cox, M. (eds.), *Forensic Archaeology: Advances in Theory and Practice,* pp. 137–158. Oxford: Routledge.

35

FORENSIC ANTHROPOLOGY AND ARCHAEOLOGY IN GUATEMALA

Ambika Flavel and Caroline Barker

In Guatemala, the application of the techniques and methods of forensic anthropology and archaeology was born out of an overwhelming need. Civilian victims of extrajudicial arbitrary executions, killed during the civil war that ended in 1996, were disposed of in clandestine graves throughout the country; these graves needed to be located and the human remains identified. In the early 1990s, survivors groups contacted experienced forensic anthropologists from North America and existing forensic teams in Latin America and requested assistance in locating and identifying the dead. It is from these early beginnings that the first Guatemalan forensic anthropology team was formed, trained by the international experts in order to develop an in-country capacity to deal with the forensic identification of the deceased.

Several forensic exhumation teams were formed in Guatemala, both during the latter stages of the conflict and after the signing of the Peace Accord in 1996. They were formed as part of the humanitarian response to requests from families of victims. Such organizations include the Human Rights Office of the Archbishopric of Guatemala (ODHAG), Center for Forensic Anthropology and Applied Science (CAFCA), and The Guatemalan Forensic Anthropology Foundation (FAFG, formerly EAFG). These organizations are largely run and staffed by Guatemalan nationals, although on occasions European, North American, and Latin American volunteers and employees have been either permanently or temporarily involved. The three aforementioned teams collaborated with the Department of Public Prosecutions (DPP) to publish a manual for forensic investigations in Guatemala (FAFG, CAFCA, & ODHAG 2004). The aim of the manual was to document a series of protocols on how forensic exhumations and post-mortem analyses should proceed and how they fit into the Guatemalan judicial process.

The history of the Guatemalan forensic teams is well documented in Stover and Shigekane (2002). The teams contribute to four purposes (Kirschner and Hannibal [1994]): returning remains to relatives, historical documentation, legal proceedings, and deterring continued violations. The Guatemalan Historical Clarification Commission (CEH) concluded: "The existence of clandestine and hidden cemeteries, as well as the anxiety suffered by many Guatemalans as a result of not knowing what happened to their relatives, remains an open wound in the country. They are a permanent reminder of the acts of violence that denied the dignity of their loved ones. To heal these particular wounds requires the exhumation of secret graves, as well as the definitive identification of the whereabouts of the disappeared" (CEH 1999).

Of all the massacres documented in Guatemala, a total of 669 have been attributed to the State and five to the Guerrilla forces. However, this figure is only a minimum, owing to the large number of new cases being investigated and exhumations that are undertaken every year. To date, only four have been successfully taken to court. These cases were recognized and tried by the Inter-American Commission on Human Rights (CIDH) based in Costa Rica.

Historical Context of the Internal Armed Conflict

Since its colonization by the Spanish in the early 16th century, Guatemala, like many countries in Latin America, has had a tumultuous history. A lack of social cohesion between the different ancestral and socioeconomic groups prevailed even after independence from Spain in 1821. This led to the division of the people and periods of political and social unrest, the most recent being the 36-year internal armed conflict. Suffice it to say that it was not a simple two-sided discord between two recognizable and opposing factions. Although the conflict can be defined as non-international in nature, the foreign policies of external countries facilitated the actions of the state-sponsored repressive regime and allowed human rights violations to be committed with impunity (CEH 1999 Chapter 4 p23 Paragraph 13).

The State is defined in the CEH report (CEH 1999) as those public servants and state agencies that were complicit in the human rights violations. Those recognizable state forces that witnesses and survivors testify to having perpetrated crimes against noncombatants are the State's National Army, Military Commissioners,[1] Civil Patrols (PACs)[2] and Death Squads, and other armed groups.[3] Moreover, these state-sanctioned forces acted collectively and separately throughout the duration of the conflict. The State as an aggressor waged a war against the "internal enemy," a broad and all-encompassing classification that could be anyone involved in either legal or illegal activities of which the State disapproved. Armed confrontation occurred between the State and the armed insurgency forces of the Guerrilla. There were four principal left-wing guerrilla groups, each with its own military command structures: the Guerrilla Army of the Poor (EGP), the Revolutionary Organization of the People (ORPA), the Rebel Armed Forces (FAR), and the Guatemalan Labor Party (PGT). These groups eventually combined in 1982 to form the Guatemalan National Revolutionary Unity (URNG), which became the political wing of the various guerrilla organizations.

The Guerrilla Forces were also found by the CEH to be responsible for human rights violations. There are documented incidences of arbitrary executions of private individuals and PAC members, and the forced conscription of individuals into the Guerrilla Forces. But the scale of these atrocities (3% of all CEH recorded human rights violations) was much less than that of the State Agents and is indicative of the overall disparity among the level of organization, number of forces, and access to military hardware between the State and the Guerrilla Forces.

During the conflict, an estimated 200,000 people disappeared or were the victims of extrajudicial arbitrary executions. The peak of the violence occurred from 1978–1983 during the presidential regimes of Generals Lucas García and Ríos Montt. The figure is not the actual recorded number of missing persons but the presumed number of missing extrapolated from the combined collected data from the three investigations by the CEH, The Recuperation of Historical Memory by the Catholic Church in Guatemala (REHMI), and CIDH. All three investigations attempted to determine the human and national impact of this violent period in Guatemala's history. They concluded that the majority of the atrocities and human rights violations were committed against those who were ethnically Mayan (83%) and that the major perpetrator of these crimes was the State (93%).

Figure 35.1 demonstrates the correlation between the conclusions of the CEH and FAFG that State Agents are responsible for the majority of the cases of mass executions in Guatemala. The comparison is based on the number of recorded cases by the CEH and number of exhumed cases by the FAFG.

All the human rights violations and abuses committed by all parties to the conflict were carried out with impunity, owing to the ineffective judicial system in place at that time. This deficiency of an available system of legal recourse, for the victims of all crime, gave rise to and enabled a regime of State social control through the use of military intelligence, military force, and internationally sanctioned counterinsurgency techniques.

The conclusions of the CEH and other reports provide the facts and figures of the violations and names of the missing based on witness and survivor testimony. Although this process endeavors to make the truth available, the prima facie evidence is the physical human remains and associated artifacts interred in clandestine graves. Such evidence has the potential to provide the link between a suspect(s) and a victim in death-related criminal investigations.

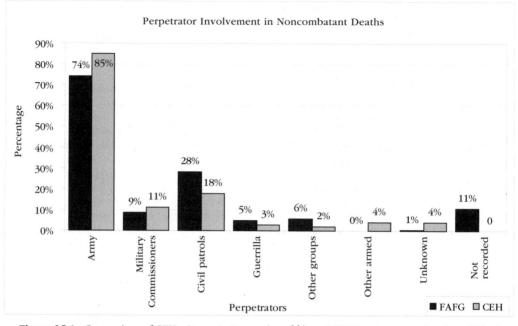

Figure 35.1 Comparison of CEH witness testimony ($n = 664$) and FAFG antemortem data ($n = 191$) of perpetrator involvement in cases of noncombatant deaths during the Guatemalan internal armed conflict.

Additionally, the recovery and identification of the remains of the missing have humanitarian, legal, and economic ramifications. Next of kin are given closure, and the burial preferences of the individual and next of kin can be honored. In addition, identifications are necessary for the inheritance of goods and property, collection of insurance policies, pensions, and the settlement of business matters and remarriage of spouses.

The conflict in Guatemala officially ended in December 1996 with the signing of the United Nations-brokered peace agreement in Oslo, Norway. The two parties to the Peace Accord were the URNG and the Government of the Republic of Guatemala. The complex historical context and the various parties involved in the conflict are covered in great detail in the CEH report "Guatemala: The Memory of Silence" (CEH 1999). The CEH was established to fulfill a ruling of the Oslo Accord with a mandate to determine the truth about the conflict. Fulfilling this obligation would enable the reparation process between the State and its people and assist Guatemala in its development from military dictatorship and social injustice to an authentic and functioning democracy.

The Judicial System of Guatemala

The judicial system of Guatemala is based on an inquisitorial system and the legal premise that the

State has a "duty to guarantee." The State's duty to guarantee is their obligation to all citizens under its jurisdiction and is established in Articles 1 and 2 of the Political Constitution of the Guatemalan Republic (Guatemala 2004). Article 1, Protection for the individual: The State of Guatemala, is organized to protect the individual and the family; its principal aim is the achievement of the common good. Article 2, Duty of the State, describes the duty of the State to guarantee the people of the Republic life, liberty, justice, security, and personal development.

The Constitution grants the Supreme Court of Justice the authority to judge, and secondary laws establish the specific capability of judges to determine an individual's complicity and responsibility for a crime. The authority to judge and to execute judgments rests with the courts of justice. The other agencies of the State, such as national civilian police (PNC), must offer the courts of justice any assistance that may be required to carry out their decisions (Guatemala 2004). To be able to administer justice, the Department of Public Prosecutions (DPP) is charged with the responsibility of investigating a crime and accusing those persons suspected of committing such acts. It is under the authority of the DPP that the forensic work takes place.

International Humanitarian Law is also directly applicable to the former conflict in Guatemala in addition to Protocol II of the 1949 Geneva

Conventions. This protocol applies in all situations of non-international armed conflict and serves to protect those people directly or indirectly involved in the conflict, especially civilians. Guatemala signed this protocol in 1977 but did not ratify it until 1987. Although the conflict would continue for a further nine years after the ratification of this treaty, the majority of the forced displacements, disappearances, and arbitrary executions occurred during the period between its signing and ratification.

The Forensic Process within the Guatemalan Judicial System

During Guatemala's internal armed conflict, many people died in suspicious circumstances and were buried in clandestine graves. Often the location of these graves was known only to relatives and neighbors; in other cases, only to the perpetrators. When community members buried their loved ones, it was invariably at great personal risk to them and accompanied by fear of reprisal. As a consequence, they often buried their relatives or friends in fairly inaccessible places, in shallow graves, or wherever the deceased were discovered. In contrast, when perpetrators buried the bodies, only they knew the location of the graves. It was often not until years later that perpetrators provided this information to relatives.

For families to recover the bodies of their relatives, they must request the permission of the DPP to exhume a presumed clandestine grave. As previously stated, the DPP is the institution in charge of investigating cases of suspicious death and must follow up any substantial accusation against a person or group with a criminal investigation. This accusation can be made by victims, relatives of victims, and human rights or legal organizations such as the Mutual Assistance Group (GAM),[4] the National Coordination of Guatemalan Widows (CONAVIGUA),[5] and Relatives of the Detained-Disappeared of Guatemala (FAMDEGUA).[6] To complete the investigation, the DPP may require the assistance of experts. In cases involving clandestine graves and unidentified human remains, forensic expertise will be necessary and will include the specialist skills of social anthropologists (skilled in antemortem data collection), physical anthropologists, and archaeologists.

The forensic archaeological work begins with an initial site inspection of the suspected location of clandestine graves. This assessment is undertaken with a DPP public prosecutor, the forensic anthropologists (physical and social), archaeologists, witnesses, relatives, and human rights and legal organizations representing the community.

Before initiating a forensic investigation, the presiding forensic expert in charge of the case[7] must sign a declaration for the public prosecutor or judge. The expert is required to compile a report on completion of the investigation. This report includes the social anthropological phase (obtaining antemortem information by interviewing the families of victims); the archaeological phase (excavation, exhumation, and on-site recording); and the laboratory phase (skeletal analysis to establish a biological profile and identification of individuals, perimortem trauma, and the cause and manner of death signed off by the pathologist). The report is presented to the public prosecutor and can be used as evidence in any further criminal proceedings.

To ensure transparency of process and the integrity of the recovered evidence, experts are required to maintain the chain of custody at all times. During the archaeological phase, the area under investigation is defined and cordoned, and those archaeologists that work within the grave are responsible for maintaining the chain of custody. At night, the maintenance of the chain of custody is handed over to Officers of the PNC, who guard the area to prevent any tampering with the crime scene or corruption of the evidence.

When the date to begin excavation and exhumation has been agreed to by all parties, the presence is requested of DPP, relatives and neighbors, legal and psychosocial support organizations, and human rights and legal organizations. All the information gleaned from the excavation of the context, condition of the site, status of the remains, and associated evidence must be recorded and thoroughly documented. Photographic, drawn, and written records are created to enable the reconstruction of the scene and postmortem depositional events. These records and the postmortem analysis findings and conclusions are used to produce the final report for submission to the presiding judge in the case.

The expert report given to the DPP provides the technical foundation of the investigation. With information from witnesses, the public prosecutor can potentially determine who was arbitrarily executed, by whom and in what circumstances. The physical evidence (exhibits) of ballistics, clothing, ligatures, and bindings are also submitted. All this evidence can be used to support the accusation that human rights violations have been committed. When a case is taken to court, the forensic expert witness may be called to give expert testimony, to clarify any doubts the court may have about the forensic evidence, or to explain their conclusions and findings to a lay audience.

The Forensic and Psychosocial Impact of the Exhumation

The exhumation of clandestine graves is usually a community event in Guatemala, with traditional Mayan and Christian ceremonies being carried out during the exhumation process, in accordance with the spiritual beliefs of the people. This collective gathering also provides an opportunity for psychosocial organizations such as the Community Studies and Psychosocial Action Team (ECAP)[8] to provide support and advice. Trained psychologists are charged with helping relatives or communities face the fear and pain they may have suffered from losing relatives and friends and having to interact with those people alleged to have been involved in these crimes and still living in their communities (Rivera Fernández 2004).

In addition, the exhumation provides an opportunity for the witnesses and survivors to give statements through informal but structured interviews with the social anthropologists. Their version of events is recorded along with the biological details of the presumed deceased, such as age, sex, stature, ancestry, and individuating criteria such as known or visible pathological conditions and details of dentition.[9] The antemortem data provides the basis for the contextual[10] and presumptive identification[11] of the remains. This is often the first occasion where the "missing" are legally acknowledged as deceased.

Ideally, techniques such as comparative DNA analysis would be used to positively identify individuals. Such scenarios are resource specific. In Guatemala, local DNA laboratory facilities and funding are not presently available. It is worth noting that forensic organizations such as the FAFG routinely collect bone samples and comparative blood samples from presumed relatives for future DNA analysis. Such samples are collected with the understanding and permission of the community and family members and are stored observing chain of custody procedures. The aim of this program is to ensure that positive identification through the use of DNA can be made in future for all those remains that have been reburied after the completion of the forensic analysis. When funding is secured, this program can commence and the results of any positive identifications can be submitted to the DPP.

Comparison of Witness Testimony and Physical Evidence

Reconciling the memories of witnesses and survivors of historical crime and the physical evidence is not an easy process. There often exists inconsistencies among the expected number of victims as detailed by witness testimony, antemortem data of named missing, and the physical evidence. This inconsistency is due, in part, to the problems of collecting information from witnesses over 20 years after the event, while the rural, ethnic Mayan communities still feel oppressed and fear reprisal should they surrender information about the perpetrators. Nevertheless, there is an 89% ($n = 170$) success rate (location and recovery of human remains) in all the exhumations carried out by the FAFG (2006) from 1992 to 2005 ($n = 191$), a testament to the cooperation and commitment of survivors and living victims to the reconciliation process. In general, the fewer the number of individuals present, the higher the correlation among the physical evidence, witness testimonies, and antemortem data of the missing. This situation can be attributed to the tendency of people to overestimate in cases of mass trauma and confusion. There is also the difficulty of keeping track of people, some of whom may have "disappeared" to another region and are still alive. Needless to say, when information about a case is inaccessible, or witnesses do not wish to talk, the difficulty in discovering the location of clandestine graves increases and often results in no graves being located at all.

Results of the Exhumations in Guatemala

As previously stated, the figures published by the CEH are comparable to those determined from the physical evidence by the FAFG.[12] The FAFG has carried out exhumations in 18 of the 22 departments of Guatemala, with human remains located and recovered in 17 of these departments (Figure 35.2). The five municipalities most commonly visited by exhumation teams correspond to the geographical and proportional distribution of the massacres recorded by the CEH (1999) who report that "during the most violent and bloody period of the entire armed confrontation, 1978–1985, military operations were concentrated in Quiché, Huehuetenango, Chimaltenango, Alta Verapaz and Baja Verapaz, the south coast, and the capital—the victims being principally Mayan and to a lesser extent Ladino. During the final period, 1986–1996, repressive action was selective, affecting the Mayan and Ladino population to a similar extent. The Communities of Population in Resistance (CPRs) were principal targets of military operations in rural areas."

The exhumations undertaken by the FAFG include human remains buried in either single

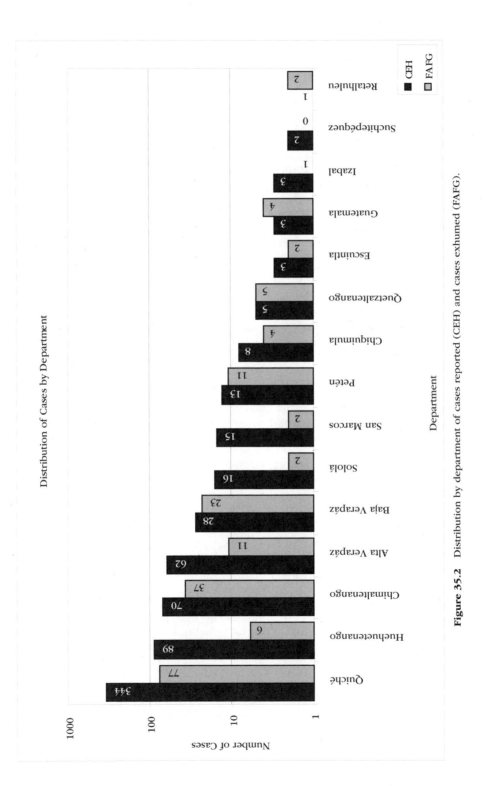

Figure 35.2 Distribution by department of cases reported (CEH) and cases exhumed (FAFG).

(minimum number of individuals—MNI 1), multiple (MNI 2), or mass (MNI 3+) graves. By far, the majority of cases (80.5%) were primary graves, with less than 4% of all graves showing evidence of secondary disturbance and 15.7% being secondary graves.[13]

Multiple graves were exhumed in almost 49% of 175 cases analyzed[14] by the FAFG, and single graves were encountered in approximately 37% of cases. Those remains not buried in graves were often recovered from naturally occurring deposition sites such as caves or on the surface, as well as from pre-existing disposal sites such as wells (or sumps).

The general trend seen by exhumation teams in Guatemala affirms that single interments (15%) are encountered as often as multiple interments (16%), but mass graves are most prevalent. Graves have been exhumed containing between 3 and 9 individuals, and these predominate (34%); those containing 10–19 individuals (15%) and 20–39 individuals (12%) are common, and graves containing over 40 individuals (7%) are least often encountered. These patterns are repeated throughout all the affected regions and support the testimony of the witnesses and survivors.

The antemortem testimony of witnesses and relatives reveals that burial of the deceased was often carried out clandestinely by members of the community, family, and friends. This pattern of small graves is mirrored in East Timor with the victims of the 1999 massacres. In contrast, other conflicts, such as in the war in the former Yugoslavia and the disappearances and arbitrary executions under the Saddam Hussein regime in Iraq, resulted in graves containing large numbers of people buried by organized groups (usually perpetrators) using heavy machinery. Archaeological signatures present in the graves of these different historical crime scenes can be used to show consistencies between the physical evidence and witness testimony.

In Guatemala, evidence of people being buried in coffins (1%) or wrapped in blankets, plastic, or tarpaulin (4%) is rarely encountered. Physical evidence that indicates human rights violations, such as binding of the hands, feet, neck, and combinations of these and/or blindfolds, is associated with 12.5% of all individuals recovered, with some form of binding of hands most commonly encountered, followed by ropes around the neck. Of the 1,809 individuals exhumed and analyzed by the FAFG, only 9.7% had no clothing, personal effects, bindings, or other items buried with them. The majority (1,601 individuals) were recovered with personal effects or associated accessories. Of these, 95%

were recovered with clothing and often personal effects such as jewellery (beaded necklaces, bracelets, and earrings) or coins and documents in the pockets of clothing. In 20% of cases, those burying the dead placed personal items or grave goods with the deceased in the grave. Such items include cups and plates, blankets, clothing, medicines, and weapons. These items hold no individual evidential value, unlike items such as ballistics or bindings, but can be used as contextual evidence to corroborate witness testimony and assist in the development of contextual identifications.

Results of the Forensic Anthropology Analyses

The following sections detail the results of the forensic anthropology analyses including the determination of biological profiles, assessment of trauma, and the identification process.

Biological Profile

It has been established that the use of population-specific standards to determine the biological profile of skeletonized victims increases the accuracy of the conclusions. The development and publication of these standards becomes more pertinent when large groups of a minority population are being assessed over a long period of time and it is likely that multiple analysts will perform the assessments.

The majority of work undertaken on the Guatemalan population, either modern or archaeological, has been related to stature estimations (Danforth 1994; Genovés 1967; Haviland 1967; Wright and Vásquez 2003) or sex identification (Ríos Frutos 2002, 2003, 2005). Published material relating to forensic anthropology in Latin America, as İşcan and Olivera (2000) state, has increased over the last decade but falls short of covering the diversity of the population within Latin America. Furthermore, there is a demand for relevant literature to be available in Spanish. There is a distinct need for the development of population-specific standards in Guatemala. an objective that one hopes will be realized once positive identifications can be made using DNA comparison. Previously recorded data can be revisited to determine the applicability of the osteological techniques presently available.

Despite this limitation, the trends and patterns of the biological profile of individuals recovered by the FAFG can be observed. There are distinct morphological variations between adult male and female skeletal remains, and, although not empirically tested within this population, they are deemed reliable within the Guatemalan forensic anthropological community. It is likely that the age ranges determined might not truly reflect those of the population but that the chronological seriation of groups of remains is correct. Consequently, the overall shape of the demographic profile is also correct. It is well known that factors such as chronic malnutrition or stress[15] experienced by individuals during the growth and maturation period affects the timing of dental and skeletal development (Scheuer and Black 2000). The development and maturation of skeletal features may be retarded, but the sequence of those changes remains the same.

The remains analyzed by the FAFG from 1992 to mid-2005 (FAFG 2006) correlate with the conclusions of the CEH (Figure 35.3). They indicate that women were the victims of the violence owing to their political or social activities or ideals, and they represent a minimum of 15% of the total number of victims. The physical evidence indicates that although adult females make up a considerable proportion, adult males represent the highest number (minimum of 55%) of skeletal remains recovered. Of the 30% of remains where sex could not be identified, the majority is non-adult (19% of all remains). Furthermore, age distribution indicates that no age group was spared. Adults (aged 26 + years) represent 64% of those recovered; young adults (18–25 years) represent almost 14%; adolescents (13–17 years) 7%; children (4–12 years) 6%; and infants (0–3 years) 5%, and foetal remains account for 1% of the total, indicating that pregnant women were targets.

Perimortem Trauma

The CEH does not publish figures relating to cause and manner of death, reporting only that "state terror was applied to make it clear that those who attempted to assert their rights, and even their relatives, ran the risk of death by the most hideous means. The objective was to intimidate and silence society as a whole, in order to destroy the will for transformation, both in the short and long term."

It is in this area that the anthropological analyses not only confirms the historical record but enhances it. Data gathered from 1,809 sets of remains analyzed by the FAFG show that after over 20 years of burial and varying degrees of preservation, perimortem trauma is still visible in 52% of the remains. Some 923 individuals exhibited visible perimortem trauma, categorized as gunshot wounds (GSW), blunt-force trauma (BFT), sharp-force trauma (SFT), and trauma of unknown

cause; 884 individuals (49%) displayed no visible perimortem trauma on the remains.

It is clear that many individuals exhibited multiple and different types of lesions. A single set of remains may exhibit perimortem signatures of GSW, BFT, and SFT that may affect the same or different regions of the body. Although 923 of the 1,809 individuals (51%) displayed evidence of perimortem trauma, a total of 1,635 trauma types and locations were recorded for these individuals. Such cases may indicate multiple perpetrators, torture prior to arbitrary execution, or the mechanism of death and body disposal (see case history at the end of the chapter). It is unlikely that the physical evidence itself, unless perimortem trauma lesions can be sequenced, would allow such conclusions, but it may provide corroborative evidence that is consistent with witness testimony.

By far, the most common areas of the body to be affected by perimortem trauma were the skull (45%, $n = 731$) and torso (35%, $n = 567$), with upper extremities accounting for 12% ($n = 202$) and lower limbs 8% ($n = 135$). Defense injuries are less common in all wound categories. Of all the lesions recorded ($n = 1,635$), GSW were present in 50% ($n = 924$), BFT in 29% ($n = 481$), and SFT in 11% of cases (179).

GSW to the skull (43% of the 923 individuals with visible trauma) ($n = 395$) is the most prevalent type of perimortem trauma, indicative of the prevalence of execution-style killings. This is consistent with the CEH conclusions that the prevailing perpetrator group was the Army, and it was they who had unlimited access to guns and ammunition. It is interesting to note that a relatively small number of cases (6.8%, $n = 123$) (committed by all parties to the conflict) display evidence of heat modification or burning. Such evidence perhaps indicates that it was felt unnecessary to destroy evidence, because the perpetrators felt themselves to have impunity and could act without the fear of future legal reprisal. Alternatively, this was another method of inducing fear.

Nineteen percent of all individuals recovered had associated ballistics[16] evidence. However, 6% of those with associated ballistics evidence did not display evidence of perimortem GSW trauma on the skeleton. This is usual in cases where only the soft tissue is affected by perimortem trauma; no manner of death can be stated in these cases. As a result, the number of injuries on the remains in all injury categories is underestimated and represents a proportion of the actual number of injuries sustained by the victims. Almost 14% of individuals were recorded as having GSW but no recovered ballistics evidence. In a relatively small number

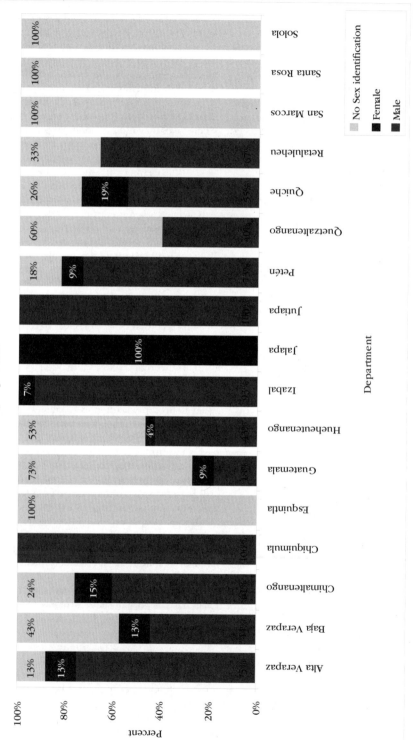

Figure 35.3 Sex distribution by department of skeletal remains recovered by the FAFG (1992 to 2005).

of cases (13%), ballistics were recovered and also trauma recorded. The majority of cases were recovered without any discernible signs of trauma, and without ballistics.

Identification

The reality in Guatemala is that in most cases there are no antemortem medical records available for comparison with the postmortem remains and the results of the forensic anthropological analyses. It has been internationally recognized by the International Committee of the Red Cross (ICRC 2003) that comparing antemortem data (collected during interviews with relatives or acquaintances of the deceased) with postmortem data is a fully acceptable method of ascertaining a presumptive identification. The forensic anthropologist should primarily explore this route and, when possible and necessary, employ other scientific methods such as DNA comparison. The lack of antemortem medical records is the reason why in Guatemala only presumptive and contextual identifications can be made. As a result, all available evidence must be used including the results of the anthropological analyses, circumstantial data from witness testimony and information gleaned from the exhumation. This is a difficult task; it relies on the memory of witnesses or relatives to identify possible individuals through the recognition of clothing or personal effects at the time of exhumation and post-analysis reburial.

The available data indicate that 51% of skeletonized remains exhumed by the FAFG are identified in the field, at the time of exhumation or reburial. The postmortem data collected in the laboratory are compared to the antemortem data collected during interviews, and where there is no clear discrepancy between the two, or there is an overall consistency among all the pieces of evidence (both circumstantial and biological), the identification stands. A prosecutor or the judge can sign off on the presumed or contextual identification and give a legal ruling on the death of a named individual or group. Relatives often recognize clothing during the exhibition of clothing prior to reburial of the remains.[17] Conversely, only 5% of the remains are first identified in the laboratory; the remaining 44% never being identified. The unidentified remains are returned to the community for reburial alongside those that have been identified. All the remains exhumed are reburied collectively, in accordance with the wishes and the cultural beliefs of the community.

This action is considered to be part of the healing and reparation process. Psychosocial support is offered to the community at this time, and reburials serve as an opportunity for all the survivors' and victims' families to remember all the deceased, even if their loved ones have not been identified. Facilities and resources do not exist to store the remains indefinitely, and long-term retention of remains would be unacceptable to the community.

A contextual identification of the deceased can potentially be obtained by the presence of a closed context (burial)—that is, one that shows no signs of secondary tampering—and by the consistency between the witness descriptions of the graves goods interred at the time of burial and the items recovered during exhumation. Bodies were often visually identified at the time of the killing when they were still fleshed, and thus personal items and grave goods were placed in the grave along with the bodies. Contextual identification is not a presumptive identification in itself, but where scientific techniques are unavailable (a situation often encountered in many postconflict environments) multiple pieces of circumstantial evidence may be packaged together to demonstrate to a presiding judge that the probability of the deceased being someone else is extremely unlikely.

Despite the obvious potential legal problems and consequences associated with the presumptive and contextual identifications and non-identifications, it is worth remembering that the humanitarian component of this work is often fulfilled in the eyes of the survivors' and victims' families. The indigenous Maya of Guatemala often live in small, tight-knit communities. Missing persons within a community are grieved for by all its members. The grief and experience are shared and forms part of the community's collective history. Moreover, the legal identification is not the primary concern to many within the community. Observation of burial practices and recognition of the missing as found are felt to be more important, giving them closure.

Two Cases

Two cases exhumed by the Guatemalan Forensic Anthropology Foundation (FAFG) in 1999 and 2000 illustrate the indiscriminate targeting by the State during the conflict, and how the physical evidence supports the conclusion of the CEH report (CEH 1999) that the State was actively engaged in genocide. Both cases presented similar challenges for the exhumation forensic team, owing to the method of disposal of the bodies in wells.

Case 1: The Exhumation of the Well at Zacualpa

The National Army of Guatemala routinely commandeered buildings or premises in locations throughout Guatemala for use as strategic bases of operations. Under the guise of administrative and operational centers, they were often used as forced detention, torture, and interrogation centers. One such example is the Army's occupation, from 1981 to 1984, of the compound belonging to the Catholic Church of the parish of Zacualpa in Zacualpa, Quiché. Incidentally, the department of Quiché was viewed by the State as the primary location of the Guerrilla Forces and was where the largest number of documented human rights violations was committed. Witnesses alleged that cases of torture, disappearances, and arbitrary executions were associated with the Army's occupation of the compound and that the victims had been disposed of in a disused well within its walled grounds (an area of 250 m²). Human remains had also been recovered in the grounds of the compound during the digging of a water-pipe trench in the late 1990s.

Under the authority of the DPP, the FAFG did a complete survey of the grounds using trial trenching techniques, and a grave truncated by a pipeline was discovered containing a minimum number of seven (complete and incomplete) sets of human remains. The witness testimony describing bodies being disposed of in a well needed further investigation but required a suitable archaeological strategy for use in what Rivera (2004) has defined as a perpendicular context. The stratigraphic depositional sequence, the discrete anatomical relationship of each set of remains, and the relationship of the remains to one another needed to be established. At the same time, the team must observe the appropriate health and safety strategies for those experts tasked with exhuming the remains. These circumstances required the forensic team to develop a suitable methodology using the available resources to ensure that all of these criteria were met.

The well was easily located in the grounds of the compound, presenting a circular ring of mortared bricks of approximately 1 m in diameter, with a visible fill of soil, rubble, and other extraneous building material. The initial phase of the well exhumation required the claims of the witnesses to be firmly established and the presence or absence of human remains to be determined. Local professional well diggers were employed and tasked with removing the upper fill from the disused well. They were instructed to cease digging should any bones or artifacts be encountered. Because the well diggers were not experienced physical

anthropologists capable of discriminating between human and nonhuman remains, this was a suitable strategy. Nevertheless, the experience of the well diggers (*poceros*) was vital at this stage because of their knowledge of the local soft geology and the well-digging methods used throughout the region. Any skeletal remains encountered were checked by one of the forensic team. The material removed from the well was also sieved and checked for human remains and other potential evidence. The human remains at Zacualpa were located at a depth of 9.4 m; at this point, excavation of the well was stopped and the remains were appropriately covered to protect them and Phase Two was implemented.

At Phase Two, the *poceros* dug an adjacent perpendicular shaft, with the common wall between it and the well removed. The purpose of this stage was to create an adjacent workspace from which the archaeologists could excavate and recover the remains, similar dimensions to the well proper were deemed appropriate, and a shaft adjacent to the well of approximately 1 m in diameter and 10.4 m deep was excavated. A brick and mortared upper rim around the well and the shaft was created to ensure against collapse of the upper walls and to act as a barrier to any potential material that might drop into the well and harm those excavating. Safety equipment such as safety helmets and harnesses were also used throughout the excavation. Periodically the remains would be covered and the adjacent shaft deepened to allow appropriate access to the deeper remains. A secure bucket, rig, and pulley system was set up over the shaft to remove the fill, remains, and evidence. Light was provided using an on-site generator and lighting system. Because illumination was needed at all times, and the work space available in the adjacent shaft was large enough only for one person, the archaeologists were rotated for fixed time periods, but the work could continue during the hours of darkness. Once the adjacent shaft was in place, the exhumation of remains and associated evidence and the in-situ recording of these features could proceed with the same archaeological rigor as used for the more commonly encountered graves.

The final result of the exhumation was that 33 bodies were recovered within 3 m at depths of 9–12 m from the ground surface. When it was presumed that the last of the bodies had been reached, the *poceros* were tasked with removing the black soil fill in the well, which contrasted with the white sand natural geology, to the reach the original bottom of the well, testing the claim that the well was disused at the time of disposal by ensuring no more human remains were present at the lower depths. The same stipulations as Phase One were applied, should remains be uncovered during this process. However, no further remains were encountered, and the final depth of the well was established at 23 m. In the course of the work, approximately 18 m³ of material were removed by hand using the bucket, rig, and pulley system.

All the stratigraphic depositional events evident in the well allow the development of a chronology of use: from its original digging, to its abandonment and backfilling, to its use as a clandestine burial location, and use as a dumping ground for soil and building material, through to the time of the exhumation (Figure 35.4).

The success of this methodology can be measured by the integrity of the remains and evidence recovered. A total of 33 almost complete sets of skeletal remains were recovered from the well: 28 adults, 3 adolescents, and 2 juveniles. Of these, 25 were identified as male, 4 female, 3 probable male, and 1 of unidentified sex, the probable and unidentified sex identifications belonging to either the adolescent or juvenile groups. Of all the perimortem trauma injuries present on the bones, there were 13 GSW, 28 BFT, and 3 SFT, and 12 causes of death were determined.

Many of the individuals were missing some of the smaller bones of the hands and feet and bone fragments. Bones were classified as commingled when an association between bones and bone fragments and a discrete single set of remains could not be made during the exhumation. The basic principle of the downward movement of commingled bones throughout the well during the postdeposition phase (approximately 20 years) can be safely assumed within this particular perpendicular context. Therefore, recovered commingled bones can belong only to those remains located at the same or a lesser depth. Since the bodies were deposited at depths of 9–12 m, it is unlikely that they were disturbed by burrowing animals, and no evidence of such activity was found in the walls of the well. No nonhuman remains were found among the human remains, so it is safe to assume that no animals had entered the interment depths from above. The movement of these bones is therefore more likely to have occurred after the decomposition of the soft tissues of the body. The diverse positions and overlapping of adjacent bodies also created small voids between the bodies where bones could fall. This is consistent with the bodies having being thrown in from the top. Limbs and torsos were often excavated resting on the walls, and the location of blunt-force trauma fractures was frequently encountered in those body regions in direct contact with the sides of the well.

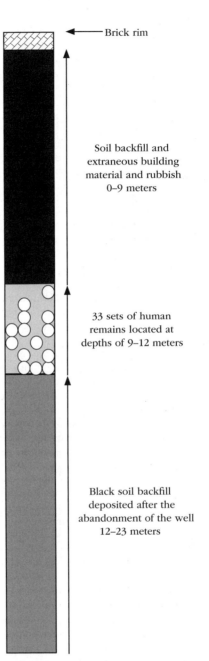

Figure 35.4 Profile of the well at Zacualpa.

It must be remembered that some of the injuries on the bodies may have been due to torture prior to execution, the timing between the infliction of the injury and death insufficient to show evidence of perimortem healing.

Within the controlled confines of the laboratory environment, where possible, a match of commingled bones and bone fragments to a set of remains could be made based on physical fit or morphological comparison. Those bones that could not be matched were included in the overall bone inventory to establish the minimum number of individuals present within the well.

Case Two: The Exhumation of the Well at Chuguexá II B

The methodology employed at the exhumation of the well at Zacualpa proved so effective, within the limits of the available resources, that it was utilized again in the exhumation of a well in February 2000. The well was associated with a massacre in 1982 in the small village of Chuguexá II B, in the municipality of Chichicastenango in the department of Quiché. The perpetrators and the method of disposal of the bodies were the same as at Zacualpa, but the circumstances were radically different. Witness testimony states that the community feared the Army would enter the village and take away or massacre the men and boys of fighting age. Thus the men and boys left the village and hid in the surrounding mountains. On entering the village, the Army encountered predominantly women and children and subsequently massacred multiple families and dumped their bodies in the well.

The well at Chugeuxá II B was circular and similar in diameter to the well at Zacualpa. The major difference between the two exhumations was that the well at Chugeuxá II B continually filled with water at a depth below 5 m, a depth consistent with ground-water level. Therefore, the adjacent shaft not only was employed to access the remains but also served to drain water from the well, which was subsequently pumped to the surface. A total of 26 bodies were recovered from the well at a depth of 5.0–6.1 m, 6.1 m corresponding to the original well bottom (Figure 35.5). This is consistent with the witness testimony that the well was in use at the time of the massacre.

The anthropological analysis of the remains determined that the overall demographic profile of the group is very different to that seen at Zacualpa. Of the 26 bodies recovered only 3 were male, 11 were female, and 12 were of unidentified sex, belonging to juveniles and infants. Execution-style gunshot injuries to the back of the cranium were seen on many of the remains. A set of female remains recovered from the well contained a neonatal set of remains wrapped within a large sheet of fabric used to carry feeding infants (a *peraje*). It is likely that the mother of the infant was the victim of arbitrary execution and both mother and child were then thrown into the well.

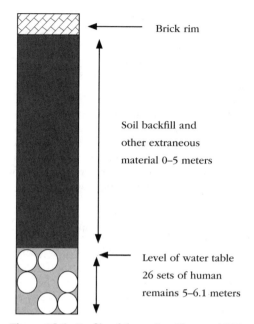

Figure 35.5 Profile of the well at Chuguexá II B.

The exhumations at Zacualpa and Chugeuxá II B illustrate the indiscriminate targeting of victims during the Guatemalan conflict by the major perpetrator, the State Forces. In addition, they also demonstrate that the effective stratigraphic exhumation of human skeletonized remains can be carried out in challenging depositional environments even with limited resources.

Acknowledgments

This chapter is dedicated to all the victims, victims' families, and survivors of the human rights violations carried out over three decades of internal armed conflict and those who dedicate their lives working to establish the truth lest we forget. Many thanks are extended to Claudia Rivera, Richard Wright, and Tim Loveless for their help and editorial input.

Notes

1. Retired military personnel acting under the authority of the State and the coordinated control of the army, responsible for command and control in rural areas.

2. Civilian military adjuncts to the Guatemalan army formed in 1981 under the Presidency of General Lucas García, tasked with controlling and reporting to the army any insurgency activities.

3. Civilian gangs incorporating military personnel that later evolved into clandestine military units acting under the coordinated control of the Army.

4. Organization of family members of the disappeared, founded in June of 1984.

5. Organization of Mayan widows of the armed conflict, formed in 1988.

6. Organization of relatives of the disappeared formed in 1994.

7. A team leader will be assigned as the forensic expert in a case and represent the forensic effort. This person is charged with maintaining the chain of custody, leading the forensic team, and producing the expert scientific report. The expert may also be required to represent the forensic effort in court as an expert witness.

8. Established in 1997 to provide psychosocial services to the victims of torture and their communities.

9. It is common for people in Guatemala to have dental work that may be uniquely identifiable. This includes gold crowns to the anterior teeth for cosmetic and decorative purposes. Such dental work, however, is seldom carried out by trained dentists, and antemortem records are rarely kept.

10. Contextual identification of a group or individual set of remains details contextual consistencies between the remains, artifacts, and burial context and the antemortem data. A presiding judge will determine whether the identification is legally valid.

11. Presumptive identification of an individual is based on the consistencies of biological profile and individuating criteria and antemortem data.

12. All figures and other information relating to exhumations and forensic anthropology are taken from the authors' personal experience and data collected by the FAFG between 1992 and 2004 (FAFG 2006).

13. Graves that contain human remains removed from their primary interment site.

14. A case refers to each commission the DPP consigns to the forensic team. Each case may contain single or multiple graves and single or multiple sets of remains, depending on the petition to the DPP.

15. Stress can be defined as physiological factors, such as disease or diet, or sociological factors, such as living under the pressures of a conflict, that exert an effect on the living individual.

16. Associated ballistics evidence is invariably copper jackets or copper jacket fragments from spent rounds, found on or immediately adjacent to the remains or within associated clothing.

17. Clothing of Mayan people, especially of indigenous women, is distinctive from Ladino clothing, and there is a high degree of individuation in colours and patterns. Women often wove their own clothing and made that of their husbands and children. Therefore, the combination of *huipil* (blouse), *faja* (belt), and *corte* (skirt) can often be recognized as that of a distinct individual.

References

CEH. 1999. *Guatemala: Memoria Del Silencio, Informe de La Comisión para el Esclarecimiento Histórico.* Guatemala: United Nations Office of Project Services (UNOPS).

Danforth, M. E. 1994. Stature change in Prehistoric Maya of the Southern Lowlands. *Latin American Antiquity* 7: 61–79.

FAFG Website. 2006. *Listado de Investigaciones Antropológas Forenses Del Año 1992–2005.* www.fafg.org/ cifras.php (accessed 01/09/06).

FAFG, CAFCA & ODHAG 2004. *Manual de Procedimientos para Investigaciones Antropológico-Forenses en Guatemala.* Embajada de Canadá en Guatemala: Ministerio Público de Guatemala.

Genovés, S. 1967. Proportionality of the long bones and their relation to stature among Mesoamericans. *American Journal of Physical Anthropology* 26: 67–77.

Guatemala, C. A. 2004. Constitución Política de la República de Guatemala. *Reformada por la Consulta Popular Acuerdo Legislativo*: 18–93.

Haviland, W. 1967. Stature at Tikal, Guatemala: Implications for ancient Maya demography and social organization. *American Antiquity* 32: 316–325.

ICRC. 2003. ICRC report: The missing and their families. *Summary of the Conclusions Arising from Events Held prior to the International Conference of Governmental and Non-Governmental Experts.* Geneva: ICRC.

İşcan, Y., and Solla Olivera, H. E. 2000. Forensic anthropology in Latin America. *Forensic Science International* 109: 15–30.

Kirschner, R., and Hannibal, K. 1994. The application of forensic sciences to human rights investigations. *Medicine Science and Law* 13: 451–460.

Ríos Frutos, L. 2002. Determination of sex from the clavicle and scapula in a Guatemalan Contemporary rural indigenous population. *The American Journal of Forensic Medicine and Pathology* 23: 284–288.

———. 2003. Brief communication: Sex determination accuracy of the minimum supero-inferior femoral neck diameter in a contemporary rural Guatemalan population. *American Journal of Physical Anthropology* 122: 123–126.

———. 2005. Metric determination of sex from the humerus in a Guatemalan forensic sample. *Forensic Science International* 147: 153–157.

Rivera Fernández, C. E. 2004. Estudio Comparativo de Excavaciones Perpendiculares en Investigaciones Antropológico Forenses en los departamentos de Chimaltenango, Quiché, Suchitepéquez y Baja Verapaz (1996–2002): Propuesta metodológica. Unpublished Bachelors thesis. Guatemala: Universidad de San Carlos de Guatemala.

Scheuer, L., and Black, S. 2000. *Developmental Juvenile Osteology*. London: Academic Press Limited.

Stover, E., and Shigekane, R. 2002. The Missing in the aftermath of war: When do the needs of victims' families and international war crimes tribunals clash? *International Review of the Red Cross* 84(848): 845–866.

Wright, L. E., and Vásquez, M. A. 2003. Estimating the length of incomplete long bones: Forensic standards from Guatemala. *American Journal of Physical Anthropology* 120: 233–251.

36

GRAVE CHALLENGES IN IRAQ

Derek Congram and Jon Sterenberg

... the potential information contained in human burials is far greater than is usually extracted from them. (Willems 1978: 88, cited Sprague 2005: 5)

This chapter discusses the new and limited role that forensic archaeology and anthropology have had in Iraq, focusing on events since the 2003 overthrow of the Iraqi government by the United States and allies. There are three background issues that have resulted in major problems for investigating and researching the situation of forensic archaeology and anthropology in Iraq:

1. The variety of contexts that may constitute the focus of forensic work (for example, various offenders, victims, time periods, and so on);

2. The lack of organized and available information and data on forced disappearances, killings, and clandestine burials;

3. The disorganized approach and ability to investigate alleged crimes to date.

Both of us have forensic experience in Iraq and several other countries and will draw on this to comment on these three issues. We also discuss

the work that has taken place recently investigating mass graves in Iraq. Finally, we address several other issues, including some social and ethical considerations that pertain to the practice of forensic archaeology and anthropology in Iraq in particular, but also in other countries. For reasons related to confidentiality regarding cases currently under investigation or on trial and contractual obligations, this chapter takes a broader perspective to describe past investigations and make recommendations for future work.

Background Issues

Definition of Context

In many cases, contemporary mass graves are an expression of the maximum effort required to dispose of persons considered unworthy of proper burial (let alone the right to life) who have been executed by the authorities that carry the responsibility of protecting these same people. In Iraq, such graves were dug long before Saddam Hussein. In fact, recent accusations by British politicians of the barbarity of chemical weapons use against the Kurds in the 1980s are hypocritical. In 1920, during the Iraqi revolution against British rule "at Winston Churchill's suggestion, the RAF (Royal

Air Force), used poison gas against the rebellious Kurds" (Simpson 2003: 28).

State-sponsored criminal events resulting in mass death, however, appear to have increased dramatically under Saddam Hussein. There is a very broad range of events, the evidence of which

may or does lie in mass graves throughout Iraq (Table 36.1).

Each of these different events has a unique context, relating to a different period of time and circumstances, diverse offenders and victims. Some graves hold evidence of crimes-against-humanity

Table 36.1 Summary of modern-era events in Iraq from which victims may be buried in mass graves and therefore subject to forensic archaeological and anthropological investigation.

Date	Victims	Perpetrators	Source
1920	6,000 Iraqis	British colonial government	Tripp 2007: 44
1933	Thousands of Kurds and Assyrians	British colonial government (RAF); Iraqi military; Kurdish tribesmen	McDowall 2000; Simpson 2003: 38; Tripp 2007: 80
Oct. 1935	Hundreds of Yazidi Kurds	Iraqi military	Tripp 2007: 87
1968–1971	2,000 political prisoners	Iraqi military	Simpson 2003: 50
1979	500+ political conspirators against Saddam Hussein	Iraqi military	Simpson 2003: 59
1980–1988	Thousands of Iranian prisoners of war	Iraqi military	McMahon 2004
Jul. 1983	Up to 8,000 members of Barzani clan	Iraqi military	Amin 1994; Human Rights Watch 2004; Recknagel 2006
1987–1989	50,000–200,000 Kurds	Iraqi military	Cordner 2005; McDowall 2007: 357–360; Middle East Watch 1993
Mar. 17, 1988	5,000+ Kurds at Halabjah	Iraqi military	Barber and Epstein 2004; Simpson 2003: 88
Aug. 2, 1990	Up to 600 Kuwaiti POWs	Iraqi military	AP 2005a; Barber and Epstein 2004; Recknagel 2003
Jan.–Mar., 1991	100,000+ Iraqi military	U.N.-sanctioned military forces	Fisk 2005: 849; Pilger 2003: 18; Simpson 2003:1, 99, 200
Feb. 13, 1991	Up to 1,600 Iraqi civilians	U.S. military, Stealth plane bombs	Keeble 1997: 166; Simpson 2003
Feb.–Apr., 1991	30,000–180,000 Shia and Kurds	Iraqi military; possibly Iranian government	Barber & Epstein 2004; Bouckaert 2003; Burns 2006; Cordner 2005; McDowall 2000; Tripp 2007
1999	1,000 Shia in Najaf	Iraqi military	Cordner 2005
Mar. 2003–October 2008	88,000–96,000 noncombatants	Coalition military forces; other military and paramilitary	www.iraqbodycount.org

and/or genocide, others of war crimes, the so-called "collateral damage" of misdirected or errant missile attacks, political purges, intra- or international fighting. Experience from other countries has shown that the comprehensive and wide-scale interviewing of witnesses, prospection for graves, planned and controlled excavation of graves and exhumations and careful analysis of remains towards identification and cause of death determination is possible (e.g., see EAAF annual reports (http://eaaf.typepad.com/eaaf_reports/), Haglund 2002; Ramey Burns 1999).

Data Sources

Archaeological evidence suggests that Mesopotamia is the birthplace of written language. The 2,500-year literary history has resulted in reams of documents and related artifacts outlining significant (and also mundane) events in human history (Bahn 1999). This tradition of recording has continued through the modern era and has resulted in documents pertaining to events of the recent past, of particular interest here those authorizing and describing mass arrests, detentions, executions, and burials of victims of the Ba'ath Party regime under Saddam Hussein (Human Rights Watch 2004). In 1991, in the Kurdish area of Iraq alone, 18 tons of regime documents on prisoners and executions were seized following the first Gulf War (McIntosh 2002). This preliminary evidence brings hope to grave investigators, despite the claim by Stover and associates (2003: 664) and Human Rights Watch (2004) that the secrecy under which the Iraqi military and police operated means that some graves are simply undiscoverable. One must also remember that mass executions and burials are not discreet events and inevitable witnesses, confessing participants, satellite imagery and able archaeologists will all assist in the discovery and analysis of graves in Iraq.

Currently there is a broad array of different sources of information, mostly mass media or the United States and Iraqi government reports. The objectives of each of the organizations responsible and the filter through which much information must pass to reach the researcher and investigator require serious consideration. Likewise, much information gathered by governments and militaries in particular is simply unavailable. Despite both of us having worked in Iraq, there is much that is unknown as a result of the disorganized state of the country and authorities operating within. There is a very wide disparity in numbers of missing persons and deaths according to the source being cited, whether Human Rights Watch, Iraqi Special Tribunal judges, or others. For this reason, ranges and sources are cited and the reader must judge for themselves what they choose to believe. For those conducting formal investigations, it is our experience and it is foreseeable in the future that under the current administration of Iraq only information pertaining to crimes committed by the Ba'ath Party under Saddam Hussein will be available.

Operational Organization

Limited forensic and related work on mass graves in the country has already been conducted by various groups and in different ways. The security and political situation limits control, coordination, and enactment of any large-scale national program. Baraybar and associates (2007) cite the negative example of poorly planned exhumations and autopsies in Kosovo to accentuate the need for a centralized and coordinated approach to investigations in Iraq. Work conducted to date in Iraq, however, shows no sign of having accounted for such mistakes elsewhere.

Despite the disorganized state that may currently exist, the vast majority of mass graves in Iraq remain unexcavated. Most of the exceptions are graves that have been unprofessionally opened (Figure 36.1), and some of these have been well publicized in the mass media (Barber and Epstein 2004; Bouckaert 2003; Hunter and Cox 2005: 206; Recknagel 2003). For example, in January of 2004, Hess (2004) reported that:

> Eleven of the 271 suspected mass graves were exhumed by family members immediately after the war. . . . In Hillah, a scene of major atrocities against Shi'ites in 1991, the discovery of a mass grave containing at least 3,000 bodies kicked off nearly a week of digging and bone collecting by family members.

The patience of the people who have refrained from *ad hoc* exhumations and are waiting for "professional" excavations of graves is limited (Human Rights Watch 2004). The controlled and apolitical excavation and analysis of these graves and the remains within is a matter that can and should be addressed by those with appropriate education, training, and skills in archaeological excavation and biological/forensic anthropology. Greg Kehoe, an investigator for the Regime Crimes Liaison Office (RCLO), which has conducted controlled excavations of eight mass graves since late 2004, claimed that these excavations were hindered by

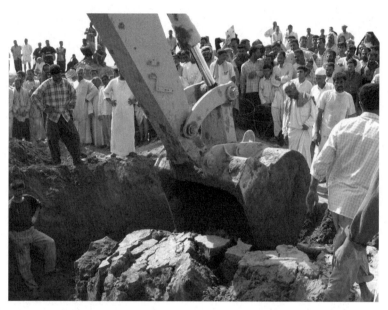

Figure 36.1   Iraqis opening a mass grave allegedly of Shia killed in 1991 (photograph Peter Bouckaert, © 2003 Peter Bouckaert/Human Rights Watch).

the failure of European experts to assist due to qualms over the possible use of the death penalty for those eventually convicted of crimes (BBC 2004a; Fairweather 2004). The main issue preventing their participation, however, is certainly the poor security situation (Figure 36.2) and it is questionable as to how serious the death penalty rates as a factor in whether or not international forensic specialists choose to participate. Nevertheless, Hunter and Cox (2005: 210) ask: "How acceptable is it, for example, for largely white middle-class, educated Westerners to 'parachute' into less-developed

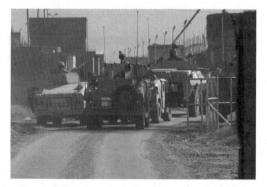

Figure 36.2   Security is the primary concern that must be resolved before any wide-scale investigation of mass graves in Iraq can occur. However, this has not improved since 2003 (photograph T. Bradshaw/ U.S. Army Corps/RCLO).

postconflict scenarios, investigate a crime to their ideal of justice, and then bail out leaving their garbage, in all its various forms, behind?"

Hunter and Cox are criticizing how operations have been conducted in the past in other countries and it is thus the methods and mandate- and not necessarily those performing the work- which is being questioned. They suggest that "in many contexts it is better to train and empower than to intervene and then walk away" (Margaret Cox, INFORCE, personal communication 2006).

Some have claimed that Iraq has no "forensic" archaeologists or anthropologists (Human Rights Watch 2004; Stover, Haglund, and Samuels 2003). This is difficult to judge as there are no universal national (or international) systems to qualify such expertise in *any* country. This stands in contradiction to the constant reference in related literature to "international standards" (e.g., Amnesty International 2004; BBC 2004a; Cordner and McKelvie 2002; Human Rights Watch 2003b; Skinner, Alempijevic, and Djuric-Srejic 2003).

The best qualified in Iraq may be those who participated in training courses with the International Forensic Centre of Excellence for the Investigation of Genocide (Inforce)[1] (see Figure 36.3, also Cox this volume) and the International Commission for Missing Persons, (ICMP).[2] Their participation in training programs involving real or simulated mass graves and their real-life experience in Iraq may make them better able to lead forensic investigations

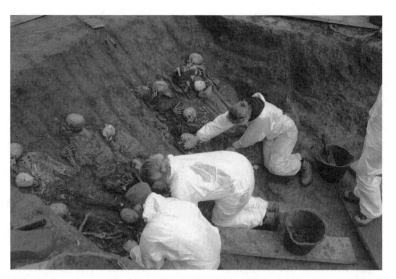

Figure 36.3   Inforce simulated mass grave with plastic teaching skeletons (photograph Inforce Foundation; used with permission by Inforce Foundation).

there than many experienced foreigners. Note that many practitioners from Western Europe or North America (including many authors in this volume) first became involved in forensic work by being "loaned" out from universities to police services without any prior education and training in forensic methods, objectives and protocols.

Developments Since 2003

Coalition Provisional Authority (CPA) Forensic Team

In June 2003, the Coalition Provisional Authority (CPA) took political control of Iraq and set about to investigate alleged mass graves. The pressure on coalition forces to protect grave sites for full forensic investigation and to prevent unregulated excavations and exhumations had to be carefully weighed against antagonizing a desperate population who had seized the moment to recover their relatives during this brief period of stability. This initial "rush to the graves" resulted in forensic evidence being destroyed, and many of the bodies claimed by families were most likely not those of the individual being sought. Many sets of remains were simply given a presumptive identification from clothing, identification documents or personal items found during these recoveries and some sets of remains were identified by such tenuous associations as the brand of cigarettes they smoked at the time of disappearance (experience of author [J.S.], Bouckaert 2003; Human Rights Watch 2004).

The objectives of the CPA forensic team included assisting in preserving forensic evidence at known grave sites, advising on procedures involved in locating grave sites, actually locating sites, and advising on a strategy for the future handling of evidence. This last aspect also involved graves that had already been disturbed. Other responsibilities included coordinating the ongoing investigation with other relevant parties; independent monitoring of the standards employed by national or international forensic teams when working within Iraq; assessment of the current Iraqi capacity to undertake forensic work and to assess the availability of training facilities within Iraq.

One major problem for the CPA was that there was no specialized equipment or identified forensic facilities suitable for use in support of the scientific investigation of mass graves. Capacity building would be one such issue that to date (September 2008), has yet to be adequately addressed.

Capacity-building involved the need to identify personnel who could be trained in forensic archaeology and anthropology in order to maintain high standards at all Iraqi-led "humanitarian exhumations" (that is, those that were *not* being conducted with a primary mandate of evidence collection for criminal trials). This involved supporting respective universities/institutes to build forensic modules into their programs. The CPA team also assessed existing forensic capacity at established professional medical institutes, (for example, the Medical Legal Institute (MLI) in Baghdad and regional mortuary facilities).

The work involved the identification of conventional archaeologists and anthropologists in Iraq, many of whom had experience with the recovery and analysis of human remains and newly graduated doctors from Medical Degree programs, where skeletal anatomy is a core subject. Although not forensic specialists *per se* it was felt that with training these people could form a core of expertise for future operations. Currently, pathologists in Iraq are under constant pressure to deal with recent cases as a result of ongoing armed conflict. Further, with only 12 pathologists throughout the country, pathology services are limited, particularly in areas such as the declaration of cause of death.

The CPA team was supported in site assessments by two satellite analysts, which helped with the positive identification of sites. Although it is believed that some aspects of satellite and aerial imagery analysis were used in Iraq prior to 1991, at present Iraq does not have the capacity to conduct its own satellite investigations.

Finally, forensic scientists capable of undertaking DNA work will be critical for establishing positive identifications. Theoretical aspects of DNA identification techniques are taught at Baghdad University, although there is currently no DNA analysis capability within Iraq. The only current possibility, then, is to have samples processed externally.

In the recent past, limited work concerning sites of atrocities had been undertaken by several NGOs including Human Rights Watch, Middle East Watch and Physicians for Human Rights (PHR). Information has since been built upon by numerous organizations and authorities, including the Human Rights Ministries in Baghdad, Basra, Erbil and Sulaimaniyah, the Anfal Organization in Sulaimaniyah, the Society for the Preservation of Mass Graves, the Free Prisoners Association, the U.S. Marine Expeditionary Force, the Criminal Investigations Division (CID) of the United States Army, and other international and local Human Rights organizations.

As a result of the multiple organizations at work, and the lack of centralization, the CPA had difficulty identifying and confirming the existence of the reported gravesites. Ongoing violence compounded this problem. The CPA forensic team therefore developed a simple database, (adapted from one developed by Ute Hoffmeister of ICMP in 2003), into which all relevant data, reports, images or site assessments could be input, including information for the comparison of antemortem and post-mortem data. Data inputting continued over an eight-month period.

Since the CPA team left Iraq in April 2004, uncontrolled excavations have continued, although as stated in Hunter and Cox (2005: 206), the frequency of these appears to have declined. Something to consider, however, is that information on these events is sparse, perhaps due to the fact that the "western" media is "embedded" with coalition forces and not in regular contact with Iraqis. The lack of Iraqi media infrastructure by which information can reach an international audience means that little about Iraqi group-led excavations becomes known outside of, or even within, Iraq. Most of the sites are not under the protection of military forces due simply to operational demands of a higher priority, such as general security, and it demonstrates how this one factor can affect all aspects of the recovery operation.

Initially, only a few incidents of atrocities were designated for detailed investigation and prosecution through the Iraqi Special Tribunal (IST) court, as determined in the CPA "Mass Grave Action Plan." A team from Denmark undertook the assessment of 20 sites across the country in a time span of nine weeks. A team from Finland undertook the first large-scale ground penetrating radar (GPR) survey of a reported site south of Baghdad. Inforce personnel also conducted geophysical surveys of graves.

Regime Crimes Liaison Office (RCLO)

In late 2003, the U.S. Government sought more physical forensic evidence for prosecution of the heads of the former regime that had been captured (approximately 22 individuals at this time). The Regime Crimes Liaison Office (RCLO) was formed and tasked with working with the CPA forensic team on the location and strategy for mass grave excavations. RCLO was charged with sampling several sites including one which had previously been partially exhumed by the United States Armed Forces Institute of Pathology (AFIP) (Sinje Stoyke, personal communication 2006[3]). In 2004, the reported RCLO budget was £55 million, or over $100 million U.S. (Fairweather 2004).

RCLO dealt primarily with evidence collection and did not specifically aim to establish the personal identification of recovered remains, although DNA samples were taken from all sets of remains exhumed. Any information was then passed on to the Iraqi Special Tribunal (IST), at that time not yet in place, and used to aid the court. By June 2005, RCLO had completed the excavation of two mass graves near Mosul, "al-Hatra" (BBC 2004a; Rubenstein 2005), and one in Muthanna

(Knickmeyer 2005; Rubenstein 2005). Rubenstein claimed that operations were "marked by the refinement of and improvement on earlier efforts conducted in Iraq and other places in Europe and Africa" (7). While a $US100 million budget inevitably facilitates a certain level of refinement, operations were, overall, on par with—although different from—many performed by ICTY in the former Yugoslavia. Between August 2004 and June 2006, RCLO had excavated six mass graves and exhumed and examined 335 sets of human remains (Daragahi 2006).

ICMP and Inforce

During 2003 and 2004, two different organizations, ICMP and Inforce, each directed teaching and training programs for Iraqi professionals with an aim of helping develop skills and knowledge towards the investigation of graves (Table 36.1). Inforce's training of 33 Iraqi professionals, (including 13 medics and six archaeologists) over 15 weeks took place in the United Kingdom and that by ICMP in Bosnia-Herzegovina, using simulated (Inforce) and real (ICMP) mass graves. One of the Inforce trainees has since gone on to lead a course in Iraq on pathology in anticipation of future work. In 2003, Inforce also seconded personnel who contributed to a CPA team and was involved in site assessments in 2003 (BBC 2004b).

Archaeologists for Human Rights (AFHR)

A German NGO, Archaeologists for Human Rights (AFHR), was founded in June 2003 by members who had archaeological experience in northern Iraq and elsewhere in the region. They deployed two archaeologists to Ainkawa, Erbil, in Northern Iraq to work with the local communities and the Kurdish Ministries in order to assist them in the recovery of remains. The group collaborated with government and other representatives including those of the United Nations Assistance Mission for Iraq (UNAMI), UN High Commission for Refugees (UNHCR) offices, the CPA and representatives of PHR and Human Rights Watch in Iraq. Coordination with South Korean Coalition Forces resulted in that country supplying excavation and mortuary equipment for the Ministry of Human Rights in Erbil. The equipment and supplies are being stored for future investigations.

One member of AFHR also took part in the excavations of the Regime Crime Liaison Office (RCLO) at al-Hatra between August-November 2004 as a representative for the Ministry of Human Rights in Erbil.

Looking to the Future

"Humanitarian" versus "Forensic" Excavations

What will be the focus of grave investigations in Iraq—humanitarian or evidentiary? Must these be distinguished? The Coalition Provisional Authority (CPA) has suggested that a limited number of sites have been selected for evidentiary examination, while the rest of the graves would be left to others, mainly Iraqi groups, for "humanitarian" investigation (Barber and Epstein 2004, U.N. 2004; U.S. Department of State 2003). This decision seems pragmatic—a way of protecting and examining only a limited number of graves and of allowing anxious and willing Iraqis to open up all the rest of the graves. The damage toward the so-called humanitarian mission of excavations by those untrained in technical methods, by those without osteological and archaeological knowledge, however, cannot be repaired. Commingling of remains and postmortem excavation fractures, the removal of commingled remains by families making presumed identifications (and the unreliability of those identifications) result in a situation in which proper identifications of these victims will almost surely never happen. Neither justice nor humanitarian aims are being served in this way.

Cordner (2005) also groups investigations into two types, which he labels "Justice" and "Humanitarian." This dichotomy is unnecessary, however, and there is no reason why both ends cannot be served at the same time. It is true that, legally speaking, genocide or war crimes may require only group identification (for example, ethnic group or civilian status), rather than individual, but even identification at the group level also serves the "humanitarian" needs of the origin community and families. Indeed, justice could be called a humanitarian need and is a Human Right. To divide mass grave excavations into two mutually exclusive groups suggests that the work can serve only one end, which is simply not true. Careful excavation, documentation, and analysis leading to identification of victims and the events that led up to their deaths and burials serve multiple purposes.

To a small degree, uncontrolled excavations serve the "humanitarian" aims of answering some questions about the fate of unidentified individuals, although information related to the timing and circumstances of their deaths is lost. Some resolution may come from the recovery of an identification document found in a grave, but if it has been separated from a set of remains, the ability to associate is gone. Is the discovery of identification papers in a grave enough to satisfy the grieving family of the death of that missing person? It would be significantly better if the sex of an associated body could be determined, if dental characteristics could be confirmed, or if clothing could be used to corroborate the suspicion that that person was killed and buried in that place. It would also be significantly better for the families if they could organize a proper burial for those remains with confidence that they actually belong to their family member and that they are complete. DNA identification would be ideal.

In many cases, it is reasonable to assume that the discovery of skulls with what appear to be gunshot trauma from a grave in this context means that the victims could all have been executed. Evidence of this type is likely to be generalized in an assumption that the remains in a grave all shared this fate. There is great danger, however, in generalizing, because bodies in a single mass grave may represent distinct events and types of victims. Perhaps some Iraqi soldiers refused to commit executions and were in turn killed and thrown in with the others. Distinctions between prisoners of war, enemy combatants, and innocent civilians can be made but may be missed without the appropriate analyses. Witnesses of executions may also become victims in the same grave. An innocent civilian, missing since the time of the execution of prisoners, may continue to be sought by family members after a declaration has been made stating that those in a grave are prisoners of war, based on limited evidence of, for example, three victims seen wearing military clothing. Although unprofessional excavations in Iraq clarify the existence of graves, there remains potential for misinterpretation about the complete contents of the graves and the circumstances surrounding the deaths of those interred.

Cultural Considerations

A significant challenge that must be recognized in Iraq is the very different social and cultural context from past projects in other countries. Religious concerns regarding treatment of the dead may affect the way work is conducted. Although there may be few differences between, for example, Shia and Sunni treatment of the dead (M. Yasin, personal communication 2006;[4] Gatrad 1994), there are certain considerations that range from "obligation" (*halal*) to "forbidden" (*haram*) (Jonker 1996). Understanding cultural and religious norms enables one to better interpret the context of the works being undertaken. The ability, for example, to distinguish different types of head garments (which may have different names according to each ethnic group) from blindfolds, or head garments *used as* blindfolds, is crucial in the interpretation of events. The idea that martyrs are buried in the clothing in which they died will be important in the assessment of criminal and clandestine burials. There is clearly a place for cultural anthropologists with knowledge of local practices.

Other considerations may involve the use of "cadaver" dogs. Such dogs are used with some regularity in missing person investigations, for mass disasters such as landslides and earthquakes, and have been used for the detection of single clandestine graves (e.g., Lasseter et al. 2003; Owsley 1995; Rebmann, Edward, and Sorg 2000: 2). They are also used to detect unexploded ordinance as has been done by the UN ICTY to search for booby traps around graves. Although in Islam dogs are considered "unclean," the *Hadith* (sayings of the prophet Mohammed) illustrate that human interaction with dogs is not strictly forbidden. As explained by one Imam (Yasin, personal communication 2006), there are two types of dogs: clean and unclean. The type considered "clean" is that which we train to help people (for example, seeing-eye or search and rescue dogs), and they may be viewed as acceptable in searches for bodies in clandestine graves. The investigator must understand these views and discuss them with those in an affected community that may have an interest in, and connection with, the victims. In light of prisoner abuse by U.S. forces, involving dogs, at the Abu Graib prison, one must also consider the possible reaction of locals if similar-looking dogs are used to find graves.

Perhaps the most contentious issue, although one that is notoriously quiet in the anthropological literature, is that of bone sampling of victims of known identity. The challenges of developing population-specific standards for anthropological aging are well-known. Although sample-taking and research deriving from known-age victims can be used to better age those in the future, there remains the inevitable question of the ethical rightness of doing so, with or without permission from the next of kin (Skinner, Alempijevic, and Djuric-Srejic 2003). Ethical standards exist within confined contexts such as universities or regional or national jurisdictions. Operating as part of an international team in a foreign country without such standards or related legislation, however, presents a number of unanswered questions that must be resolved before work proceeds.

Grave Sampling

Another issue to consider is the partial excavation of mass graves, as suggested by Skinner in 1987, whereby only a portion of a grave is excavated and possibly some (though probably not all) bodies exhumed (for example, "grave sampling"). The idea of such an undertaking does not necessarily suggest that it would only ever be partially excavated. As with conventional archaeology, sampling via partial excavation allows one to better understand what one is facing. It provides limited information to better judge what approach to take if full excavation were to be carried out. The experience of one of us (D.C.) suggests that some people do not want their relatives exhumed for further investigation and autopsy. With preliminary information gleaned from testing a grave, investigators can then proceed to seek the advice of the affected community as to how they wish to proceed.

Another type of sampling may be related to sites where there are multiple mass graves (for example, "site sampling"). It may be naïve to think that all the mass graves in Iraq will be excavated and all the victims found and identified, because of the resources required. It should be for the Iraqis and specific communities related to victims within Iraq to decide the extent to which excavations and exhumations should occur, and the idea of sampling graves—in the sense that only some will be excavated (for instance, those believed to be representative)—may provide a pragmatic, perhaps temporary, solution.

While sampling is commonplace in conventional archaeology, the forensic context introduces more serious ethical concerns. It is hard to imagine that families would be content with the exhumation of 10 of their community members from a grave of 1,000 victims, or of a single mass grave at a site with 10 mass graves. With the group or individual identification of the smaller sample, however, decisions can be made as when and how a grave will be approached. Certain communities may decide simply to erect a memorial in that place. Others may wish to pursue full excavation and exhumation.

There is a significant risk, however, in sampling graves or sites that may circumvent its use. Although in general, mass graves contain bodies, victims of genocide that belong to one particular ethnic or national group and of a single event, this is not necessarily so. Both of us, along with others (e.g., Wright, Hanson, and Sterenberg 2005), have participated in excavations where the nature of the evidence strongly suggested that bodies in graves arrived at different times, from different places, and events surrounding their deaths may have varied. These events may be both criminal and noncriminal, the victims of which are all in the same mass grave. Site and/or grave sampling could result in

incorrect premature conclusions that affect decisions to exhume or not. If members of one community are opposed to exhumation, their decision to leave a grave may affect the members of other communities whose members remain undiscovered in the same grave. The search for those members would then continue indefinitely on the false assumption that they must be elsewhere.

Who Will Lead?

One problem of mass-grave investigations from other countries as a model for Iraq, such as the former Yugoslavia, is the unlikely involvement of the United Nations if large-scale violence continues. Political and military/security capability of the U.N. are extremely limited in this context, and thus the challenge of protecting sites and personnel from armed aggression practically rules out their present participation.

A possible future scenario incorporates a multinational/multi-organizational effort, involving teams from different governments and NGOs under centralized Iraqi government coordination. The scale and the cost of potential operations mean that one organization alone will not be able to properly address the situation. Despite early inter-organizational cooperation in Iraq—such as the Inforce contribution to the CPA team and that of Archaeologists for Human Rights—such events have been isolated.

What is required to coordinate several groups, however, is a standard operating procedure and an oversight group that can monitor and instruct individual groups. A similar situation has been used in the former Yugoslavia with U.N. monitors, advising and assisting national teams. A national system of monitors would help ensure consistent standards and coordination of information as well as enable other groups and countries to assist with the burden of resources. Given current political instability in Iraq, an organization such as International Commission of the Red Cross (ICRC) could play a role. The ICRC have experience in conflict and postconflict countries and a general trust-position with governments, and their current program, "The Missing," could be used as a platform for the launch of a mass-grave investigation coordination system. Until now, however, ICRC's Missing program has generally not conducted grave excavations, exhumations, and autopsies (Tidball-Binz 2006).

The suggestion made by Cordner (2005) and by ICRC (Human Rights Watch 2004) of local community-led exhumations is certainly an option for Iraq, but we must keep in mind that many mass graves are located in remote areas. Furthermore, because many victims were transported to other parts of the country before being executed and buried, local communities may not be interested in investing their resources in recovering the dead of other groups. Indeed, this situation could affect the integrity of such investigations, given mounting ethnic rivalries.

There has been great reservation in the anthropological community about participating in any sort of work in Iraq in light of the fact that many consider the war, invasion, and occupation to have been illegal and immoral (Concerned Anthropologists, http://concerned.anthropologists. googlepages.com/). For this reason, practitioners may consider that work in Iraq may be acceptable, but working for foreign or even Iraqi governments is unacceptable. The idea that forensic practitioners (and forensic archaeologists specifically) can take the initiative in proposing and leading investigations (that is, be *proactive*, rather than *reactive*) has been suggested by Blau and Skinner (2005). This action could easily be foreseen as coming into conflict (although not necessarily) with the advice given by Hunter and Cox (2005: 217) when they suggest that one should "refrain from working with non-police or other formal investigative agencies." This advice is diluted by their later statement, true though it may be, that "justice means different things to different peoples: the meaning of justice varies culturally, and can be multi-faceted and complex" (Hunter and Cox 2005: 207). Given the current political instability and uncertainty in Iraq, the large presence of foreign military powers and the institution of a judiciary funded and actively "advised" by a foreign power, then, one must wonder what qualifies as an Iraqi formal investigative agency.

In other countries, such as Argentina, Guatemala, Colombia, and Kosovo, the perpetrators of crimes have included the military and members of active and continuing governments. Thus, exhumations have been led by nongovernment organizations (NGOs) despite disinterest or actual opposition of formal investigative bodies. With time, and change of government, the information gathered by these groups has been used for trials against the perpetrators of crimes and continued to serve the humanitarian need of the families of the missing, arguably a responsibility of the state (Castiglione 2004: 133, 134).

For whom one works or with which objectives are issues that have been raised about work in Iraq. It is very possible that a funding organization would provide resources for the exhumations of only one ethnic group. Is the exhumation of some victims better than none? In Kosovo, after NATO entry, access to ethnic Serb witnesses of crimes, many of whom had fled as refugees to Serbia, was limited, meaning that much more information was available on other victims, thus affecting which crimes were investigated and which bodies exhumed. The deliberate focus on only certain groups in Iraq would clearly exacerbate ethnic tensions (unless specific groups deliberately chose not to support exhumations of *their own* people) and therefore would be unacceptable.

There are, of course, many other social and ethical issues that warrant discussion. Given the limitations of this work, they will be addressed only in brief with the hope that they will initiate further discussion. Although the comments of RCLO investigator Kehoe about Europeans not participating in forensic work out of fear of the death penalty were generally dismissed previously, there may be some truth to them. Some may claim that a forensic scientist has no right to judge the sentencing process and should merely stick to his or her job. Inevitably, however, we are not only scientists and may have competing concerns based on the multiple identities of each practitioner. It is not difficult to foresee that those concerned with human rights may also be strongly opposed to the death penalty in some or all circumstances.

The level of participation in projects is also an issue to be decided. If one is told that she may simply observe exhumations, does she then give implicit approval to the process, regardless of how it is managed and performed? By posting coalition soldiers at the graveside of uncontrolled excavations in 2003, or by providing the locals with water, shelter, and shovels, are the military authorities implying that the work is being done to an acceptable level? If advice on how to excavate more carefully is given and ignored, should the advisor leave in protest (see also Skinner, Alempijevic, and Djuric-Srejic 2003)?

The consequences of not engaging and sharing experience and knowledge is that the grave-excavation process may be taken up and performed by those *completely* unqualified to do it. This situation has been seen in other countries, where people who had no experience or training in archaeology, anthropology, or pathology were leading mass-grave excavations and exhumations, not taking notes and not making any records of the process. Given the early stages of mass-grave work in Iraq, this problem can be avoided by continuing to engage Iraqi professionals with related experience and pressuring governments to support the work.

Conclusion

Three major challenges face those investigating graves of missing persons and alleged atrocity crimes in Iraq: the variety of contexts of crimes, the lack of organized and available information on victims and killings, and the disorganized and disabled approach employed to date to investigate. Although a very small proportion of mass burials have been excavated in Iraq in recent years, it has been done by different local community and nongovernmental groups and also U.S.-sponsored groups, each with different objectives and employing different methodologies (including *ad hockery*) with varying results and little or no communication or coordination among them. The number of victims from recent decades is in the hundreds of thousands, and their bodies surely lie in thousands of unmarked graves throughout the country.

Currently, because of the security situation, excavations appear to be possible only in the Kurdish-controlled north. The Regime Crimes Liaison Office appears to have ceased U.S.-government-sponsored excavations. It is possible that local Iraqi groups are active, but there is no evidence in the Western press or literature of this. With increasing awareness of the contribution of archaeologists and anthropologists to grave investigations greater interest by Iraqi and other governmental and nongovernmental organizations is likely but feasible only on any significant scale once improved security has been established across the country.

There are many broader challenges that face the development and employment of forensic archaeology and anthropology in Iraq and elsewhere, some of which we have addressed here. We believe that this volume is a major event toward this development and will act as a catalyst for further thought, discussion, and service.

In the 1980s in Latin America and the 1990s elsewhere, we saw *Forensic Generation One*: students who went straight into forensic archaeology and anthropology as a career after graduating. Despite decades of experience and development of these forensic disciplines, we still lack standard protocols, professional organization, and accreditation systems. In many countries, other more traditional forensic or police practitioners still play the role of archaeologist or anthropologist at the crime scene and in the lab. The tremendous interest and experience of conventional archaeology and anthropology in Iraq, indigenous and from abroad, means that the transition to a forensic context can be easily foreseen. For the purposes of accurate historical records, criminal investigations, and identification and repatriation of victims, the central organization of this forensic context is a significant, primary task.

Lessons from work in other countries in many ways enable us to learn from mistakes and build on successes. Given past neglect of these types of investigations in the region, it is a new context that warrants special treatment and not a simple transference of a system from another country. Engagement with the Iraqi population toward methodologically sound investigations is the only proper way to proceed. Working in association with Iraqis, learning from them, and teaching what some of us have learned in our experience elsewhere are the only practical ways of achieving any measure of success in the enormous challenge of investigating modern, unmarked graves in Iraq.

Acknowledgments

D.C. gives particular thanks to the other authors of this long-awaited book. The majority have taught and inspired him either as formal teachers or as exemplary colleagues. He also wishes to thank Sarah Karmi for her thoughtful comments.

Notes

1. International Forensic Centre of Excellence for the Investigation of Genocide, a U.K.-based charity.

2. An international organization based in Sarajevo, Bosnia-Herzegovina, operating largely in the former Yugoslavia.

3. This information and that related to Archaeologists for Human Rights, below, was provided by Sinje Stoyke, formerly of AFHR and later Programme Co-ordinator, Iraq with ICMP, with a contribution from Ursula Janssen, founding member of AFHR.

4. Majid Yasin, Imam, Bournemouth Islamic Centre, personal interview May 3, 2006.

References

Amin, R. 1994. Plight of the Kurdish people. Letters; *British Medical Journal* 309: 875–876.

AP (Associated Press). 2005a. Excavators find mass grave in Iraq, Sunday, April 17, www.foxnews.com/story/0,2933,153676,00.html (accessed 29/05/06).

———. 2005b. Mass grave in Karbala thought to date from '91. *Stars and Stripes* 3(261) December 28: 3.

Bahn, P. G. (ed.) 1999. *Cambridge Illustrated History of Archaeology.* Cambridge: Cambridge University Press.

Baraybar, J. P., Brasey, V., and Zadel, A. 2007. The need for a centralized and humanitarian-based approach to missing persons in Iraq: An example from Kosovo. *International Journal of Human Rights*: 11(3): 265–274.

Barber, B., and Epstein, S. 2004. *Iraq's Legacy of Terror; Mass Graves.* U.S. Agency for International Development (USAID), www.cpa-iraq.org/human_rights/iraq_mass_graves.pdf (accessed 14/08/06).

BBC. 2004a. *Babies Found in Mass Grave*, http://news.bbc.co.uk/go/pr/fr/-/2/hi/middle_east/3738368.stm. Published 13 October (accessed 14/08/06).

———. 2004b. *Archaeologists Play Key Role in Iraq*, http://news.bbc.co.uk/1/hi/world/middle_east/3378931.stm. Last updated Thursday, 8 January. (accessed 14/08/06).

Blau, S., and Skinner, M 2005. The use of forensic archaeology in the investigation of human rights abuse: Unearthing the past in East Timor. *The International Journal of Human Rights* 9(4): 449–463.

Bouckaert, P. 2003. *The Mass Graves of al-Mahawil: The Truth Uncovered.* Human Rights Watch report, 15(5)(E), May 2003. http://hrw.org/reports/2003/iraq0503/ (accessed 14/08/06).

Burns, J. F. 2006. Uncovering Iraq's horrors in desert graves. *New York Times*, June 5, www.nytimes.com/2006/06/05/world/middleeast/05grave.html?ex=1307160000&en=f61682fbc3536b01&ei=5088&partner=rssnyt&emc=rss (accessed 08/09/06).

Castiglione, S. 2004. Legal aspects, in *Management of Dead Bodies in Disaster Situations*, Disaster Manuals and Guidelines Series, No. 5, pp. 129–147. Washington, D.C.: Pan-American Health Organization.

Cerkez-Robinson, A. 2007. 131 bodies exhumed from Bosnian grave. *USA Today*, July 27, www.usatoday.com/news/topstories/2007-07-27-3941419480_x.htm (accessed 17/10/07).

Cordner, S. 2005. The Missing: Action to resolve the problem of those unaccounted for as a result of armed conflict or internal violence, and to assist their families. *VIFM Review* 3(1): 2–6.

CNN. 2005. *Experts Combing through Mass Grave in Iraq*, Saturday, April 30, www.cnn.com /2005/WORLD/meast/04/30/iraq.main/ (accessed 14/08/06).

———. 2006. Bush: "I'm the decider" on Rumsfeld, Tuesday, April 18, www.cnn.com/2006/POLITICS/04/18/rumsfeld/ (accessed 26/04/08).

Daragahi, B. 2006. Victims in mass graves hid clues in clothing. *Los Angeles Times*, June 27, www.borzou.com/stories/2006/20060627.mht (accessed 08/09/06).

EAAF (Equipo Argentino de Antropologia Forense, [Argentinean Forensic Anthropology Team]) annual reports, http://eaaf.typepad.com/eaaf_reports/ (accessed 14/08/06).

Fairweather, J. 2004. *Lack of EU support "is hindering pace of inquiry,"* www.telegraph.co.uk/news/main.jhtml?xml=/news/2004/10/14/wirq314.xml&sSheet=/news/2004/10/14/ixnewstop.html, Telegraph Group Limited (accessed 4/08/06).

Fisk, R. 2005. *The Great War for Civilisation: The Conquest of the Middle East.* London: Fourth Estate.

Gatrad, A. R. 1994. Muslim customs surrounding death, bereavement, postmortem examinations, and organ transplants. *British Medical Journal* 309: 521–523.

Haglund, W. D. 2002. Recent mass graves: An introduction, in W. D. Haglund and M. H. Sorg (eds.), *Advances in Forensic Taphonomy: Method, Theory, and Archaeological Perspectives*, pp. 243–261. Boca Raton, FL: CRC Press.

Hess, P. 2004. Evidence to be unearthed from mass graves. *The Washington Times*, January 7, www.house.gov./hasc/issues/Hussein/04-01-07washtimes.htm (accessed 14/08/06).

Hiel, B. 2003. Iraqis train for gruesome task. *Tribune-Review*, Tuesday, December 16, 2003, www.pittsburgh live.com/x/tribune-review/specialreports/iraqgraves/s_170172.html (accessed 14/08/06).

Human Rights Watch. 2003. Iraq: US unresponsive on mass graves. *Human Rights News,* http://hrw.org/english/docs/2003/05/14/iraq6046.htm (accessed 14/08/06).

———. 2004. Iraq: State of the evidence. *Human Rights Watch report* 16(7).

Hunter, J., and Cox, M. 2005. *Forensic Archaeology: Advances in Theory and Practice.* London: Routledge.

Jonker, G. 1996. The knife's edge: Muslim burial in the diaspora. *Mortality* 1(1): 27–44.

Keeble, R. 1997. *Secret State, Silent Press.* Bedfordshire: John Libbey Media.

Knickmeyer, H. 2005. 113 Kurds are found in mass gave. *Washington Post*, April 30: A09.

Lasseter, A. E., Jacobi, K. P., Farley, R., and Hensel, L. 2003. Cadaver dog and handler team capabilities in the recovery of buried human remains in the Southeastern United States. *Journal of Forensic Sciences* 48(3): 1–5.

McDowall, D. 2000. *A Modern History of the Kurds.* New York: I. B. Tauris and Co. Ltd.

McMahon, R. 2004. *Iraq: Who Is Buried in Hussein's Mass Graves?* (Part 2). Radio Free Europe, www.rferl.org/features/2003/07/07072003165402.asp (accessed 14/08/06).

Middle East Watch Report. 1993. *Genocide in Iraq; The Anfal Campaign against the Kurds.* New York: Human Rights Watch.

News24. 2006. 1000 bodies found in Iraq. *News 24,* South Africa, June 4, 2006, www.news24.com/News24/World/Iraq/0,,2-10-1460_1912229,00.html (accessed 14/08/06).

Owsley, D. W. 1995. Techniques for locating burials, with emphasis on the probe. *Journal of Forensic Sciences* 40(5): 735–740.

Pilger, J. 2003. The lies of old, in D. Miller (ed.), *Tell Me Lies*, pp. 18–22. London: Pluto Press.

Ramey Burns, K. 1999. *Forensic Anthropology Training Manual.* Upper Saddle River, NJ: Prentice Hall.

Rebmann, A., Edward, D., and Sorg, M. H. 2000. *Cadaver Dog Handbook.* Boca Raton, FL: CRC Press.

Recknagel, C. 2003. *Iraqis Open Saddam Hussein's Mass Graves, Demand Justice* (Part 1). Radio Free Europe, July 7, www.rferl.org/features/2003/07/07072003163318.asp (accessed 14/08/06).

———. 2006. *Iraq: Kurds Collect Evidence for More Cases against Hussein.* Radio Free Europe/Radio Liberty, January 24, www.rferl.org/featuresarticle/2006/01/a5bf8e58-f53e-4143-83c6-dd20fe7c1a53.html (accessed 14/08/06).

Rosenfeld, N. 1991. Buried alive. *Lies of our Times,* October: 12–13.

Rubenstein, P. 2005. The Iraq mass graves team: USACE leads a team of scientists to learn the truth about the killing fields of Iraq. *Planning Ahead,* June 8(6), U.S. Army Corps of Engineers.

Simpson, J. 2003. *The Wars against Saddam; Taking the Hard Road to Baghdad.* London: Macmillan.

Skinner, M. 1987. Planning the archaeological recovery of evidence from recent mass graves. *Forensic Science International* 34: 267–287.

Skinner, M., Alempijevic, D., and Djuric-Srejic, M. 2003. Guidelines for international forensic bio-archaeology monitors of mass grave exhumations. *Forensic Science International* 134: 81–92.

Sprague, R. 2005. *Burial Terminology: A Guide for Researchers.* Walnut Creek, CA: AltaMira.

Stover, E., Haglund, W. D., and Samuels, M. 2003. Exhumation of mass graves in Iraq; Considerations for forensic investigations, humanitarian needs, and the demands of justice. *Journal of the American Medical Association* 290(5): 663–666.

Straziuso, J. 2005. *Iraq Remains Thought to Be from 1991 Grave.* ABC News International, http://abcnews.go.com/International/wireStory?id=1445699&page=1 (accessed 24/05/06).

The Seattle Times. 2003. *The History of Iraq.* http://seattletimes.nwsource.com/news/nation-world/usiraq/timeline/03.html (accessed 14/08/06).

Tidball-Binz, M. 2006. Forensic investigations into the missing: Recommendations and operational best practices, in A. Schmitt, E. Cunha, and J. Pinheiro (eds.), *Forensic Anthropology and Medicine: Complementary Sciences from Recovery to Cause of Death,* pp. 383–407. Totowa, NJ: Humana Press Inc.

Tripp, C. 2007. *A History of Iraq.* Cambridge: Cambridge University Press.

United Nations (U.N.). 2004. *Iraq: Focus on Mass Graves.* United Nations Office for the Coordination of Humanitarian Affairs, OCHA. Integrated Regional Information Network (IRIN), 7 January, http://iys.cidi.org/humanitarian/hsr/iraq/04a/ixl7.html (accessed 26/05/06).

UNSC1, United Nations Security Council Report. 2005. *Twentieth Report of the Secretary General Pursuant to Paragraph 14 of Resolution 1284 (1999),* 8 August, S/2005/513.

UNSC2, United Nations Security Council Report. 2005. *Twenty-First Report of the Secretary General Pursuant to Paragraph 14 of Resolution 1284 (1999),* 8 December 2005, S/2005/769.

U.S. Department of State. 2003. Mass graves in Iraq: Uncovering past atrocities. Publication Number 11106. *Bureau of Democracy, Human Rights and Labor with the Bureau of Public Affairs.* Washington, D.C.: December 19, www.state.gov/g/drl/rls/27000.html (accessed 26/05/06).

Wright, R., Hanson, I., and Sterenberg, J. 2005. The archaeology of mass graves, in J. Hunter and M. Cox, M. (eds.), *Forensic Archaeology: Advances in Theory and Practice,* pp. 137–158. London: Routledge.

FIVE

THE PROFESSIONAL
FORENSIC ANTHROPOLOGIST

MORE THAN JUST BARE BONES: ETHICAL CONSIDERATIONS FOR FORENSIC ANTHROPOLOGISTS

Soren Blau

Forensic anthropology is the field of study concerned with the identification of suspected or known human remains from medico-legal contexts. Traditionally, forensic anthropologists dealt with dry, complete, and fragmentary skeletal remains, but they now commonly work with fleshed, decomposed, burnt, and dismembered remains. In addition, forensic anthropologists assist in answering questions of identification in clinical cases, such as those related to the age of an individual, and investigations involving missing persons and victims of crimes, accidents, mass disasters, and war crimes. Because of the emotive nature of the material that forensic anthropologists work with and the diversity of contexts in which they may work, the ethical issues practitioners have to consider span social, cultural, and political realms. The aim of this chapter is to consider a number of ethical issues a forensic anthropologist may face, and, in doing so, it seeks to raise questions rather than provide answers about the plethora of ethical matters that should and do concern the practice of forensic anthropology.

Following a brief discussion of the nature of ethics, this chapter examines why ethics are important for the practice of forensic anthropology with particular reference to training, accreditation, the development of anthropological techniques, limitations of evidence, and research. Finally, individual versus professional ethical questions are considered.

What Is Ethics, and Why Is It Important?

Ethics is defined as a body of principles or standards of human conduct that govern the behaviour of individuals and groups (Bottorff 2005). Most professions adhere to an agreed code of conduct, commonly referred to as a "code of ethics," with the intention that all practitioners should strive toward principles of "good practice." In addition to rules of conduct, ethics is seen as "the science of morals, that branch of philosophy which is concerned with human character" (*Chambers English Dictionary* 1990: 490). Ethical considerations therefore apply to the profession *and* to the individual (Hunter and Cox 2005; Sapir 2001).

In the 18th century, the philosopher Kant argued that system-wide consistency was a logical requirement of ethics. He stated that ethics begins with the rejection of non-universal principles and that any adopted ethical principle must be a desirable universal law applied by everybody (Urmson and Rée 1991). However, the nature of an ethical dilemma stems from what has more recently been acknowledged as part of the "postmodern condition"—namely, that there is not one correct way to engage with the world. We are conditioned by our environment and culture, and therefore we are socialised as to what actions and behaviour are "reasonable" and / or "appropriate."

Ethics generally is deemed important essentially because there are multiple value systems. Different cultures, societies, and groups have different value systems—their own definitions of what is considered right and wrong (*appropriate*) (Walker 2000: 20; White 2000: 319). This fact is clearly borne out by peoples' differing attitudes to death, the deceased, and human skeletal remains. For example, in some Western countries, physical contact with the dead is rejected, and events surrounding death and dying are often suppressed (e.g., Blaauw and Lahteenmaki 2002: 772). In contrast, in some Muslim societies, there is close contact with the body of the deceased, which must be washed by a family member prior to burial. While some cultures actively and openly display human remains, as in the case of the All Saints Cemetery Chapel in the Czech Republic, other cultures—for example, some Indigenous Australian and Maori communities—are highly offended by the display of their ancestors (for further discussion on the different values placed on human skeletal remains see Hubert 1992: 117–118; Walker 2000: 12–18).

Sociocultural attitudes toward the dead should have an impact on the conduct of practitioners dealing with the deceased. Although the living body is usually regarded as a person, some have argued that after death the body becomes merely an object (e.g., McEvoy and Conway 2004: 540). In the forensic context, the body (object) is regarded at one level as empirically unchallengeable evidence.[1] This is perhaps more the case when one is dealing with human skeletal remains. Attitudes toward the human body, death and dying in the contemporary world were anecdotally surveyed for students undertaking a Master of Science degree in forensic and biological anthropology in Bournemouth University (U.K.). Only half of the cohort (*n* = 16) who had excavated human skeletal remains identified with them as once having been a living person (see also McEvoy and Conway 2004: 540). Such views, however, contradict the fundamental ethical principle for modern research in the biomedical and social sciences: respect for human dignity based on "the belief that it is unacceptable to treat remains solely as . . . objects or things" (Walker 2000: 20).

Death is biological; however, it is also an inherently social process (McEvoy and Conway 2004: 541; Prior 1989: 13), particularly given the "premise that human rights continue at death" (Vizenor 1996: 653). It is the dichotomy between human remains as utilitarian objects of scientific interest and human remains important for their cultural, symbolic, and spiritual value that raises many ethical questions for the forensic anthropologist.

Ethics and Forensic Anthropology

Ethics is fundamentally about behaviour. To obtain general guidance on how to *behave* in a professional setting, most practitioners have a code of conduct or a code of ethics provided by their profession. In the case of forensic anthropology, however, there are relatively few national and international associations with formal codes of ethics. Relatively recent exceptions include the American Board of Forensic Anthropology (ABFA) and, in the U.K., foundations such as the International Forensic Centre of Excellence for the Investigation of Genocide (INFORCE) (Hunter and Cox 2005: 217). Such codes provide relatively broad guidance about behaviour with little attention given to the specifics of practice.

The practice of forensic anthropology includes a range of analyses that may include determining whether the material is actually osseous, the bone is human or nonhuman, and the human bone is of forensic significance. Analyses may also include describing the condition and the preservation of skeletal remains; developing an inventory of recovered remains; determining the ancestry, sex, age, and stature of the individual; and describing any individualising characteristics or pathological and/or traumatic injuries. Each of these specific practices, including the formation of the final report, has associated ethical considerations. If we take, for example, the analysis of trauma to the skeleton, how far is it appropriate for the practitioner to go to describe the trauma? In the case of a 35-year-old female homicide victim who exhibited extreme perimortem soft-tissue trauma to the head and neck, how much more information will be gained from decapitating the head, macerating and cleaning the remains (e.g., Marks, Hudson, and Elkins 1999: 263)? Is it necessary to have a code of practice that stipulates the extent to which the practitioner can be invasive, or "is it just better to let the . . . anthropologist work to their conscience on the principle of 'best practice'" (Hunter and Cox 2005: 220)?

Obviously, it is important for forensic anthropologists to understand the appropriate conduct at a scene of crime (for example, their relationship with the pathologist and their position in the investigative structure); however, forensic anthropologists also have an ethical responsibility to understand relevant legislation and how this relates to domestic casework. Cases may, for example, involve attending scenes where the recovered skeletal remains turn out to be non-human or archaeological but are obviously part of an assemblage of historic interest. Despite the fact that such cases are of no forensic significance, does the forensic anthropologist have an ethical responsibility to be aware of the legislation covering Indigenous remains or historic sites?

A further role of the forensic anthropologist is to determine the forensic significance of any recovered human remains. If the skeletal remains are determined to be archaeological *and* of no forensic significance, does the forensic anthropologist have the ethical responsibility to provide further information about the remains? It has been argued that "due dignity and respect should be afforded in the recovery, storage, investigation and reburial of human remains regardless of their context" (Hunter et al. 2001: 176).

Much has been written about the politics associated with Indigenous human remains (e.g., Cantwell 2000; Hubert 1992; Jones and Harris 1998; McEvoy and Conway 2004: 542–547; Pardoe 1992; Vizenor 1996; White 2000: 323–326). Fundamentally, it is important to appreciate that the results of an ancestry determination may have serious political, social, and ultimately economic implications (Cantwell 2000: 92). Such implications perhaps support the proposal that training for forensic anthropologists should remain under the four-field approach, which incorporates the importance of being both scientifically competent in addition to culturally and politically sensitive (ibid.: 99) (see below for discussion on international work).

Typically, in countries with a colonial history, it is vital that forensic anthropologists are aware of the potential social and political concerns and debates surrounding Indigenous remains. In addition, practitioners must know the appropriate agencies with which to liaise. In Australia, for example, forensic anthropologists make a concerted effort to reinforce a rapport between State Coroners and Aboriginal Affairs Offices. This can be done by contacting the relevant agencies when skeletal remains of suspected Indigenous origin are discovered, and by contributing to training courses for heritage officers.

Training

Training in forensic anthropology has traditionally been associated with education in archaeology. Given that forensic anthropology is no longer merely dealing with skeletal material, there has been increasing discussion about the

appropriateness of viewing anthropology/archaeology as simply the transference of anthropological/archaeological principles and methods to the crime scene. In the late 1980s and early 1990s in the U.K., for example, nothing was published on the legal framework of forensic archaeology and anthropology. There was no educational provision to inform anthropologists/archaeologists of the requirements of the subject (Cox 1998: 22). As a result, there are some anthropologist/archaeologists who are self-appointed experts, who inappropriately call themselves "forensic anthropologists" or "forensic archaeologists." The implications of individuals labelling themselves as forensic experts without the appropriate training and qualifications have been highlighted (Cox 1998; 2001; Hunter and Cox 2005). The standard of training in forensic anthropology is critical to ethical practice.

The quality of training in forensic anthropology is of concern, because both forensic anthropology and archaeology have been affected by the increase in fascination for anything "forensic" (e.g., Fraser 2003; Thompson 2003). This situation has resulted in institutions appending the term *forensic* to courses merely to increase student numbers, with little concern for the detail of the course content. Many courses offer a cursory introduction to the principles of forensic anthropology/archaeology, but few of them provide an in-depth education in both practical skills as well as the legal and moral responsibilities and serious implications of the work (Cox 2001; Hunter 2002; Hunter et al. 2001; Thompson 2001).

In the case of forensic anthropology in the U.K., there is emerging debate about the need for practitioners of forensic anthropology to obtain training in medical schools (anatomy departments) rather than from Arts faculties (archaeology departments) (Professor Sue Black, University of Dundee, personal communication 2006). In contrast, attitudes toward training in forensic anthropology in the U.S. tend to advocate training with an Arts background, because it provides the relevant broad social and technical skills to undertake ethical practice (see Ubelaker this volume).

Given the range of attitudes toward the dead in contemporary societies (e.g., Adams 2000; Baudrillard 1993: 181–182; Richardson 1987; Walker 2000: 5), such debates are associated with discussions about how students of forensic anthropology are appropriately prepared for exactly what it is they will be dealing with: it is far more that just the "bare bones." Whatever training one chooses to undertake, forensic anthropologists (and archaeologists) have the professional and therefore ethical responsibility to be, and remain, competent. The nature of how this competence is assessed relates to issues of accreditation and standards.

Accreditation

A wide range of courses is offered in forensic anthropology across the world, which has resulted in a broad variation of expert credentials. The potential impact on the courts of this variable expert credibility has resulted in calls for accreditation. Acceptance and implementation of accreditation for forensic anthropologists vary, not surprisingly, among countries and according to the extent to which the discipline is established. For example, the American Board of Forensic Anthropology (ABFA) offered certification to American forensic anthropologists as early as 1977 (Reichs 1998: 14–15).

Although there is no association of forensic anthropologists in the U.K., the Council for the Registration of Forensic Practitioners (CRFP) has provided forensic anthropologists with the opportunity of obtaining formal accreditation (Black 2003). At present, there are eight registered forensic anthropologists in the U.K. (Professor Sue Black, University of Dundee, personal communication 2006; see also Cox this volume).

With the increasing recognition in Australia of the role forensic anthropology can play in the identification process, issues of accreditation have begun to be addressed. A symposium on standards and accreditation involving Australian forensic anthropologists (and forensic entomologists and forensic odontologists) was held at the Centre for Human Identification (Victorian Institute of Forensic Medicine) in December 2006. Practitioners identified the need for minimum standards for forensic practitioners. However, as was, and to some to extent continues to be, the case in the U.K., Australian forensic anthropologists may well face a situation in which formal registers are deemed by some to create a "closed shop." Such concerns are not, of course, restricted to the discipline of forensic anthropology (Beloff 2003: 15).

Reference Collections and Forensic Anthropological Techniques

The accuracy and precision of the forensic anthropologist in identifying an unknown individual from their skeletal remains or providing an age assessment of a living person depends not only on the preservation of the remains but also on the techniques employed. Forensic anthropologists have an ethical responsibility to consider the reliability and acceptability of techniques being employed.

The majority of techniques used by forensic anthropologists today were developed using descriptions and measurements collected either from archaeological collections where age and sex were unknown (e.g., Molleson and Cox 1993) or from anatomical samples (e.g., The Huntington, Terry and Hamann-Todd Collections) where independent records of these biological attributes exist (Hunt and Albanese 2005). While these reference collections have been invaluable for both forensic and archaeological research, it is now widely recognised that there are problems with the standards developed from these collections.

In the case of archaeological collections, the majority of demographic data are inferred rather than independently known. Many modern reference collections exhibit socio-economic and genetic biases that may affect biological trends. Many reference collections were small, some had skewed age distributions, disproportionate representation of the sexes and ancestry, and some were subject to the specific removal of biological outliers (Cox 2000: 63; Ubelaker 2000: 51–51). In addition, accurate recording of biological information was not always undertaken. In the case of the Hammon-Todd Collection, for example, there was doubt about the reliability of the documented ages for the skeletons. In some cases, ages were estimated by anatomists on the basis of the external appearance of the cadaver rather than on known age. Also, to date, studies that have compared dental age with skeletal age have been based on small archaeological samples of known chronological age (Bowman, MacLaughlin, and Scheuer 1992).

Some of the factors affecting human growth and health (including diet and medical intervention) have changed since the collection of data in the early 20th century, and it is now recognised that many aspects of skeletal morphology have markedly changed over the past century and a half. With the recognition that existing standards are becoming outdated, research is increasingly being undertaken to provide contemporary population-specific data in order to develop relevant reference standards (e.g., in South America: Frutos 2002, 2005; South Africa: Patriquin, Loth, and Steyn 2003; Steyn and İşcan 1997). It is no longer appropriate to say that "it is only something in the anthropologist's experience that tells him [sic] there is an undefinable something about the skeleton that suggests one race over another" (Stewart 1979: 231). As outlined in the Daubert Guidelines (see Ross and Kimmerle this volume), it is imperative that techniques are readily accepted and employed with known error rates, empirically tested, and subjected to review (Rogers and Allard 2002; White 2000: 322).

Limitations of Evidence

Even if appropriate standards exist, the forensic anthropologist has an ethical responsibility to differentiate between objective observations and subjective interpretations (Lucas 1989: 724) and to know the limitations of the evidence they are dealing with. If findings cannot be supported and justified, should they be included in a report? Can, for example, cause of death be attributed to drowning as a result of examination of human skeletal remains alone (e.g., Cantwell 2000: 85)?

Another poignant example of conclusions going far beyond the physical evidence is provided by White (2000: 321). The case involved the analysis of some 50,000 pieces of bone resulting from the death of 13 American men in plane shot down over Laos in 1987. From an analysis of the bone fragments, most of which had a maximum dimension of 1 cm (with the largest being 13 cm) long, it was announced that positive identification had been made and that all 13 men were accounted for. The remains were returned to the families for burial, but when the relatives questioned the issue of identification resulting in an independent investigation of the skeletal remains it became clear that the conclusions about age, sex, and ancestry and individualisation went far beyond the actual evidence (Getlin quoted in White 2000: 321).

Research

To qualify for accreditation, practitioners must demonstrate a certain level of education, training, and professional contribution (Mario 2002: 104). One way to contribute to the profession is by undertaking research and publication. However, forensic anthropologists have an ethical responsibility to carefully consider both the context of their reference material and the ramifications of their research findings and publications (e.g., Thompson 2001). For example, is it appropriate for practitioners to base their research on collections of human skeletal remains curated in museums, particularly when such collections are viewed as a violation of fundamental human rights by some Indigenous groups (Walker 2000: 19)? Such questions take on a different dimension when the remains are archaeological (Donlon 1994; Thompson 2003; Webb 1987), and there

are concerns about who "owns" or controls the past. There is further complexity in cases such as the analyses of the human skeletal remains from Spitalfields (the site of a former Medieval priory and hospital in London), where individuals were of known age and sex and often had living relatives (Molleson and Cox 1993).

Although assessment of the utility of forensic anthropology methodologies as applied to specific populations certainly has a place in terms of addressing the relevance of standards (as discussed above) (e.g., Schaefer and Black 2005), exactly how data are collected to develop population specific standards must be scrutinised (for example, examples cited in Hunter and Cox 2005: 215). Consider research aimed at using cranial morphology to differentiate between a Croatian and a Bosnian (Griffis 2001). Does such research take into account the complicated politics resulting in the 1992–1995 Bosnian war? Is it appropriate to undertake research based on human remains exhumed for evidence in war crime trials? If it is considered appropriate, has consent from the relatives of victims been sought and given (Hunter and Cox 2005: 215)? Such questions raise the importance of the need for cultural and ethical awareness and invite the larger question: what limits should one put on the expert's right to information (Meskell and Pels 2005: 5)?

Given the sensitive nature of the material that forensic anthropologists examine, all research and publications using skeletal material must be undertaken with the appropriate ethics research committee approval. This approach will also help avoid notions that forensic anthropologists can undertake any research *they* feel is appropriate.[2] It is not, however, enough to "do the paperwork": the broad ethical implications must be considered throughout and beyond the lifespan of the project (Loff and Black 2004).

The use of human remains (physical or illustrative) for research, teaching, lecturing, or demonstration purposes should be undertaken only if the activity has a specific point to address (O'Sullivan 2001: 130). When it comes to publishing research results, the forensic anthropologist has to consider ethical problems associated with both publishing and suppressing text and images of human remains. Whether a domestic case or one involving international assistance, the main parameter should be the definition of what is appropriate and what is relevant to specific audiences.

Is it ethical to undertake research but never publish the findings? For example, one of the issues raised by some Australian Aboriginal groups in discussions about the return of a prominent skeletal collection was the fact that despite the museum in question having held the remains for over 70 years, the researchers had published relatively little on their findings. What benefits, therefore, could be gained from the continued curation of these remains (Associate Professor Chris Briggs, The University of Melbourne, personal communication 2005; see also Hubert 1992: 116)?

Representations of the Dead

The propensity for humans to have a fascination with the macabre has seen a dramatic increase in the West in the portrayal and representation of the dead. This is evidenced by the number of photographs of human skeletal remains that appear on the front pages of newspapers and academic and fictional books and by the popularity of public exhibitions such as *London Bodies* or *Body Worlds*. *London Bodies* was an exhibition in which the human remains were the "star attractions" (Ganiaris 2001: 267) used to display the effects of urban living on Londoners from the prehistoric times to the present day (ibid.). Approximately 70,000 visitors attended the exhibition, which was the highest number for a temporary exhibition at the Museum since 1992 (ibid.: 271). *Body Worlds* consisted of 200 plasticised human beings, organs, and body slices and has attracted 6.5 million visitors in three years (Biehl and Gramsch 2001: 271).

In addition, and perhaps most powerful, is the media's depiction of the dead and those associated with death investigations (Black 2000: 491). Although some television shows claim to have consulted with forensic practitioners in the making of such shows (e.g., Lester n.d.), the impact of such "entertainment" cannot be underestimated. There has been significant discussion about the effect of such shows on the judicial process (e.g., ABC News 2005; Tyler 2006), and the influence on education is evidenced by the significant increase in demand for courses with a "forensic tag."

The ethics of such depictions in terms of the impact on the community must, however, be questioned. It is possible that increased (and possibly over-) exposure to fictional death and dying in the media has created a certain immunity (or blasé reaction) to the *idea* of the corpse. In reality, however, we know that there is limited correspondence between reality and images (Bartov 1996: 10). We may be subjected to numerous accounts of death through the media, but accounts of death are obviously very different from the actual experiences and even from personally witnessing the scene (Taylor 1998: 4). The ability to regard the human corpse (that is, soft tissue as well as hard skeletal tissue)

merely as an object that contains evidence for the court represents a "cultural detachment of no small dimension" (Richardson 1987: 31; see also Hockey 1996: 57). Whether students choose to undertake degrees in subjects such as forensic anthropology and archaeology because of the increasing search for sensation (Taylor 1998: 84; Wholley 2001: 276) or for a genuine desire to learn a skill, educators have a responsibility to ensure that students are clear about the reality (as opposed to the fiction) of what is involved in forensic anthropology investigations and are well equipped both with practical and social skills (Moss 2000).

Personal Ethical (Moral) Dilemmas

As discussed above, most professions have a code of conduct with which the practitioner must comply. It has been argued that "the cornerstone of . . . professional ethics is private morality" (Schroeder quoted in Lucas 1989: 727; see also Jones 2000: 29 for a discussion on professional vs. personal ethics). Although practitioners must consider and comply with organisational/professional ethics, it is impossible for them to ignore individual (personal) ethical (moral) issues in everyday practice. The potential for individual and professional ethical approaches to conflict must be considered (e.g., Lucas 1989), which raises a number of moral questions. It has been argued that a true ethical code should exist not to judge expertise per se but to "facilitate the negotiation of expertise within as well as outside of the profession" (Meskell and Pels 2005: 3), that is, to explicate responsibilities rather than rights.

Practice and Meaning

It may be argued that the role of the forensic anthropologist and/or archaeologist is simply to undertake a scientific investigation for service provision; the practitioner turns up, excavates and/or analyses the remains, and returns home. The occasional lecture may subsequently be presented using images taken from casework. However, as Weber (1948) pointed out, scientific investigations tell us nothing about the *meaning* of the world or the objects within it. Can practice really be undertaken in a cultural and philosophical vacuum (Jones 2000)? As forensic anthropologists (and archaeologists), we document the body and contribute to understanding issues related to manner of death. Is it, however, necessary to take into account the social aspects of death?

Although on the one hand, the body has to be treated objectively (in terms of the law, it is evidence), on the other hand, there are social and emotional attachments to the body that may require cultural flexibility. Since forensic anthropologists are now involved in both domestic and international casework, should such ethical concerns be expanded to include both the dead and the living? Is it important for practitioners to have training in the ways in which different societies view the dead and the body? Is it appropriate to encourage those working overseas to obtain an understanding of the language and culture (including burial practices) of the destination country? Such information may be important in recognising what is and is not normal for a particular culture's burial practice (Burns 1998: 66; Congram and Sterenberg this volume).

In addition to practical considerations, to what extent do practitioners have an ethical responsibility to consider the political dimensions of the work they undertake (Blau 2006; Congram 2005a; Hunter and Cox 2005: 208)? For example, how appropriate is it to accept employment from a military organisation that is willing to provide an inflated salary for services but has originated in a country that participated in questionable international military intervention? Such questions also relate to issues of objectivity. How does the anthropologist (or archaeologist) stay objective when she receives payment from a particular group, whether military or humanitarian?

Also, how ethical is it to undertake work in a country for a finite (usually relatively short) period of time, without leaving any infrastructure (both in terms of resources and knowledge) for Indigenous people to undertake future investigations for themselves (e.g., Hunter and Cox 2005: 210, 222)? The answers to such questions hinge on personal views and reflect one's own political stance, thus emphasising that forensic anthropology is political and, consequently, must have an ethical dimension.

Standards of Work

When engaged in overseas investigations (whether humanitarian or judicial), consultants will experience varying working conditions. The physical environment may be different both in terms of climate and landscape, but also in terms of available resources. Should limited resources dictate the standards of the work of the forensic anthropologist? In theory, we know the answer to this should be "no"; all remains from any context should be treated with the same respect. The challenge to forensic anthropologists is to ensure that in practise this is the case. The next logical question involves whose standards should then apply (Hunter and Cox 2005: 220). What if the choice is

between undertaking work limited in quality and undertaking no work at all?

The Rights of the Families

The benefits of including families when undertaking exhumations have been raised in the literature (Blaauw and Lahteenmaki 2002: 777; Fondebrider 2002: 887; Hunter and Cox 2005: 221; McEvoy and Conway 2004: 560). If families of victims are present during the excavation of human remains, to what extent is it ethically (in)appropriate to familiarise yourself with the families? Does familiarity affect your professional ability to undertake work to the best of your ability? Further, although International Criminal Tribunals believe they are acting professionally by employing experts to excavate and analyse remains, this approach may cause unhappiness or unrest in situations where local people do not want "outsiders" touching the remains of their relatives.

Do forensic anthropologists need to consider the potential impact of their work on families of victims (Hunter and Cox 2005: 221)? Although excavating remains may provide closure for some, others are less than content with the knowledge that, in addition to disturbing the dead, the analysis of remains may result in confronting the reality that a relative is actually dead and no longer "missing" (e.g., Blaauw and Lahteenmaki 2002: 776; Williams and Crews 2003: 256). Further, "what level of predicted success for identification is necessary to justify exhumation and identification procedures" (Williams and Crews 2003: 225).?

Death Penalty

If forensic anthropologists (and archaeologists) participate in the excavation of mass graves and the analysis of the interred human remains for collection of evidence to prosecute war crimes, the evidence may be used to help convict an alleged perpetrator. In some countries, those convicted of such crimes are subject to the death penalty. If practitioners find the death penalty personally abhorrent, is it ethical to engage in work in such countries (e.g., Congram 2005b; Cordner 2005: 4; Hunter and Cox 2005: 222)? Alternatively, the decision not to engage in international work raises a number of social dilemmas that have potential social and economic ramifications (e.g., Blaauw and Lahteenmaki 2002: 769).

Personal Safety

To what extent is it ethically appropriate to undertake work where one's personal safety is at risk?

Consider, for example, the death threats posed to the Guatemalan Forensic Anthropology Foundation and its team (Anon. 2006). But, again, to not engage in such work poses ethical dilemmas.

Questions of Justice

Forensic anthropologists will often be involved in the analysis of remains for judicial purposes. The aim is provide evidence so that justice can be served. One of the ethical dilemmas is justice for whom? The recovery and analysis of a victim of homicide may contribute to solving a crime and delivering punishment to the perpetrator but devastate those associated with the convicted offender. Consider the example provided by Cox (2001) in which a man is convicted of killing his wife after having led his three children to believe their mother had left them some 25 years ago. At one level, justice was served; the father was convicted of the crime he committed, and the mother of the victim could lay to rest her daughter whom she had believed abandoned her family. At another level, the lives of the children were traumatised; their father had not only lied to them but killed their mother, and their mother had, in fact, not abandoned them as their father had led them to believe (ibid.: 151).

At the international level, one must consider the ethical issues associated with participating in the analysis of human remains where the priority is given to determining the cause and manner of death rather than identifying the deceased (e.g., Fondebrider 2002: 889; United Nations 1991). Although legal justice may prevail, issues of social justice may remain unaddressed (McEvoy and Conway 2004: 558; Stover and Shigekane 2002). Conversely, if the investigation is undertaken for humanitarian purposes only, how appropriate is it to participate where immunity for alleged perpetrators prevails?

Conclusion

Traditionally, texts on forensic anthropology have often provided cursory considerations of ethics. The preceding discussion, however, illustrates that ethical issues are paramount in day to day practice and deserve greater attention. A set of ethical principles that specify a code of conduct is essential for the discipline of forensic anthropology to progress. However, ethics go beyond codification. Because of the implications of their work, forensic anthropologists must consider what is "reasonable" and/or "appropriate" for their profession and

the people it serves, both at a personal and professional level.

Acknowledgments

I am grateful to Tim Denham and Melanie Archer for their comments on drafts of this chapter.

Notes

1. The idea of the corpse as an object is, however, contrasts with the interpretation of a corpse under Anglo-Australian law, whereby the corpse "cannot be the subject of property so cannot be stolen" (Frekelton 1988: 259) and is therefore, not considered an object (Hubert 1992: 119).

2. See Beloff 2003 for a discussion on notions of appropriateness, cf. Bahn's conclusions "archaeologists have the right to do just about anything in the name of scholarship" (1984: 127). Bahn's conclusions differ little from some medical practitioners in the 19th century who believed "they were entitled to make whatever uses of the dead they wished" (MacDonald 2005: 189).

References

ABC News. 2005. *"CSI Effect" Making Cases Hard to Prove: Lawyers,* www.abc.net.au/news/newsitems/200509/s1467632.htm (accessed 02/02/07).

Adams, P. 2000. Death and contemporary popular culture, in A. Kellehear (ed.), *Death and Dying in Australia,* pp. 105–115. Oxford: Oxford University Press.

Anon. 2006. Guatemalan Forensic Anthropology Foundation again facing death threats. AAAS Human Rights Action Network, http://shr.aaas.org/aaashran/alert.php?a_id=316 (accessed 18/01/06).

Bahn, P. 1984. Do not disturb? Archaeology and the rights of the dead. *Oxford Journal of Archaeology* 3(2): 127–139.

Bartove, O. 1996. *Murder in Our Midst: The Holocaust, Industrial Killing and Representation.* Oxford: Oxford University Press.

Baudrillard, J. 1993. *Symbolic Exchange and Death.* London: Sage Publications.

Beloff, H. 2003. Medical ethics in professional conduct. *International Journal of Human Rights* 7(1): 9–15.

Biehl, P. H., and Gramsch, A. 2001. Reviews. *European Journal of Archaeology* 4(2): 271–273.

Blaauw, M., and Lahteenmaki, V. 2002. "Denial and silence" or acknowledgement and disclosure. *International Review of the Red Cross* 84: 767–783.

Black, S. 2000. Forensic osteology in the United Kingdom, in M. Cox and S. Mays (eds.), *Human Osteology in Archaeology and Forensic Science*, pp. 491–503. London: Greenwich Medical Media.

———. 2003. Forensic anthropology: Regulation in the United Kingdom. *Science and Justice* 43(4): 187–192.

Blau, S. 2006. The powerful evidence of the bodies: Ethical considerations for the forensic anthropologist involved in the investigation of mass graves. *Indian Journal of Physical Anthropology and Human Genetics* 25(2): 247–258.

Bottorff, D. L. 2005. What is Ethics? www.ethicsquality.com/about.htlm (accessed 2/12/02).

Bowman, J. E, MacLaughlin, S. M., and Scheuer, J. L. 1992. The relationship between biological and chronological age in the juveniles from St. Brides Church, Fleet Street. *Annals of Human Biology* 19: 216.

Burns, K. 1998. Forensic anthropology and human rights issues, in K. J. Reichs (ed.), *Forensic Osteology: Advances in the Identification of Human Remains* (2nd ed.), pp. 63–85. Springfield, IL: Charles C. Thomas.

Cantwell, A. 2000. "Who knows the power of his bones": Reburial redux. *Annals of the New York Academy of Sciences* 925: 79–119.

Congram, D. 2005a. Spinning in their graves; The political spin and parameters of mass grave exhumation and the archaeologists who dig them. Paper presented at the Theoretical Archaeology Group Conference, Sheffield.

———. 2005b. Intentional limitations on identifications. Paper presented at the Theoretical Archaeology Group Conference, Sheffield.

Cordner, S. 2005. The Missing: Action to resolve the problem of those unaccounted for as a result of armed conflict or internal violence, and to assist their families. *Victorian Institute of Forensic Medicine Review* 3(1): 2–6.

Cox, M. 1998. Criminal concerns: A plethora of forensic archaeologists. *The Archaeologist* 33: 21–22.

———. 2000. Ageing adults from the skeleton, in M. Cox and S. Mays (eds.), *Human Osteology in Archaeology and Forensic Science*, pp. 61–81. London: Greenwich Medical Media.

———. 2001. Forensic archaeology in the UK: Questions of socio-intellectual context and socio-political responsibility, in V. Buchli and G. Lucas (eds.), *Archaeologies of the Contemporary Past*, pp. 145–167. London: Routledge.

Donlon, D. 1994. Aboriginal skeletal collections and research in physical anthropology: An historical perspective. *Australian Archaeology* 390: 73–82.

Fondebrider, L. 2002. Reflections on the scientific documentation of human rights violations. *International Review of the Red Cross* 84(848): 885–891.

Fraser, S. 2003. Colleges add "forensic" tag to market course. *Scotland on Sunday*, 18 May.

Frekelton, I. 1988. Identification and the law, in J. G. Clement and D. L. Ranson (eds.), *Craniofacial Identification in Forensic Medicine*, pp. 257–265. London: Arnold.

Frutos, L. R. 2002. Determination of sex from the clavicle and scapula in a Guatemalan contemporary rural indigenous population. *American Journal of Forensic Medicine and Pathology* 23(3): 284–288.

———. 2005. Metric determination of sex from the humerus in a Guatemalan forensic sample. *Forensic Science International* 147(2–3): 153–157.

Ganiaris, H. 2001. London bodies: An exhibition at the Museum of London, in E. Williams (ed.), *Human Remains: Conservation, Retrieval and Analysis*, pp. 267–274. BAR International 934. Oxford: Archaeopress.

Griffis, L. 2001. *Investigating Bones: The Work of the C. A. Pound Human Identification Laboratory*. CLASnotes 15(3). http://clasnews.clas.ufl.edu/news/clasnotes/0103/pound/html (accessed 02/07/06).

Hockey, J. 1996. Encountering the "reality of death" through professional discourses: The matter of materiality. *Mortality* 1(1): 45–60.

Hubert, J. 1992. Dry bones or living ancestors? Conflicting perceptions of life, death and the universe. *International Journal of Cultural Property* 1(1): 105–127.

Hunt, D. R., and Albanese, J. 2005. History and demographic composition of the Robert J. Terry Anatomical Collection. *American Journal of Physical Anthropology* 127(4): 406–417.

Hunter, J. 2002. Foreword: A pilgrim in archaeology: A personal view, in W. D. Haglund and M. H. Sorg (eds.), *Advances in Forensic Taphonomy: Method, Theory and Archaeological Perspectives*, pp. xxv–xxxii. Boca Raton, FL: CRC Press.

Hunter, J., and Cox, M. 2005. Social and intellectual frameworks, in J. Hunter and M. Cox (eds.), *Forensic Archaeology: Advances in Theory and Practice*, pp. 204–225. London: Routledge.

Hunter, J. R., Brickley, M. B., Bourgeois, J., Bouts, W., Bourguignon, L., Hubrechts, F., de Wine, J., van Haaster, H., Hakbijl, T., de Jong, H., Smits, L., van Wijngaarden, L. H., and Luschen, M. 2001. Forensic archaeology, forensic anthropology and human rights in Europe. *Science and Justice* 41(3): 173–178.

Jones, D. G. 2000. *Speaking for the Dead: Cadavers in Biology and Medicine*. Dartmouth: Ashgate.

Jones, D. G., and Harris, R. J. 1998. Archaeological human remains: Scientific, cultural and ethical considerations. *Current Anthropology* 39(2): 253–264.

Lester, S. N.d. The body behind CSI: Anthony Zuiker. www.fhmonline.com/articles-3208.asp (accessed 02/02/07).

Loff, B., and Black, J. 2004. Research ethics committees: What is their contribution? *Medical Journal of Australia* 181(8): 440–441.

Lucas, D. M. 1989. The ethical responsibilities of the forensic scientist: Exploring the limits. *Journal of Forensic Sciences* 34(3): 719–729.

MacDonald, H. 2005. *Human Remains: Episodes in Human Dissection*. Melbourne: Melbourne University Press.

Mario, J. R. 2002. A review of Anglo-American forensic professional codes of ethics with considerations for code design. *Forensic Science International* 125: 103–112.

Marks, M. K., Hudson, J. W., and Elkins, S. K. 1999. Craniofacial fractures: Collaboration spells success, in A. Galloway (ed.), *Broken Bones: Anthropological Analysis of Blunt Force Trauma*: 258–286. Springfield, IL: Charles C. Thomas.

McEvoy, K., and Conway, H. 2004. The dead, the law, and the politics of the past. *Journal of Law and Society* 31(4): 539–562.

Meskell, L., and Pels, P. 2005. Introduction: Embedding ethics, in L. Meskell and P. Pels, P. (eds.), *Embedding Ethics*, pp. 1–26. Oxford: Berg.

Molleson, T. I., and Cox, M. J. 1993. *The Spitalfields Project Vol 2. The Anthropology: The Middling Sort*. Research Report 86. York: Council for British Archaeology.

Moss, B. R. 2000. Death studies at university: New approaches to teaching and learning. *Mortality* 5(2): 205–214.

O'Sullivan, J. 2001. Ethics and the archaeology of human remains. *The Journal of Irish Archaeology* 10: 121–151.

Pardoe, C. 1992. Arches of radii, corridors of power: Reflections on current archaeological practice, in B. Attwood and J. Arnold (eds.), *Power, Knowledge and Aborigines*, pp. 132–141. Melbourne: La Trobe University Press.

Patriquin M. L., Loth, S. R., and Steyn, M. 2003. Sexually dimorphic pelvic morphology in South African Whites and Blacks. *Homo* 53(3): 255–262.

Prior, L. 1989. *The Social Organisation of Death: Medical Discourse and Social Practice in Belfast*. London: Macmillan Press.

Reichs, K. J. 1998. Forensic anthropology: A decade of progress, in K. J. Reichs (ed.), *Forensic Osteology: Advances in the Identification of Human Remains* (2nd ed.), pp. 13–38. Springfield, IL: Charles C. Thomas.

Richardson, R. 1987. *Death, Dissection and the Destitute*. London: Routledge.

Rogers, T. L., and Allard, T. T. 2002. Expert testimony and positive identification of human remains through cranial suture patterns. *Journal of Forensic Sciences* 49(2): 1–5.

Sapir, G. I. 2001. Review of Ethics in forensic science and medicine: Guidelines for the forensic expert and the attorney. *Journal of Forensic Sciences* 46(5): 1268.

Schaefer, M. C., and Black, S. M. 2005. Comparison of ages of epiphyseal union in North American and Bosnian skeletal material. *Journal of Forensic Sciences* 50(4): 777–784.

Stewart, T. D. 1979. *Essentials of Forensic Anthropology*. Springfield, IL: Charles C. Thomas.

Steyn, M., and İşcan, M. Y. 1997. Sex determination from the femur and tibia in South African Whites. *Forensic Science International* 90(1–2): 111–119.

Stover, E., and Shigekane, R. 2002. The missing in the aftermath of war. *International Review of the Red Cross* 84(848): 845–865.

Taylor, J. 1998. *Body Horror: Photojournalism, Catastrophe and War*. Manchester: Manchester University Press.

Thompson, T. 2001. Legal and ethical considerations of forensic anthropological research. *Science and Justice* 41(4): 261–270.

———. 2003. The quality and appropriateness of forensic anthropological education in the UK. *Public Archaeology* 3: 88–94.

Tyler, T. R. 2006. Viewing *CSI* and the threshold of guilt: Managing truth and justice in reality and fiction. *The Yale Law Review* 115: 1050–1085.

Ubelaker, D. H. 2000. Methodological considerations in the forensic applications of human skeletal biology, in M. A. Katzenburg and R. Shelley (eds.), *Biological Anthropology of the Human Skeleton*, pp. 41–67. New York: Wiley-Liss.

United Nations. 1991. *Manual on the Effective Prevention and Investigation of Extralegal, Arbitrary and Summary Executions*. New York: United Nations.

Urmson, J. O., and Rée, J. (eds.). 1991. *The Concise Encyclopedia of Western Philosophy and Philosophers*. London: Routledge.

Vizenor, G. 1996. Bone courts: The rights and narrative representation of tribal bones, in R.W. Preucel and I. Hodder (eds.), *Contemporary Archaeology in Theory: A Reader*, pp. 652–663. Cambridge: Blackwell.

Walker, P. L. 2000. Bioarchaeological ethics: A historical perspective on the value of human remains, in M. A. Katzenberg and S. R. Saunder (eds.), *Biological Anthropology of the Human Skeleton*, pp. 3–39. New York: Wiley-Liss.

Webb, S. 1987. Reburying Australian skeletons. *Antiquity* 61: 292–296.

Weber, M. 1948. Science as a vocation, in H. Gerth and C. W. Mills (eds.), *From Max Weber: Essays in Sociology*, 129–156. London: Routledge.

White, T. 2000. *Human Osteology* (2nd ed.). New York: Academic Press.

Wholley, A. L. 2001. The attraction of the macabre: Issues relating to human soft tissue collections in museums, in E. Williams (ed.), *Human Remains: Conservation, Retrieval and Analysis*, pp. 275–281. BAR International 934. Oxford: Archaeopress.

Williams, E. D., and Crews, J. D. 2003. From dust to dust: Ethical and practical issues involved in the location, exhumation and identification of bodies from mass graves. *Croatian Medical Journal* 44(3): 251–258.

38

How to Do Forensic Archaeology under the Auspices of the United Nations and Other Large Organizations

Richard Wright and Ian Hanson

Fancy what a game at chess would be if all the chessmen had passions and intellects . . .: if you were not only uncertain about your adversary's men, but a little uncertain also about your own; if your knight could shuffle himself on to a new square by the sly; if your bishop, in disgust at your castling, could wheedle your pawns out of their places; and if your pawns, hating you because they are pawns, could make away from their appointed posts that you might get checkmate on a sudden. . . . You might be the longest-headed of deductive reasoners, and yet you might be beaten by your own pawns. You would be especially likely to be beaten, if you . . . regarded your passionate pieces with contempt. (George Eliot Felix Holt, *The Radical* [1866])

Achieving a successful outcome in forensic archaeology is like playing a game of chess—but the game of chess as described by George Eliot. The organization that you work for has a mind of its own. You have a mind of your own. Your team members have minds of their own. Any human piece on the chessboard may move to checkmate the most technologically and logistically prepared of missions.

This chapter is a guide to achieving a successful outcome for those who are employed as forensic archaeologists by large organizations such as the United Nations (UN). More specifically, it targets the needs of forensic archaeologists directing investigations of mass graves.

We have already written about technical matters relating to the archaeology of mass graves (Wright, Hanson, and Sterenberg 2005). There, we merely touched on the psychosocial matters that we now bring to the fore in this chapter. In fact, a meld of both technical and social planning is necessary. Only with this can a team deliver the evidence of criminal activities and personal identifications in such an impeccable manner that no challenge to the team's work will succeed.

It might be thought that attention to technical matters suffices. To think this is a mistake, akin to thinking that people are pieces on a chessboard that have fixed moves and that cannot move themselves. To consider only technical matters and protocols is not enough. There is also a psychosocial environment for successful forensic field-work. The team must be supported physically and psychologically. Complex relationships will develop among members of the team, between the director and the team, and among the sponsoring organization, other agencies, and the director.

These complexities must be managed, particularly in a stressful environment. Bad relationships will make the field experience unpleasant—and, unfortunately, things may get worse than merely unpleasant. At the very worst, the evidence itself might become prejudiced by noncooperation between agencies or by dissident team members writing letters of denigration that fall into the hands of the defense.

One might concede that psychosocial problems need attention but assume that a large sponsoring organization that employs many staff and has policies on occupational health and staff welfare will so nurture the team that problems will not arise. One might also assume that the dedication of the team to the mission will prevent selfish dissidence. However, we assume in this chapter that the director will prepare, manage, and intervene proactively. Therefore, this chapter attends to both the director's downward management of forensic archaeological teams and the upward "management" of large sponsoring organizations.

Why an Archaeologist as Director?

We have elsewhere discussed our specific technical reasons for having an archaeologist as director of the excavation team "within the tapes" and working with a crime scene manager (Wright, Hanson, and Sterenberg 2005). Our comments are not intended to devalue the role of other forensic professionals; however, we disagree with Snow's opinion that a forensic anthropologist can practice forensic archaeological work after reading a few articles and perhaps attending a summer school (Snow 1982). More experience than this is required to evaluate what occurred at spatially and chronologically complex crime scenes and mass graves, and to bring work to successful completion.

Furthermore, it is dangerous for the prosecution to present an anthropologist as an expert witness concerning mass graves when the defense has the ability to call an archaeologist experienced with stratigraphy to test that evidence. Disturbance, in particular graverobbing, creates an intricate stratification, and the evidentiary danger is acute if there is a dispute in court about whether graves have been disturbed. In our experience, disturbance is a common occurrence at mass graves in the Balkans, Guatemala, and Iraq, because communities search for the missing and perpetrators hide and destroy evidence. The management of area surveys and excavations is a specialized but everyday professional undertaking of stratigraphically aware rescue/salvage and academic archaeologists. They should be used as experts.

There are additional psychosocial points for an archaeologist to direct the team that go beyond the technical. One point must be emphasized, because

it bears on style of leadership. An experienced archaeologist will be familiar with managing large teams of people who have disparate experience and disparate egos—and with managing them under stress (Wright, Hanson, and Sterenberg 2005: 138). We have argued that:

> Some professions are hierarchically ordered, with attendant hierarchically ordered privileges and comforts. This culture does not transfer productively to the more egalitarian fieldwork scene. Making sense of the novel properties of each mass grave favours a seminar environment at the site rather than an unquestioning command structure, although a protocol for decision-making is still essential. (ibid.: 157)

To develop this point, we note that each grave is unique in its size, number of bodies, condition of bodies, soil environment, and drainage and engineering requirements. The director, as an experienced field archaeologist, must come up with a unique plan of excavation that integrates all these interacting variables of the mass grave. Members of the team will hopefully have specialized archaeological knowledge that may not be part of the director's compendium of experience. The director must tap that experience and incorporate it into the unique plan of excavation of a novel site.

By contrast, procedures in forensic anthropology, although requiring a great degree of skill and experience, have become formalized. Apart from needing to develop population-specific standards, most anthropology team members likely will not offer something that requires a rewriting of a plan of analysis of sex, age, ancestry, and cause and manner of death. It is the director of anthropology's duty to be wary of innovation and to ensure that standard protocols are followed. Consequently, a managerial structure is required for the anthropological laboratory that is more hierarchical than the looser structure that will prove beneficial on an archaeological excavation.

Leadership and Style

Directors will initially have authority because of their appointment by the organization and their prior experience. At first, leadership should be easy. However, as time proceeds, especially in an exotic environment, hierarchical leadership tends to weaken because of rotation and mixing of personnel, isolation, and the hardships that must be shared. An autocratic leader will have problems with this sapping of authority. A sign of a breakdown of leadership is when a director starts living in a hotel, spends a large amount of time away from the team and site, or turns up at the site only when it is visited by important people or the media.

Essentially, there are three styles of leadership:

- *Laissez-faire*: members of the team make the decisions
- *Autocratic*: the director decides, and members of the team do not participate in the decision making
- *Consultative*: the director consults and interacts with members of the team but then decides unilaterally

Laissez-faire leadership on forensic excavations can be dismissed immediately as ineffective, since it is too anarchic for evidentiary purposes and risks producing work that the director could not speak to in court.

Autocratic leadership is also maladaptive for a successful outcome. It isolates the director from the collective experience of members of the team, who may have ways of solving technical problems. Unless the director's experience exceeds that of the combined experience of the team, autocratic leadership encourages dissidence. This may even break out after the fieldwork is over and prejudice the evidence.

Consultative leadership is the most successful method and leads to a better technical outcome. Some members of the team may have uniquely relevant experience that the director does not have. Consultative leadership will tend to keep the team cohesive and free from dissidence.

Nevertheless, there must be some management of this consultative style of leadership. In a multicultural team, for instance, some members may not even be familiar with the concept of consultative leadership. They may not speak the lingua franca of the team, they may be too embarrassed to express their views at a team discussion, and they may fear that offering advice will be seen as subversive. In these situations it may be necessary for the director explicitly to seek such members' opinions privately, until they become more accustomed to the culture of consultative leadership.

It should go without saying that the director should take the time to brief each new member of the team on arrival. Unfortunately, this practice is not always followed in general archaeology, and there are tales of persons working in a hole for weeks, having never been informed about what

is being done and why. People treated in this way are likely to become disaffected and work in a manner that is incompatible with the planned process.

In forensic archaeology, such neglect of new team members is not so likely, since each team member will have to be taken through the very necessary risk assessments, safety briefs, and protocols for the excavation. It is the director who should take them through the protocols. A forensic excavation is not General Motors: there is not a long line of management that prevents the director from dealing directly with each new team member.

The excavation will benefit from the director doing the rounds of the site, checking on the logging of finds, the surveying, and the security and safety of the site. Informal chats coupled with watchful eyes can discover what might be going wrong in matters as diverse as undermining of section walls, deviation from protocols, and inadequate backing up of excavation logs.

In brief, the purpose of consultative leadership is not to make everybody feel good. The purpose is to produce the best outcome and to forestall dissidence that might prejudice the evidence.

Exotic Environments

Much forensic excavation will be done in environments that are exotic to members of the team. Appointing locals to the team would obviously reduce the effects of the exotic nature of the environment, but for evidentiary reasons appointing locals may not be acceptable. Harrison and Connors analyze the special relationship between exotic environments and small teams (1984: 53). They found that published studies analyzing this relationship are virtually restricted to groups in submarines and in polar and outer space settings. Among the groups they mention as ignored are archaeologists.

So far as we know, there is still no literature on the psychosocial dynamics of archaeological teams in exotic environments, although some attention has been paid to tensions in small teams in non-exotic environments (Moore 1986) and large teams in exotic environments ameliorated by massive infrastructure (Hamilton 2000). The problems associated with the work undertaken by forensic archaeologists have perhaps more in common with disaster management and mass-fatality incidents. These have been written about in depth (Haddow and Bullock 2006; Levinson and Granot 2002; Pan American Health Organisation 2004).

To adapt the comments of Harrison and Connors to forensic teams, we would say that the climate may be harsh or unfamiliar; there may be physical danger from local perpetrators, unexploded ordnance, contamination, unfamiliar wildlife; facilities and supplies may be poor; the team will be isolated from family and friends, and members of the team will be forced to interact with one another. The team must cope with "accelerated acquaintance processes, limited personal space, an inability to escape companions who have annoying traits or mannerisms, and an inability to keep conflicting individuals apart" (Harrison and Connors 1984: 54).

It is critical that head office does not force domestic arrangements on the team (for example, barrack style accommodation) that exacerbate these social tensions. The head office should be encouraged to provide a postal service and international phone calls and internet access and discouraged from interfering with domestic living arrangements. Whenever possible, members of the team should be left to their own devices outside working hours.

Working hours should vary according to the length of the mission. For 2 weeks, people can work 12 hours a day for all 14 days—even under stressful conditions. However, they cannot work like this on a project that lasts 6 months and is likely going to be disgusting and possibly dangerous. Head office probably works a 5-day week, so the director can use that information when countering pressure for the team to work physically and psychologically damaging hours.

Working under pressure will encourage errors, thus prejudicing the quality of the evidence. Working under pressure will also create tensions in the team that may lead to dissident complaints that prejudice the evidence. Members of the team may benefit from reading handbooks devoted to working in exotic environments. A very practical guide is provided by Ehrenreich (2005).

Composition of the Team

The team may embark with a strong sense of mission. This promising start makes it all the more distressing when tensions start to develop within the team—as they most certainly will. The director must manage these tensions lest they adversely affect the quality of the work and the integrity of the evidence.

The director should choose the team members. However, advice should be taken from others about "who's who" in the world of forensic fieldwork, so that there is a proper mixture of nationalities and experience. A multicultural team is unlikely to be accused of being subservient to the prosecutors and the lawyers or, worse still, of fixing the evidence.

Ensure that the personnel division at head office requires a medical examination of team members, certifying fitness to travel and to undertake fieldwork. As a precaution on the psychological side, try to get people who have already handled soft tissue, if that is anticipated at the excavations. Emphasize to head office that human remains may cause feelings of disgust, shock, distress, and/or anger in team members. A forensic exhumation is no place for an unproven person that somebody in head office would like to provide with work experience.

Harrison and Connors (1984: 61) discuss the type of people suitable for working in small groups in exotic environments. The team needs people who are technically competent to achieve a successful outcome, but also people who contribute to the overall quality of the team's social life. On its own, obsessive attention to technical matters can cause social stress in the team. However, an orientation that is too socio-emotional may cause the team to fall short of the required high performance standards.

People who are socially versatile—not so introverted that they provide little stimulation to the group and not so extroverted that they force themselves on others—make up a successful team (ibid.). In the light of our experience, those who are paid on contract, not volunteers, make a better team. Volunteers tend to be restless in exotic environments. They may resent having to miss the sights and decide to wander off. If having volunteers is inevitable, then make sure that there is a core team of paid and trusted people under contract. A core team provides the advantage of continuity through the whole project and a fund of experience from which the team as a whole can draw. In particular, try to get a Scene of Crime Officer (SOCO[1]) to manage the handling of evidence throughout the whole project. Do not rely on SOCOs volunteered by a friendly country, but who are rotated every two weeks. However good the individual SOCOs are, the lack of continuity creates a burden of induction and a threat to the admissibility of evidence owing to changes of style and record keeping.

Dealing with the Organization

The team will depend on the employing organization for its survival. Members therefore cannot avoid dealing with its bureaucracy. The problem is that the team will have very little time to learn how to deal with the organization's bureaucracy. The mission's success or failure may take place over a period of only three weeks, so fulminate against the organization's bureaucracy later and concentrate on winning in the short term.

Paradoxically, major problems often relate to the fact that a particular bureaucracy may literally not work. It does not attend to its "bureaus." Cash for maintenance expenses may not be delivered in a cash-only economy. Crucial equipment may not be repaired or replaced. Flights for team rotation may not be booked.

In our experience, a major cause of such paralysis is administrators going on leave. If somebody goes on leave in a business, then their desk is attended to by somebody else—lest the business's inefficiency makes it go bankrupt. Such continuity may not be provided in an organization such as the UN, where going bankrupt is an irrelevant prospect. Nor is dismissal much practiced. The best the team can hope for, if a particular person repeatedly lets it down, is that the person will be shifted over to some non-operational section, such as "policy."

Dealing with Bureaucracy

It may be aggravating that an organization that employs a team to do its critical work should then act as if the team is a nuisance. The remainder of this section contains advice on how to succeed with the bureaucracy. The team must succeed if the work is to be satisfactorily completed. The points are disparate and not listed in order of importance.

- Ensure that the team is provided with an experienced project manager to attend to the logistics and to remain with the team, who is familiar with the organization and the local country of operation.

- The director should become acquainted with senior people in the organization, who can advise on its organizational structure and policy. At times of emergency, the director can appeal to these people to deal with a recalcitrant bureaucracy. The director should insist on a visit to head office well before the fieldwork starts and be introduced to the critical people in the legal section, personnel, finance, and the section that deals with procurement of supplies. Regularly contact the manager at head office. Give good news about the fieldwork first and bad news and requests second.

Head office may decide that fieldwork will start on a particular date. It probably will not. In fact, the work may be repeatedly delayed. Some of the delays will be due to bureaucrats not doing their work. Some delays, however, will be legitimate and caused by unforeseen changes in the weather or security. Whatever their origin, these delays can damage the finances of the self-employed who are sitting at home waiting and conflict with the leave arrangements of the employed. The team can try to mitigate the problem by getting contracts on a fixed date regardless of the delays, but the chances for doing this are not good.

The contracts the team members are asked to sign when they turn up in the field may differ from the draft contracts they were sent when at home. Invariably, we have found that these differences favored the organization. Sometimes the potential reductions in pay were severe. For example, a team had for three years worked for a monthly flat rate of pay. Suddenly, a novel clause was inserted that set the same monthly rate but abolished pay for days off. In other words, you could make the same money as before only by working seven days a week instead of the established five. This novel clause was discarded when it was made plain to the administration that they would have no team for the fourth year.

Has the employing organization taken into account the possibility of accident? Is it possible to prepare a helicopter landing area near the site? Does the team know where to go in the case of a medical evacuation? How will the team communicate with medical people if there is an emergency? Has the organization provided a satellite phone that can be operated from anywhere, and round the clock, in the case of emergency? Has the organization properly considered whether the work is to take place in a potentially hostile social environment? What kind of protection will the team need? If the director concludes that the team needs armed protection, who can authorize its use and who will provide it?

There may be a puzzling refusal by the organization to provide goods. To take an extreme example, for three years we were not provided with drinking water at the work on mass graves in Bosnia. Team members had to bring dubious town water in bottles, drink chemically sterilized washing water at the site, or hope for bottles of water to drop off the back of the trucks of their military escort. Bottled water was unobtainable in the shops. There was a simple bureaucratic reason for the organization not providing drinking water—they gave us a living allowance and could not work out how to get the money back from us if they provided drinking water. We were slow to solve this one. Victory over the accounting conundrum came only when we were able to show that the organization was in breach of the International Labour Laws by not providing drinking water at the workplace. We solved the problem by making it no longer an accounting issue. The moral is to get these basic issues resolved before deployment.

Beware of having forensic protocols inflicted on your team by the archaeologically ignorant. The protocols may be unworkable, and your lack of compliance may then be used in court to question the value of your evidence. Be proactive and work out your own protocols. Keep them simple yet essential, so as not to prejudice the evidentiary value of your work because of non-compliance.

Likewise, beware of having physically harmful health and safety procedures inflicted on you. Make sure that the procedures are workable. In summer, in most parts of the world, excavation cannot proceed if the team is required to wear impermeable body suits, face masks, and arm-length gauntlets. We have argued elsewhere that mass graves are not, in our experience, inherently unhealthy environments (Wright, Hanson, and Sterenberg 2005). The key is to identify risks and to mitigate them in a flexible and practical way.

Consider how you and the team have dealt with matters of insurance and legal liability. Does the organization cover its contracted team for injury at work? Does it compensate dependent relatives for death? The contracts with the UN stated that contractors were treated as if they were UN staff from the point of view of compensation. Does your organization explicitly adopt that proper attitude and comforting provision? The provision must reflect the potentially hazardous nature of working environments. If team members are made to provide their own insurance (necessarily through brokers because of the nature of the work and its location), they may find insurance premiums are so financially prohibitive as to deter them from taking on the job. Alternatively, they may not insure themselves.

You need to plan for sensible occupational health arrangements. Be wary of accepting counsellors. In fact, counsellors can be a disruptive nuisance when managers inflict them on a professional forensic team. Their very presence implies that members of the team have undergone some sort of appalling stress. Usually they have not. Paradoxically, counsellors may make the team feel guilty, because they have not felt upset, because they have found the work interesting, because they have enjoyed camaraderie with others in the team and have enjoyed the occasional black humor. Persuade head office that counsellors are intended for those that have experienced out-of-the-ordinary, sudden, and unexpected emotional trauma. Your team is unlikely to experience professionally out-of-the-ordinary, sudden, and unexpected emotional trauma. Members of your team have started the job prepared for the worst.

One good protection against stress at mass graves is an obvious one: that the people recruited should at the very least have already worked closely with skeletal remains. They will thereby have already put behind them the disturbing "intimations of mortality" that first contact with any human remains can induce. So, ideally your team will already be professionally inured. Nevertheless, you cannot be careless about the psychology of your team. In particular, ensure that the team environment is supportive—and be supportive yourself. Look after those who have no friends and will be returning home to a place where they live on their own with loss of team contact. Constrain, isolate, or get rid of any damagingly aggressive team members.

Encourage members of the team to bring as much cash as they can if you are operating in a cash-only economy. The contract may specify that you will be paid a living allowance in cash in advance, but work on the assumption that you may not see the cash for a few weeks. During this time of paralysis at head office you must pay for your accommodation and food. We were members of a team of which several were reduced to penury, and had to rely on the others, because of the persistent incapacity of head office to provide the promised cash.

Stress to those who procure equipment that your specifications about equipment must be followed to the letter. We have experienced altered specifications leading to refrigerated vans whose doors could not be opened when they were mounted on their flatbed trailers; a dumpy level that swung on a 400-unit base, instead of the 360-degree base that our survey software required; trowels that had blades the size of an A4 sheet of paper (chosen perhaps from an armchair notion that it would allow us archaeologists to shift more soil than the conventional namby-pamby 4-inch blade); a laptop computer that had its operating system altered by an information technology section that thought it knew better than Microsoft, with the result that it could not run our specialized laboratory-style DOS programs. All these deviations were discovered once equipment was delivered to the operations' base. So explain in advance to the procurement section that some items are technically vital and cannot therefore have their specifications altered.

This may mean writing such a precise procurement description that no brand or model other than the one you require can be purchased.

Ask the organization to discourage the media. In dangerous situations, the presence of the media may aggravate the perpetrators into attacking the team. Some members of the team may not want their faces to appear on internationally distributed public media (they may have worked on politically sensitive excavations elsewhere). Members of the team may be caught off their guard, being filmed smiling in a scene that includes a corpse. Media presence must be tightly managed, and therefore infrequent. This necessity may be at odds with your organization's desire to publicize its work and the political need to demonstrate to local and international communities that work is being carried out. A balance needs to be negotiated.

Do not rely on the organization's head office to provide the director with critical personal details that may be required in an emergency. An accident may happen over a weekend. So ensure that the members of the team provide information about their blood group, specialist medical details (such as anaesthetic or antibiotic allergies), names and contact details of next of kin, and their own contact details for the immediate post-excavation period.

Team members should be reminded they are ambassadors for the team and may need to restrain their behavior in public. To reduce the chance of accident or incident, tell your team where they can and cannot go on their days off. Warn them not to talk shop with people whom they do not personally know.

After working for an organization for some weeks, a caste system may develop. Administrators in head office work in clean, airconditioned comfort. The team is doing such inexplicably disgusting work that it is unclean. Head office may distance itself from having to think about the polluted team to such an extent that inadequate support is given. People at the level of mass-grave diggers could not possibly have dependent families and mortgages, so what do delays in paying them matter? A prior visit to head office should help to dispel these prejudicial notions. More importantly, encourage administration to visit the excavations.

Dealing with the Dead

The team may be doing its fieldwork at the point of a gun and with the backing of a Security Council resolution. Or the continuity of its humanitarian work may require negotiations, renegotiations, and cooperation with the authorities and relatives.

Dealing with the dead, in contrast with the archaeology of artifacts, creates specific risks and responsibilities. The director will ultimately be held responsible if dealing with the dead and the living is clumsily handled. We have included below a suggested checklist of what to consider. This list covers only the context of dealing with the dead, not general matters of the mission or the archaeological work.

Finally, we have discussed a number of problems in this chapter. However, on the positive side, we agree with Harrison and Connors that exotic environments can provide substantial rewards for team members (1984: 69). These include:

1. an opportunity to become totally immersed in one's work;
2. an opportunity to be judged on the basis of performance rather than on the basis of extraneous factors such as age or race;
3. a socially uncomplicated existence;
4. a financially uncomplicated existence;
5. an opportunity to build self-esteem;
6. adventure.

All this rings true. To the points of Harrison and Connors we add:

7. an opportunity to contribute to international justice;
8. an exciting and exotic experience in a short time;
9. opportunities to develop new methods, techniques, and research;
10. interaction with diverse regions and communities.

At the end of a forensic field season, many of us have said "never again" only to remember the enjoyment and return the next year.

Conclusion

In summary, remember that all the team's actions should be directed to maintaining the integrity of the evidence. The integrity of the evidence is necessary for both the successful identification of the dead and for prosecutions. Ultimately, it is the team's work that may be the key to gaining convictions and repatriation of remains to families.

Without the materialized evidence of killings, the perpetrators, their defenders, and revisionists can set up a contest whereby we argue over the meaning of lines of text in historical documents or phrases in an investigator's intercepted telephone call and argue over the integrity of a person's memory. Of course, scholarship, investigations, and memories are critical. But we also need to look at the powerful evidence of the bodies. They are there; somebody shot them. They demand an explanation.

And explanations must come through the eyes of the unbiased forensic professionals in a team. That is why the sometimes recalcitrant organization will have hired the team. The organization may see members of the team as pieces on a chessboard, but you must make the organization work for you by playing the style of chess that George Eliot's quotation describes at the start of this chapter.

Checklist for Preparing to Excavate Human Remains

This checklist draws on personal experience and literature. Some sources of advice that may be consulted are Historic Scotland (1997), N.S.W. Heritage Office (1998), and Williams (2001).

Prior considerations:

- Can you honestly estimate the time the work will take? Whom are you going to consult and from whom must permissions be sought?

  Consider:

  —owners, managers, and tenants of the land

  —police

  —coroner

  —governments at various levels (for example, state and federal)

  —tribunals and commissions

  —health authorities

  —those claiming to be relatives and friends

  —religious authorities

  —heritage authorities if graves are in important areas of heritage

  —ethnic and other community groups that claim a direct interest in the particular dead

  —local historians/archaeologists/anthropologists and their societies, if graves are in areas of cultural significance

- Do you need a court order?

- Should you conduct and advertise a public meeting before starting work?

- How will 7-day/24-hour protection be provided for the human remains at the site, to guard against animal scavenging, looting, and tampering with evidence?

- What special health and safety considerations do the particular remains call for?

- Have you considered allowing relatives to perform religious rites on the site before and during the excavation/exhumation?

- What are the dress codes that locals will expect your team to follow?

- How much local involvement is allowed in the examination and recovery of the remains? In some cultures, local people may want to take part. You may be able to accommodate their wishes, although questions of legal liability may need to be explored with your organization. However, at crime scenes, and at other evidential exhumations, no local involvement is likely to be permitted—regardless of local wishes—owing to the risk of accidental or deliberate contamination of evidence.

- How will you shield sensitive work from the unwanted view of the public and media? Shielding human remains may intensify public excitement and rumor. So it could be appropriate to have some skeletal remains on view. It is probably not appropriate to have bodies with soft tissue on view.

- Where will the remains go immediately after excavation, and are storage facilities there adequate and permanent enough for the requirements of the project?

- What transport and packaging requirements are needed for samples and remains?

- Do arrangements need to be made for reinterment, and, if so, when will reinterment happen, and how will the bodies be treated? Will they be put in their original graves, in new individual graves, or in a mass grave?

- What ceremonies will be required at reinterment, and how will you resolve competing claims for rituals?

- What will the site look like after restoration?

- Will a monument or monuments be required?
- Who will require reports on the work, and what will they need to know?
- Importantly, who will finance all these requirements?
- In briefing the team, have you discussed why human remains are publicly sensitive items? For example:
  —they remind people of their own mortality;
  —they may disturb those who have lost loved ones;
  —seeing and disturbing the dead may be celebrated in some cultures but taboo in others;
  —the public may be concerned about whether relatives and friends have given consent to what you are doing;
  —young children may find the sight of human remains traumatic;
  —human remains may stimulate morbid curiosity and macabre behavior in some people.

In briefing the team, have you asked them to:

- tell you if they are reacting badly to the task of handling the remains, with a view to being assigned more general duties;
- show tact and respect in dealing with human remains;
- follow appropriate dress codes—codes may be different for men and women, but the aspects to consider usually relate to covering the head, covering the shoulders, and wearing trousers rather than shorts;
- ensure that the work of excavation is not presented as a spectacle;
- encourage visitors not to see the remains as bizarre but (where appropriate) to feel empathy with the dead and their former lifestyles;
- treat fellow team members with respect and understanding—the more so if the work is physically and psychologically disturbing;
- realize that emotionally disruptive behavior may lead to a person being asked to leave the team;
- enter into voluntary after work activities (for example, a meal, outings) so that off-site interaction among members may help counter stress.

Some human remains may have to be excavated at the point of a gun in a socially hostile environment, for example, in gathering evidence for an international tribunal. If this is the scenario, have you prepared your team for the abandonment of the channels of getting permission (channels that they will see as customary) and the consequent surrender of many of the ethical considerations included in these notes?

Protocols during and after Excavation

- Who can handle the remains during excavation and removal?
- Who can see the remains during excavation and removal?
- Have you assigned somebody to answer questions from the public?
- Would it be useful to have a leaflet about the work to give to interested persons?

Prepare for Dealing with the Media before They Turn Up

- Decide what you will communicate to the media, and how.
- If necessary, get prior agreement from the media for restricting identity of victims and witnesses or team members, and for a moratorium on sensitive information.
- Assign somebody to answer questions from the media.
- Advise the rest of the team to politely decline answering questions from the media and to refer the media to the assigned person.
- Tell team members to watch what they say if approached by strangers (both on and off site).
- Make it plain to the media that any photography or filming must be restricted to specific periods; if the media is allowed to film at any time, then it places too much strain on the behavior of the team, who may, for example, be caught off their guard laughing or engaging in the relief of stress by dark humor.
- Assure yourself that you know the context in which information given to the media will be used.
- Do not assume the media is on your side; do not assume the media will be well-disposed in the representation of your

work, regardless of what they say when they approach you.

- Have you located clean areas of the site for eating, chatting, and smoking?
- Are the ablutions a respectful distance away from the remains?
- Where can the remains be taken?
- Can remains be put on public exhibition, if, for example, aggrieved relatives want this?
- Would this conflict with your organization's mission statement?

Photographs

- Who can photograph the human remains, including video and film?
- Your team members will want to take their own photographs. If they are forbidden, they will feel aggrieved when they see others taking unofficial photos. Consider the pragmatic guideline that what is open to the public and media to photograph is also open to team members to photograph.
- Who can look at the photographs?
- Is enhancement of photographs allowed?
- Where can photographs be published? For example:
  —in the media?
  —in scientific papers or scientific books?
- Where can photographs be publicly exhibited?
- If photographs are to be included in a report to local individuals, have you considered including a statement on the front cover along the lines of: "Warning—this report contains pictures of human remains."

Research

- Who authorizes any research on the human remains?
- What permissions are required and from whom: families, communities, authorities, agencies, judiciaries?
- Is the research being undertaken restricted to assisting in the identification of the victims, or is research allowed for more general scientific advancement?
- Who is allowed to undertake the research?
- Are researchers required to lodge copies of their field and laboratory notes?

- Can the results be published?
- What kind of research will be undertaken? For example:
  —invasive;
  —parts of the body temporarily removed for nondestructive analysis such as measurement;
  —parts of the body permanently removed for nondestructive analysis, for example, to a Museum of pathology;
  —parts of the body removed for destructive analysis, for instance, DNA, radiocarbon dating, or stable isotope analysis.

Note

1. A Scene of Crime Officer (SOCO), also referred to as a Crime Scene Examiner, is responsible for recording, photographing, sampling, and recovering evidence (Hunter and Cox 2005: 6).

References

Ehrenreich, J. H. 2005. *The Humanitarian Companion*. Rugby: ITDG Publishing.

Eliot, G. 1866. *Felis Holt: The Radical*. Edinburgh: W. Blackwood.

Haddow, G. D., and Bullock, J. A. 2006. *Introduction to Emergency Management*. Oxford: Butterworth Heinemann.

Hamilton, C. 2000. Faultlines: The construction of archaeological knowledge at Catalhoyuk, in I. Hodder (ed.), *Towards Reflexive Methods in Archaeology: The Example at Catalhoyuk*, pp. 119–128. Oxbow: McDonald Institute of Archaeological Research/British Institute of Archaeology at Ankara.

Harrison, A. A., and Connors, M. M. 1984. Groups in exotic environments, in L. Z. Berkowitz, (ed.), *Advances in Experimental Social Psychology*, pp. 49–87. New York: Academic Press, Inc.

Historic Scotland. 1997. *The Treatment of Human Remains in Archaeology*. Operational Policy Paper (Historic Scotland) 5. Edinburgh: Historic Scotland.

Hunter, J., and Cox, M. 2005. Introduction, in J. Hunter and M. Cox (eds.), *Forensic Archaeology: Advances in Theory and Practice*, pp. 1–26. London: Routledge.

Levinson, J., and Granot, H. 2002. *Transportation Disaster Response Handbook*. San Diego: Academic Press.

Moore, L. 1986. Patterns without Rhythm: Social Structure Ambiguity in an Archaeological Field Camp. M.A. thesis, University of Montana.

N.S.W. Heritage Office. 1998. *Skeletal Remains: Guidelines for the Management of Human Skeletal*

Remains under the Heritage Act 1977. Sydney: N.S.W. Heritage Office.

Pan American Health Organisation. 2004. *Management of Dead Bodies in Disaster Situations*. Disaster Manuals and Guidelines Series, No 5. Washington, D.C.

Snow, C. 1982. Forensic anthropology. *Annual Review of Anthropology* 11: 97–150.

Williams, E. (ed.). 2001. *Human Remains: Conservation, Retrieval and Analysis*. Oxford: Archaeopress.

Wright, R., Hanson, I., and Sterenberg, J. 2005. The archaeology of mass graves, in J. Hunter and M. Cox (eds.), *Forensic Archaeology: Advances in Theory and Practice*, pp. 137–158. London: Routledge.

39

CONTRIBUTION OF QUANTITATIVE METHODS IN FORENSIC ANTHROPOLOGY: A NEW ERA

Ann H. Ross and Erin H. Kimmerle

The emergence of any new field of study begins with a description of what it is and what it may become.

In the United States, the first methods for estimating the biological profile of unknown individuals in a forensic context were developed in the 19th century by Thomas Dwight (1843–1911). Dr. Dwight, a Harvard anatomist, used "inverse regression"[1] to estimate stature, sex, and age from skeletal remains. While the field of forensic anthropology would not become officially recognized in the United States by the forensic sciences as its own discipline until after 1972,[2] the methods produced by Dwight set the stage for the early development of the field and established its quantitative basis (İşcan 1989; Stewart 1979).

The need to identify war dead during World War II and the Korean War ignited a surge of research on methods for biological profiling and human identification. This body of work included methods for age (Brooks and Suchey 1990; Hoffman 1979; İşcan, Loth, and Wright 1984, 1985; Lamendin et al. 1992; McKern and Stewart 1957; Moorees, Fanning, and Hunt 1963; Stewart 1979; Todd 1920; Ubelaker 1989), sex (Giles and Elliot 1963; Krogman 1962), ancestry (Giles and Elliot 1962), and stature (Trotter 1970; Trotter and Gleser 1952, 1958) estimation—which have become known as the *four pillars of forensic anthropology.*

Statistical methodology for biological profiling has been largely based on descriptive and univariate statistical methods, such as regression, discriminant function analysis, and principal components analysis. In addition to univariate statistics, the concept of *descriptive methodology* appropriately characterizes much of the research in forensic anthropology. A qualitative approach, as evidenced through published technical notes, case studies, and the annual American Academy of Forensic Sciences (AAFS) academy meeting presentations, has even lead to the idiom that forensic anthropologists are lower on the academic food chain, lest they present 'gee whiz' cases in place of scientifically rigorous research. This problem is not unique to anthropology, but has plagued all areas of forensic science to such a degree that scientific evidence has been called into question and at times excluded from trial (Lynch and Jasanoff 1998; Robertson and Vignaux 1995; Saks and Koehler 2005; Waits, Luikart, and Taberlet 2001). This paradox has even lead some skeptics to question the very use of the term *science* with *forensic.*

In the past, forensics has been viewed as an *applied science*, relying on research and methodology from established disciplines such as biology and medicine, which in turn 'apply' expertise to legal and social problems. Statistical analyses have been largely descriptive (Gullberg 1993). As the forensic sciences have developed in recent years, there is an emerging trend for each discipline to be more research driven, including anthropology. The complex problems facing investigators today requires specialized knowledge and scientific pursuits directed towards answering a variety of specific legal and medical questions. In other words, the legal issues that arise during the process of a trial are now steering the direction of scientific research directed towards answering medico-legal questions (Christensen 2004; Rogers and Allard 2004; Steadman, Adams, and Konigsberg 2006; Kimmerle and Jantz 2008; Kimmerle et al. 2008a, 2008b).

One only needs to look at challenges to the presentation of scientific evidence in court to realize that a legal context changes the role and responsibilities of the scientist (Wilson 2005). Rogers and Allard (2004) outline the American and Canadian standards for the scientific presentation of evidence in court. The qualifications of a scientific expert witness and the admissibility of scientific evidence in the United States are defined in *Frye v. United States, 54 App. D.C. 46, 47, 293F. 1013, 1014, 1923;* Federal Evidence Rule 702, 2001; and *Daubert v. Merrell Dow Pharmaceuticals, Inc. 509 US 579, 199.* The U.S. Federal standard is based on the Supreme Court ruling of *Daubert v. Merrell Dow Pharmaceuticals, Inc.* (1993), which requires a scientific method to be more than "generally accepted" and to have known or potential error rates associated with it, thus putting pressure on the forensic community to standardize and test their methods. Much of the driving force behind the push for quantitative methods and research driven methodology, stems from challenges to DNA and fingerprint evidence (Robertson and Vignaux 1995; Rogers and Allard 2004; Waits, Luikart, and Taberlet 2001). Culminating from this trend, current research in forensic anthropology is largely focused on the use of quantitative methods, Bayesian statistical modeling, probability and maximum likelihood theory, and the use of new technologies such as virtual modeling of 3D imaging. The following chapter delineates the contribution of quantitative methods to the field of forensic anthropology.

Quantitative Methods for the Four Pillars of Biological Profiling

The question of human variation, as it pertains to biological profiling for unknown victims in medico-legal cases, is paramount for the increasing number of anthropologists working globally investigating crimes against International Humanitarian Law. Human variation was once an academic pursuit of interest to skeletal biologists, demographers, and palaeoanthropologists—not lawyers. However, the question of whether methods for estimating biological profiles are reliable universally is now a legal question. Consequently the focus of forensic anthropologists on the identification of unknown individuals, has contributed significantly to the study of human skeletal remains, especially in developing the standards used by the discipline as a whole. Aykroyd and coauthors (1997: 261) wrote:

> . . . there is still a case to be made in favour of the "forensic" approach in situations where there may be a limited number of individuals available for study, such as the prehistoric tumuli of Western Europe, or whenever the anthropologist needs to know the age of a specific individual. The "forensic" approach should be seen as complementary to the emerging techniques of estimating population age structure.

As a result, forensic anthropology is at the forefront of innovative and modern quantitative methods for the study of human variation. In the last decade, we have seen a transformation from indiscriminately and inappropriately utilizing equations developed from American populations on other populations to the development of population-specific identification standards (e.g., Del Angel and Cisneros 2004; Ross and Konigsberg 2002; Ross et al. 2004; Schaefer and Black 2005; and Indriati this volume). Further, Kemkes-Grottenthaler (2002: 64) provides a brief review of various studies that have found significant population variation in "biologically induced differences in the aging mechanisms." In fact, this transformation can be unmistakably seen in the quality and nature of the papers being presented at the Academy[3] meetings with much more attention being given to the "large-scale" issues that we have been criticized for lacking in the past. Multivariate statistical analysis and probability theory are essential to understanding human variation, improving existing methods, and developing new identification methods.

Sex and Ancestry

The estimation of sex and ancestry are key components when rendering a biological profile from skeletal or badly decomposed remains. The precise estimation of sex and ancestry are critical in the identification process, because they can narrow the search for an unknown individual, which can lead to identification. The estimation of sex and ancestry is the first step in a biological profile; other analyses such as age and stature are sex- and ancestry-specific and cannot be adequately determined without this information.

A key component to expediting the identification process is the ability to most accurately determine race or ancestral information from skeletal remains. Knowledge of the ethnic origins of an individual drastically narrows the search for missing persons, and this can ultimately increase the speed and likelihood of successful victim identification and facilitate the reconstruction of the events surrounding a crime.

Traditional Craniometric Methods. Since the 1960s, forensic anthropologists have utilized their knowledge of population variation to develop measurement standards and discriminant functions to estimate ancestry from human remains (Giles and Elliot 1962; Ubelaker, Ross, and Graver 2002). In the mid-1980s, Richard Jantz, from the University of Tennessee, created the Forensic Data Bank using traditional techniques of size and shape analysis based on linear measurements to assemble skeletal data for improving identification methods (Jantz and Moor-Jansen 1988; Moore-Jansen, Ousley, and Jantz 1994). This effort resulted in the computer program FORDISC 2.0 (Ousley and Jantz 1996) (recently upgraded to FORDISC 3.0), which is widely used by forensic practitioners and derives custom discriminant functions for up to 21 cranial measurements to classify unknown crania into 7 possible racial groupings (White, Black, Amerind, Japanese, Hispanic, Chinese, and Vietnamese) dependent on the sex of the individual. The utility of the software is dependent on the similarity of the unknown skull to one of the reference populations within FORDISC (Ubelaker, Ross, and Graver 2002).

Historically, methods of size and shape analysis, such as those employed by FORDISC, have relied on the application of multivariate statistical methods (for example, multivariate analysis of variance, discriminant function analysis) to sets of caliper measurements that correspond to linear distances, and sometimes to angles (Lynch, Wood, and Luboga 1996; Rohlf and Marcus 1993; Ross, McKeown, and Konigsberg 1999). One of the major limitations of this type of data acquisition and analysis is that the measurements or angles are ultimately based on the positions of the endpoints, or anatomical landmarks, by which they are defined, yet they encode only incomplete information about the relative positions of these defining points (Bookstein 1991; Slice 2005). In many such cases, for instance, information on biological variation crucial for ancestral determination may not be conveniently oriented along the span of such caliper measurements as are commonly recorded in a traditional analysis (e.g., Ross, McKeown, and Konigsberg 1999).

3D Methods: Geometric Morphometrics. Modern methods of size and shape analysis, called *geometric morphometrics*, address the potentially serious problems of traditional methods by focusing on the analysis of landmark coordinates (Rohlf and Marcus 1993; Slice 2005). Such data completely and efficiently archive the geometric information available in the landmarks, and any traditional measurement based on the same points can easily be recovered by using elementary geometric formulae. Furthermore, since these methods retain the geometric relationships between the points throughout an analysis, graphical depictions are possible that allow one to more easily relate the results of abstract multivariate procedures directly to the morphology of interest.

Once sets of coordinate data have been superimposed in a common coordinate system, using the method of Generalized Procrustes Analysis (GPA) (see Rohlf and Slice 1990; Slice 2005 for methodological details), they can be treated as multivariate shape variables and subjected to familiar statistical procedures such as principal components analysis, the construction of multigroup classification functions, and canonical variates analysis. These newer morphometric methods using 3D landmark coordinates can provide considerably more anatomical information than their traditional counterparts, but they have received little to no application in forensic anthropology or victim identification (Ross, McKeown, and Konigsberg 1999).

The value of these newer methods in the forensics setting is illustrated by the results of Ross and colleagues (1999), who found that although the geometric morphometry classification results for an American Black and an American White sample were comparable to traditional discriminant analysis, the newer methods outperformed traditional methods in their ability to locate specific regions of variability that would otherwise have remained undetected. In addition, because geometric morphometry was able to detect the specific regions of variation, individuals could be classified according to a reduced set of landmarks instead of the whole suite of measurements necessary with traditional caliper methods. Using a reduced set of landmarks can also extend the utility of this method to the identification of fragmentary remains.

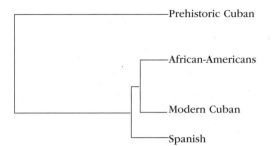

Figure 39.1 Phenogram showing the morphological affinity of modern Cuban crania to modern African-American and European Spanish samples and dissimilarity of the modern and prehistoric Cubans. Results based on UPGMA clustering of squared Mahalanobis distances between sample means computed from GPA-superimposed, 3D landmark coordinates (see Ross and coworkers [2004] for details).

This technology would be particularly useful in geographic regions where large ethnically diverse populations predominate. In a recent study, Ross and associates (2004) demonstrated that modern Cubans show a strong African affinity followed by a Spanish component while lacking an indigenous Amerindian biological affinity (Figure 39.1 and Figure 39. 2). Figure 39.2 depicts the mean difference in relative landmark location of cranial landmarks in Mexican and Cuban populations. Here, differences in mean landmark locations are shown as difference vectors magnified by a factor of 2. The Mexican crania are shown to be characterized by more lateral zygomaxillare, more inferiorly placed opisthion, more superiorly placed eurions, and more posteriorly positioned landmarks throughout the upper face.

A study presented by Rosas and Bastir (2002) investigating allometry through 3D morphometrics

and sexual dimorphism among a Portuguese population demonstrated that size and sex had a significant influence on shape of the craniofacial region. In a more recent study, Pretorius and coworkers (2006) report preliminary findings that the shape of the eye orbits are more sexually dimorphic than the commonly used mandibular ramus. Morphometric techniques may help us better understand the relationship between the size and the shape of craniofacial features. They may help to quantify the shape variables forensic anthropologists routinely use and additionally, point out new areas of the skeleton to use for estimating sex from human remains. More recently, cross-populational studies of sexual dimorphism also illustrate the importance of secular trends (Kimmerle, Ross, and Slice 2008). Therefore, the creation of population standards should take into account secular trends, as well as genetic diversity. This again highlights the importance of choosing the right reference sample for the creation of international parameters for estimation.

We do not anticipate that geometric morphometric methods will immediately replace more traditional methods, but they can be viewed as the next logical step in developing new tools for victim identification. As an added benefit, these new methods conveniently utilize the same standard craniofacial landmarks known to most forensic scientists and can thereby address all the shortcomings associated with the analysis of sparse linear measurements in a familiar context.

Stature

Stature is one of the initial parameters of the biological profile used to confirm or exclude presumptive identifications. Traditionally, stature equations developed from U.S. skeletal samples have been inappropriately and indiscriminately applied to

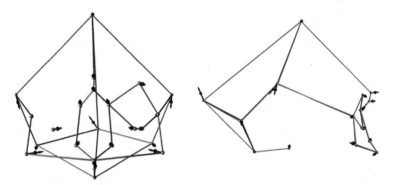

Figure 39.2 Morphological differences (x2) between modern Mexicans and modern Cubans.

different populations. In the past decade, however, the identification efforts in the Former Yugoslavia underscored the inappropriateness of applying nonlocal standards for sex, age, and stature estimation (Komar 2003; Ross and Konigsberg 2002; Schaefer and Black 2005; Steadman and Haglund 2005). Although the absence of antemortem medical and dental records was the major problem, in the Former Yugoslavia it was evident early on that stature equations based on Trotter and Gleser underestimated stature in the Balkan populations.

Although a Bayesian approach for estimation or the preservation of evidence has been utilized in the forensic sciences, it has received little attention in forensic anthropology (Konigsberg, Ross, and Jungers 2006). Historically, a Bayesian approach to data analysis has been criticized by classical statisticians, who do not accept the use of informative or known priors, arguing that this method produces biased estimates (Ross and Konigsberg 2002). However, Konigsberg and colleagues (1998) discuss the arguments for applying a Bayesian versus a maximum likelihood approach to stature estimation and contend that, in forensic anthropology, the Bayesian model should be the preferred method.

Basically, Bayesian inference is based on the idea of using both unconditional (the *prior probability* of a particular stature in the target sample) and conditional (the probability from the reference sample of obtaining the observed long-bone length conditional on a given stature) probabilities to produce informed parameters. Bayes's theorem states that the probability of s is equal to s, given

$$P_T\left(s|lb\right)= \frac{P_R\left(lb|s\right)\times P_T\left(s\right)}{\int\left\{P_R\left(lb|s\right)\times P_T\left(s\right)\right\}ds}$$

where $P_T\left(s|lb\right)$ is the posterior distribution for s. Ross and Konigsberg (2002) presented a Bayesian solution to stature estimation where the reference sample provided information about the relationship between long-bone length and stature [shown above as $P_R(lb|s)$], but the prior for stature originated from the known stature distribution for the living population from which the forensic case was drawn [shown above as $P_T(s)$]. Because it is known that Eastern Europeans are taller than American Whites, they used this information as a known prior in their analysis.

Age-at-Death

Statistical methods for estimating age-at-death from skeletal remains consist of univariate and multivariate statistical models that cover both morphological and metric data for teeth and bones. Therefore, a number of models have been used for continuous and discrete traits, among both juveniles and adults. Age parameters are generally based on descriptive statistics or regression (inverse calibration). Investigations into the accuracy and reliability of various techniques have also employed diverse statistical methods. Multivariate methods have been used to statistically combine multiple age indicators. Owing to individual variation and the wide age parameters associated with aging technique, it is imperative that multivariate trait analysis be used to establish the biological age-at-death of skeletons. Yet, the estimation of an age-at-death interval based on numerous criteria from a variety of skeletal traits is often problematic because of the suite of possible trait combinations at each age, the strong association between age-progressive skeletal features, and the lack of standardization among skeletal biologists in determining age parameters. Often, osteologists rely on experience to "average" the aging information for each individual and establish the age interval.

Increasingly, the need for anthropological methods to be based in probability statistics is being addressed. Probability theory establishes the outcomes that are possible and the likelihood of achieving each of those outcomes. In other words, probability theory informs investigators if their conclusions are random and the result of chance or due to an actual treatment (that is, a correct identification).

In a Bayesian model, phase (i) is regressed onto age (t): $i = a + b * t$. Phase is assumed to be dependent on age to calculate the maximum likelihood estimate of age conditional on phase: Pr(age – phase). Hoppa and Vaupel (2002: 2) point out that the probability of being a certain age, given a particular skeletal characteristic Pr(age |phase), must be calculated from the probability of obtaining the characteristic through Bayes's Theorem. Hoppa and Vaupel (2002: 2) wrote:

> Even the most experienced and intelligent osteologists cannot make this calculation in their heads. Pencil and paper or a computer is required, as well as information concerning f(a), the probability distribution of ages-at-death (i.e., life span) in the target population of interest.

A Bayesian approach requires the distribution of age, f(age), which must be estimated or taken from a reference sample of identified age.

Studies demonstrating the need for this methodological approach and several methods that actually offer a multitrait approach with aging parameters have been put forth to improve the accuracy of age estimation (i.e., Acsádi and Nemeskéri 1970; Boldsen et al. 2002; Gustafson 1955; Holman, Wood, and O'Connor 2002; Kongisberg and Frankenberg 1992; Kongisberg and Holman 1999; Lovejoy, Meindl, and Barton 1985). However, multitrait methods are rarely applied in practice and pose their own statistical challenges.

Kimmerle and Konigsberg (2004) presented an example of how a multivariate statistical approach may be applied to age estimation. This test used a set of Bayesian statistical methods, maximum likelihood estimates, and a Gompertz-Makeham hazard model (Wood et al. 1992) and demonstrated that a multiple-trait approach, in combination with an informed prior, produces the most accurate age estimates.

Three aging techniques were investigated, the sternal rib (İşcan, Loth, and Wright 1984, 1985), tooth wear (Ubelaker 1989), and tooth root translucency (Lamendin et al. 1992). The full conditional (on age) distribution of indicators using a "maximum weight dependence tree" was approximated (Chow and Liu 1968; Lucy, Aykroyd, and Pollard 2002). This approach uses a trivariate distribution:

$$\Pr\left(\text{rib, wear, trans}\,|\,\text{age}\right) \cong$$
$$\Pr\left(\text{rib}\,|\,\text{age}\right) \times \Pr\left(\text{wear}\,|\,\text{trans, age}\right) \times f\left(\text{trans}\,|\,\text{age}\right)$$

Second, Bayes's theorem was used to estimate age:

$$f(\text{age}\,|\,\text{rib, wear, trans}) = \Pr(\text{rib, wear, trans}\,|\,\text{age})\,f(\text{age})$$

$$f\left(\text{age}\,|\,\text{rib, wear, trans}\right) =$$
$$\frac{\Pr\left(\text{rib, wear, trans}\,|\,\text{age}\right) \times f\left(\text{age}\right)}{\displaystyle\int_{t=15}^{\omega} \Pr\left(\text{rib, wear, trans}\,|\,t\right) \times f\left(t\right) dt}$$

In this equation, $f(\text{age})$ is a probability density function (pdf) for age, starting at age 15 years (the minimum possible age) and running to, the maximum possible age (100 years).

To demonstrate the advantage of using an informed prior, two methods for estimating the pdf of age were used. The first used a uniform prior, such that the pdf at any age between 15 and 100 is $1/(100 - 15)$. This approach is akin to "classical calibration"[4] and should have been immune to the problem of "regression to the mean";[5] however, it unrealistically assigned equal probability to all ages at death (Figure 39.3).

The second approach was based on a Maximum Likelihood (ML) derived hazard model, for which separate Gompertz-Makeham models

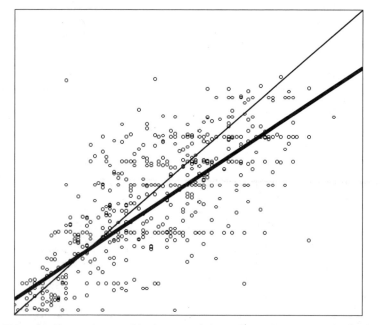

Figure 39. 3 Using a uniform prior, a multitrait approach is used to estimate age-at-death. The thinner diagonal line represents perfect prediction, and the heavier line represents the regression of estimated on actual age. Although this approach is based on "classical calibration," using a uniform prior inappropriately assumes an equal likelihood of age for all individuals. As a result, the age estimate for most individuals is misclassified. (This example and figure were taken from Kimmerle and Konigsberg [2004].)

were calculated from a population of identified individuals. This approach demonstrated that using a standard multiple-trait estimate to calculate skeletal age intervals does improve the accuracy of age estimation. Through the use of maximum likelihood estimates, the predicted ages were nearly identical to the actual ages-at-death (Figure 39.4).

As forensic anthropology becomes more global, one should exercise caution when applying current aging methods to diverse populations. Because many adult aging techniques rely on degenerative changes of the skeleton, one must understand the population for which these methods are being applied to. Even within the U.S., these aging techniques can produce less than satisfactory results. A case in point occurred in the identification efforts in the aftermath of Hurricane Katrina, when forensic anthropologists were consistently under-aging the elderly from Louisiana.

Innovative Technology for a New Era

The computer revolution of the 1980s, coupled with technological advancements in computer digitizing, laser scanning, computerized tomography

(CT), and magnetic resonance imaging (MRI), has empowered the anthropological and medical communities to enter a new era of research and methodology. As a result, multivartiate statistics are used by anthropologists to compute metric and shape variables in all areas of human identification with sophistication and ease.

Innovative advancements in 3D imaging have enabled the use of computerized tomography (CT) and geometric morphometric techniques to analyze and implement biometric variables for personal identification and trauma analysis (Meyers et al. 1999). CT technology is a powerful tool for identifying useful internal structures that are not externally visible, describing biological form quantitatively in three dimensions, and visually displaying such evidence to a jury or court. 3D-CT technology (Figure 39.5) is being used by forensic anthropologists to establish a baseline for understanding human variation as well as the various aspects of the biological profile of unknown, unidentified victims of criminal activity, natural disasters, terrorist attacks, and armed conflicts. CT technology is being used for facial reconstructions and to determine the sex, age, ancestry, and height of an individual from skeletal tissue. The accurate application of 3D imaging technology is a leading

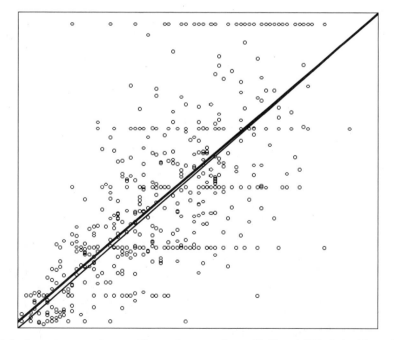

Figure 39.4 In contrast to using a uniform prior, a maximum likelihood (ML) derived hazard model is shown, for which separate Gompertz-Makeham models were calculated based on identified individuals. Note that the predicted ages are nearly identical to the actual ages-at-death. (This example and figure were taken from Kimmerle and Konigsberg [2004].)

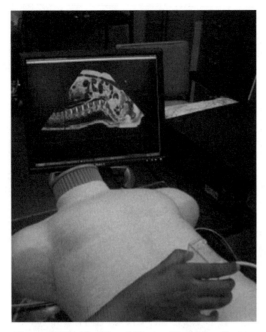

Figure 39.5 The Virtual Human Navigation System enables visualization and navigation of biometric image data in real time. Metric, shape, and volume metric data may be obtained, making this system the latest tool for investigative research in the biomedical and anthropological fields.

tool for investigators and has the potential to dramatically enhance the identification of missing children and adults. In addition, data from clinical CTs also would have the advantage of currency and quantity, since hundreds are produced at any given geographical location curtailing the issue of appropriate sample sizes. This is potentially important since significant secular changes have been documented in the cranial morphology in the U.S. over the past 200 years. Jantz and Meadows Jantz (2000) for example, noted considerable increase in heightening, narrowing, and lengthening of the vault along with heightening and narrowing of the face of American white crania within the last 135 years (see also Angel 1976, 1982; Jantz 2001; Kimmerle and Jantz 2005; Wescott and Jantz 2005).

The *Virtual Human Navigation System* (Hilbelink 2005a, 2005b; Hilbelink and Lothe 2005) is at the forefront of cutting edge technology and is a leading tool for teaching anatomy and virtual surgery to medical students. This system also has the potential to become an important teaching and analytical tool for forensic anthropologists for whom anatomy and osteology are critical. The *Virtual Human Navigation System* permits the import of any volumetric medical image data set for use in

the system and its registration in 3D space using the Cartesian coordinate system. The precise location and orientation of the pciBird tracker relative to the volumetric data can be followed in real time and can be used to obtain specific feature measurements of the structures contained within the image volume. This system offers the opportunity for a virtual classroom where the culmination of osteology, human anatomy, human variation, trauma analysis, and human identification are explored for instruction or for multivariate-based research for any biometric data.

Conclusion

Trotter's work on WWII casualties has formed the basis of stature estimation for several generations of forensic anthropologists. To discard vital information from war victims would be a disservice to those who seek identification of the victims. The development of local identification standards would be impossible without preservation of skeletal information. This approach has been used to good effect in forensic cases resulting in the Forensic Anthropology Data Bank.

The burgeoning field of forensic anthropology has come full circle as the methods and studies produced to answer medico-legal questions are being applied to more traditional areas of study such as in human biology, bioarchaeology, and palaeoanthropology. The subfield of biological anthropology, once viewed as merely an application of knowledge, is now a dynamic and innovative field of study where problem-oriented questions are a driving force in medico-legal research, even setting new standards for biological anthropology as a whole.

Acknowledgments

We would like to thank Lyle Konigsberg and Richard Jantz for forcing us to take many years of statistics courses and ensuring that our research approach was through rigorous quantitative methods. We would also like to acknowledge Lyle for use of Figures 39.3 and 39.4 and the associated research example, extracted from a 2004 presentation. We also thank Dennis Slice for introducing us to and training us on the use of *Geometric Morphometrics*—his software made such research possible. We also thank Don Hilbelink for use of the Figure 39.5.

Notes

1. "Inverse regression" is one means of establishing a relationship between variables. In inverse

calibration, the y variable is predicted from the x variable. Continuous y variables in this example include age, sex, or stature.

2. The first section of Forensic Anthropology organized for the American Academy of Forensic Science annual meeting was in 1972 (Rhine 1998).

3. "Academy" refers to the American Academy of Forensic Sciences, which publishes abstracts for the Annual Meeting Program.

4. "Classical calibration" is an alternative approach to "inverse calibration." In "classical calibration," y is regressed onto x. The results are used to estimate the unknown parameters of x from the known parameters of y. "Classical calibration" is considered a superior form of calibration and is recommended for forensic methods, particularly in formulating aging estimates (Aykroyd et al. 1997; Konigsberg, Frankenberg, and Walker 1994).

5. "Regression to the mean" is a common problem when using regression or "inverse calibration" techniques. It refers to the phenomena of age estimates over-aging young individuals and under-aging old individuals (Konigsberg and Frankenberg 2002).

References

Angel, J. L. 1976. Colonial to modern skeletal change in the U.S.A. *American Journal of Physical Anthropology* 45: 723–736.

———. 1982. A new measure of growth efficiency: Skull base length. *American Journal of Physical Anthropology* 58: 297–305.

Acsádi, G., and Nemeskéri, J. 1970. *History of Human Lifespan and Mortality*. Budapest: Akademiai Kiado.

Aykroyd, R. G., Lucy, D., Pollard, A. M., and Solheim, T. 1997. Technical note: Regression analysis in adult age estimation. *American Journal of Physical Anthropology* 104: 259–265.

Bookstein, F. L. 1991. *Morphometric Tools for Landmark Data: Geometry and Biology.* Cambridge: Cambridge University Press.

Boldsen, J. L., Milner, G. R., Konigsberg, L. W., and Wood, J. W. 2002. Transition analysis: A new method for estimating age from skeletons, in R. D. Hoppa and J. W. Vaupel (eds.), *Paleodemography: Age Distributions from Skeletal Samples*, pp. 73–106. Cambridge: Cambridge University Press.

Brooks, S. T., and Suchey, J. M. 1990. Skeletal age determination based on the os pubis: A comparison of the Ascáadi-Nemeskéri and Suchey-Brooks methods. *Human Evolution* 5: 227–238.

Christensen, A. M. 2004. The impact of Daubert: Implications for testimony and research in forensic anthropology (and the use of frontal sinuses in personal identification). *Journal of Forensic Sciences* 49: 427–430.

Chow, C. K., and Liu, C. N. 1968. Approximating discrete probability distributions with dependence trees. *IEEE Transactions on Information Theory* 14: 462–467.

Daubert v. Merrell Dow Pharmaceuticals. 1993. 113 S.Ct. 2786; U.S. LEXIS 4408.

Del Angel, A., and Cisneros, H. B. 2004. Technical note: Modification of regression equations to estimate stature in Mesoamerican skeletal remains. *American Journal of Physical Anthropology* 125: 264–265.

Giles, E., and Elliot, O. 1962. Race identification from cranial measurements. *Journal of Forensic Sciences* 7: 147–157.

———. 1963. Sex determination by discriminant function analysis of the mandible. *American Journal of Physical Anthropology* 22: 29–135.

Gustafson, G. 1955. Age determination on teeth. *Journal of the American Dental Association* 41: 45–54.

Hilbelink, D. R. 2005a. Human spatial morphometrics. *Clinical Anatomy* 18: 627.

———. 2005b. Three-dimensional Cartesian coordinate system for the human body. *Clinical Anatomy* 118: 627.

Hilbelink, D. R., and Lothe, A. 2005. Virtual human navigation system. *Clinical Anatomy* 18: 627–628.

Hoffman, J. M. 1979. Age estimations from diaphyseal lengths: Two months to twelve years. *Journal of Forensic Sciences* 24: 461–469.

Holman, D. J., Wood, J. W., and O'Connor, K. A. 2002. Estimating age-at-death distributions from skeletal samples: A multivariate latent-trait approach, in R. D. Hoppa and J. W. Vaupel (eds.), *Paleodemography: Age Distributions from Skeletal Samples*, pp. 193–221. Cambridge: Cambridge University Press.

Hoppa, R. D., and Vaupel, J. W. (eds.). 2002. *Paleodemography: Age Distributions from Skeletal Samples*. Cambridge: Cambridge University Press.

Howells, W. W. 1973. *Cranial Variation in Man*. Papers of the Peabody Museum of Archaeology and Ethnology Harvard University, Vol. 51.

İşcan, Y. M. 1989. *Age Markers in the Human Skeleton*. Springfield, IL: Charles C. Thomas.

İşcan, Y. M., Loth, S., and Wright, R. 1984. Age estimation from the rib by phase analysis: White males. *Journal of Forensic Sciences* 29: 1094–1104.

———. 1985. Age estimation from the rib by phase analysis: White females. *Journal of Forensic Sciences* 30: 853–863.

Jantz, R. L. 2001. Cranial change in Americans: 1850–1975. *Journal of Forensic Sciences* 46: 784–787.

Jantz, R. L., and Meadows Jantz, L. 2000. Secular change in craniofacial morphology. *American Journal of Human Biology* 12: 327–338.

Jantz, R. L., and Moore-Jansen, P. H. 1988. *A Data Base for Forensic Anthropology: Structure, Content and Analysis.* Report of Investigations No. 47, Department of Anthropology, The University of Tennessee.

Kemkes-Grottenthaler, A. 2002. Historical perspectives on age indicator methods, in R. Hoppa and J. W. Vaupel (eds.), *Paleodemography: Age Distributions from Skeletal Samples*, pp. 48–72. London: Cambridge University Press.

Kimmerle, E. H., and Jantz, R. L. 2005. Secular trends in craniofacial asymmetry studies by geometric morphometry and generalized procrustes methods, in D. E. Slice (ed.), *Modern Morphometrics in Physical Anthropology:*, pp. 247–263. Dordrecht: Kluwer Academic Publishers.

———. 2008. Variation as evidence: Introduction to a symposium on international human identification. *Journal of Forensic Sciences* 53(3): 521–523.

Kimmerle, E. H., Jantz, R. L., Konigsberg, L. W., and Baraybar, J. P. 2008a. Skeletal estimation and identification in American and East European populations. *Journal of Forensic Sciences* 53(3): 524–532.

Kimmerle, E. H., and Konigsberg, L. 2004. Estimating individual age-at-death parameters through multitrait Bayesian analysis. Poster presentation to the American Association for Physical Anthropology Annual Meeting, Dallas, TX.

Kimmerle, E. H., Konigsberg, L. W., Jantz, R. L., and Baraybar, J. P. 2008b. Analysis of age-at-death estimation through the use of pubic symphyseal data. *Journal of Forensic Sciences* 53(3): 558–568.

Kimmerle, E. H, Ross, A. H., and Slice, D. 2008. Sexual dimorphism in America: Geometric morphometric analysis of what matters most. *Journal of Forensic Sciences* 53(1): 54–57.

Komar, D. 2003. Lessons from Srebrenica: The contributions and limitations of physical anthropology in identifying victims of war crimes. *Journal of Forensic Sciences* 48: 713–716.

Konigsberg L. W., and Frankenberg, S. R. 1992. Estimation of age structure in anthropological demography. *American Journal of Physical Anthropology* 89: 235–256.

———. 2002. Deconstructing death in paleodemography. *American Journal of Physical Anthropology* 117: 297–309.

Konigsberg, L. W., Frankenberg, S., and Walker, R. B. 1994. Regress what on what? Paleodemographic age estimation as a calibration problem, in Paine R.R. (ed.), *Integrating Archaeological Demography: Multidisciplinary Approaches to Prehistoric Population*, pp. 64–88. Carbondale: Southern Illinois University.

Konigsberg, L. W., Hens, S. M., Jantz, L. M., and Jungers, W. L. 1998. Stature estimation and calibration: Bayesian and maximum likelihood perspectives in physical anthropology. *Yearbook of Physical Anthropology* 41: 65–72.

Konigsberg, L., and Holman, D. J. 1999. Estimation of age at death from dental emergence and implications for studies of prehistoric somatic growth, in R. D. Hoppa and C. M. FitzGerald (eds.), *Human Growth in the Past: Studies from Bones and Teeth*, pp. 264–289. Cambridge: Cambridge University Press.

Konigsberg, L. W., Ross, A. H., and Jungers, W. L. 2006. Estimation and evidence in forensic anthropology: Determining stature, in A. Schmitt, E. Cunha and J. Pinheiro (eds.), *Forensic Anthropology and Forensic Medicine: Complementary Sciences from Recovery to Cause of Death*, pp. 317–331. Totowa, NJ: Humana Press.

Krogman, W. M. 1962. *The Human Skeleton in Forensic Medicine.* Springfield, IL: Charles C. Thomas.

Lamendin, H., Baccino, E., Humbert, J. F., Tavernier, T., Nossintchouk, R. M., and Zerilli, A. 1992. A simple technique for age estimation in adult corpses: The two criteria dental method. *Journal of Forensic Sciences* 37: 1373–1379.

Lovejoy, C. O., Meindl, R. S., and Barton, T. J. 1985. Multifactorial age determination of skeletal age at death: A method and blind tests of its accuracy. *American Journal of Physical Anthropology* 68: 1–14.

Lucy, D., Aykroyd, R. G., and Pollard, A. M. 2002. Nonparametric calibration for age estimation. *Applied Statistics* 51: 183–196.

Lynch, M., and Jasanoff, S. 1998. Introduction. Contested identities: Science, law and forensic Social Studies of Science, Special Issue on *Contested Identities: Science, Law and Forensic Practice* (Oct.–Dec., 1998) 28(5/6): 675–686.

Lynch, J. M., Wood, C. G., and Luboga, S. A. 1996. Geometric Morphometrics in Primatology: Craniofacial Variation in Homo sapiens and Pan troglodytes. *Folia Primatologia* 67: 15–39.

McKern, T., and Stewart, T. D. 1957. *Skeletal Age Changes in Young American Males, Analyzed from the Standpoint of Identification.* Technical report EP-45. Headquarters, Quartermaster Research and Development Command, Natick, MA.

Meyers, J., Okoye, M., Kipple, D., Kimmerle, E. H., Reinhard, K. 1999. Three-dimensional (3-D) imaging in post-mortem examinations: Elucidation and identification of cranial and facial fractures in victims of homicide utilizing 3-D computerized imaging reconstruction techniques. *International Journal of Legal Medicine* 113: 33–37.

Moore-Jansen, P. M., Ousley, S., and Jantz, R. L. 1994. *Data Collection Procedures for Forensic Skeletal*

Material. Report of Investigations 48, University of Tennessee, Anthropology Department, Knoxville, TN.

Moorees, C. F. A., Fanning, E. A., and Hunt, E. E. 1963. Formation and resorption of three deciduous teeth in Children. *American Journal of Physical Anthropology* 21: 205–213.

Ousley, S. D., and Jantz, R. L. 1996. [computer program] FORDISC 2.0. Knoxville: Department of Anthropology. The University of Tennessee, Knoxville.

Pretorius, E., Steyn, M., and Scholts, Y. 2006. Investigation into the usability of geometric morphometric analysis in assessment of sexual dimorphism. *American Journal of Physical Anthropology* 129: 64–70.

Robertson, B., and Vignaux, G. A. 1995. DNA evidence: Wrong answers or wrong questions? *Genetica* 96: 145–152.

Rohlf, F. J., and Marcus, L. F. 1993. A revolution in morphometrics. *Tree* 8: 129–132.

Rohlf, F. J., and Slice, D. E. 1990. Methods for comparison of sets of landmarks. *Systematic Zoology* 39: 40–59.

Rogers, T. L., and Allard, T. T. 2004. Expert testimony and positive identification of human remains through cranial suture patterns. *Journal of Forensic Sciences* 49:1–5.

Rosas, A., and Bastir, M. 2002. Thin-plate spine analysis of allometry and sexual dimorphism in the human craniofacial complex. *American Journal of Physical Anthropology* 117: 236–245.

Ross, A. H., and Konigsberg, L. W. 2002. New formulae for estimating stature in the Balkans. *Journal of Forensic Sciences* 47: 165–167.

Ross, A. H., McKeown, A. H., and Konigsberg, L. W. 1999. Allocation of crania to groups via the "New Morphomtry." *Journal of Forensic Sciences* 44: 584–587.

Ross, A. H., Slice, D. E., Ubelaker, D. H., and Falsetti, A. B. 2004. Population affinities of 19th century Cuban crania: Implications for identification criteria in South Florida Cuban Americans. *Journal of Forensic Sciences* 49: 11–16.

Saks, M. J., and Koehler, J. J. 2005. The coming paradigm shift in forensic identification. *Science* 309(5736): 892–895.

Schaefer, M. C., and Black, S. M. 2005. Comparison of ages of epiphyseal union in north American and Bosnian skeletal material. *Journal of Forensic Sciences* 50: 777–784.

Slice, D. E. 2005. Modern morphometrics, in D. E. Slice (ed.), *Modern Morphometrics in Physical Anthropology*, pp. 1–45. Dordrecht: Kluwer Academic Publishers.

Smith, B. H. 1984. Patterns of molar wear in hunter-gatherers and agriculturalists. *American Journal of Physical Anthropology* 63: 39–56.

Steadman, D. W., Adams, B. J., and Konigsberg, L. W. 2006. Statistical basis for positive identification in forensic anthropology. *American Journal of Physical Anthropology* 131(1): 15–26.

Steadman, D. W., and Haglund, W. D. 2005. The scope of anthropological contributions to human rights investigations. *Journal of Forensic Sciences* 50: 23–30.

Stewart, T. D. 1979. *Essentials of Forensic Anthropology*. Springfield, IL: Charles C. Thomas.

Todd, T. W. 1920. Age changes in the pubic bone: I, the male white pubis. *American Journal of Physical Anthropology* 3: 285–334.

Trotter, M. 1970. Estimation of stature from intact long limb bones, in T. D. Stewart (ed.), *Personal Identification in Mass Disasters*, pp. 71–84. Washington, D.C.: NMNH, Smithsonian Institution.

Trotter, M., and Gleser, G. C. 1952. Estimation of stature from long bones of American Whites and Negroes. *American Journal of Physical Anthropology* 10: 463–514.

———. 1958. A re-evaluation of estimation of stature based on measurements of stature taken during life and long bones after death. *American Journal of Physical Anthropology* 16: 79–123.

Ubelaker, D. H. 1984. Positive identification from the radiographic comparisons of frontal sinus patterns, in T. A. Rathbun and J. E. Buikstra (eds.), *Human Identification: Case Studies in Forensic Anthropology:*, pp. 399–411. Springfield, IL: Charles C. Thomas.

———. 1989. *Human Skeletal Remains* (2nd ed.). Washington, D.C.: Taraxacum Press.

Ubelaker, D. H., Ross, A. H., and Graver, S. M. 2002. Application of forensic discriminant functions to a Spanish cranial sample. *Forensic Science Communication* 4: http://fbi.gov/hq/lab/fsc/backissu/july2002/ubelaker1.htm.

Waits, L., Luikart, G., and Taberlet, P. 2001. Estimating the probability of identity among genotypes in natural populations: cautions and guidelines. *Molecular Ecology* 10: 249.

Wescott, D. J., and Jantz, R. L. 2005. Assessing craniofacial secular change in American Blacks and Whites using geometric morphometry, in D. E. Slice (ed.), *Modern Morphometrics in Physical Anthropology*, pp. 231–245. Dordrecht: Kluwer Academic Publishers.

Wilson, R. 2005. Judging history: The historical record of the International Criminal Tribunal for the Former Yugoslavia. *Human Rights Quarterly* 27: 908–942.

Wood, J. W., Holman, D. J., Weiss, K. M., Buchanan, A. V., and LeFor, B. 1992. Hazard models for human population biology. *Yearbook of Physical Anthropology* 35: 43–87.

40

THE EXPERT WITNESS AND THE COURT OF LAW

Maciej Henneberg

Most professionals are unprepared for the rigors of the courtroom and have no formal training in providing effective courtroom testimony. Aggressive cross-examination can often make the courtroom experience stressful and anxiety producing. By knowing what to expect, professionals will better manage their courtroom presentation and thereby become more effective witnesses. (Brodsky 2004)

Expert witnesses are engaged to determine specific facts of a case that may be ruled by civil or criminal law. The vast majority of the cases that archaeologists and biological anthropologists are involved in are criminal cases. Although I limit this chapter to description of actions of an expert witness in criminal cases, most of what I write about applies also to civil cases.

Expert witnesses usually start their involvement in a case by examining the evidence and providing a written report to the crime investigating authority. This report starts with a statement on the expert's qualifications, proceeds to describe facts, and ends with an opinion. Particular jurisdictions have specific rules determining the format of a report and types of information to be included. There are even specific forms to be used for witness reports. Depending on the case, the report may need to be supplemented by additional materials, such as detailed notes from an examination of

evidence, radiographs or CT scans, photographs, video illustrations of superimpositions, or photographic boards comparing video evidence from the crime scene (security closed circuit television systems) with photographs of the accused. If crime-investigating authorities, usually the police, decide to press charges, the prosecution uses determinations made by an expert witness to prepare a formal charge to be laid in the court of law. If the accused pleads guilty to the charges, sentencing follows and the case ends; thus ends the involvement of an expert witness.

If the plea of not guilty is entered, an expert witness oral testimony may be needed in court. At this stage of a case, another expert witness may also be engaged by the defence. Testimony of this expert witness will be presented in court, too. Whether an expert is engaged by the prosecution or by the defence, her or his first responsibility is to help the court to establish the facts of the case objectively, not to advocate for or against the accused. In many clear-cut cases in which an expert witness established material facts without the need for expressing specific opinion—for example, when sex and age of a skeleton were identified—there may be no need for the witness to appear in court. In my experience, court appearances are not common in the practice of forensic anthropology and archaeology, because written expert witness reports are considered sufficient in some cases. Thus many forensic anthropologists and archaeologists may be unfamiliar with the environment of courts of law and their procedures.

The court of law must hear testimony in the case rather than just read the reports, because each witness's testimony is subject to scrutiny by the court and to cross-examination by the prosecution or the defence. If the case is heard before a jury, then the jury must hear all testimonies as a series of witnesses' answers to specific, clearly formulated questions. Members of the jury come from all sectors of society and do not need to be able to understand technical details provided in the experts specialised reports. However, they must take the statements and opinions of expert witnesses into account when formulating their verdict.

Although expert witnesses may be called either by prosecution or by defence, the role of such witnesses is to determine objectively and impartially all facts falling into their area of expertise and to formulate a professional opinion that may help the court. Presenting an opinion is a task specific to an expert witness. Testimony from other witnesses, such as eye witnesses, for example, is limited to helping the court to establish facts only.

It is very difficult for anyone to remain completely impartial, especially if one is engaged, and often remunerated, by the police, prosecution, or defence. The way expert witness evidence should be presented both in written reports and in the court is regulated by Practice Directions issued from time to time by the courts (e.g., Federal Court of Australia 1998; Supreme Court of South Australia 2002). The precise role of expert witnesses and rules of their ethical conduct are subject to continuing debates (Freckleton, Reddy, and Selby 1999; McAbee and Freeman 2006). Such debates have a bearing on the conduct of an expert witness in court. Detailed advice on how an expert witness should act may vary from one area of expertise to the next and may depend on particular positions preferred by legal practitioners and experts with respect to fine points of ethics and interpretations of specific laws. Below I give my own view of how witnesses should act. This is based on experience gained during my successful appearances before courts in Poland, the United States of America, Republic of South Africa, and in various Australian jurisdictions.

Duties and Rights of an Expert Witness

Like any participant in legal proceedings, an expert witness has duties and rights. These duties and rights may be regulated by specific Practice Directions in different jurisdictions, but generally they follow similar rules. Adherence to these rules ensures that the testimony is clear and helpful to the court. The witness testifies under oath (or an affirmation, if nonreligious) and is thus liable to prosecution for perjury for making deliberately false statements.

Duties of an Expert Witness

Summary of the duties of an expert witness:

- Use all available knowledge and skills to determine the facts of the case. This normally calls for a peer-review of expert's findings before they are presented.

- Remain impartial and truthful in formulating an opinion.

- Provide information as required to prosecution, defence, and the court but to no one else. This includes not talking to the media before the case is complete.

- Explain findings fully and clearly so that they can be understood unequivocally by laypeople.

- Do not venture beyond one's area of expertise.

- Do not judge guilt or innocence.

- Appear in court when called (usually under subpoena).

- Disclose any conflict of interest that may produce bias.

Rights of an Expert Witness

Summary of the rights of an expert witness:

- To examine all exhibits and information related to the case (but only that which is relevant to the specific area of expertise).

- To request technical assistance.

- To be fairly compensated for time, expenses, and equipment used.

- To ask for an adjustment of dates/times of court appearances to expert's availability. Adjustment is not always possible, because the witness is under subpoena and must appear as directed.

- To ask to be excused after cross-examination is completed. This is not always possible, because the parties may wish to call the witness again at a later stage of the case.

Sequence of Events When the Case Comes to Court

There are several steps in the process of criminal justice. The involvement of an expert witness may be terminated after any of these steps.

Conference with Prosecution and Defence

Before a court hearing the witness may be asked to meet with both prosecution and defence legal teams simultaneously. This meeting takes place irrespective of which side engaged the witness, but it is not always required. The meeting has an informal format of a conversation between the witness and the parties. Conference is usually held on the day of the trial in a separate room in the court building. Lawyers for both sides have the expert's written report available to them and during the conference may question the witness on anything relevant to his/her role in the case. They usually probe details of the witness's qualifications, experience, and statements made in the report. The opposing side will try to gather information useful for weakening the importance of future testimony by the witness. The side that engaged the witness will listen carefully to questions asked by the opposing side and to the witness's answers in order to modify their future line of questioning in the court. This will bring out important aspects of the witness's findings that were not stated clearly enough in the written report.

During the conference, the expert must remain meticulously truthful and answer questions precisely but as briefly as possible, in order not to volunteer any peripheral information that may be used by the opposing side against the testimony. All answers will be scrupulously analysed by both sides, and any information additional to the written report will be scrutinised by the lawyers after the conference with the aim of bringing it out during cross-examination. Most experts, not being trained in the practice of the law, and being naturally enthusiastic about their expertise, tend to volunteer information beyond what is necessary for the case. This should be avoided.

Barristers who question witnesses in court are skilled at using psychology and sometimes even theatrical effects in order to win the case. During the conference, they will try to assess the personality of the witness to gain future advantage by choosing an appropriate style of questioning. Thus the demeanour of the expert during the conference should be calm, composed, self-assured, and helpful, but reserved. Expert witnesses should be careful about what they say during the conference:

they should not deviate from the truth and should avoid offering what is not asked for.

Layout of the Courtroom

The rest of the case is heard in the courtroom. The layout of a courtroom reflects the way a case is conducted. Size of the public gallery and some details may differ, but the essential elements of all courtrooms remain the same.

The bench for the presiding judge is located at the head of the courtroom on an elevated dais opposite the main entrance. The box for the jury is on one side of the bench; a dock for the accused is located on the other. The witness stand is near the jury's box or the dock. A table for stenographers, secretaries, judge's associates, and sheriffs is below the bench. Barristers' tables are located in the centre of the courtroom facing the bench. Each barrister is accompanied by a legal team usually comprising a solicitor, a junior lawyer, and sometimes an expert witness or a clerk. Seats for the public are at the back of the room in the space between the barrister's tables and the main entrance. The bench is the focal point of the courtroom and, when occupied by the judge, requires all persons present in the courtroom to face it and bow toward it when entering and leaving.

Admissibility of Evidence Hearing

The admissibility of evidence hearing (*voir dire*) is the first enquiry to be held in court and allows the judge to determine whether the evidence of an expert witness is good enough to be presented at the trial. This is not a public hearing. Only the judge, defence, prosecution, and accused are present. The witness appears under oath/affirmation, and proceedings are recorded. Questioning concentrates on establishing the qualifications of an expert and on the quality and relevance of the witness's findings. At the conclusion of the hearing, the judge rules whether the witness may be called during the trial. The judge uses specific rules of evidence in each legal system to determine the admissibility of a witness. The rules of evidence are being periodically altered in response to progress in specialist areas and in legal theories and practice (e.g., Federal Court of Australia 1998; Supreme Court of South Australia 2002).

The Committal Hearing

The aim of this hearing is to determine whether the case should proceed to a trial. A committal hearing is held in a lower court, such as a magistrate's court. It is a formal court hearing, normally open to the public, presided over by a magistrate but with no jury. The witness appears under oath/affirmation. The party that brought the witness leads in questioning the witness, and cross-examination by the other party follows. The magistrate may interject to clarify the expert's answers or to rule on objections raised by one barrister with regard to the line of questioning by the other party. When all evidence has been given by witnesses and followed by cross-examinations, a magistrate makes a determination whether to commit the case to trial. This is based on the plea the accused makes (guilty or not guilty) and on the strength of evidence in the case. If the accused pleads not guilty but the evidence of guilt seems to be strong enough to be considered by the court, the case proceeds to trial. If the accused pleads guilty, there is no need for the trial and the case goes directly for sentencing. In such cases, there is no further need for witness' testimonies.

The Trial

The trial is normally held in an open court, often with a jury that determines whether the accused is guilty. The prosecution leads the case and presents its witnesses. The defence then cross-examines these witnesses. Next the defence calls its witnesses, who are subject to cross-examination by the prosecution. All witnesses testify under oath/affirmation. Examination and cross-examination proceed in a way similar to that at a committal hearing. Greater attention is paid to the facts and opinions of an expert. The examination starts with establishing the qualifications of the expert. Details of the expert's formal education and professional experience are presented with special attention to the relevance to the case. Questions about the facts discovered by the witness and witness's opinions follow. Various exhibits may be shown to the witness, the judge, and the jury at this stage. The witness may present and discuss exhibits (for example, photographs, videos, photo-comparison boards) as needed. Cross-examination follows. The presiding judge may interject instructing a witness or ruling on objections to various questions. If the objection is raised after the witness has already answered a question, the judge may instruct the jury to disregard the answer. Formally, the jury must do so, but they have already heard the answer and the information provided may influence their thinking. Such situations happen, for example, when an expert speculates beyond the factual evidence and his area of expertise (Kassin, Williams, and Saunders 1990).

The witness should answer questions clearly and succinctly. If in any doubt about the meaning of a question, the witness must ask for clarification. Although the jury is not playing any active part in the proceedings, it is the jury who will make a decision. Thus the witness must give evidence in a way that will be clearly understood by members of the jury. It is difficult to assess how a jury receives a witness's evidence, but sometimes a pointed answer from a witness makes the jury react spontaneously by smiling, or even laughing. The witness should provide answers directly addressing specific questions and avoid longer lecture-style presentations, or complex qualifications of answers, such as "yes, but only if one considers that the degree of certainty of the method applied under circumstances. . . . " Simple "yes" or "no" is usually sufficient. If a qualification of an affirmative or negative answer is necessary, it should be started as "possibly, but I am not certain."

During cross-examination barristers use a technique of making a statement and then asking the witness—"do you agree?" If the witness does not agree with the statement made, the answer must be very clear—"no, I disagree." Any "well, yes, but not really . . ." will confuse the jury. All questions must be answered truthfully. The witness may refuse to give an answer to a question outside his/her area of expertise or to speculate if there is not enough evidence. The witness's opinions are treated very seriously and thus must be expressed responsibly. The opposing party may try to discredit the witness by quotations from the literature or by testimony of another expert witness showing that the original opinion was based on inadequate knowledge. Thus a witness should not make statements that cannot be supported by professional literature or by well-established specialist practice. The attitude "trust me, I am an expert" is dangerous. If an expert witness becomes discredited in an open trial, he or she will not likely be approached again to work on new cases. Modesty, reliability, clarity, and truthfulness are the best tools of an expert witness. It is much better to say "I do not know" than to make a statement that can be shown to be false. In summing up the case, the prosecution and the defence will refer to statements made by the witness under oath.

Each case proceeds in the majesty of the law. Time is taken to fully explore all aspects of the case. The conduct of all persons in the courtroom is serious and polite even if diametrically opposing views are expressed. Witnesses should act and express themselves accordingly. Displays of emotion or use of strong language must be avoided. The judge makes all decisions concerning how the case proceeds, and he or she must be deferred to. The judge is addressed as "Your Honour," and if in any doubt about what to do, the witness must turn to the judge for decision. "May I stand up Your Honour?" or "Your Honour, may I show this photograph to the jury?" are correct ways of action, rather than just getting up or showing a picture to jurors.

After both sides exhaust their lines of questioning and the judge is satisfied that the witness gave full evidence, the witness is excused. In most cases this ends the witness's involvement in the case, and he/she is free to go. The witness, however, can be recalled later in the case, depending on how the trial proceeds. There is no need for the witness to be present during the entire trial. In certain cases, a witness may testify by telephone or video link.

Although it is not required, in the interest of objectivity, experts should abstain from following details of the case that are not relevant to their area of expertise. These details may influence a witness's personal feelings about the case and lead to bias in his/her opinions. It happens that witnesses try to influence the outcome of the case by stressing some facts beyond their actual significance or by formulating their opinions categorically instead of presenting them cautiously (Crawford et al. 2005). Such behaviours must be avoided, because they will eventually undermine the expert's reputation.

Conclusion

The role of expert witness is extremely important; a person undertaking this function must do so with a full understanding of responsibilities and commitments. To accept the task of an expert witness in a particular case, one must ensure that up-to-date professional knowledge relevant to the case is available. The expert must have skills necessary to apply this knowledge, demonstrate integrity and independence, and ensure that the time and resources necessary to carry out all tasks, including court appearances, will be available. Given the complexities of procedures of various legal systems, the extent of an expert's involvement may be much greater than initially estimated. Responsible behaviour at all stages of the case, integrity and truthfulness, in addition to excellent professional knowledge and skills, are hallmarks of a good expert witness.

References

Brodsky, S. L. 2004. *Testifying in Court Workshop: Survival Skills for Professionals.* Specialized Training Seminars, June. Columbus, OH.

Crawford, M., Davis, P., Herbison, J., Mok, J., Mott, A., Payne, H., Postlethwaite, R., Price, J., Samuels, M., Sibert, J., Sills, J., and Speight, N. 2005. Expert witness: Opinion and dogma are pitfalls in medical journalism as well as in reports. *Archives of Disease in Childhood* 90: 218–219.

Federal Court of Australia. 1998. *Practice direction: Guidelines for expert witnesses in proceedings in the Federal Court of Australia.* 15th September.

Freckelton, I., Reddy, P., and Selby, H. 1999. *Australian Judicial Perspectives on Expert Evidence: An Empirical Study.* Melbourne: Australian Institute for Judicial Administration.

Kassin, S. M., Williams, L., and Saunders, C. L. 1990. Dirty tricks of cross-examination: The influence of conjectural evidence on the jury. *Law and Human Behavior* 14: 373–384.

McAbee, G. N., and Freeman, J. M. 2006. Expert medical testimony: Responsibilities of medical societies. *Neurology* 65: 337.

Supreme Court of South Australia. SCR 38.01 A. 2002. Practice Direction 46 A.

41

LEGAL ASPECTS OF IDENTIFICATION

David Ranson

All death investigation takes place in a medical, scientific, administrative, and legal environment that is specific to the type of community and legal jurisdiction within which the death occurred. The differences among jurisdictions arise from a variety of interrelated factors including social, religious, political, and legal influences, as well as the development of the medical profession and its specialties. At the most mechanical level, records are generated and retained about who has died. A cause of death is assigned within a registry office inside government bureaucracy, generally by recording on a death register the cause of death given in the report or certificate of the treating doctor. The maintenance of a death register and a birth register has important social implications. A community needs to know information regarding those who make up its population. From a practical perspective, this is needed in order to ensure that community services are appropriate to the size and makeup of the population. However, at a deeper level our concerns about threats to our safety generate a desire to find out more about deaths that occur in our community and to understand their causes so that we can feel less threatened. Community and personal grief involve important emotions that can have deep effects on the functioning of individuals, families, and in some cases the whole community. In this environment,

a society's ability to independently investigate critical deaths from a perspective that is focused beyond that of any individual professional group, such as scientists, the medical profession, or the police, is important.

Our popular media seem to be obsessed by death, disaster, and accident, responding to, and fanning, our community's seemingly insatiable drive to know the details and profiles of both victims and perpetrators of homicide, lethal error, and catastrophe. Cases involving the discovery of hidden bodies, terrorist attacks, pandemics, tsunamis, uncontrolled bushfires, homicidal medical practitioners, toxic spillages, gangland killings, and dangerous workplaces are just some of the deaths that particularly concern the community and as a result receive the attention of the public media. This focus places death investigators directly in the public eye, which for many is a radical departure from their traditional quiet and private scientific role.

Those involved in death investigation should never lose sight of the social importance of the work they undertake. It is all too easy to become involved in the technical and scientific aspects of solving the death puzzle and as a result fail to be aware of the personal, family, and community loss. Similarly, it is easy to become enmeshed in the often complex administrative and bureaucratic processes that surround death investigation with the result that the human aspects of grief and loss become invisible.

Broadly, the European and Scandinavian systems, as well as a number of medical examiner systems, focus on whether criminal behaviour has brought about a death. By contrast, coroners' death investigations in the Anglo-Australian jurisdictions take a broader and more public health perspective, inquiring in a wide variety of circumstances whether the conduct that gave rise to a death could or should have been different and whether alternative processes might in the future avoid such deaths. Put another way, at the heart of the distinctive systems of coronial investigation is accuracy in both the public record about deaths and prophylaxis— learning from deaths so as to minimise the risks of recurrence, where possible. This means in practice that the purview of the coroner extends into noncriminal matters such as deaths in natural and man-made disasters, workplace and transport accidents, and unsatisfactory medical treatment events, to identify just a few examples.

From a legal perspective the coroner functions as an "inquisitorial" oasis in the broader "adversarial" legal system. In the death investigation court hearing or inquest, the coroner functions as both an investigator assembling the evidence he or she needs and as a decision maker, working without the constraints of the rules of evidence and formal procedure. This is quite different from the systems in place in the criminal and civil courts in the same jurisdiction that operate in an adversarial fashion. In these courts, the judge sits as an impartial observer and decision maker but is not involved directly in the management of the investigation process. In addition, coroners are not Royal Commissioners. They do not have an open mandate to investigate at large. A question that is regularly posed in specific inquests is this: Where do the lines need to be drawn, beyond which a coroners' investigations, findings, and recommendations should not trespass?

Death and the Coronial Investigation

Before instituting an inquest, a coroner must be persuaded that a dead body is within the jurisdiction or that a person died an unnatural death within the jurisdiction. The definition of *death* is relatively wide, and in some jurisdictions a coroner's investigation can be commenced in relation to a suspected death but when no body has been found. Establishing that a death has occurred by reference to remains is sometimes not altogether straightforward. The presence of disembodied parts of a human body may not be determinative. A severed arm or leg has been held not to constitute conclusive evidence that the body from which it comes is dead. Thus, it was held in *Ex parte Brady; Re Oram* (1935) 52 WN (NSW) 109 that the finding of a tattooed arm, severed from a human trunk by a sharp knife, was not sufficient to constitute a body for the purpose of giving the coroner jurisdiction to hold an inquest, since an arm may be removed from a body without loss of life (Clark 1936). However, it is recorded in *Jervis on the Office and Duties of Coroners* (Matthews and Foreman 1993) that in an English case

> . . . portions of human lung were found in the sea at the point at which an aircraft had crashed, without any trace of the pilot being found. [T]he person from whom the lung material had come was shown to have had the same blood group as the missing pilot. The coroner held that the lung material constituted a body and accordingly he had jurisdiction because of its presence in his area. Similarly, in another case the coroner held that he had jurisdiction to hold an inquest where the lower half only of a girl's body was found in the street, and the rest was not recovered.

The question, then, is whether the separate parts of the body that have been located are necessarily inconsistent with the person still being alive whose potential death is being investigated.

With their responsibility to investigate deaths, coroners are often required to investigate the finding of suspected human remains, which permits them to control the scene and order specialist investigators to attend and carry out their work. In the case of skeletal remains, they may well be subsequently identified as those of a nonhuman animal. At this point, the jurisdiction of the coroner ceases, and there is no basis for further coronial involvement in the incident. Essentially, the role of the coroner in investigating the suspected death at this stage is an administrative one, consequent on the coroner's legal jurisdiction.

Latitude has traditionally been extended to the coroner to enable him or her to investigate a death even when no body has been found, provided the death has some real connection with the relevant jurisdiction. Likewise, the fact that a body has been destroyed or is not recoverable does not preclude the holding of an inquest. A local coroner may investigate the deaths of persons ordinarily resident within the jurisdiction that have occurred overseas as a result of a man-made or natural disaster. Today international travel is far more common than when much coronial legislation was formulated. As a result, the need to investigate the sudden and unexpected death of a traveller overseas is not an uncommon requirement of the modern coroner's jurisdiction.

In addition to the presence of a body, a coroner must be satisfied that the body is dead. In terms of coronial practice, obtaining proof of death is usually not a problem. Coroners have tended to take the view that a person is dead if an appropriately qualified medical practitioner has stated that he or she is dead. Definitions of death have become more complex with the development of organ transplantation and the ability to artificially sustain the circulation of blood and breathing.

However, as a matter of practice, coroners' inquests do not take place while a body is hooked up to life support systems, even though a persistent vegetative state may have commenced and a person may be wholly brain-dead (Matthews 2002). This does not mean that the coronial jurisdiction into a reportable death has not been initiated. The death of a person who has been officially declared brain-dead and whose death is reportable to a coroner should be reported even if his or her somatic organ systems are being medically supported and maintained. Such a death comes under the coroner's jurisdiction, and in principle the coroner has legal control of the body. It could be said that the clinical medical staff managing the brain-dead patient is acting under an implied authority of the coroner.

The question as to which deaths must be investigated by a coroner is answered by reference to the legislation in the given jurisdiction. A distinction exists between the holding of an inquiry or an investigation, and the holding of an inquest. Today, in Anglo-Australian jurisdictions, as well as in other countries, the legislation varies as to when a coroner is obliged to conduct an inquiry and when an inquest must be held. In general, where there is reasonable cause arising out of an inquiry or investigation for the coroner to suspect that a person has died a violent or unnatural death or died in circumstances that are unclear, or in a prescribed facility, such as a prison, police cell, juvenile facility, or psychiatric hospital, then an inquest must be held.

The endpoint of a coroner's investigation, whether or not an inquest is held, involves the setting out of a finding and the delivery of a verdict. The transition from a coroner's *verdict* to that of a discursive, structured set of *findings* is a particular feature of the modern development of the coronial jurisdiction as it has moved away from its English

origins in Australia, New Zealand, and Canada. Traditionally, coroners have to determine the identity of the deceased, when and where he or she died, the cause of death, and how he or she died. The identification of individuals who have contributed to a death may also form part of a coroner's finding. Indeed, in some jurisdictions the coroner has the power to refer individuals to the Director of Public Prosecutions when the coroner believes a criminal action may have been involved.

Modern legislation often permits coroners to make specific recommendations in matters affecting public health and safety and the administration of justice. The power to make a recommendation as part of a finding is not unfettered. Indeed, there should be a clear nexus between the comments or recommendations made and the circumstances surrounding the death into which the coroner inquires. In the context of an inquest into the deaths of prisoners in a jail fire in Victoria, in the case of *Harmsworth v. State Coroner* [1989] VR 989, 996, Nathan J. noted the power to make comments and recommendations but held unequivocally that the "power to comment is incidental and subordinate to the mandatory power to make findings related to how the deaths occurred, their causes and the identity of any contributory persons." The cause and circumstance of death together with recommendations regarding death prevention are perhaps the most important outcome of a death investigation and inquest. However, the key administrative outcome of an inquest is the determination of the particular items of information required to register the death. This information is essential in order for the public record to be made complete and if necessary "set straight."

The Coronial Investigation Process

The legal requirements regarding deaths that must be reported to a coroner differ from jurisdiction to jurisdiction. Legally reportable deaths must be reported to a coroner. However, the legislative reporting requirement is often satisfied where the death is reported to the police, who in turn have a duty to inform the coroner and assist in the coroner's investigation. Although the whole community has a responsibility to report reportable deaths to the coroner, this duty is usually made a specific statutory responsibility of the medical profession and the police. This is for purely practical purposes, in that these two groups are most likely to be involved following a death.

When a death or the discovery of unknown human remains is reported to the coroner by a person other than a police officer, the coroner's office will usually contact the police station closest to the site and request that a police officer attend and obtain the necessary details. This effectively identifies a particular officer as the reporting officer attached to that case, so that subsequently, if the coroner requires further information about the circumstances of the death, there is a local police contact point that allows for additional information to be collected. Regardless of who takes the initial report of death, the basic principles are the same. Relevant demographic details are recorded, including the name (if it is known) of the person who has died and the name and contact details of the person reporting the death.

The quality of the initial investigation that takes place within the first 48 hours after a death sets the scene for all subsequent investigations and is crucial in ensuring that a thorough overall investigation takes place. Errors and omissions in the initial processes of investigation often cannot be corrected later. The coordination of the initial investigation process is therefore a task that is essential. Involvement of the coroner in this coordination process is variable. In some jurisdictions, the coroner will leave the initial coordination of the investigation to police and clerical staff. In other jurisdictions, the coroner may insist on being informed of each and every death regardless of the time of day. In jurisdictions with centralised coroner services, the coroner may set out protocols that determine which cases he or she should be directly informed about, so that he or she can attend the scene and coordinate the initial death investigation. Scenarios where the coroner may wish to step in and direct the investigation include deaths in custody or during a police response, incidents involving mass loss of life, work-related fatalities, and aviation or marine fatalities.

The organisation of a coroner's investigation is dependent on the administrative structures that are in place to manage and support the coroner's jurisdiction. In some jurisdictions, such as England and Wales, the coroner's administrative structure is provided by local government and lies outside the administrative services of the civil and criminal courts. In other jurisdictions, it may be that the central justice ministry or the police provide most of the support and investigative services for the coroner. Regardless of the exact administrative structure of the organisation of a coroner's office, the tasks that are carried out are remarkably similar from jurisdiction to jurisdiction. In some small offices, one person may carry out many roles, whereas in larger organisations each role may be taken by an individually trained member of the coroner's staff, seconded government administrative staff, external medical staff, or independent contractors.

The tendency for recent coronial legislation in Australia has been to create centralised offices headed by a State Coroner (or Chief Coroner or Territory Coroner, as the case may be) with Deputy Coroners to assist him or her. Generally, legislation provides in reasonably short form for the role of the State Coroner. Section 71 of the *Coroners Act 2003* (Qld) is an example:

> The State Coroner's functions are:
> (a) to oversee and coordinate the coronial system; and
> (b) to ensure the coronial system is administered and operated efficiently; and
> (c) to ensure deaths reported to coroners that are reportable deaths are investigated to an appropriate extent; and
> (d) to ensure an inquest is held if
>> (i) the inquest is required to be held under this Act; or
>> (ii) it is desirable for the inquest to be held; and
> (e) to be responsible, together with the Deputy State Coroner, for all investigations into deaths in custody; and
> (f) to issue directions and guidelines about the investigation of deaths under this Act; and
> (g) any other function given to the State Coroner or a coroner under this Act.

As can be seen, the role of the head of the coronial service is principally administrative. However, this administrative role exists in addition to the specific responsibility of any coroner to investigate reported deaths.

Much of the day-to-day aspects of a coroner's death investigation is carried out by a variety of individuals, some of whom are directly employed by the coroner's office and others are external contractors.

Court Clerks

Within the coroner's office, administrative officers or coroner's clerks manage the day-to-day case work and ensure, through liaison with the coroner, that an appropriate level of investigation has been carried out. The coroner's clerk must ensure that the investigation of the death is sufficient to meet the needs of the coroner in dealing with an inquest or arriving at an appropriate chamber finding or verdict. It is usually the coroner's clerk who receives the information about a reportable death from the police, a medical practitioner, or member of the public. The clerk will evaluate the case and, after discussion with the coroner or by applying general coronial guidelines, organise the administrative matters resulting in the performance of an autopsy by an appropriately qualified pathologist.

While most of the day-to-day administrative procedures in a coroner's office are delegated to court clerical and administrative staff, office procedures in many jurisdictions require that the coroner be contacted directly for particular types of cases, in order to attend the scene of a death and to initiate special investigations.

When an inquest is to be held, the coroner's clerk has a similar duty to that of other court clerks in organising the listing of hearings and ensuring that all interested parties including the family are informed of the proceedings. The court clerk manages the administration of the hearing, including the liaison with legal representatives. At the completion of the inquest, the clerk ensures that the finding or verdict is appropriately recorded and that the death is formally registered with the registrar of births, deaths, and marriages. The clerk will ensure that records of the inquest are kept and cross-referenced with any other material relating to the death, including any criminal justice processes that may also be under way in other courts.

Police Assistants

In some jurisdictions, police officers seconded from other duties may perform some of the court clerical duties. Often they act in a combined liaison/operational role between the coroner and operational police units, including general duty police and detectives. Police on general duties have a limited involvement in death investigations, whereas coroners' police assistants deal with the issues on a daily basis. Indeed, coroners' police assistants help in the investigation of many more deaths than a specialist police homicide investigation unit. The investigation of deaths occurring in the setting of medical care as well as transport-related deaths involving aircraft, marine craft, and trains is often supervised and managed by coroners' police assistants. However, when a death involves police operations, such as a death in custody, there is the potential for allegations of conflict of interest. In such cases, the coronial service needs to have special procedures in place for the appointment of other investigators, legal counsel, or independent supervisors who can oversee the police investigation. Such cases are a minority within coronial practice; for the most part, the advantages of the

close working relationship between coroners and the police outweigh the disadvantages.

Bereavement Support Staff

The introduction of a counselling service based at a coroner's court has the capacity to greatly enhance the services for clients and also to improve the efficiency of the coroner's process. These counselling services are not usually designed to provide long-term bereavement care. They are usually fashioned around acute intervention services to provide initial support, counselling, and information in an environment that maximises the autonomy of the family. Inevitably, many families require far longer periods of support and counselling. To enable this, counselling services at coroners' courts usually have close working relationships with other community support services and health services to which families can be referred.

Specialist Investigators

Many deaths involve complex investigations that lie outside the knowledge of the general police or the coroner's staff. Issues involving medical treatment, pathological processes, homicide investigation, death and crime scene investigation, engineering, military procedures, fire services, maritime matters, accountancy, and the wide range of forensic sciences may arise in cases from time to time. It is appropriate that these issues are comprehensively addressed. To this end, the coroner may well contract out this part of the investigation by commissioning external experts in the relevant field and providing them with relevant information from the coroner's case file.

The most common external medical investigation service used by a coroner is the autopsy service provided by forensic pathologists (see below). Death investigation systems, such as those operated by a coroner, usually have the power to order that an autopsy be carried out to assist in the determination of the manner, circumstances, and cause of death.

Although pathologists are the group of medical practitioners most closely involved in the work of coroners, increasingly other medical specialists are also utilised by coroners in death investigation. Deaths occurring in the setting of medical treatment may require investigations by nonpathology medical specialists. Experts in anaesthetics, intensive care, and accident and emergency services, as well as specialist physicians and surgeons, may have an important role to play in the evaluation of such deaths. Today, the advent of the use of alternative death investigation processes, in addition to or as a replacement for the autopsy, demonstrates the need for a wider range of medical specialists to be engaged by a coroner.

Death Scene Investigation and Retrieval of Human Remains

A coroner's jurisdiction in respect to death investigation starts with the report of a death. This death will have occurred at a particular location that may not necessarily be the location where the dead body was found. In many cases, these locations will have a direct or indirect relationship to the death. Indeed, the place in which the death occurred may contain evidence in the environment that can suggest what the cause of death might be or help explain the circumstances in which the death occurred. Detailed evaluation of the death scene may help identify environmental hazards that contributed to the death, and the recognition of these may even assist in future death prevention. From a criminal perspective, when homicide is suspected, the death-scene environment may contain important physical evidence that can link an offender with the scene. It follows, therefore, that the steps taken in the initial phases of the investigation of the scene of death lay the foundation for the whole of the death investigation. Mistakes made in the initial examination of the scene often cannot be rectified later. Once a body has been moved and multiple people have walked in and out of the death scene, objects within the death scene have been touched or moved, or the scene has been affected by environmental factors such as rain or extremes of temperature, permanent damage may have been caused to the investigation. Consequently, it is critical that sound procedures are put in place to ensure an adequate examination of the scene of death.

Clearly, the nature and scope of a death-scene examination that occurs in the case of a suspected homicide or the finding of skeletal remains will be different from that required in the case of an individual dying at home in bed from apparently natural causes. Because of the variability in the types of death reported to a coroner it is difficult to be precise about the scope and depth of death-scene investigation that may be required. Although most deaths investigated by a coroner do not involve crimes, crime-scene management principles form a solid foundation that should underpin all death-scene investigations. Indeed, because one of the roles of a coroner in investigating a death is to consider the possibility of criminal acts associated with it, the investigation must proceed in a manner

that allows for the possibility that a criminal charge may be laid, and the evidence-gathering process must be sufficiently rigorous to withstand forensic scrutiny in due course in the coroner's court and the criminal courts. A "crime scene" can be considered to be any venue that has the potential to reveal evidence of the commission of an offence or to rule out the commission of an offence. Such a scene is capable of revealing considerable information regarding the behaviour of individuals and objects in and around the scene both before and after a death.

Locard's theory of interchange underlies the principles of crime-scene investigation. Although the theory can be described in many ways, in practical terms it means that a contact between objects or individuals and objects will leave evidence of that contact through the transfer of trace evidence from one object or individual to the other. Such traces may be visible or invisible. They may be stable and permanent, or temporary. The identification, analysis, and documentation of this trace evidence can be critical in determining what happened at a death scene.

The identification, collection, transportation, and documentation of trace evidence is a responsibility of all investigators at a death scene. However, the crime-scene examiner plays the major role in this respect and takes responsibility for ensuring that the appropriate evidence is collected or suitably sampled. It is also the examiner's role to take steps to avoid loss of potentially useful evidence by destruction at the scene in the course of a careless examination or by contamination during the process of transportation from the scene to the laboratory. In many cases, specialised techniques may need to be employed to preserve material evidence, and this can involve taking impressions of the material, such as tire tread marks in mud, and ensuring that biological trace evidence is appropriately refrigerated or dried so as to preserve its character.

There are a number of general considerations regarding the investigation of a death scene. One of the most important is the determination of the extent of the death scene and what limits should be set on the range and scope of the investigation. In many straightforward death scenes, the immediate environment constitutes the appropriate boundary of the death-scene examination. However, where there is evidence of blood, other bodily fluids, or human remains in other locations, it may be necessary to include all these locations as separate scenes.

To ensure that evidence collected from a crime scene or a death scene can be used in court, it is necessary to be able to show that the evidence is reliable and truly reflects the material present at the death scene or involved in the death. There must be continuity of evidence or a clear "chain of evidence." To this end, it is essential that the death scene is effectively secured and controlled. There should be no possibility that evidence from the scene could have been interfered with, altered, or adulterated. As noted above, a key factor in planning the security measures is the identification of the boundaries of the death scene. This is a combination of physical practicality and scientific or investigative necessity. Some death scenes are composed of multiple small scenes within a defined area, whereas others, such as those involved in a mass disaster, may be spread over tens of kilometres.

Managing the media is an important aspect of death-scene investigations. Simply keeping journalists out of the way is an inappropriate response to these issues. The media can in fact be very useful in a death investigation. By making the community aware of a death that has occurred in particular circumstances, additional new information may be gained from unanticipated sources within the community. However, this advantage must be balanced against the risk of confidential forensic information being deliberately or inadvertently distributed by the media in a way that prejudices the investigation. The provision of timely information to media personnel present at a death scene is an important task. Police departments regularly employ public relations personnel in the form of media liaison officers who can assist in this work.

The recording of evidence is a critical aspect of any forensic investigation. In the case of death scenes, particularly those that are thought to be suspicious, it is essential that a complete, thorough, and timely record be made of the appearance of the area. The usual way in which death scenes are recorded initially is by means of video-recording and photography. However, detailed drawings, sketches, and plans are also useful ways of recording a scene. Some investigators, particularly forensic pathologists, rely on textual descriptions of a scene rather than visual records. This is usually because a visual record is already being made by police investigators for the coroner, and it would be a duplication of effort for the pathologist to make a further visual record. Notes taken at a death scene will vary depending on the nature of the scene and the environment. The initial assessment of the nature of the death scene will also determine the range and scope of the investigation and the quantity of notes recorded. Clearly, in the case of a suspicious death where criminality

may be involved, there will be a higher standard expected for recording of data and collection of material. In such a case, there will usually be extensive use of video and photographs, as well as detailed written notes and sketches.

The medical examination of the body at a scene is necessarily limited by the resources available and by the physical restrictions posed by most death-scene environments. Factors such as lighting, physical access to body surfaces, and difficulties in moving a dead body all limit the scope of the medical examination of the body at the scene. Despite these difficulties, a pathologist may attempt to ascertain whether there are any significant wounds to the body and look for signs that suggest a possible mechanism for the death. This examination should be limited, however, so that procedures are not undertaken that would compromise the later examination that can be carried out in the context of a full forensic autopsy.

On completion of the medical examination of the body at the scene of death, the pathologist should consult with the coroner and the investigating police about an appropriate time for the removal of the body from the scene, its transportation to the mortuary, and the subsequent forensic autopsy. When these matters have been agreed on, the pathologist should supervise the collection of the body in order to ensure that there is no damage or inadvertent loss of evidence from the body as a result of extracting it from the scene or its transport. When a body is moved, other evidence may come to light beneath the body or from the clothing. It is important for pathologists to be aware of this, because it may alter the scope of the subsequent examination at autopsy. It may be important for the pathologist to document and collect objects left by ambulance officers on and around the body. These can include drug administration sets, intravenous fluids, and airways and other resuscitation devices. Analysis of these objects may help in reconstructing what occurred during resuscitation, including what drugs were administered to the patient.

Exhumations

Exhumations are a special example of a complex death scene. Exhumations may be required particularly where allegations are made, some time after a death, that an unnatural process was involved, such as negligent injury, incompetent medical treatment, or most particularly, homicide. Homicide investigations are sometimes undertaken many years after a death, because new information has come to light as a result of other criminal investigations.

The coroner will usually seek the advice of a forensic pathologist regarding the feasibility of conducting the exhumation and the relative likelihood that a postmortem examination of the exhumed remains will reveal information pertinent to the allegations that made the death reportable. In order to provide the coroner with this information about the potential for the autopsy to materially assist in the death investigation, the pathologist needs detailed information about the time interval since death and the funeral procedures and processes, including the nature of any embalming procedures performed and the type of coffin. Information about the depth of burial, the soil composition, and the drainage of the cemetery may also be required in order to assess whether pathological and toxicological examination of the exhumed remains is likely to lead to new evidence.

If the coroner concludes that an autopsy may provide useful information, he or she will inform the cemetery authorities (and, depending on the circumstances, the family of the deceased) that an exhumation is to be performed. Usually a funeral director and the staff of the cemetery will work with coroner's investigators, including the police and the forensic pathologist, to determine an appropriate time for the exhumation. Frequently, exhumations are performed early in the morning, prior to the arrival of members of public at a cemetery, in order to minimise the impact on the local community. The exhumation of a body needs to be carried out with considerable care so as not to disturb nearby graves. Occasionally, when a plot contains more than one body or plot markings are unclear, an exhumation may result in the uncovering of other bodies, in which case the issue of identity needs to be very carefully addressed. In such situations, it may be necessary to bring more than one body to the mortuary for detailed identification processes as well as pathological examination.

The exhumation of a body from a grave can easily result in damage to the remains if special precautions are not taken. Although a mechanical digger may be used to expose the upper levels of a grave, its use close to the coffin may result in damage to it and/or to the body inside. For this reason a degree of manual digging (sometimes involving a forensic anthropologist and/or archaeologist) is usually required toward the end of the mechanical exhumation process. Some coffins are prone to disintegration, particularly those made of veneered chipboard, and in such cases additional support of the coffin may be required during the lifting process, through the use of a stretcher-type device. If the coffin has completely collapsed or disintegrated, the fabric or plastic lining of the coffin containing the body may be removed directly from the grave, acting as a body bag. If this, too, has been destroyed, a more archaeological approach to the removal of individual portions of human remains from the grave may need to be considered.

The process of exhumation needs to be clearly documented with photographs that include images of the plot site prior to exhumation, any identification markers present on the plot, the exposure of the coffin, the state of the coffin, and any identification markers on the coffin itself. During the removal of the coffin and the body from the grave it may be necessary to take samples or specimens from the vicinity of the grave site. These may include samples of soil from above and below the coffin or from the substance of the coffin itself. Drugs and toxins that were present in the body at the time of death may be identified in the soil adjacent to the coffin rather than in the bodily remains. In some exhumations, there will be a visible body fluid drainage area present in the soil adjacent to the coffin. Samples from this region may prove valuable for toxicological analysis. Control samples of soil from some distance away from the grave site must also be taken to ensure that the soil in the cemetery is not generally contaminated with some suspicious chemical substance.

With the completion of the medical examination of exhumed remains and the collection of samples for forensic scientific testing, the body is usually returned to the cemetery within a few days and buried in the same grave plot. It may be necessary for the coroner to assist the family in arranging a further funeral service at the time of reinterment.

The Autopsy

The autopsy can be considered a "highly invasive" and "all-encompassing" pathology test that, using a combination of both screening and diagnostic analyses, surveys the body for the presence, nature, and extent of disease or injury. It also represents the most comprehensive type of medical examination or procedure performed on an individual. Because the autopsy is a "one-off" procedure and is followed by the disposal of the body by burial or cremation, repeating parts of the procedure if mistakes or omissions are made is difficult or impossible.

In jurisdictions that employ pathologists to carry out medico-legal autopsies, it is the coroner who must determine whether the death investigation requires an autopsy and, if so, formally order that it be undertaken. Within certain limits, the coroner can control the extent of the examination and choose who performs the autopsy. In practice, there are many agencies, individuals, and groups who may have an interest in an autopsy. Each might reasonably expect to be consulted regarding the extent of an examination. For example, police officers, occupational health and safety inspectors, treating medical practitioners, and the family of the deceased may all have a view as to the extent of the autopsy.

There are two types of "autopsy": the clinical autopsy and the medico-legal autopsy. A clinical autopsy, sometimes referred to as a hospital autopsy, is distinctly different from the medico-legal autopsy ordered by a coroner. Clinical autopsies in Australia, and in many other jurisdictions, require the consent of the next of kin and can be performed only for the purpose of contributing to our understanding of disease and the effects of medical treatment. They must not be performed to determine the cause of death; if the cause of a death is unclear to the treating clinician, the death must be reported to the coroner, in which case a medico-legal autopsy may be undertaken.

A variety of autopsy procedures and associated scientific techniques can assist with a coronial investigation. In terms of the medical examination of deceased persons or unknown human remains, the pathologist usually acts as the coordinator and team leader of the medical, dental, anthropological, and scientific units involved. In addition, during the autopsy the pathologist can provide information on the injuries, diseases, and individual physical characteristics of a body, going far beyond the features that could be observed by superficial inspection.

The aims of the autopsy (forensic and clinical) include:

- confirmation or determination of the identity of the deceased
- identification of injuries and natural disease
- reconciling events in life with the presence of anatomical and pathological features
- determination of the extent of injuries and natural diseases
- evaluation of the effect of medical treatments
- assessment of the mode of death
- determination of the cause of death
- comprehension of the mechanisms involved in the death
- provision of an educational resource for the medical profession
- provision of tissues for use in medical research and therapeutic procedures

- retrieval of trace evidence and other samples for use as evidence in court
- reconstruction of the circumstances surrounding the death

The autopsy alone cannot meet all these aims. Indeed, the autopsy is an examination carried out to identify pathological processes and anatomical abnormalities at "a point in time," namely, at death. It is only when these findings are integrated with information about the death scene and the individual's medical history and lifestyle that the information obtained from the autopsy can be put into a proper context.

Whether undertaken for clinical or a medico-legal purposes, the autopsy has three elements:

1. Initial contact with the family, outlining the autopsy procedures and the family's rights with respect to the extent of the autopsy, and the use of any tissues and organs retained, as well as the potential implications the autopsy information may have for family health.

2. Conduct of a detailed macroscopic and microscopic examination of the body, including all medical and scientific tests necessary to meet the wider purposes of the autopsy, including but not restricted to determining the cause of death.

3. Postautopsy consultation with the family, providing information about the findings with respect to the death and its implications for the health of family members. This consultation would also include any appropriate medical or legal referral.

In theory, a complex autopsy could take months to complete. However, in practice most physical autopsies take a few hours. This means that the performance of an autopsy, whether for medical or medico-legal reasons, should not introduce any significant delay to a family's funeral arrangements.

Information obtained from autopsies conducted in an environment of open communication with the family and the community have the capacity to be of enormous private and public benefit. It is the responsibility of coroners and forensic pathologists to ensure that the community is made aware of the value of the autopsy and that families are included in the decisions surrounding the medical examination and able to benefit from the information that the autopsy provides.

Identification of Human Remains

The identification of the dead is essential for the lives of others to return to normal. From an emotional standpoint, the uncertainty and anguish suffered by families who have a missing loved one who they fear may be dead can be tremendous. From a practical standpoint, if the identification of the deceased is problematic or proves to be impossible, the consequence can be that many others suffer real hardship. For example, the family may not be able to wind up the financial affairs of the deceased, and disbursement of property according to the deceased's wishes may be significantly delayed.

Ultimately, it is the coroner who must determine identity on a legal basis. To do so, he or she relies on statements of identification provided by witnesses and on the results of specialist medical and scientific investigations. The weight that the coroner places on different types of information uncovered in relation to identity is a critical factor in accurate human identification. The circumstances of a death may suggest the probable identity of the deceased, but this information is rarely sufficient on its own for a coroner to make a formal legal determination of identity.

There are several identification methods available to investigate human remains. They include:

- visual identification
- fingerprint identification
- serological identification
- molecular biology (DNA identification)
- dental identification
- craniofacial reconstruction
- medical and anthropological identification
- radiological identification

Visual Identification

The identification of someone who was a friend or a relative is almost invariably a very stressful ordeal for the witness. Even in the best of circumstances, where the body is fresh, intact, clean, and unmutilated and when it is displayed in a clean, bright, nonthreatening environment, such as a modern mortuary, with the support of an enlightened and sensitive staff, the family of the deceased may still find it difficult to identify the body. Inevitably mistakes will be made, occasionally frauds will be perpetrated, and in some cases bodies will be unrecognised and remain visually unidentifiable. There are a variety of reasons why this may be so. The most obvious (and overstated) is "denial" on the part of the relatives, who just cannot accept that it is a member of their family who has died. However, a dead body may bear much less similarity to the person in life than might be anticipated.

In more difficult cases, bodies may have significant injuries and be disfigured. They may remain bloodstained from the events in which they were killed or may be so damaged that the general configuration of the body is lost. At some stage, a decision has to be made as to the degree of psychological stress and trauma that may have to be inflicted on witnesses in order to achieve a "visual identification." The decision to proceed with a visual identification has to be balanced against the likelihood of a reliable outcome and the distress to the family.

Some bodies are completely unrecognisable by any conventional visual criteria as a result of gross decomposition, severe burning, or other gross disruption. Visual identification given in such circumstances must be treated with a high degree of suspicion.

Fingerprint Identification

The taking of fingerprints from a deceased person is well established as a technique for confirming identity. It is one of the mainstays of the identification procedures in mass disasters, in part because a record of fingerprints can be stored as a paper record, as an electronic image, and as a coded database entry. In addition, where a fingerprint record is not available for a deceased person, latent prints can be lifted from objects that are likely to have been handled by that person. This ability to use latent fingerprints from a person's normal environment greatly enhances the utility of fingerprints for the identification of deceased persons. Most people whose deaths are investigated by a coroner do not have a criminal record and therefore are unlikely to have their fingerprints recorded on a police database. However, where the identity of the deceased person is suspected and fingerprints can be collected from the body, a comparison can be made between those fingerprints and latent prints lifted from various objects and surfaces at the person's home and place of work.

Such a form of identification is less accurate than a comparison with fingerprints taken from a known individual in life. In the case of multiple fatalities occurring in the same family or workplace, the use of this type of latent fingerprint comparison will not provide sufficient discrimination among individuals.

Before taking fingerprints from a deceased person, one must ensure that the procedure will not interfere with other examinations of the body. In some cases, this may mean that the fingerprints will have to be collected after the completion of the autopsy. If photographic recording of injuries to the hands or fingers is an essential part of the autopsy, then the presence of fingerprint ink may obscure the photographic appearances. In addition, trace evidence in the form of hairs, paint flakes, bloodstains, and so forth could be lost or contaminated in the process of inking the fingers.

Where the body is decomposed or severely desiccated, the taking of fingerprints may be particularly problematic. The early processes of decomposition are associated with the lifting and degloving of the superficial layers of the skin that retain the friction ridges or fingerprints. A careful operator can remove the separating layer of superficial skin and ink and fingerprint it by placing this over his or her own gloved finger. If the tissue is too friable, a photographic method can be used to record the fingerprint pattern. Even the tissue beneath the degloved finger retains the friction ridge pattern, but this may be more difficult to record.

Molecular Biology (DNA Identification)[1]

The study of the genetic basis of disease was the foundation for the technology of DNA analysis that is now widely used in criminal investigations. However, the role of DNA analysis for human identification by the coroner is still relevant. When DNA analysis is required in coroners' investigations, it is usually applied in circumstances quite different from those in criminal case work.

Identification of deceased persons subject to a coroner's investigation does not require the use of DNA technology. Indeed, molecular biological techniques are usually employed only when other methods of identification have failed. The only exception is in the case of a mass disaster, when the use of multiple individual means of identification for each and every body or body part may be required.

Dental Identification[2]

The application of forensic odontology to human identification involves two main methods of comparison. The first relates to the anatomical structures of the teeth, the jaws, and associated facial regions. Genetic and developmental factors influence the structure and relationship of teeth to various oral structures; as a result, there is enormous variation among individuals in dental anatomy. The second method of comparison relates to identification and documentation of dental treatment, including the effects of restorative dentistry and other forms of dental treatment. With the improvement in oral hygiene in recent years, many young people show no evidence of having received restorative dentistry. However, the advent of modern radiographic techniques to assess dental structures in the living for the purpose of orthodontics has provided a means of comparison with postmortem forensic odontological radiological examination.

Craniofacial Reconstruction and Superimposition[3]

The recovery and identification of human skeletal remains may pose particular challenges to investigators. Forensic anthropological assessment of the human skeleton can provide important information regarding general features of the deceased including ancestry, sex, age, and height. This information can be useful in narrowing the field of individuals who might be the deceased—that is, in creating a biological profile. When it comes to actual identification of skeletal remains, some of the newer techniques of craniofacial reconstruction and comparison may be of considerable use (see, for example, Clement and Ranson 1998). However, these techniques tend to be more useful in exclusion than in confirmation of identity. Nonetheless, where limited material is available for identification, craniofacial reconstruction and facial superimposition techniques may be extremely valuable.

Medical and Anthropological Identification[4]

Medical information about the presence of disease, together with the description of general characteristics of a body, can form important information about identity. As part of the routine process of autopsy, the external characteristics of a body are described. These include hair and eye colour, the presence of tattoos, scars relating to surgery or previous injury, and "birthmarks" or skin lesions. External characteristics on the body can provide useful information that can assist with at least a general classification or group into which the deceased can be placed. In the case of mass disasters where there are many dead, information about previous surgery such as an appendectomy can be highly useful when added to other data. In individual case identification, information about tattoos or scars from prior surgery may narrow the field of possible missing persons who could be the deceased.

Internal examination of the body can reveal evidence not only of current disease but of previous disease processes. This information can prove useful when compared with antemortem records that include notes of prior medical history. Effects and alterations of anatomy caused by previous surgery identified at autopsy can also be important for identification. Sometimes prosthetic devices have been left in the body, for example, from orthopaedic surgery whereby replacement joint surfaces or internal fixator devices are used. Some of these devices will have serial numbers or batch numbers, and it may be possible for the manufacturer's records to be used to identify where the device was dispatched. Review and assessment of such devices by an orthopaedic surgeon may be helpful. When it comes to evidence of other types of surgery, it may be appropriate to obtain the advice of a surgeon from that field of practice, because styles of surgery and techniques employed may differ over time and between schools of surgical practice. The information that the deceased perhaps underwent a surgical procedure more than 20 years ago in Europe may be a useful discriminator in the process of human identification.

Although a pathologist records details of anatomy during the course of autopsy, a specialist anatomist or anatomical anthropologist, experienced in the analysis of a range of differentially preserved human remains, is regularly involved in examination of skeletal remains and may provide far more detailed information about the remains (see Part 3 this volume). They can also provide very useful assistance in cases requiring exhumation and in the examination of decomposed and disrupted remains. In the case of persons who have been involved in explosions, there may be considerable fragmentation of the body, resulting in the need to identify grossly distorted body parts among commingled remains (see for example, Briggs and Buck this volume).

Radiological Identification

The use of radiology in human identification is a useful adjunct to the work of many medical and scientific professionals engaged in the task of human identification. Radiographs taken of people in life may be compared with postmortem radiographs taken at the time of autopsy. Even if there has been subsequent severe bone damage at the time of death, reconstruction of bone fragments and subsequent radiology may still provide enough information to enable a direct comparison. If the skeleton is widely fragmented, it may be possible to match up the characteristic micro-architecture of a bone fragment with a small region of a radiograph taken in life.

A number of areas of the human skeleton show very individual characteristics; the skull is a good example. The pattern of the air sinuses, particularly the frontal sinuses of the skull, may provide enough information to confirm identity. As discussed above, this is usually carried out through the use of two-dimensional X rays of a skull specimen that is positioned to match the orientation of the original antemortem X ray. The use of 3D computerised tomography scans of the skull can assist with this: a virtual 2D slice can be made of the 3D data set in any plane or position, to allow computerised manipulation of the image to match the orientation of the 2D radiograph taken in life.

One of the advantages of radiology in assessing the human skeleton is that it can provide a record of the skeletal structures of the remains, which can be retained even following disposal of the body. Because the specimen is close to the X-ray film when postmortem radiographs are taken, measurements of the bone can be taken from the radiograph directly. Such measurements can be used by anthropologists and radiologists in estimating the deceased's height or measuring key features that can be used to suggest the ancestry or sex of the individual. Computerised tomography (CT) scans of the body provide an ideal 3D record of the remain, which allows for detailed measurements of the morphology of individual skeletal structures.

In addition to bone shape and size, radiographs of skeletal structures can also identify the existence of current or previous disease. This is not limited to disease of the bone but can include information about other systemic disease markers that can be seen in bone changes. People who have been subject to debilitating diseases in early life may show lines of maturation arrest in irregularities of bone formation that occurred during childhood bone development.

In skeletal remains of young persons, radiological assessment can assist in determining the probable age of persons at the time of their death from a variety of factors, including the appearance and closure pattern of epiphyses (the ends of long bones). In older people, radiological assessment of age-related changes and wear patterns may again assist in determining the person's probable age at the time of death, although this is likely to be less precise than the age estimation that can be calculated for younger individuals.

Disaster Victim Identification[5]

Among the major death-investigation and death-scene management processes involved in a mass-casualty scenario, the identification of deceased persons is usually the foremost consideration for the community. Coroners have overall responsibility for this function in addition to their broad death investigation role. Although in some mass-casualty events visual identification of the victims will be possible, when fire or explosion is involved the bodies may not be identifiable without recourse to special scientific and medical techniques. It is essential that the process put in place to investigate the cause of a major disaster causing multiple loss of life does not interfere with the process of identification of the victims. Identification and incident investigation should go hand in hand; indeed, each relies on the other for information. For example, in the case of a bomb blast, identification of the most fragmented body can assist in determining the location of the bomb and perhaps the identity of the "bomber."

For a coroner who has ultimate legal responsibility for both incident investigation and human identification, the coordination of all phases of a mass disaster investigation is an important responsibility. In most cases, a coroner delegates individual tasks to various specialists, and the coordination of the identification of victims is often handled for the coroner by a senior police officer. When the circumstantial, scientific, medical, and dental information that establishes the identity of a victim has been collected to the police officer's satisfaction, this information is presented to the coroner during the process of reconciliation. The identity of the individual is not confirmed until the coroner is satisfied with the information provided.

The Inquest

In traditional coroners' jurisdictions based on the English model, the inquest is the legal hearing that finally determines those matters that the coroner is required to state publicly. An inquest is an investigative process concerned with setting the public mind at rest when there are unanswered questions about a reportable death. The process of inquiry is principally inquisitorial but has been described as containing both inquisitorial and adversarial elements. In this way, it differs from a fundamentally investigatory process such as a Royal Commission. The coroner receives evidence in the form of documentary statements, certificates, and expert reports as well as oral testimony. It may well be that the coroner has personally visited the scene of death and been directly involved in the more practical aspects of the investigation. The role of the coroner is fundamental to the inquest process. In a number of respects, it is more significant to the outcome of hearings than is the role of the judge in standard civil and criminal hearings. This is

because inquests are coroner-driven: the coroner is principal investigator in the sense of generating the search for evidence to be taken into account in the decision-making phase. The coroner also has a range of administrative responsibilities that must be discharged and, in most contemporary jurisdictions, is the judge of the facts and of the law.

The most important product of an inquest is the decision. Traditionally, the formal decision of the coroner's court was termed the "inquisition." Currently, it is variously referred to as the "findings" or the "verdict" of the coroner or the coroner's jury.

Coroners' court decisions are unique among decisions by judicial officers in two respects: they are the result of an inquisitorial inquiry (as opposed to an adversarial process), and they often attract the attention of media to a degree not encountered by any other courts. For this reason, they can devastate reputations, can generate very strong emotions, and can have major ramifications for affected persons and bodies in terms of both commercial and vocational viability. They can also have an indirect effect on secondary criminal, civil, and disciplinary actions.

Coroners' court decisions also place on the public record a formal determination of the circumstances in which a person has died and the causes of the death. Although the finding as to how a death occurred or as to the circumstances of death is perhaps the most important outcome of an inquest, the key administrative outcomes, including the particular items of information required to register the death, are an important aspect of the coroner's role. This information is essential for the public record to be made complete and, if necessary, "set straight."

Another aspect of the inquest is that it is traditional for coroners and coroners' juries, when they deem it appropriate, to add to the findings a "rider" in which recommendations or suggestions are made, directed toward reducing the likelihood that similar circumstances will occur and lead to avoidable deaths. Technically, riders are not part of an inquisition; they are comments or recommendations arising out of the findings. Riders can be contentious and can have major pecuniary ramifications for institutions, employers, and government.

Riders were abolished in 1980 in England and Wales and replaced with a very limited power on the part of coroners to make suggestions to government. In other jurisdictions, in particular in Australia, New Zealand, and Canada, the potential for formal recommendations to be made as part of the outcome of the inquest has broadened the focus of coronial practice.

Today the benefits of the broader form of the coronial inquest process include:

- determining the medical cause of death, including social and psychological factors
- advancing medical knowledge, including facilitating accurate statistical information on causes of death
- investigating deaths to allay rumours or suspicion, and thereby to ensure that no foul play or wrongdoing slips through the net
- making recommendations to avoid future fatalities
- checking on the death registration system
- enabling family and friends to find out how the deceased died
- assisting in personal and community grieving processes
- providing an independent review and investigation of the deaths of individuals in the care or custody of state agencies
- providing families with medical information that may have direct relevance to the maintenance of their health and well-being

Conclusion

Death investigation systems commonly involve a combination of medical, legal, and administrative structures. The differences among jurisdictions arise from a variety of interrelated factors including social, religious, political, and legal influences, as well as the development of the medical profession and its specialties. Balanced perspectives in assessing death can be difficult. It is not easy to come to terms with the fact that sometimes people simply pass away—that deaths just happen. It is very tempting to expect or insist on having someone to blame when a loved one passes away. This is so whether the person is young or of advanced years. Could not something have been done? If someone had intervened, would not the person still be alive? If more care had been taken, would not the likelihood of death have been reduced? Lives lost in such a manner call for explanation, and there is a temptation that someone must be found to blame.

Grief can readily lead to guilt, frequently unwarranted but nonetheless burdensome to survivors and to careers left behind. This means that there is a constant pressure for investigation into circumstances of death and a need to evaluate whether conduct that brought about death should not have occurred. The other inquiry is into what needs to be done to avoid repetition of the events

that caused the death. Sometimes, there are ready answers, such as criminal prosecution of the homicidally culpable. Sometimes there are complex, systemic responses that might reduce the potential for other fatalities.

The focus on the role of the coroner in preventing injury and death has become a prominent characteristic in the evolution of coronial law in Australia and Canada, particularly since the mid-1980s. Recognition has increased that the value of death investigation goes beyond resolving legal issues and simple identification of facts surrounding a death. Although even today coroners' inquests are largely directed toward ascertaining direct causes of death, such as accidents or a deficit in provision of care, natural-disease deaths (which comprise the majority of coroners' death investigations) are acknowledged as having significant public health implications.

As risk management, occupational health and safety, and preventive medicine have grown into important vocations, together with integrated systems for coroners' inquiry, the application of these disciplines as part of a coroner's death investigation has assumed a greater importance. This represents a significant departure from the traditional role of the coroner's jurisdiction and is an example of expansion in response to perceived community needs.

Notes

1. See Baker this volume.
2. See Clement this volume.
3. See Stephan this volume.
4. See Sauer and Wankmiller, Braz, Rogers, and also Willey, all this volume.
5. See Sledzik, Black, Briggs, and Buck, all this volume.

References

Clark, H. R. 1936. The law and the coroner 2. *Medical Journal of Australia* 565.
Clement, J. G., and Ranson, D. L. (eds.). 1998. *Craniofacial Identification in Forensic Medicine*. London: Edward Arnold.
Matthews, P. 2002. *Jervis on the Office and Duties of Coroners* (12th ed.). London: Sweet and Maxwell.
Matthews, P., and Foreman, J. C. 1993. *Jervis on the Office and Duties of Coroners* (11th ed.). London: Sweet and Maxwell.

42

CONCLUSION: GLOBAL PERSPECTIVES ON ISSUES IN FORENSIC ANTHROPOLOGY

Douglas H. Ubelaker and Soren Blau

This volume presents diverse perspectives on the very nature of forensic anthropology, its history as played out in different regions of the world, its applications to various medico-legal issues, and the background and training of personnel. With increasing frequency, forensic anthropologists are involved in domestic criminal cases and law enforcement initiatives thought to involve human remains, international investigations of atrocities and humanitarian missions directed toward victims of such atrocities, recovery and identification of war dead, mass-fatality incidents, and training at a variety of levels. In addition, forensic anthropologists contribute to what has been termed "judicial anthropometry" (identification of the living), scene management, and interaction with family members. Those practitioners with a background in social anthropology have also proven useful in forensic contexts working with communities in assembling antemortem data on missing persons, especially in areas where medical and dental records are rare.

Clearly, definitions of *forensic anthropology* and *forensic anthropologists* vary considerably (see Blau and Ubelaker this volume), and to a large extent they are regionally determined. Although the forensic anthropology practitioner may hold a Ph.D. in physical anthropology or a medical degree or come from a variety of other educational backgrounds, the science applied is universal, rooted

in experience, casework, research experimentation, and the vast and rapidly growing scientific literature. In the investigation of mass disasters and international events involving mass casualties, those involved bring a variety of experiences ranging from specialists with worldwide perspectives and formal training to those working locally with communities involved and who have abundant experience and knowledge of working conditions. All these perspectives are important, and all are needed in forensic investigations.

This volume provides regional historical perspectives on the development of forensic anthropology from the United Kingdom, France, Italy, Spain, South America, United States, Canada, Australia, and Indonesia. Although particular regional developments are noteworthy, many common historical developments exist, specifically: (1) deep roots in anatomical studies with early anatomists, physicians, and anthropologists becoming involved in forensic casework; (2) similar trajectories in the growth and development of the field of forensic anthropology as measured by the formation and increased enrollment in organizations, publications, teaching, and the incorporation of anthropological perspectives in investigative efforts. Decisions about which personnel become involved in casework and what academic perspectives are followed usually are made not by anthropologists but by judges, magistrates, and others who have such responsibility by law. Clearly, extensive educational efforts have improved the nature of anthropological involvement worldwide, especially in the inclusion of archaeological perspectives in recovery efforts and the addition of anthropological skillsets to identification teams.

A variety of case studies are presented in this volume to reflect on the diversity of applications in what has become forensic anthropology and forensic archaeology. These cases range from involvement in domestic homicides and routine investigations of what are believed to be human remains to large-scale mass disasters and victims of atrocities. Many common issues emerge throughout the discussions of these case studies. These include the nature and the extent of involvement of forensic anthropologists and archaeologists at critical steps in the investigation, the nature and thoroughness of recovery efforts, accuracy of identifications, consideration of health issues, approaches to complex sites (including secondary deposits), and debates over the bureaucratic classification of sites as either judicial or humanitarian and how such classifications affect the use of resources. Throughout the discussion of all the various cases, the important role of family and community is paramount, not only as a key source of antemortem information for identification but also for their continued involvement in case resolution and commitment to justice and closure. Insight is provided in this volume on the realities of site investigation and on working within large organizations. Other perspectives examine the value of including those working locally, of familial involvement, and the trade-offs involved in the selection of personnel with extensive local experience versus those with advanced degrees and international perspective.

Search and Detection

Many of the authors in this collection of papers speak to the key issue of anthropological involvement in search and detection efforts, especially those involving recovery efforts that include excavation. It has been argued that these areas of forensic anthropology/archaeology have a greater likelihood of bringing the anthropologist to court as an expert witness. Even in geographic regions where forensic anthropologists/archaeologists by training are not involved in analysis of recovered remains, they become involved in recovery because of their unique qualifications.

In spite of the availability of forensic anthropologists/archeologists to assist or to direct recovery efforts, actual participation varies considerably. In the case studies reported here, factors dictating whether anthropologists or archaeologists are involved in investigations (which in turn affect the quality of recovery efforts) are the perceived need for rapid results to press charges against the accused, limited goals of identification of the deceased rather than full understanding of the events involved, perceptions of the pace of recovery and how it might be affected by careful excavation, and lack of institutional control of sites. Examples are also presented regarding how much can be learned about relative events through careful excavation and documentation. Such examples illustrate how limiting the factors listed above can become. Clearly, proper location and recovery are important and are enhanced through proven techniques such as the use of probes, coring, limited and extensive excavation, and remote sensing—the last including soil resistivity studies, magnetometry, and the use of ground-penetrating radar. All sites involving human remains are complex, but those including secondary deposits reflecting multistage behavior can be resolved only through careful anthropological excavation and analysis.

Skeletal Analysis

Skeletal analysis begins by determining if the recovered elements are human or not. If remains are extremely fragmented, it first may be necessary to ascertain if bone and/or tooth are represented, since many particles of other materials can resemble these tissues. To determine if remains are of human or nonhuman origin, morphology, histology, and even protein radioimmunoassay can provide solutions.

Usually, it also is important to determine as accurately as possible the time since death, especially in the case of suspicious deaths. In the types of cases requiring an anthropological perspective, this can be problematic to accomplish from morphological indicators alone, since so many variables affect tissue alteration. Other approaches include chemical analysis, immunology, analysis of fat content, colorimetry, and ion-exchange chromatography. The most promising techniques, however, appear to be radioisotope studies, especially those involving radiocarbon and strontium-90, isotopic variables influenced by atmospheric testing of thermonuclear devices in the 1950s and 1960s. The aim of future research will be to produce a user-friendly method that provides results in a timely and cost-efficient manner.

The estimation of sex is an important element in establishing the biological profile as part of the identification process. Bone morphology usually allows successful estimation for adults, especially if the pelvis is well preserved. Size-related differences are apparent throughout the skeleton but, except for those of the pelvis, usually are not of sufficient magnitude to allow sex estimation with great certainty. Of course, molecular approaches are now available, and especially useful are those techniques that evaluate the amelogenin gene and/or detect indicators from the Y chromosome. Molecular approaches have the advantage of allowing sex determination for subadults whose sex cannot be determined reliably from morphological assessment.

Estimation of age at death has become complex with many methods available. The general age (neonate, infant, child, adolescent, young adult, old adult) determines which methods should be employed. This area of forensic anthropology has been augmented with statistical advances, as well as rigorous testing of multiple techniques on documented samples. There is a continued need for further population-specific research to be undertaken in order to improve the contribution that forensic anthropology can make to statements about age.

Ancestry determination continues to represent an important contribution to the biological profile and can prove pivotal within mass-disaster investigations in distinguishing local residents from tourists and other foreigners. Discussions in this volume make the important distinction between race and ancestry and recognize the importance of terminology in this complex issue. Methodologies involving measurements and visual assessment are available, but proper use of databases and recognition of the social factors involved remain critical. Such factors include, for example, the practitioner's need to understand the underlying assumptions inherent in the development of a dataset and the fact that physical skeletal manifestations do not always equate to the deceased individual's social identity in life.

Techniques of facial approximation and craniofacial superimposition are available to assist identification efforts. The former is utilized only in cases in which standard attempts at identification have failed and the need exists to reach out to the general public in search of leads aimed at identification. Superimposition techniques are used primarily for exclusion in cases for which both skulls of a deceased and photographs of the possible living individual represented are available. A diversity of approaches to these techniques exists with a continued need for additional research, testing, and evaluation.

Methodology aimed at the estimation of living stature can be traced back to the very beginnings of the field of forensic anthropology. Today, a variety of approaches are available involving formulae requiring measurements of individual as well as groups of bones. Contributors to this volume discuss the caveats of utilizing antemortem stature records. Although formulae are now available for both sexes and different ancestral groups, additional research is needed on body proportions among different populations from around the world.

Techniques involved in estimating age at death, ancestry, and stature all have profited enormously from advances in quantitative methods. The large databases that can be accommodated with modern computer technology enable new types of research not possible only a few years ago. Geometric morphometrics conducted utilizing 3D methodology and advances in Bayesian statistics enable new approaches to traditional topics in forensic anthropology, enhancing accuracy.

New approaches in the study of forensic taphonomy facilitate greater understanding of the relationships of evidence to environment, particularly in reference to the postmortem history of human remains. Taphonomic indicators can provide key clues to time since death determination, trauma assessment, and reconstruction of postmortem history. An important component of taphonomic study consists of the study of burned bone. Although terminological issues abound in this area, research initiatives utilizing X-ray diffraction, small-angle X-ray scattering, and study of human albumin blood proteins all show promise in recognizing the evidence of burning and in teasing out related information on temperature, duration, and the timing of events within the perimortem/postmortem window.

Although forensic anthropologists usually do not make the call on cause and manner of death, they frequently find and interpret the evidence that allows such determinations to be made. Before interpretations of perimortem trauma can be advanced, antemortem and postmortem alterations must be evaluated. A feature such as a developmental foramina can look like a gunshot injury, for example, while postmortem animal tooth marks can mimic sharp force trauma. Trauma interpretation is complex and calls for the experience and techniques of forensic anthropology.

Identification of deceased individuals from skeletal remains represents the goal of much of the effort and methodology discussed above, yet discussions in this volume reveal considerable variation in definitions and degrees of identification. At one extreme, positive identification is accomplished when unique features found on the deceased are known to have existed on a missing person. Such identifications are most likely to occur in cases for which the antemortem information includes medical and/or dental records, fingerprints, and/or suitable DNA samples. At the other extreme, "presumptive" identifications are made through family recognition, clothing comparisons, and general attributes shared with a missing person. The latter type of identifications are all that may be possible in cases for which prints are not preserved, medical and dental records are not available, and DNA technology does not exist or samples are not sufficiently preserved. Clearly, molecular technology has revolutionized the identification process, but issues of preservation and contamination remain. Technological advances promise to increase the accuracy even with severely degraded samples. For example, the polymerase chain reaction methodology has enabled identifications of very small samples, including relatively ancient ones.

Professional Conduct

Who is qualified to work as a forensic anthropologist in cases such as those presented in this volume? Clearly, forensic science continues to struggle with this issue—individuals with widely varying academic degrees, training, and experience are involved. Although accreditation efforts have been made, no worldwide standard yet exists for the field. The American Board of Forensic Anthropology, sponsored by the American Academy of Forensic Sciences, is frequently cited as being noteworthy in this regard. This Board grants certification to those who have the necessary qualifications, experience, and letters of recommendation and who pass an examination. However, such certification is only available to residents of the United States and Canada.

The Forensic Anthropology Society of Europe (FASE), a subsection of the International Academy of Legal Medicine, was formed in 2003 and in 2006 includes 47 members from 10 countries. This relatively new organization offers training, communication, and academic advancement of the practice of forensic anthropology in Europe.

More recently (September 2007) the Senior Managers of Australian and New Zealand Forensic Laboratories (SMANZFL) agreed to support the formation of a Medical Sciences Specialist Advisory Group (SAG), which includes forensic anthropology, forensic odontology, forensic entomology, and mortuary managers.[1] The formation of a SAG, the aim of which is to promote science excellence, provides a forum for practitioners from across Australia and New Zealand to discuss and improve technical skills, undertake research and training, and develop quality issues (including proficiency tests/trials, development of standards, databases and reference collections, and validation studies). The formation of the Medical Sciences SAG is the first time that forensic anthropology has been formally recognized by forensic service providers in Australia. Overall, the growth and development of these societies and groups across the world reflect the increasing interest in forensic anthropology/archaeology and the accompanying need for improved standards. Their formation provides an excellent opportunity for the development of the discipline.

Forensic anthropologists work closely with practitioners from other disciplines, especially forensic pathologists and forensic odontologists. As indicated above, forensic anthropologists leave determinations of cause and manner and death to the pathologists but frequently find and interpret the evidence that underlies the opinions expressed. Forensic anthropologists do not interpret dental restorations but overlap with forensic odontologists regarding interpretations of age at death and ancestry from dental evidence and the interpretation of craniofacial features in regard to identification and trauma.

Forensic applications continue to lure students and professionals alike in anthropology. Many who become involved in forensic endeavors are not prepared for some of the complex new situations they encounter, such as court testimony. Advice offered in this volume to tell the truth, to stay within professional expertise, to answer questions directly, and to avoid the natural tendency to lecture is well founded. Those practicing forensic anthropology not only have to follow courtroom procedures but also must pay attention to ethical issues as well. Such issues include being informed of appropriate laws and sociopolitical concerns, maintaining appropriate standards of training and accreditation, using reliable, accepted methodologies, writing concise readable reports that are objective and not speculative, receiving appropriate permissions for research attempted, and respecting the rights and concerns of families and descendants.

Clearly, forensic anthropology represents a diverse, complex, challenging, and rapidly expanding field. Practitioners (both up and coming and established) have a number of responsibilities, including the need to be

- *Technically competent*: knowledgeable in human and nonhuman anatomy, have experience working with a range of differentially preserved human and nonhuman remains, and fully versed in the advantages and limitations of the appropriate methodologies
- *Inquiring*: mindful of the potentially different approaches to a casework problem
- *Innovative*: developing research questions which address the problems raised by casework
- *Socially aware*: both in terms of working with other practitioners from other disciplines and in terms of the responsibility to the families of victims, the courts, and the media

The combination of these responsibilities makes the profession of forensic anthropology and forensic archaeology exciting disciplines to be part of. The methodologies summarized in this volume are state of the art but hardly the last word. As this volume goes to press, innovative research is being pursued in all of the areas within the field. Much of this involves applications of new technology and/or new applications of existing technology. However, many of the most significant advances will likely not involve new technology but rather the acquisition of samples from around the world in areas not well represented now. Such samples are needed for a more complete understanding of how human variation affects determinations in forensic anthropology. Clearly, forensic anthropology/archaeology will continue to be practiced worldwide; our science needs to reflect all humanity to meet that challenge.

Note

1. Other established SAGs include Biology, Chemical Criminalistics, Document Examination, Field and Identification Sciences, Toxicology, Illicit Drugs, and Electronic Evidence.

CONTRIBUTORS

Bradley J. Adams, B.A., M.A., Ph.D. Dr. Adams is currently a forensic anthropologist for the Office of Chief Medical Examiner (OCME) in New York City. He is also Adjunct Lecturer at Hunter College and Pace University, holds a faculty position at the New York University Medical Center, an affiliation with the NYU Anthropology Department, and frequently lectures in the New York City area on topics relating to forensic anthropology. In his present position with the OCME, Adams has responsibilities that include supervision and analysis of World Trade Center remains. He serves as a critical member of the OCME disaster response team.

From 1997 to 2004, Dr. Adams was a forensic anthropologist and Laboratory Manager at the Central Identification Laboratory (CIL) in Hawaii, where he directed large-scale recovery and investigation operations in Burma, Indonesia, Vietnam, Cambodia, Laos, Papua New Guinea, Kiribati, South Korea, North Korea, Nicaragua, and Panama. These operations were conducted in order to recover the remains of missing U.S. military personnel.

Melanie Archer, B.Sc. (Hons.), Ph.D. Dr. Archer has made four visits to the Solomon Islands to assist Malcolm Dodd with autopsies. She is the only forensic entomologist in Victoria and is one of three in Australia. She is Honorary Lecturer in the Department of Forensic Medicine, Monash University. She is also Vice President of the Victorian branch of the Australian and New Zealand Forensic Science Society. Melanie works at the Victorian Institute of Forensic Medicine primarily as a forensic entomologist and also as a forensic technician.

Eric Baccino, M.D. Dr. Baccino is Head of the Medico-Legal and Prison Medicine Unit at University Hospital, Montpellier. He is also president of the Forensic Anthropology Society of Europe (FASE) and Secretary General of the Société de Médecine Légale et de Criminologie de France.

Lori Baker, B.A., M.A., Ph.D. Dr. Baker is Assistant Professor in the Department of Anthropology, Forensic Science, and Archaeology at Baylor University. She obtained her doctorate from The University of Tennessee, Knoxville, where she conducted DNA analysis from hair shafts collected by Franz Boas and colleagues for the World's Columbian Exposition in 1893. Currently, Dr. Baker oversees the DNA section of Sistema de Identificación de Restos y Localización de Individuos (SIRLI), a database established by the Government of Mexico designed to locate living and to identify deceased Mexican nationals abroad. Her research interests lie in molecular analysis of ancient and modern bone, teeth, and hair samples in order to better understand population variation. Dr. Baker has numerous publications regarding mitochondrial DNA sequences analysis and molecular sex identification from forensic and ancient specimens.

Caroline Barker, B.Sc. (Hons.), Pg.Dip., Dip. FHID. Ms. Barker has worked internationally as a forensic practitioner since 1997. She was a member of the international forensic exhumations team for the United Nations International Criminal Tribunal for the Former Yugoslavia (ICTY). In Guatemala, she was employed as a forensic anthropologist for the Fundación de Antropología Forense de (FAFG) and assisted the team in the recovery and identification of human remains believed to be the victims of human rights violations from more than three decades of civil war. As the Senior Forensic Anthropologist and expert witness for the Serious Crimes Unit (SCU) of the United Nations Mission of Support in East Timor (UNMISET), she worked on the identification of human remains believed to be the victims of human rights violations and arbitrary executions from the 1999 referendum on Independence. She was employed as a consultant forensic anthropologist and technical advisor with the Inforce Foundation, U.K., and designed and implemented multiple forensic-training and capacity-building programs for Iraqi nationals. Caroline is currently based in Colombo, Sri Lanka, employed as the Forensic Expert for the support team for the International Independent Group of Eminent Persons (IIGEP) assigned to observe the activities of the Sri Lankan Commission of Inquiry (CoI) tasked with investigating alleged human rights violations.

William Basler, B.A. William Basler received his Bachelorette degree in business from University of Northern Iowa before joining the Iowa Division of Criminal Investigation (DCI) in 1975 as a Special Agent. He has worked over 500 cases in northern Iowa and testified in more than 100 trials. In 2003, he became the Special Agent in Charge and held this position until he retired from the DCI in 2006. Since then he has been the Criminal Justice Program Leader at North Iowa Area Community College.

Sue Black, OBE, B.Sc., Ph.D., D.Sc., FRSE Professor Black is Head of Anatomy and Forensic Anthropology at University of Dundee. She is a founding member and director of the Centre for International Forensic Assistance and a founder of the British Association for Human Identification. She was awarded an OBE for her services to forensic anthropology in Kosovo and is a Fellow of the Royal Society of Edinburgh. She is lead assessor for forensic anthropology with the Council for the Registration of Forensic Practitioners and is a registered expert with the National Centre for Policing Excellence.

Soren Blau, B.A.(Hons.), M.Sc., Ph.D. Dr. Blau has worked in the Centre for Human Identification (now Human Identification Services - HIS) at the Victorian Institute of Forensic Medicine (VIFM) as a forensic anthropologist since January 2005 and is currently the manager of the HIS. She is an honorary Senior Lecturer in the Department of Forensic Medicine at Monash University. Soren is involved in local and international casework as well as contributing to international Disaster Victim Identification (DVI) training courses. During her time at the VIFM, Soren has developed an interest in using computerized tomography (CT) data to establish population specific standards for forensic anthropology in Australia. She is currently coordinating a project in East Timor investigating alleged human rights abuses.

Kristina Bowie, B.A. Kristina Bowie is a graduate in physical/biological anthropology from University of Victoria (2004) and has a certificate in International Human Rights Law from Oxford University (2005). She has worked for the American Museum of Natural History in the High Arctic islands of the Northwest Territories of Canada prospecting for Late Pleistocene vertebrates. She also worked as a forensic archaeologist for the Royal Canadian Mounted Police Major Crimes Section, Missing Persons Unit. She currently works for a Victoria, B.C., archaeological consulting firm, contracted out over the province of British Columbia to lead field crews in the surveying and testing for archaeological sites. She plans on continuing with graduate studies to follow her interests in the recovery of missing or disappeared persons, drawing on her background in human osteology and human rights violations.

Valeria Silva Braz, B.A., M.Sc. Valeria Braz is Associate Researcher in the Department of Anthropology, Museu Nacional, Universidade Federal do Rio de Janeiro, Brazil. She has a M.Sc. in morphological sciences from Institute of Biomedical Sciences, Universidade Federal do Rio de Janeiro, Brazil. Her thesis examined the taphonomic processes in skeletal remains from the Moa and Beirada shell mounds, Saquarema, Brazil. Valeria also has a Specialist qualification in Palaeopathology, History and Evolution of Diseases, from the National School of Public Health (FIOCRUZ), Rio de Janeiro, Brazil. Valeria has experience related to gross and microstructural postmortem alterations in human skeletal tissues, structural evaluation of trabecular bone quality using imaging techniques, and Fast Fourier Transform and osteobiographic studies of human remains.

Christopher A. Briggs, B.Sc., M.S., Ph.D. Associate Professor Briggs is Lecturer in the Department of Anatomy and Cell Biology at University of Melbourne and currently Deputy Head of Department. Since 1991, he has been Staff Anatomist and Consultant in Forensic Anthropology at the Victorian Institute of Forensic Medicine. He is also

Honorary Associate Professor in the Department of Forensic Medicine at Monash University. Chris has assisted in crime scene examination and investigation of skeletal and otherwise unidentified remains and, in cases of homicide has presented expert evidence in court. He worked as consultant forensic anthropologist with the United Nations in East Timor in 2000 and with the Australian Federal Police in Bali in 2002. He has also participated in the recovery of skeletal remains from archaeological sites in Turkey and Britain.

Alanah M. Buck, Dip.Teach., B.App.Sci., Ph.D. Dr. Buck has worked as a forensic anthropologist with Forensic Pathology, PathWest (Australia) since 1992. She was part of the Australian DVI team and the first forensic anthropologist that attended the 2002 Bali Bombings and Australian Embassy Bombing in 2004. Alanah is the author of the current DVI Forensic Anthropology Guidelines in the Australasian DVI Standards Manual and is also the Forensic Anthropology representative for the Western Australian DVI Committee. She is currently working as a consultant for the delivery and development of Forensic Services to the Cambodian Criminal Justice Assistance Project.

John Byrd, B.A., M.A., Ph.D., DABFA Dr. Byrd's expertise is in the fields of forensic anthropology and archaeology. He is currently a laboratory manager and forensic anthropologist for the Central Identification Laboratory, Joint POW/MIA Accounting Command in Hawaii. He serves as a member of the Editorial Board of *Journal of Forensic Sciences*. Dr. Byrd's research interests include the science of identification, morphometrics, and statistics in forensic anthropology, zooarchaeology, and North American archaeology.

Cristina Cattaneo, M.D., Ph.D. Dr. Cattaneo graduated from McGill University (Canada) in biomedical sciences, received her M.A. and Ph.D. in osteology and anthropology at University of Sheffield (U.K.), and later graduated in medicine and specialized in forensic pathology (Medicina Legale) at Università Statale di Milano (Italy). She is now Associate Professor of Legal Medicine in the Faculty of Medicine of University of Milano and teaches anthropology at the Faculty of Sciences and of Arts of the same university. In 1996, she founded and now heads the Laboratorio di Antropologia ed Odontologia Forense (LABANOF) of the Institute of Legal Medicine of the University of Milano, is Secretary of FASE (Forensic Anthropology Society of Europe, a subsection of the International Academy of Legal Medicine [IALM]), and is currently Associate

Editor for the Osteology section of *Forensic Science International*.

Paul N. Cheetham, B.Sc. Hons. Paul Cheetham is Senior Lecturer in Archaeological Science at Bournemouth University and currently leads the Field Archaeology and the Archaeological and Forensic Sciences degree programs. He is also involved in running and teaching an M.Sc. program in forensic archaeology at Bournemouth. Graduating from the School of Archaeological Sciences, University of Bradford, in 1985, in the 1990s he worked closely with John Hunter and Rob Janaway on promoting awareness of and developing forensic archaeology through education, research, and involvement in cases throughout the U.K. He is a founding member of the U.K. Forensic Search Advisory Group, promoting the effective use of geophysical techniques in a forensic archaeological context, and is also founding member of the International Society for Archaeological Prospection. Paul has now worked on almost 40 U.K. cases, has been involved in international mass-grave investigations, and is an Inforce advisor on ground-based remote sensing.

John Gerald Clement, B.DS., Ph.D. (Lond.), LDS RCS (Eng.), FFFLM RCP (Eng.), Dip. for Odont. (LHMC), FICD Professor Clement holds the Inaugural Chair of Forensic Odontology at the School of Dental Science at University of Melbourne. He is also Honorary Associate Professor at Monash University in the Department of Forensic Medicine. Professor Clement is past President of the British and Australian societies for Forensic Odontology (BAFO and ASFD) and a founding member of the International Dental Ethics and Law Society (IDEALS) and The International Association for Craniofacial Identification (IACI). He contributed to the identification of the victims of the 2004 Tsunami. He has also served on an expert advisory panel to the International Committee of the Red Cross (ICRC) dealing with the problem of the identification of missing persons and human remains following conflicts and civil strife. He is a member of the Scientific Steering Committee on Forensic Science Programs to the International Commission on Missing persons (ICMP).

Derek Congram, B.A. (Hon.), M.Sc., M.A. Derek Congram worked with the United Nations in the former Yugoslavia between 1999 and 2003. He has also contributed to medico-legal investigations in Costa Rica, Iraq, and Canada. He is currently undertaking a Ph.D. at Simon Fraser University (Canada) in archaeology, researching aspects of clandestine mass graves from the Spanish Civil War.

Samuel V. Connell, Ph.D. Dr. Connell received his Ph.D. from University of California, Los Angeles. He has published in *Antiquity* and *Latin American Antiquity* and has co-edited a volume on Ancient Maya Rural Complexity. From 2002 to 2005 he was a member of the Department of Defense Central Identification Laboratory, where he led missions to Southeast Asia and worked with geophysical instrumentation to search for, recover, and identify missing U.S. military dead. Dr. Connell is Assistant Professor of Anthropology at Foothill College, Los Altos Hills, California. His current research focuses on fortresses of the Ecuadorian highlands. Dr. Connell has presented at numerous conferences worldwide and is a member of the Institute of Andean Studies Society for American Archaeology, American Anthropological Association, and Register of Professional Archaeologists.

Margaret Cox, B.A. (Hons.), B.A. (Open), Ph.D., FSA, FRSA, MIFA Dr. Cox is currently Professor of Forensic Archaeology and Anthropology at Cranfield University. Before taking up this position she was Head of Forensic and Bioarchaeological Sciences at Bournemouth University, U.K. until September 2006, where, with her colleagues, she developed and led their forensic programs. Margaret is founder and Chief Executive of the Inforce Foundation and has worked in Kosovo, Rwanda, Iraq, and Cyprus. She has published extensively in peer-reviewed journals and produced two significant textbooks about forensic archaeology in the U.K. and the scientific investigation of mass graves.

Christian Matthew Crowder, B.A., M.A., Ph.D. Dr. Crowder is a forensic anthropologist for the Office of Chief Medical Examiner (OCME) in New York City. He is also Adjunct Lecturer at Hunter College and holds a faculty position at the New York University Medical Center. Dr. Crowder received his B.A. from Texas A&M University (1996), his M.A. from The University of Texas, Arlington (2001), and his Ph.D. in anthropology from University of Toronto (2005). Before accepting the position at the OCME in 2006, he completed a one-year postdoctorate at the Joint POW/MIA Accounting Command—Central Identification Laboratory (JPAC-CIL) in Hawaii. He has published papers in *Journal of Forensic Sciences* and *American Journal of Physical Anthropology*.

Eugénia Cunha, Ph.D. Dr. Cunha is Full Professor of Physical Anthropology at the Faculty of Sciences and Technology, University of Coimbra, and National Consultant for Forensic Anthropology for the National Institute of Forensic Medicine, in Portugal (since 1997), where she is responsible for the forensic anthropology cases. She is the coordinator of the forensic anthropology modules in the courses of legal medicine in Portugal. She also teaches regularly abroad in other postgraduate courses, for example, in Spain, Italy, Tunisia, and Hungary. She is founding member and vice president of the Forensic Anthropology Society of Europe (FASE). Among other publications, she is one of the editors, and author and/or co-author, of three chapters of *Forensic Anthropology and Medicine: From Recovery to Cause of Death* (2006).

Malcolm J. Dodd, MBBS, FRCPA, DMJ (Path.), Assoc. Dip. MLT, MACLM, AAIMLT, FACBS, Grad. Cert. Health. Prof. Ed. Dr. Dodd is a senior forensic pathologist at the Victorian Institute of Forensic Medicine. He has visited the Solomon Islands 12 times, both to perform autopsies and give evidence for Operation RAMSI. He has also worked for the UN in East Timor and Kosovo and was part of the first Australian response team following the 2005 Boxing Day Tsunami. Malcolm was part of a group of RAMSI and RSIP personnel who received the 2005 Founders Award of the International Homicide Investigators Association for their contribution to investigating the Marasa Village killings (see Archer and Dodd this volume). He has particular expertise in ballistics and is the author of *Terminal Ballistics: A Text and Atlas of Gunshot Wounds* (2005). Malcolm's experiences as a forensic pathologist involved in overseas operations are also documented in *Justice for the Dead: Forensic Pathology in the Hot Zone* (2006).

Denise Donlon, B.Sc., Dip.Ed., B.A. (Hons.), Ph.D. Dr. Donlon is curator of Shellshear Museum of Physical Anthropology and Senior Lecturer in the Department of Anatomy and Histology, University of Sydney. She has a Ph.D. in physical anthropology and a B.A. (Hons.) in archaeology. She coordinates courses in comparative primate anatomy and forensic osteology and supervises postgraduate students. Research interests include forensic anthropology of the Sydney region, dental and postcranial skeletal variation and Australian Aboriginal burial archaeology. Denise has published on topics including forensic osteology, nonmetric traits, and dental metrics. She is a consultant to the New South Wales Department of Forensic Medicine and a member of the RAAF Specialist Reserves.

Ambika Flavel, B.Sc. (Hons.), M.Sc. Ambika Flavel has worked in Bosnia-Herzegovina (for the International Tribunal for the Former Yugoslavia—ICTY) and Guatemala (for the Fundación de Antropología Forense de Guatemala [FAFG] and Equipo de Exhumaciones de la Oficina de Derechos Humanos del Arzobispado de Guatemala—ODHAG) locating and excavating mass graves and analyzing and repatriating human skeletal material. Ambika has also been involved in capacity building and training both field and laboratory techniques to university students, Iraqi nationals, and law enforcement agencies with Inforce and Bournemouth University. In the capacity of forensic consultant, she was invited to Iraq by Inforce on behalf of the Coalitional Provisional Authority to advise on the location and exhumation of war graves. Subsequently, Ambika participated in the mass-grave investigations for the Regimes Crime Liaison Office (RCLO) in Iraq.

Luis Fondebrider, Licenciado Luis Fondebrider is a forensic anthropologist, cofounder and current Director of the Argentine Forensic Anthropology Team, Equipo Argentino de Antropologia Forense (EAAF). As a member of EAAF, Luis has participated in forensic investigations in Argentina, Chile, Brazil, Bolivia, Peru, Paraguay, Colombia, Venezuela, Guatemala, El Salvador, Haiti, Croatia, Bosnia, Kosovo, Romania, Iraq, Philippines, Indonesia, Cyprus, Georgia, South Africa, Zimbabwe, Ethiopia, Sudan, Kenya, and Namibia. He worked as a consultant for Truth Commissions of Argentina, El Salvador, Haiti, Peru, and South Africa; International Tribunal for the Former Yugoslavia, Committee of Missing Persons of Cyprus; UN Secretary General Investigation Team for Democratic Republic of Congo; UN Commission of Inquiry on Darfur; Special Commission search of Che Guevara remains; Panel of Experts for Chile; Special Prosecutor Office of the Transitional Government of Ethiopia; International Committee of the Red Cross (ICRC) for the project "The Missing"; and the Medico Legal Institute of Colombia, among others.

Shari Forbes, B.Sc., Ph.D. Dr. Forbes received her B.Sc. (Hons.) in Applied Chemistry-Forensic Science and Ph.D. from University of Technology, Sydney, Australia. She is currently Assistant Professor at University of Ontario Institute of Technology (UOIT), where she coordinates and teaches the undergraduate forensic science program. Her research is focused on the processes of decomposition, particularly in burial environments, and employs a multidisciplinary approach involving forensic chemistry, taphonomy, and anthropology. The significance of the research is the potential to assist forensic and human rights investigations involving clandestine grave sites.

Julia C. Goodin, M.D. Dr. Goodwin is Chief State Medical Examiner for Iowa. She graduated from Western Kentucky University in Bowling Green (1979) and earned her Doctorate of Medicine from University of Kentucky (1983). Dr. Goodin received her training in anatomic and clinical pathology at Vanderbilt University Medical Center and was a fellow in forensic pathology at the Office of the Chief Medical Examiner in Baltimore, Maryland. She has held positions in the medical examiner's offices of Nashville, Tennessee, Albuquerque, New Mexico, and the Alabama Department of Forensic Sciences in Mobile. Dr. Goodin is certified by the American Board of Pathology in Anatomic Pathology, Clinical Pathology, and Forensic Pathology. She is licensed to practice medicine and has been certified as an expert in the field of forensic medicine in courtrooms in several states.

Ian Hanson, B.A., M.Sc. Ian Hanson is Senior Lecturer in Forensic Archaeology at Bournemouth University. A graduate in archaeology from University of Southampton and forestry and business management from University of Aberdeen, he has worked as a professional archaeologist on rescue and research projects, excavating and directing sites from the Neolithic to post-Medieval in Europe, Africa, Australasia, and the Middle East. In the forensic context, he has spent over 24 months in the field consulting, training, and teaching in the areas of search, location, and recovery of burials and the investigation of genocide, war crimes, and human rights, for various police forces as well as UNDPKO, UNICTY, FAFG, INFORCE, and CMP Cyprus in the U.K., U.S.A., Bosnia, Croatia, Guatemala, DR Congo, Iraq, Cyprus, and Sudan.

Maciej Henneberg, M.Sc., Ph.D., Dsc. Dr. Henneberg is a human biologist educated in Poland. Maciej worked at the universities of Texas at Austin (1978, 1984–1986), Cape Town (1986–1990), and Witwatersrand, Johannesburg (1990–1995). He is currently Wood Jones Professor of Anatomy and Head of Anatomical Sciences at The University of Adelaide (since 1996). Maciej's research interests include human evolution, anatomical variation, and population genetics.

Michael J. Hochrein, B.A. Mike Hochrein has been a Federal Bureau of Investigation Special Agent since 1988. He is currently assigned to the

Laurel Highlands Resident Agency within the FBI's Pittsburgh Division, where he investigates a variety of federal violations including violent crimes, computer crimes, public corruption, and financial crimes. Before joining the FBI, Agent Hochrein was a field archaeologist and analyst on salvage and research projects. Specializing in historical archaeology, he worked for Carnegie Museum of Natural History and University of Pittsburgh Cultural Resources Management Program. As an FBI Evidence Response Team member, Agent Hochrein develops and conducts research, teaches, publishes articles, and testifies in areas of geotaphonomy and forensic archaeology, as well as crime-scene mapping and general evidence collection. As an FBI certified police instructor, he has traveled to the Middle East, Africa, and Southeast Asia to assist in crime scene investigation training for national police organizations.

Thomas D. Holland, Ph.D., DABFA Dr. Holland received his Ph.D. from University of Missouri, Columbia. He has published in *American Journal of Physical Anthropology, American Antiquity, Journal of Forensic Sciences, Current Anthropology, Studies in Archaeological Method and Theory, Quaternary Research*, and *Plains Anthropologist*. Since 1992, Dr. Holland has been Scientific Director of the Department of Defense Central Identification Laboratory and is responsible for the recovery and identification of U.S. military dead. He has supervised excavations of aircraft crash sites and burial sites in China, North Korea, South Korea, Iraq, Kuwait, and Southeast Asia. Dr. Holland is Diplomate of the American Board of Forensic Anthropology, Fellow of the American Academy of Forensic Sciences, and a member of the American Society.

John Hunter, B.A., Ph.D., FSA, FFSSoc. Dr. Hunter was appointed Professor of Archaeology and Ancient History at University of Birmingham in 1996. Following an extensive scheme of research excavation and survey in Scotland, he began to develop forensic archaeology in 1988, cowrote the first textbook on the subject, and has routinely lectured to police and forensic groups ever since. He helped found the Forensic Search Advisory Group and is a lead assessor for the Council for the Registration of Forensic Practitioners (CRFP) and member of CRFP's Incident Investigation panel. He works actively on police and war crime missions throughout the world and has recently returned from the Balkans as a consult to the International Commission on Missing Persons (ICMP). He has recently been appointed Royal Commissioner on the Ancient and Historical Monuments of Scotland.

He is co-author of a new book on forensic archaeology published in late 2006.

Etty Indriati, Ph.D. Professor Indriati practiced dentistry for several years before obtaining a Ph.D. in anthropology at The University of Chicago (1998). She is currently Head of the Laboratory of Bio and Paleoanthropology at the Faculty of Medicine, Gadjah Mada University. Etty was awarded the Albert A. Dahlberg Prize as a dental anthropologist (1996); the Kenneth Holland Award as a Fulbright scholar (1998); and the Women's International Science Collaboration from the American Association for the Advancement of Science, New York (2002). She has published in *American Journal of Physical Anthropology* and *Proceeding of the National Academy of Sciences*, among others, and is the author of *Antropology Forensik*, a textbook on forensic anthropology in Indonesia.

Erin H. Kimmerle, B.A., M.A., Ph.D. Dr. Kimmerle has worked as a forensic anthropologist for the United Nations, International Criminal Tribunal for the Former Yugoslavia as on missions in Kosova, Croatia, and Bosnia-Herzegovina. She has also worked as an osteologist for the National Museum of Natural History, Smithsonian Institution, in Washington, D.C. Erin currently holds a Visiting Assistant Professor position in the Department of Anthropology at the University of South Florida. Her current research areas include medicolegal investigations of human rights abuses and the application of virtual technologies to study skeletal biology and variation such as geometric morphometric analysis of craniofacial shape variation, facial reconstructions, and 3D imaging of skeletal trauma.

Dennis F. Klein, B.A., M.D. Dr. Klein is Deputy State Medical Examiner at the Iowa Office of the State Medical Examiner. He is also Adjunct Clinical Assistant Professor at The University of Iowa School of Medicine and Adjunct Associate Professor of Forensic Pathology at Des Moines University. Dr. Klein received his medical degree from The University of Vermont and his postgraduate training in pathology at Beth Israel Hospital in Boston, Massachusetts. Dr. Klein is board certified by the American Board of Pathology in Anatomical, Clinical, and Forensic Pathology.

Louise Loe, B.A., Ph.D. Dr. Loe is Head of Heritage Burial Services, Oxford Archaeology. Following undergraduate studies in archaeology at University of Bristol, Louise worked for several years with Dr. Juliet Rogers on the analysis and reportage of human skeletal remains from archaeological sites. Since completing a Ph.D.

in biological anthropology at the University of Bristol, Louise has lectured on forensic programs at University of Bournemouth and has assisted the Inforce Foundation in capacity-training programs. Her main research interests lie in biocultural perspectives on health and socio-economic status and peri- and postmortem modification of human remains, focusing particularly on prehistoric archaeological assemblages from Britain.

Dawn M. Mulhern, B.Sc., M.A., Ph.D. Dr. Mulhern received her Ph.D. in anthropology from University of Colorado at Boulder. She is Assistant Professor of Anthropology at Fort Lewis College in Durango, Colorado. Her primary research areas are skeletal histology and palaeopathology. She has extensive laboratory experience in the biological analysis of Native American skeletal remains prior to repatriation. She has also conducted fieldwork and skeletal analyses at Giza, Egypt. She is currently Research Associate for the National Museum of Natural History, Smithsonian Institution, and is also a forensic anthropologist for the Disaster Mortuary Operational Response Team (DMORT), a national emergency response team.

Stephen P. Nawrocki, B.A., M.A., Ph.D., DABFA Dr. Nawrocki received his B.A. from The University of Maine and his M.A. and Ph.D. from State University of New York at Binghamton. He has taught at University of Indianapolis since 1991. Stephen has archaeological experience examining 19th-century trash pits and scatters of prehistoric artifacts and burials particularly within historic Euroamerican cemeteries. In 1996, Stephen became certified as a Diplomate of the American Board of Forensic Anthropology. Current research interests include the statistics of age estimation from the skeleton, forensic archeology, and human decomposition.

Kimberly Nugent, BH.Sc., M.Sc. Kimberly Nugent received both of her degrees from University of Toronto, where she studied in the department of Physical Anthropology. She is an active member of the Canadian forensic community and is currently designing forensic science curricula and instructing in the forensic science undergraduate program at Ontario Institute of Technology. Her interests involve undergraduate education and curricula development in a forensic context. She aims to motivate student learning and foster critical-thinking skills through the development of hands-on instructional exercises.

João Pinheiro, M.D., M.Sc. Dr. Pinheiro is a medical doctor with a master's degree in occupational health. Besides being a forensic pathologist for 16 years he is the Director of the Thanatology Service at the National Institute of Forensic Medicine in Coimbra and Professor of Human Anatomy at a High School of Medical Technology. He also teaches forensic pathology and anthropology to postgraduate students of legal medicine and forensic anthropology in Portugal, Spain, and Kosovo. He took part in international missions investigating human rights violations in Kosovo, Bosnia, and Colombia. He has published in the fields of forensic pathology and is one of the editors, as well as author and/or co-author, of three chapters, of *Forensic Anthropology and Medicine: From Recovery to Cause of Death* (2006). João is a founding member of Forensic Anthropology Society of Europe (FASE).

José L. Prieto, M.D., D.D.S. Dr. Prieto earned M.D. and D.D.S degrees from Complutense University of Madrid, Spain, took up the post of Forensic Doctor in 1988, and is currently Head of the Laboratory of Forensic Anthropology and Odontology at the Forensic Institute of Madrid, as well as Professor of Legal Medicine at the Complutense University. Dr. Prieto is, among others, a founding member of the Asociación Española de Paleopatología, Asociación Española de Antropología y Odontología Forense, and Forensic Anthropology Society of Europe, as well as a member of the American Academy of Forensic Sciences and Asociación Latinoamericana de Antropología Forense. He has published widely in the fields of forensic medicine and forensic anthropology.

David Ranson Professor Ranson is a medical practitioner and specialist anatomical pathologist (histopathologist) and forensic pathologist with qualifications in both medicine and law. He is Deputy Director of the Victorian Institute of Forensic Medicine, Director of the National Coroners Information System, and heads the specialist death investigation unit at the Institute. He has published widely in the field of forensic medicine and medical law and is the author and editor of a variety of texts in this area. He has produced medico-legal policy and research reports for government and private agencies and has given evidence to parliamentary and senate inquiries on matters relating to forensic medicine. Internationally, he has taken part in the investigation of mass fatalities occurring in civil and military contexts and has been a visiting International Expert in Forensic Pathology at the Health Sciences Authority in Singapore.

Tracy L. Rogers, B.A., M.A., Ph.D. Dr. Rogers is a forensic anthropologist and Assistant Professor at University of Toronto at Mississauga. She completed her undergraduate degrees at McMaster University in Hamilton, Canada (1989, M.A. 1992), and her Ph.D. at Simon Fraser University, British Columbia, Canada (2000). Tracy has been a consultant to the British Columbia Coroner's Service, local police agencies in British Columbia and Ontario, and the Royal Canadian Mounted Police (RCMP), most recently in conjunction with the largest serial killer investigation in Canadian history. Tracy's research interests include aspects of scene investigation, personal identification (including skeletal age estimation, sex determination, and assessment of ancestry), and expert testimony.

Ann H. Ross, B.A., M.A., Ph.D. Dr. Ross is Assistant Professor of Anthropology at North Carolina State University. She is a physical anthropologist with a subspecialty in forensic anthropology and bioarchaeology and a specialty in human identification and trauma analysis. She received her education from The University of Tennessee. Her research focus includes developing population-specific identification standards using traditional measurement techniques and modern 3D methods. She has participated in Human Rights missions in Bosnia and the Republic of Panama and also consults on a regular basis for the Republic of Panama Institute of Legal Medicine and occasionally on local cases in North Carolina.

Norman J. Sauer, Ph.D. Dr. Sauer is Professor of Anthropology and Director of the Forensic Anthropology Lab at Michigan State University. He is past Chair and Secretary of the Physical Anthropology section of the American Academy of Forensic Sciences and is on the Executive Board for the American Board of Forensic Anthropology. Dr. Sauer has lectured in forensic anthropology throughout the United States, Europe, and China. A regular consultant to a number of local, state, and federal law enforcement agencies, he has been interested in the concept of "race" in anthropology throughout his career.

Mark Skinner, B.A. (Hons.), Ph.D. Dr. Skinner received his doctorate in palaeoanthropology from University of Cambridge (1978). In 1982, he became the first Canadian board-certified Diplomate of the American Board of Forensic Anthropology. By June 2006, he had been consulted in Canada on 358 instances involving 144 forensic cases, of which 56 were homicides and 13 involved court appearances. In the last 10 years, he has worked for various agencies investigating allegations of mass graves in Afghanistan (1997), Bosnia (1998), East Timor (1999), and Yugoslavia (2001). In 2002,

he received the Bora Laskin National Fellowship in Human Rights Research. He was Director of the Forensic Sciences Department for the International Commission on Missing in 2004–2005. He continues to teach as Full Professor in the Department of Archaeology at Simon Fraser University, where he consults on forensic anthropology cases in Canada and Kosovo.

Paul S. Sledzik, B.A., M.Sc. Paul Sledzik manages victim recovery and identification efforts for the National Transportation Safety Board in Washington, D.C. Previously, he served as a forensic anthropologist and museum curator at the Armed Forces Institute of Pathology (AFIP). From 1998 to 2003, he oversaw the Region 3 U.S. Disaster Mortuary Operational Response Team and responded to cemetery floods in Missouri, Georgia, and North Carolina and to the Oklahoma City bombing, Egyptair 990, and the crash of United 93 on September 11, 2001. While at AFIP, he assisted in forensic efforts for Operation Desert Storm, USAir 427, and Iraqi Freedom. He has consulted for the Joint POW/MIA Accounting Command, the National Center for Forensic Science, the National Center for Missing and Exploited Children, and the U.S. Soldier Biological and Chemical Command.

Dawnie Wolfe Steadman, B.A., M.A., Ph.D., DABFA Dr. Steadman received her Ph.D. from The University of Chicago and is currently Associate Professor at Binghamton University, State University of New York. Her research interests include paleopathology, bioarchaeology, taphonomy, population genetics, and forensic anthropology. Dr. Steadman is a Diplomate of the American Board of Forensic Anthropology and serves as a forensic anthropological consultant for law enforcement and medical examiners. She assisted in the identification efforts at the World Trade Center and the Tri-State Crematorium in Noble, Georgia. Dr. Steadman also is involved in forensic human rights investigations and currently collaborates with Spanish colleagues to locate and identify individuals killed during the Spanish Civil War and the subsequent Franco regime.

Carl N. Stephan, BH.Sc., BH.Sc. (Hons.), Ph.D., GCHEd Dr. Stephan is Lecturer in Anatomy and Developmental Biology at the School of Biomedical Sciences, The University of Queensland, Australia. He is an anatomist and biological anthropologist with a special interest in craniofacial identification. Since completing his Ph.D. (2003), he has published over 30 scientific articles, most of which have concerned craniofacial identification methods. Dr. Stephan has assisted international, national, and local policing bodies in numerous forensic investigations and has served as a reviewer to many leading professional journals including *Journal of Forensic Sciences, Forensic Science International, American Journal of Physical Anthropology, Journal of Forensic Odonto-Stomatology,* and *International Journal of Osteoarchaeology.*

Jon Sterenberg, B.A., M.Sc. Jon Sterenberg worked on the forensic recovery of remains from mass graves for the United Nations (UN) in former Yugoslavia between 1997 and 2001, during which time he undertook work for the UN in Sierra Leone. Since 2002, he has continued to work toward the recovery of remains from the area of the recent Balkan conflicts, where he is the current Head of Excavation and Examination Division at ICMP, based in Sarajevo, Bosnia. He worked for the United States Government in Iraq 2003–2004 on investigations of mass graves relating to the former Iraqi regime and has co-authored articles and chapters on the subject of recovery of remains from mass grave sites. He is also a member of the Forensic Search Advisory Group (FSAG), based in the United Kingdom.

Tim Thompson, B.Sc. (Hons.), M.Sc., PCHE, Ph.D. Dr. Thompson is Senior Lecturer at the Centre for Forensic Investigation, University of Teesside. He has been conducting research into the effects of burning on bone and human identification for several years while in positions in the Medico-Legal Centre, University of Sheffield, and the Unit of Anatomy and Forensic Anthropology, University of Dundee. Tim has extensively published in peer-reviewed journals and books on a range of subjects from osteology to anthropological educational frameworks, from the ethics of forensic anthropology to biometric identity cards to burned human remains. Tim is currently a fully accredited and practicing forensic anthropologist, in both the U.K. and abroad. He is also Membership Secretary and Council Member for the British Association for Human Identification.

Douglas H. Ubelaker, Ph.D. Dr. Ubelaker is a curator and senior scientist at the Smithsonian Institution's National Museum of Natural History in Washington, D.C., where he has been employed since 1971. He received a Ph.D. from the University of Kansas (1973). He has published extensively in the general field of human skeletal biology with an emphasis on forensic applications. Since 1978, he has served as the primary consultant in forensic anthropology for the FBI Laboratory currently located in Quantico, Virginia. In this capacity, he has reported on over 800 cases and has testified in numerous legal proceedings.

Jane C. Wankmiller, B.S. Jane Wankmiller is a Ph.D. candidate in the Department of Anthropology at Michigan State University. She has extensive forensic anthropology casework experience and has conducted fieldwork in bioarchaeology on a Roman site in Albania and on a pre-Classic site in western Mexico.

P. Willey, B.A., M.A., Ph.D., DABFA Dr. Willey is Professor at Chico State University, Chico, California, where he has taught courses in physical anthropology since 1989. Before being employed there, he curated the Bass Skeletal Collection at The University of Tennessee, where he also received his Ph.D. His long-term research interests are prehistoric and historic skeletal series. He has more than 80 publications and is engaged in forensic anthropology cases. He has analyzed more than 140 civil cases, served JPAC-CIL as a consultant since 1997, worked with the Regime Crimes Liaison Office on Iraqi mass graves in 2004, and been a Diplomate of the American Board of Forensic Anthropology since 1989.

Richard Wright, B.A., M.A. Emeritus Professor Wright is an archaeologist and Emeritus Professor of Anthropology at University of Sydney, Australia. His interest in forensic archaeology, mass graves, and execution sites developed in 1990–1991, when the Australian government employed him to investigate mass graves in Ukraine dating to World War II. A second major assignment was from 1997 to 2000, when Richard was Chief Archaeologist for the International Criminal Tribunal for the Former Yugoslavia (ICTY). In that role, he led an international team of archaeologists and human biologists whose job was to locate clandestine mass graves and to examine the evidence contained in them. Richard's other major interest is the application of multivariate methods to archaeological and anthropological data. He is the author of *CRANID*, a multivariate package designed to identify ancestry from craniometric data.

INDEX